Y0-CAJ-280

Southern Missionary College
Division of Nursing Library
711 Lake Estelle Dr.
Orlando, Florida 32803

NEW DIMENSIONS IN MENTAL HEALTH– PSYCHIATRIC NURSING

NEW DIMENSIONS

FOURTH EDITION

2013
DF

IN MENTAL HEALTH-PSYCHIATRIC NURSING

Editors

MARION E. KALKMAN
ANNE J. DAVIS

WY
160
K 14i
1974

6 6 2 3

McGraw-Hill Book Company
A Blakiston Publication

New York St. Louis San Francisco Düsseldorf Johannesburg
Kuala Lumpur London Mexico Montreal
New Delhi Panama Paris São Paulo Singapore Sydney Tokyo Toronto

Southern Missionary College
Division of Nursing Library
711 Lake Estelle Dr.
Orlando, Florida 32803

NEW DIMENSIONS IN MENTAL HEALTH–PSYCHIATRIC NURSING

Copyright © 1974 by McGraw-Hill, Inc. All rights reserved.
Formerly published under the title of
PSYCHIATRIC NURSING copyright © 1958, 1967 by McGraw-Hill, Inc.
All rights reserved.
Copyright 1950 by McGraw-Hill, Inc.
All rights reserved. Printed in the United States of America.
No part of this publication may be reproduced, stored in a retrieval system, or
transmitted, in any form or by any means, electronic, mechanical, photocopying,
recording, or otherwise, without the prior written permission of the publisher.

2 3 4 5 6 7 8 9 0 K P K P 7 9 8 7 6 5 4

This book was set in Optima by Black Dot, Inc.
The editors were Cathy Dilworth and Sally Barhydt Mobley;
the designer was Anne Canevari Green;
the production supervisor was Bill Greenwood.
Kingsport Press, Inc., was printer and binder.

Library of Congress Cataloging in Publication Data

Kalkman, Marion E, date
    New dimensions in mental health–psychiatric
nursing.

    "A Blakiston publication."
    First-2d ed. published under title: Introduction
to psychiatric nursing; 3d (1967) ed.:   Psychiatric
nursing.
    1. Psychiatric nursing. 2. Psychiatry.
I. Davis, Anne J., date   joint author.
II. Title. [DNLM: 1. Psychiatric nursing. WY160
K14i 1974]
RC440.K27 1974   610.73'68   73-17155
ISBN 0-07-033242-8

CONTENTS

LIST OF CONTRIBUTORS

Irene Mortenson Burnside, R.N., M.S., Coordinator for Nursing Education, Ethel Percy Andrus Gerontology Center, University of Southern California, Los Angeles, California 90007

Anne J. Davis, R.N., Ph.D., Associate Professor, Psychiatric Nursing, University of California School of Nursing, San Francisco, California 94143

Ben H. Handleman, M.S.W., Lecturer, Social Work, University of California School of Nursing, San Francisco, California 94143

Janice E. Hitchcock, R.N., M.S., Assistant Professor, Community Mental Health Nursing, California State College Sonoma, Rohnert Park, California 94928

Marion E. Kalkman, R.N., M.A., Professor Emeritus, Psychiatric Nursing, University of California School of Nursing, San Francisco, California 94143

Paula J. LeVeck, R.N., M.S., Lecturer, Psychiatric Nursing, Extended Degree Program, University of California School of Nursing, San Francisco, California 94143

Helen Pazdur Monea, R.N., Lecturer, Child Psychiatric Nursing, University of California School of Nursing, San Francisco, California 94143

Judith A. Moore, R.N., M.S., Assistant Clinical Professor, Psychiatric Nursing, University of California School of Nursing, San Francisco, California 94143

Patricia C. Pothier, R.N., M.S., Lecturer, Child Psychiatric Nursing, University of California School of Nursing, San Francisco, California 94143

Judith M. Sitzman, R.N., M.S., Assistant Clinical Professor, Cardiopulmonary Nursing, University of California School of Nursing, San Francisco, California 94143

Eugenia Waechter, R.N., Ph.D., Associate Professor, Child Development, University of California School of Nursing, San Francisco, California 94143

Eleanor M. White, R.N., M.S., Assistant Clinical Professor, Psychiatric Nursing, University of California School of Nursing, San Francisco, California 94143

FOREWORD

The phenomenal growth of psychiatric nursing since the enactment of the National Mental Health Act in 1946 is reflected in this fourth edition of Marion Kalkman's book on psychiatric nursing. The new title, *New Dimensions in Mental Health–Psychiatric Nursing*, suggests not only the recent expansion of and changes in psychiatric nursing practice but the many changes in this edition of the text as well. A new coeditor—Anne J. Davis, who has worked and studied with Miss Kalkman at the University of California—has been added. The number of contributing authors has been increased from four to ten, emphasizing the necessity for depth of preparation in specific areas of mental health–psychiatric nursing and providing freshness, variety, and new points of view from which to consider and evaluate human behavior. Eighteen chapters in this edition are totally new, and four more have been heavily revised.

In this edition the authors have provided five theoretical models from which to choose in developing content, directing programs, and giving nursing care in newly evolving areas of practice in psychiatric nursing and related health professions. The depth and scope of the content make this book appropriate not only for undergraduate nursing students but for master's and doctoral students and nursing practitioners as well. This comprehensive book is more specific than previous editions in its discussion of theory and its application to the role and responsibility of the psychiatric nurse today, regardless of the area chosen for practice. Implications for all nursing care appear throughout the book.

Marion Kalkman, Professor Emeritus, University of California, San Francisco, is an outstanding leader in the development of the clinical specialist role in psychiatric nursing and in the preparation of clinical specialists. Her psychiatric nursing experience has spanned four decades and includes extensive supervision and teaching. In addition, she has had a rich career in public service in both nursing and nonnursing organizations, nationally and locally. Anne J. Davis is currently Associate Professor at the University of California, San Francisco. She has held numerous clinical positions in psychiatric nursing in private, state, and federal facilities in this country. Abroad she has worked in Israel and Denmark, been a visiting lecturer in Nigeria, and served as a W.H.O. Fellow in Ghana and Kenya.

Esther A. Garrison, R.N., M.A., LL.D., D.Sc.
Formerly Chief, Psychiatric Nursing
Training Branch, Division of Manpower
and Training Programs, National
Institute of Mental Health, Public
Health Service, U.S. Department of Health,
Education, and Welfare

PREFACE

New Dimensions in Mental Health–Psychiatric Nursing, the fourth edition of our textbook of psychiatric nursing, has evolved from our belief that a body of advanced content in the field of mental health–psychiatric nursing exists and is necessary for the nurse practitioner who must meet the demands of the new professional roles emerging in the mental health field. This book attempts to meet this need.

We also believe that a theoretical framework for the practice of mental health–psychiatric nursing is highly desirable. However, when we reviewed the many theories currently in use in psychiatry and nursing, no one theoretical system could be found which would provide understanding of the many problems encountered by the nurse and furnish guidance for nursing practice. Therefore, we have selected five theoretical models, each of which we believe can be helpful in illuminating a particular aspect or area of the mental health field and of mental illness. These five models are the developmental, the medical, the behavioral, the psychodynamic, and the unitary or general system theory.

The developmental model seems particularly well suited for an understanding of the normal growth process, the intrinsic problems of growth which generally occur at the transition phases of the various stages of the life cycle, as well as various other causes of maldevelopment which may arise during the growth process. The whole problem of prevention of psychological and social maladjustment, the importance of family interaction, and the role of the nurse in effecting such primary prevention stem naturally from this model. In other words, this model covers that large area in the field of psychiatry formerly referred to as mental hygiene and now better known as mental health. Included in the section on mental health is a presentation of the developmental model, followed by six chapters which discuss the application of this model to the various stages of the life cycle. These discussions provide an understanding of common developmental problems which can interfere with normal development as well as indicate ways by which health professionals can help the client overcome some of the deterrents to the achievement of his maximum mental health potential.

People who suffer from emotional stress sufficiently severe to produce mental symptoms or abnormal behavior which interferes with effective functioning in society are said to have some form of mental illness or psychiatric disorder. These people come to health agencies seeking relief from their distress in the form of some kind of treatment. The responsibility for providing this help rests upon those members of the health professions trained in psychiatry and psychiatric techniques. For the nurse who specializes in the care and treatment of psychiatric patients, four models have been selected out of the many currently used because they seem to represent the most distinct and diverse points of view. Many other treatment models, such as gestalt therapy or client-centered therapy, consist of elements or combinations of these models. The four treatment models selected are the medical, the behavioral, the psychodynamic, and the unitary. Chapters 9 through 16 present these four models, together with the major types of disorders and the methods used in treatment.

A major innovation in this edition is the section on environmental influences on mental health and mental illness. Until very recently the causes of both developmental difficulties and frank psychiatric disorders were considered to be primarily factors within the body of the person such as heredity, physiological and psychological stress, conflict, and psychosomatic reactions. However, mental health professionals in increasing numbers now find that their clients are greatly affected by a whole range of external factors such as pollution, poverty, overpopulation, sexual and racial discrimination, and cultural shock. The mental health professional has only a partial understanding of his client unless he recognizes the need for a deeper awareness and knowledge of the complicated network of external forces which surround his client. This network of external forces influences such fundamental matters as his life-style, his interpersonal relationships, and his ability to obtain the necessities of life.

One of the therapeutic techniques considered essential for the mental health–psychiatric nurse specialist is initial patient assessment and evaluation, a technique rapidly becoming a requirement for two reasons. Patient assessment and evaluation is both a preliminary step for introducing a patient into psychotherapy and a technique required of the nurse who is expected to screen clients for treatment by other health professionals. Other essential

psychotherapeutic methods include individual, group, and family psychotherapy.

The expanded and extended role of the nurse, discussed in detail in the first
and last chapters, is also specifically noted in various chapters throughout the
book. We have attempted in an exploratory way to indicate trends and
directions for mental health–psychiatric nursing. We have tried to include
enough content to encourage the reader to develop his practice along the lines
of his greatest interest. By using the extensive references at the end of each
chapter, the reader can deepen his knowledge of a given subject according to
his needs and wishes.

Marion E. Kalkman
Anne J. Davis

ACKNOWLEDGMENTS

The editors wish to thank the following publishers and authors for permission to quote material from the works listed. Basic Books Inc., Publishers, from the *American Handbook of Psychiatry,* 1959, vol. II, edited by Silvano Arieti, pp. 1024, 1040, 1102, 1179–1180, 1245, 1340, 1345–1346; and from *Adolescence; Psychosocial Perspectives,* 1969, edited by Gerald Caplan and Serge Lebovici, p. 77. Williams & Wilkins Co., Baltimore, from *Comprehensive Textbook of Psychiatry,* 1967, edited by Alfred M. Freedman and Harold Kaplan, pp. 707–708, 711–715, 728, and 750. International Universities Press, Inc., from *The Severely Disturbed Adolescent,* 1969, by William M. Easson, p. 177 and references. *International Nursing Review,* vol. 18, no. 4, pp. 360–366. Harper and Row Publishers, Inc., from *Dark Ghetto,* 1967, by Kenneth B. Clark, p. 83 and Chapters VIII and X. W. B. Saunders Company from *Modern Clinical Psychiatry,* 1968, 7th ed., by Arthur P. Noyes and Lawrence C. Kolb, p. 91. National Institute of Mental Health, U.S. Department of Health, Education and Welfare, from *Suicide among the Young: A Supplement to the Bulletin of Suicidology,* 1969, by Richard M. Seiden, references and studies cited in text.

Thanks are due to the secretaries of the Department of Mental Health and Community Nursing, University of California School of Nursing, and especially to Maria Sandoval.

PART ONE

Evolution
of Psychiatric Nursing

1

THE PSYCHIATRIC NURSE—
HISTORICAL DEVELOPMENT OF THE ROLE

Marion E. Kalkman

NURSING BEFORE 1860

Nursing—the care of the young, the ill, and the helpless—has a history as long as that of the human race. But the emergence of the *nurse* as one who makes nursing her profession dates back to 1860 when the first Nightingale School at St. Thomas Hospital, London, was opened. Before then, nursing was done by members of the family, or by neighbors, servants, members of religious nursing orders or humanitarian societies, or even by convalescent patients and prisoners. For all of them, nursing was an extra task imposed in addition to their usual duties. (Patients today still worry about being a burden to their nurses.) Even for the members of the religious nursing orders nursing care was a secondary objective; the primary concern was for the spiritual welfare of the patient.

During the Crimean War, the practice of using untrained women as nurses for the wounded soldiers created many difficulties for Florence Nightingale. Therefore, when she returned to England, she campaigned for professional schools of nursing to be set up in England. However, the concept of trained nurses was in opposition to the prevailing notion that any "good" woman had an intuitive humane instinct for nursing and that no organized instruction or supervised practice was necessary. Shryock (1959) writes, "As she [Miss Nightingale] pointed out, no one claimed that good intentions alone could qualify a man to be a physician. By the same token, as demands on nurses became more complex, no one should think a woman fit to be a nurse merely because she was a nice person."

Because of Miss Nightingale's profound impact on nursing, she is considered the founder of professional nursing and nursing education. Historically, though, the first nursing schools were organized between 1782 and 1815 in Germany, by Dr. Franz May. The first was opened in Mannheim in 1782, the second at the University of Heidelberg in 1800. Of particular interest to psychiatric nurses is Dr. May's belief that the quality of nursing care could not be improved unless the nurses were themselves well treated by their superiors. He thought that only satisfied, well-trained, and faithful nurses could give good nursing care to patients. He even suggested that a servant be assigned to the nurse for her personal service. It is also interesting that Dr. May's colleagues opposed his teaching nurses to be responsible for bandaging, dressings, enemas, and the administration of medications. Nurses were not considered capable of performing these everyday medical procedures (Shryock, 1959, pp. 232–235).

THE ROLE OF THE NURSE FROM 1860 TO 1880

In 1860, when the professional training of nurses was instituted, the prevalent medical concepts were concerned with sanitation. The Industrial Revolution had brought crowded conditions in the big cities attended by poverty, dirt, and filth. Infectious diseases were rampant and infant mortality high. Yet specific pathogenic organisms for the various disease entities had not been identified. Crude research in some of the large hospitals had shown that when sanitary measures had been instituted such as clean bedding, uncontaminated water, fresh air, and wholesome diets, mortality rates decreased markedly. In 1865, Lister introduced antisepsis in surgery by the use of carbolic acid dressings and, later, carbolic acid spray. Antisepsis lowered the mortality rate associated with surgery, although Lister was not aware of the specific organisms that he was destroying. Disease entities were not clearly described or classified, etiology was usually unknown, and specific treatments were not available except empirically, as the use of quinine for malaria. Nursing care also was oriented to the principles of sanitation. Miss Nightingale, in her article "Nursing the Sick" (Seymer, 1954, pp. 335–336), describes the duties of a nurse as follows:

Nursing proper means, besides giving the medicines and stimulants prescribed, or applying the surgical dressings and other remedies ordered—(1) The providing, and the proper use of, fresh air, especially at night—that is, ventilation, and of warmth or coolness. (2) The securing the health of the sick-room or ward, which includes light, cleanliness of floors and walls, of bed, bedding and utensils. (3) Personal cleanliness of patient and nurse, quiet, variety, sympathy, and cheerfulness. (4) The administering and sometimes preparation of diet (food and drink). (5) The application of remedies. In other words, all that is wanted to enable Nature to set up her restorative processes, to expel the intruder disturbing her rules of health and life. For it is Nature that cures: not the physician or nurse. (6) Observation of the patient.

Onset of Custodial Care

There are parallels in the nursing care of the mentally and the physically ill of this period. In both fields little treatment was available. The "moral treatment" of the 1830s and 1840s which followed the humanitarian principles of Pinel and Tuke was in its decline; classical descriptive psychiatry and the psychoanalytic psychiatry of Freud were still in the future. This was a period of custodial psychiatric treatment. Custodial nursing care at its best during this period was based on Miss Nightingale's "sanitary principles," with primary emphasis on cleanliness of wards and personal hygiene, fresh air and exercise, concern for adequate food and sleep, and kindness toward patients.

In the United States this was a time of great waves of immigration. Recent immigrants who became mentally ill could not be accommodated in the small private mental hospitals, and although many new state mental hospitals were built following the reform movement of Dorothea Lynde Dix, the hospitals were overcrowded. Physicians and attendants were few and greatly overworked. Psychiatric care was poor. Miss Linda Richards, America's first professional psychiatric nurse, as well as the first American graduate nurse, also belongs in this period. Miss Richards was graduated from the New England Hospital for Women and Children in 1873. After graduation she went to England to study Miss Nightingale's methods. When she returned, she organized the nursing services and nursing educational programs in Boston City Hospital and in several state mental hospitals in Illinois as well as in other states.

THE EMERGENCE OF THE ROLE OF THE
PSYCHIATRIC NURSE FROM 1880 TO 1930

In 1882, the first school specifically for the preparation of nurses to care for the mentally ill was opened at McLean Hospital, a private psychiatric hospital in Waverley, Massachusetts. By 1890, ninety men and women were graduated from the two-year program. About that time, trained nurses were beginning to be employed on the nursing staffs of the state mental hospitals, where their superior preparation and training were recognized by the administrative psychiatrists. This recognition was demonstrated by relieving the trained psychiatric nurses of some of the more menial tasks and by employing additional men and women to do the scrubbing, bed-making, and washing of dishes and windows. Relief from menial tasks enabled the nurses to use their skills to better advantage.

Santos and Stainbrook (1949) write in their very interesting article, "A History of Psychiatric Nursing in the Nineteenth Century," that there was evidence by the end of the century of the growing appreciation of the therapeutic role of the psychiatric nurse. Her duties included carrying out or assisting the physician with the psychiatric procedures of the day; administering sedative drugs such as whiskey, chloroform, and paraldehyde; and hydrotherapeutic measures such as hot and cold douches, showers, continuous baths, and wet sheet packs. Various methods of inducing patients to take food also played an important part in the therapeutic measures practiced by physicians and nurses. However, the nineteenth-century psychiatric nurse had very few psychological nursing skills at her command.

The Role of the Nurse in Custodial Care

The therapeutic role of the psychiatric nurse did not change from 1890 until about the 1930s. It continued to be largely custodial with the primary focus still on the general physical needs of the patient according to the old precept of a sane mind in a sound body. Physical nursing care was supplemented by a limited number of psychiatric procedures such as hydrotherapy, tube-feeding, and restraint measures. Psychologically, the nurse was concerned wtih maintaining "good attitudes"; that is, kindly, tolerant, humane behavior toward the patient. This was also the period in psychiatry of the rise and decline of descriptive psychiatry. Dr. Emil Kraepelin, who published his textbook, "Psychiatrie," in 1883, was the outstanding proponent of the school of descriptive psychiatry. He was the first to describe and classify psychiatric disorders in a systematic way. Kraepelinian psychiatry, however, tended to be pessimistic in its prognosis of mental illness, and possibly for this reason did not make any noteworthy contributions to the treatment of psychiatric disorders.

The Development of Dynamic Psychiatry

The influence of descriptive psychiatry was widespread in this country as well as in Europe, especially in state mental hospitals. The dominance of this point of view in psychiatry was finally challenged by a new outlook, that of dynamic psychiatry. Jean-Marie Charcot (1825–1893), Pierre Janet (1859–1947), Eugen Bleuler (1857–1939), Adolph Meyer (1866–1950), and Sigmund Freud (1857–1939) were prominent among the psychiatrists who formulated these concepts. Of this group the greatest contribution was made by Freud with the development of psychoanalysis. Noyes (1953, p. 15) states, "It is generally considered beyond dispute that his [Freud's] concepts have contributed more to an unlocking of the secrets of the human personality and to an understanding of the psychogenesis of mental disorders than have those of any other system of psychology."

Whereas descriptive psychiatry was primarily interested in describing objectively the characteristics of a mentally ill individual by a method similar to that used in describing a specimen in the biological or physical science laboratory, dynamic psychiatry was concerned with the influences or forces at work within and without the personality which produce the pathology seen in the mentally ill person. Dynamic psychiatry also recognized that the observer could not remain aloof and detached from the observed, like a scientist observing a specimen, but that the observer himself both influenced and was influenced by the person observed.

The concepts of psychoanalysis took root slowly and encountered a great deal of opposition in both medical and nonmedical circles. Concepts such as infantile sexuality, the oedipal situation, and the origin of anal aggressive behavior shocked many people. However, in spite of dogged opposition, psychoanalytic concepts gradually supplanted the older theories of psychiatric treatment. Not only was psychoanalysis coming into use as a method of treatment, but the body of psychoanalytic theory was providing many forms of psychoanalytically oriented psychotherapy.

Nurses Slow to Utilize Dynamic Concepts

During the struggle for acceptance of psychoanalysis and psychoanalytic treatment by psychiatrists, nurses were not very much affected. There seemed to be no role for the nurse in the treatment of a patient undergoing psychoanalysis. Psychoanalytic patients were usually treated in the analyst's office as private patients. However, when psychoanalysis became the predominant method of treatment in a number of private psychiatric clinics, sanitariums, and hospitals well staffed with psychiatric nurses, these nurses became acquainted with psychoanalytic treatment and sometimes, as at Chestnut Lodge, Rockville, Maryland, became involved as participant members of the treatment team. When psychoanalytic theory became part of the curriculum in medical schools, and psychoanalytically oriented psychotherapy was being practiced in the psychiatric units of teaching hospitals, psychiatric nurses became aware of the value of this body of knowledge for psychiatric nursing education and practice.

Dissatisfaction of Nurses with the Nursing Role

For a long time nurses had been dissatisfied with the lack of psychological techniques available to them. In many of the hospitals where descriptive psychiatry was practiced nurses were dismayed and discouraged by the belief that mental illness was incurable. Many nurses were also overwhelmed by the large numbers of patients which made individualization of patient care impossible, by the severity of psychotic behavior demonstrated by patients, and by the number of patients whose illness was of many years duration. This was essentially the picture of psychiatric nursing at the end of the period from 1880 to 1930.

DEVELOPMENT OF THE ROLE OF THE PSYCHIATRIC NURSE FROM 1930 TO 1960

New Techniques in Psychiatric Treatment

Many new developments in psychiatry and psychiatric treatment profoundly influenced the evolution of the role of the psychiatric nurse. An important discovery was that certain medical treatments could be used for specific psychiatric disorders. These treatments were usually grouped together under the heading somatic therapy. The earliest application of somatic therapy for psychiatric disorders was in 1917 when Wagner-Jauregg found that paresis could be arrested by inoculating the patient with malaria organisms. The high fever produced by the malaria destroyed the spirochetes of syphilis. Later, in 1919, arsenicals were substituted for the malaria inoculations, and since 1943 penicillin has been used. However, it was not until the 1930s that a number of somatic treatments were developed and were met with widespread acceptance by psychiatric circles. These treatments included deep sleep therapy (1930), insulin shock therapy (1935), Metrazol shock therapy (1935), electroshock therapy (1937), and psychosurgery (1935–1936). Though these therapies varied greatly in their rationale of treatment and in their procedural methods, they all had several important effects on psychiatric nursing and the role of the psychiatric nurse.

Effects of New Treatments on the Nurse's Role

Because somatic therapies were medical and surgical treatments, they required the services of highly skilled nurses. It was Florence Nightingale who had first proved to the medical profession by her hospital mortality statistics that trained nurses were necessary for effective medical treatment. During the 1930s, while the psychiatric nurse was groping to find her role in psychiatric treatment, her role in caring for the patient's general physical needs was acknowledged. However, her contribution to the treatment of the patient's psychiatric disorder did not seem significant either to the psychiatrist or to the psychiatric nurse herself. With the enthusiastic acceptance of the somatic therapies by the medical profession, the technical knowledge and skills of the nurse were in great demand by the psychiatrists utilizing these methods. Thus, through her professional training as a nurse and her medical-surgical nursing skills the psychiatric nurse first achieved recognition as one having a significant role in psychiatric treatment.

The use of the somatic therapies had other important effects on psychiatric nursing. When the first flush of optimism over the successful results of somatic therapy had somewhat abated, two interesting facts emerged. One was the realization that the psychological methods of treatment which had been overshadowed by the success of the somatic therapies were still very important. At first it was thought that somatic therapy alone could treat mental disorders effectively, but later it was found that psychotherapy was needed both to reinforce the effects of somatic treatment and also to treat those patients who were not amenable to somatic treatment. Another unexpected finding was that many patients who were successfully treated by somatic therapy then, for the first time, became accessible to psychological methods of treatment. Thus, somatic therapy increased rather than decreased the demand for psychotherapy. The greatest pressure fell on the psychiatrists, but those in the other psychiatric disciplines also felt the impact, including psychiatric nurses. The nurses, however, realized that they would have to develop new and more effective psychiatric nursing techniques and that they would have to adapt psychotherapeutic techniques used by the psychiatrists to the practice of nursing.

Before new psychological techniques could be developed in nursing, nurses needed some theoretical concepts on which to base their practice. The theories which proved most helpful for clinical practice in psychiatric nursing came from three main sources—psychoanalytic theory, the interpersonal theory of psychiatry, and communication theory. All these theories either were developed or gained general acceptance during this period, from 1930 to 1960. Some of the principles derived from these theories which were most useful to nursing practice will be discussed in subsequent chapters as they apply to the various psychological techniques, including individual psychotherapy, group psychotherapy, psychological aspects of general nursing care, family therapy, and community mental health nursing.

MENTAL ILLNESS RECOGNIZED AS A NATIONAL HEALTH PROBLEM

World War II and the economic and social changes which followed deeply affected psychiatric nursing. During the war 850,000 inductees were rejected by the Selective Service system because of psychiatric defects. Psychiatric disabilities accounted for 43 percent of all Army discharges. With such a high percentage of mental disorders found among a selected portion of the population, it was reasonable to assume that the incidence of mental illness among the general population was probably much higher. For the first time the nation was made aware of the extent of mental illness as a national health problem. Another result of the war was that during military service millions of young men came in contact with psychiatrists and with a variety of psychiatric services. These contacts ran the gamut from the routine psychiatric interview during induction to emergency, brief, or prolonged psychiatric treatment. When these men returned home, many sought psychiatric help for themselves and their families regarding problems for which they previously would not have wanted psychiatric assistance.

The National Mental Health Act

The government's concern over the seriousness and magnitude of the problem of mental illness and the increased demand for psychiatric services resulted in the enactment of the National Mental Health Act in 1946. This act authorized the development of a National Institute of Mental Health and also a threefold program for (1) training psychiatric professional personnel, (2) supporting psychiatric research, and (3) providing aid to individual states for the development of mental health programs. Psychiatric nursing was one of the four professions specified in the training program. NIMH funds spurred the development of psychiatric nursing programs in accredited collegiate and university schools of nursing at both the undergraduate and graduate levels.

EFFECT OF MENTAL HEALTH ACT ON NURSING EDUCATION

The training programs provided a standard of psychiatric nursing education which was far superior to any previously available. Graduates of these programs received a professional and academic education which made it possible for them to function as colleagues on the psychiatric treatment team with members of the other psychiatric disciplines. In many instances training programs for psychiatric residents, student psychologists, and social workers were conducted in the same institutions as the psychiatric nursing training programs. Students from all four disciplines often worked with the same patients, and attended the same case conferences and ward meetings. Psychiatric nursing students learned to utilize the psychiatrist, the psychologist, and the social worker as consultants, and also to work with them on the multidisciplinary treatment team. As a result of such experiences, the other professions learned to know and appreciate the special skills which the nurse could contribute to the treatment of the psychiatric patient.

Development of New Techniques in Psychiatric Nursing

The influence of these collegiate psychiatric nursing programs extended to several other important areas. Many of the graduates of these programs helped to alleviate one of the most serious shortages in psychiatric nursing, that of well-qualified teachers. Teachers were needed not only for psychiatric programs in collegiate schools of nursing, but also for associate degree, diploma, practical nurse, and psychiatric attendant programs. New techniques in psychiatric nursing such as individual psychotherapy and nursing group psychotherapy were developed and systematically taught in these programs. These new psychiatric nursing techniques emphasized the importance of the personality and behavior of the nurse as a factor in therapeutic interaction with patients. The self-awareness demanded by conscious utilization of the nurse's personality in the service of the patient was in direct conflict with the traditional impersonal and emotionally uninvolved nurse role. Until 1960, this conflict was still raging and had spread to other areas of nursing.

Development of Graduate Psychiatric Nursing Programs

During this period (1930 to 1960), psychiatric nurses also became aware of the need to test psychiatric nursing principles and practices which had evolved from their practical experience in caring for psychiatric patients. Yet they found themselves woefully lacking in the necessary research tools and techniques. However, a beginning was made when graduate academic programs offered specialization in psychiatric nursing and every graduate psychiatric nursing student was required to do some research in the form of a thesis, dissertation, or special research study. From these graduate programs in psychiatric nursing emerged professional psychiatric nurses equipped with knowledge and skill of a more advanced level than was offered in any other nursing program. These students also received preparation which would enable them to become the future teachers, supervisors, consultants, and researchers in psychiatric nursing.

Integration of Psychiatric Principles in the Basic Curriculum

In 1956, collegiate schools of nursing began to improve the quality of their basic psychiatric nursing programs which prepare nurses for first-level positions in psychiatric nursing, the level at which the nurse gives direct patient care. This improvement was made possible when funds were made available to schools of nursing by the National Institute of Mental Health for obtaining well-prepared psychiatric teachers. Government support was also made available to promote the integration of psychiatric nursing principles throughout the curriculum so that every nurse prepared in a collegiate program would have the essential knowledge and skills not only in caring for psychiatric patients in psychiatric hospitals, general hospitals, or the community, but also for meeting the psychological nursing needs of other types of patients.

Experimental Projects for Psychiatric Aide Education

A variety of solutions to the problem of providing additional personnel for the direct care of psychiatric patients were attempted during this period. One attempted solution was to develop a category of personnel separate and distinct from nurses who would be trained primarily to care for the patients' psychological needs. The best known development of this idea was the experimental Psychiatric Aide Training Program conducted at the Menninger Foundation and Topeka State

Hospital from 1949 to 1952. This program was directed by Dr. Bernard H. Hall with funds from the Rockefeller Foundation. The report of this project, "Psychiatric Aide Education," was published in 1952. One of the results of this study showed that the duties of the psychiatric aide cannot be separated from nursing and are, in fact, nursing functions. Dr. Karl Menninger (1959, p. 716) writes, looking back on this experiment:

> In the past few years the psychiatric nurses have recognized their responsibility for participating in a program which many formerly viewed with misgivings and suspiciousness. The relationship of aides to nurses is one of the most important problems in working out methods and procedures. In my opinion the work of the psychiatric aide *is* psychiatric nursing at a level administratively subordinate to that of the psychiatric nurse. In the future, the aide will belong to the nursing team, a representative of which will function on the total psychiatric "executive team" consisting of adjunctive therapists, social workers, psychologists, and other specialized workers under the leadership of the psychiatrist.

Another result of this experimental project was the recognition that the individual who was the operative agent for giving direct patient care, to whom the patient was exposed for the longest periods of time, and upon whom the hospitalized patient was most dependent, must have better training, whether this individual be a professional nurse, a practical nurse, an aide, or an attendant. The curriculum developed for the Menninger experimental program included theory and practice far beyond what was being offered in most basic professional nursing programs, and was immeasureably beyond the apprentice type, in-service training programs generally offered in most large mental hospitals for aides and attendants. An extensive course in psychotherapy (180 hours) was included in the curriculum on the basis of a frank recognition that psychiatric nursing personnel, in this case the psychiatric aide, are engaged in a type of psychotherapy whether they and the medical personnel are aware of it or not, and that they need suitable instruction if psychiatric treatment is to be effective.

Another project which should be included in any discussion of aide education was a seminar project which was conducted for teachers of psychiatric aides. This project extended from April 1958, to September 1960, and was cosponsored by the National League for Nursing and the American Psychiatric Association. A staff of six expert psychiatric nurse educators, headed by Miss Garland K. Lewis as director, conducted eighteen seminar courses of 2 weeks each for 175 nurses who were responsible for the psychiatric nursing instruction of 5,000 psychiatric aides, attendants, and nursing assistants. The 175 nurses who participated in this intensive teacher-training program came from twenty-five psychiatric hospitals located in four Southern states—Arkansas, North Carolina, South Carolina, and Tennessee. A follow-up study conducted by a sociologist in a selected hospital a year after the seminar revealed that the project was instrumental in bringing about innovations in patient care, marked attitudinal changes, and new teaching methods in the majority of nurses who had participated in the program, two-thirds of whom were actively engaged in situational teaching. The report of this project, entitled "An Approach to Education of Psychiatric Personnel," was published by the National League for Nursing in 1961 (Lewis et al., 1961). The role of the psychiatric nurse in assuming increasing responsibility for teaching all personnel engaged in the nursing care of psychiatric patients was one which began to gain general acceptance at the end of this period.

THE THERAPEUTIC COMMUNITY

Social psychiatry gained prominence in the years after World War II and added a new dimension to the role of the psychiatric nurse. Social psychiatry covers a wide variety of methods of treatment based on the concept that man finds his fulfillment or self-realization in his interpersonal relationships with the individuals in his environment and the culture in which he lives. Goodwin Watson wrote in his foreword to Maxwell Jones's "The Therapeutic Community" (1953): "Psychiatry now verges upon another great forward step, one which may have consequences even more far-reaching than those flowing from psychoanalytic discoveries. In the field of mental health, most attention has been given to psychotherapy; some to mental hygiene, but very little as yet, to the design of a whole culture which will foster healthy personalities." The two main factors in the development of social psychiatry at this particular time in history, primarily in Great Britain, The Netherlands, and the Scandinavian countries were the great shortage of psychiatrists and other psychotherapists, which became painfully evident during the war, and the highly developed sense of social responsibility which forced therapists to seek new methods of treatment to meet the increased demands.

The Role of the Nurse in the Therapeutic Community

From Great Britain, social psychiatry spread to the United States. The methods of social psychiatry seemed to offer some solutions to the

problem of shortage of personnel combined with large patient populations in state and federal mental hospitals. The form which it most
frequently took was based on the method described by Maxwell Jones
(1953) in his book, "The Therapeutic Community." Watson writes:
"The Therapeutic Community views treatment as located not in the
application by specialists of certain shocks, drugs or interpretations,
but in the normal interactions of healthy community life. The doctor
has a vital role, but so also do the nurses, the job supervisors, and the
other patients." Nurses, in fact, have a very complex and important
role to play in the form of treatment described in Jones's book. In one
aspect of their role nurses represent the cultural norms of the
community, exerting what is referred to as positive discipline in setting
limits for patients, or using their authority to protect the therapeutic
community from antisocial elements. Another aspect of the nurses'
role is social—offering friendliness, security, stability, and individual
attention to each patient. The therapeutic aspect of the nurses' role is
to support and encourage patients in their participation in the total
treatment and to act as a clarifier and interpreter when the patient
encounters difficulties, collaborating with the doctor in therapy, and
most importantly, to serve as the transmitter of the therapeutic
community culture to the patient.

THE CHANGING ROLE OF THE NURSE

While the concept of the therapeutic community was gaining acceptance in this country, the open door policy, patient government,
group psychotherapy, mental hygiene clinics, patient social clubs,
therapeutic clubs, halfway houses, the trend toward smaller hospitals
and the division of large mental hospitals into smaller, autonomous
units, and a number of other methods of treating psychiatric patients
by influencing them through their social milieu were being introduced. All these methods demanded that psychiatric nurses change
their focus from medical treatment of the patient within the four walls
of a hospital to social treatment oriented toward reintegration of the
patient into the community. Most nurses were not enthusiastic about
participating in the new social therapies, for very little in their previous
nursing education or experience had prepared them for it. Neither
psychiatric nurses nor members of the other psychiatric disciplines
could determine just what the nurse could contribute to patient
treatment or, indeed, whether he should even be included as a
member of the psychiatric team. At the end of the 1950s, these
questions were still far from a solution of any kind.

Psychosomatic Medicine and the Nurse

The development of psychosomatic medicine from 1930 to 1960 had important implications not only for the psychiatric nurse but for all nurses. The term *psychosomatic medicine,* although not completely accepted by the medical profession, is nevertheless generally used in referring to those medical conditions in which emotional and personality factors play important roles. In his article, "General Concepts of Psychosomatic Medicine," Lidz (1955) states that it was necessity that finally forced an interest in psychosomatic conditions. As the conquest of the infectious diseases approached, the unsolved problems of chronic and metabolic disorders challenged the attention of medical scientists. Psychiatric investigative and therapeutic techniques seemed to offer a fresh approach to these so-called medical problems by emphasizing the importance of the patient's relationships to his psychological and social environment as well as to his physiologic activities.

Physicians discovered that many of the methods used in psychiatry were also effective in treating patients with psychosomatic disorders. Nurses who were not knowledgeable in psychosomatic theory or skilled in psychological nursing techniques found themselves in difficulties with both patients and physicians. Many of the skills generally used by psychiatric nurses in caring for patients with psychiatric disorders could be adapted to the care of psychosomatic patients. In some hospitals, expert psychiatric nurses were utilized as consultants to help staff nurses with problems related to patients with psychosomatic disorders. Nursing educators came to realize that many of the principles of psychiatric nursing were valid for all clinical areas of nursing and that many of the skills could be used in all aspects of nursing care.

Initially, programs for the integration of psychiatric nursing concepts into the curriculums of collegiate schools of nursing were supported by NIMH training funds. Although many attempts have been made to incorporate psychiatric nursing principles into the general nursing curriculum, none has proved completely successful. However, there is no question but that the principles of psychological nursing derived from psychiatry are profoundly influencing concepts of nursing care, nurses' attitudes toward patients, and the whole philosophy of nursing.

The Psychiatric Nurse as a Clinical Specialist

During the 1950s psychiatric nurses began to be concerned about defining their role. In 1952 the writer stated (Kalkman, 1952),

Changing concepts in psychiatry have brought changing concepts of what the psychiatric nurse should do. If the psychiatric nurse is to play a meaningful role in the treatment of the psychiatric patient, if she is to become a fully accepted member of the psychiatric team, her functions must be defined. One must consider the particular contributions which the psychiatric nurse can make to the care of the patient. What can the nurse do for the patient that cannot be done by the psychiatrist, the social worker, or the psychologist? Why is she needed to complete the psychiatric team?

The writer would like to suggest . . . the areas in which the psychiatric nurse can profitably function, and the goals toward which psychiatric nursing education should be directed. . . . These are: (1) the psychiatric nurse as a scientific observer, (2) the psychiatric nurse as the creator of a therapeutic environment, (3) the psychiatric nurse as a socializing agent, and (4) the psychiatric nurse as a psychotherapeutic agent.

The psychiatric nurse of this period felt at the greatest loss in the role of a psychotherapeutic agent. She was not considered qualified to utilize any of the then current forms of psychotherapy which could have provided a theoretical framework on which to base her practice. Then in 1952 came the development of nurse-patient relationship therapy, which provided this theoretical framework.

Nurse-Patient Relationship Therapy

Relationship therapy had been an accepted method of psychotherapy for many years. It had been used extensively by psychiatrists, psychologists, and social workers. However, psychiatric nursing is indebted to Gwen Tudor for the first use of relationship therapy as a technique applicable to the nursing care of psychiatric patients. She described her use of this form of therapy in her article, "A Sociopsychiatric Nursing Intervention in a Problem of Mutual Withdrawal on a Mental Hospital Ward." Since this paper was published in 1952, many other articles have appeared in the literature which describe the use of this method in nursing. Since that time, nurse-patient relationship therapy has been utilized by nurses not only in the care of psychiatric patients but also in the care of many other types of patients.

Maurice Levine (1952, p. 352) defines relationship therapy as:

. . . a fairly prolonged period of contact of patient and therapist in which the therapist can maintain, without much conscious effort, a good therapeutic attitude . . . . In such a growing relationship certain therapeutic experiences occur which may be listed as follows: (a) the experience of being accepted as of value, or potentially so, and of not being condemned or rejected because of defensive distortions; (b) the growth of an identification with some of the more successful techniques and adjustments of the therapist as they may fit the individual needs of the patient; and (c) spontaneous corrective emotional experiences, based on the fact that the therapist does not respond in the manner expected by the patient.

Definition of Nurse-Patient Relationship Therapy

Nurse-patient relationship therapy falls within Levine's definition of relationship therapy in that it is also a prolonged relationship between a nurse-therapist and a patient in which the patient can feel accepted by the nurse as a person of worth, is free to express himself without fear of rejection or censure, and can learn new and more satisfying patterns of behavior. The nurse in a nurse-patient relationship therapy is always a particular nurse, and the patient a particular patient. Although other nurses and nursing personnel may be involved in the total nursing care of this patient, there is only one nurse-therapist until the relationship is terminated. The relationship is a professional one, and is maintained on this level. It is a relationship mutually entered upon by the nurse and the patient for the purpose of helping the patient to get relief from his symptoms, to improve his interpersonal relationships with others, and to achieve a richer and more satisfying life by way of more effective patterns of social interaction and the development of his potentialities.

The nurse accepts a patient for nurse-patient relationship on the basis that this therapy is a prescribed part of the patient's total treatment plan. The patient's psychiatrist indicates that the patient could benefit from this type of nursing care, and that the particular nurse chosen to work with his patient is acceptable. He also expresses his willingness to confer with the nurse as seems indicated.

Nurse-Patient Relationship Therapy in the Preparation of the Psychiatric Nurse Specialist

The latter part of the 1950s saw the development of the psychiatric nurse specialist. In May 1958, at a meeting of the Graduate Seminar of the Western Council on Higher Education for Nursing (WCHEN), the deans of schools of nursing in the West where graduate programs were offered appointed faculty members to delineate the clinical content at the master's level in four areas of nursing. These areas were: maternal-child health, psychiatric nursing, medical-surgical nursing, and public health nursing. In the report prepared by the psychiatric nursing group, published in 1967, the role of the psychiatric nurse specialist was delineated. In this role delineation, it was stated that the primary function of the psychiatric nurse specialist was that of a nurse therapist, and that the basic core of this therapy was the nurse-patient relationship. This applied also to group therapy, family therapy, and milieu therapy. Other functions of the psychiatric nurse specialist were: assumption of primary responsibility for the nursing care of the psychiatric patient; the ability to make effective interventions in the treatment situation; the utilization of relevant theories as a basis for clinical practice; the acquisition of personal clinical expertise before teaching or supervising others; and the ability to practice psychiatric nursing in whatever setting the need for psychiatric services exists (Fujiki et al., 1967, p. 2).

The utilization of nurse-patient relationship therapy in the nursing care of psychiatric patients spread rapidly during the 1960s. It constituted the form of psychotherapy practiced by most psychiatric nurses who were developing the level of practice required for specialization. It came to be regarded as a psychotherapeutic method identified with nursing, comparable with that of psychiatric casework in social work. In both methods the nurse or social worker practiced as adjunctive therapists in conjunction with the more highly regarded therapy of the psychiatrist. This secondary role for both social casework and nurse-patient relationship therapy was inevitable because, in both cases, the primary responsibility for the patient's treatment resided in the psychiatrist. Nevertheless, in time, as psychiatric nurses developed depth in understanding the problems which confronted their patients, skill in the therapeutic interventions, and ability to create and utilize the interpersonal relationship for the patient's benefit, this method of therapy gained the respect of psychiatrists and other health professionals as well as that of members of their own profession. Many psychiatric patients have benefited from it, and it is still a method of treatment by nurses, especially in in-patient settings where it was first developed.

THE COMMUNITY MENTAL HEALTH MOVEMENT AND THE PSYCHIATRIC NURSE

The Community Mental Health Centers Act of 1963 had a revolutionary impact not only in changing the direction of psychiatric nursing but also in expanding the role of the psychiatric nurse. The basic concept of the community mental health movement is that mentally ill people can and should be treated in the environment in which they live and expect to function after recovery (Public Law 88–164). This concept of treating the mentally ill in their own neighborhoods had the effect of taking many psychiatric nurses into local communities and freeing them from the almost exclusive practice of psychiatric nursing in large state hospitals, where 98 percent of the mentally ill had formerly been treated. This new freedom was a frightening experience for many psychiatric nurses who left the security of their well-defined roles in the bureaucratic state hospital system for the uncharted responsibilities and ill-defined functions in such loosely structured settings as mental health centers, day treatment centers, and patients' homes. In the early days of community mental health centers many psychiatric nurses had no background in community health nursing and no knowledge of community mental health agencies. On the other hand, many community health nurses were equally uneasy about the numbers of discharged state hospital patients who became part of their case load. These public health nurses did not feel prepared to cope with the emotional problems with which these discharged patients confronted them. It quickly became obvious to both groups that each group needed some of the knowledge and skills of the other group. Hilda Richards (1970, p. 1020) writes, "The professional—nurse or otherwise—has had to modify his own role and reexamine his perceptions and value systems. He has also discovered the inadequacy of his knowledge in such areas as change theory, community organization, and the politics of institutional structures."

The Community Mental Health Nurse

The problem of finding a nurse with an adequate professional background to function in a community mental health program was ameliorated somewhat when two programs were developed for the special preparation of community mental health nurses at the post-master's level at the Maimonides Hospital (Stokes, 1969) and the University of California, San Francisco. There were also a number of university-based graduate psychiatric nursing programs at the master's level with courses in community mental health nursing (University of Maryland and National Institute of Mental Health, 1967). The Maimonides Community Mental Health Center training project for the preparation of community mental health nurses provided its students with course content of the theoretical foundations and principles basic to the practice of community mental health. This content included: normal growth and development; dynamics of human behavior; family dynamics; psychopathology; epidemiology of mental illness; group dynamics; and social sciences with emphasis on sociology, role theory, and social psychology. Williams regarded this theoretical background as essential for clinical practice in community mental health programs. She also stressed the importance of good clinical supervision and the availability of consultation when needed (Williams, 1969, p. 55). The students were also expected to develop the following skills as nursing practitioners: identification and analysis of the psycho-bio-sociological factors that influence behavior; participation in therapy and community groups as leader, coleader, or peer; decision making with patients, professionals, and nonprofessional personnel; identification of essential factors in the creation and maintenance of a therapeutic milieu; clinical supervision; mental health consultation; institutional planning and organization; community mental health administration; and community organization (Davidites and Williams, 1969, p. 123).

The Changing Role of the Nurse in Community Mental Health Treatment

Some of the concepts of community mental health treatment had important consequences for the role and functions of psychiatric nurses. One of these concepts was that of multidisciplinary team leadership. It is a fact that the original concept of a multidisciplinary treatment team consisting typically of a psychiatrist, a psychologist, a social worker, and a nurse came into being during the era of Jones's therapeutic community in the 1950s. Although the members of this treatment team were, in theory, coequals, there was never any doubt that, in practice, the psychiatrist was the head of the team and that his word carried more weight than that of any other member of the team. The nurse's opinion carried the least weight, with the psychologist and the social worker jockeying for second and third places on the team. On the community mental health treatment team, this was not the case. Any member of the team could be the team leader—leadership was based on individual skills, background, and experience rather than on the basis of traditional professional role relationships (Ullman, 1969, p. 2). This concept destroys the traditional hierarchical structure with the psychiatrist as the leader and all other professionals subservient to him. The community mental health concept also required that each health profession must assume responsibility for preparing its students to assume leadership when necessary and, perhaps equally important, to be able to relinquish leadership to a colleague when this is indicated.

Another concept of community mental health treatment which has greatly expanded the role of the psychiatric nurse is the concept that the same therapist should provide and/or be responsible for the total treatment of the patient. To develop a therapist who is capable of providing treatment during the different phases of the patient's illness and who may need to follow him through the various agencies in the system, the role of the *generic worker* was developed by the Maimonides Community Mental Health Center. As defined by Stokes (1969, p. 26):

A generic mental health worker is viewed as a "generalist" who is active in different areas and on different levels of practice. . . . A staff member in our Center is given the opportunity through engagement in practice to develop skills in addition to those he has customarily performed as an outgrowth of his professional preparation.

She adds (Stokes, 1969, p. 46):

Continuity of care is provided to the patient through the assignment of the same therapist, called the primary therapist in all the services the patient needs, from diagnosis, to cure, to rehabilitation. Increased emphasis has been placed on family involvement with treatment in the home as well as in the agency.

The generic roles for all professional mental health workers include: psychotherapist, mental health consultant, mental health community worker, mental health teacher and counselor, psychiatric practitioner in in-service units, mental health administrator, and supervisor for students of one's own discipline and also of other disciplines (Stokes, 1969, p. 132).

Another consequence of the nurse participating as a coequal with other psychiatric health professionals in the community mental health setting was that all members were expected to perform a designated number of essential services, one of which was to provide psychotherapy for the patient. This psychotherapy, it should be noted, was not a brand of nursing therapy, as is the case with nurse-patient relationship therapy, but psychotherapy per se; that is, the nurse becomes for the time being a psychotherapist and practices psychotherapy and not nursing. To do this, nurses had to upgrade their knowledge and skill in psychotherapy to attain competence equal with that of other psychiatric professionals. To attain this level of competence necessitated additional study and supervised practice. Davidites and Williams (1969, p. 122), referring to the students in their program, state,

The roles of the psychiatric nurse in community mental health are extended beyond those of other clinical specialists in psychiatric nursing. She shares the generic roles of psychotherapist, mental health educator, mental health consultant, and community worker with members of the other disciplines. . . . Psychiatric nurses with preparation at the master's level have the knowledge and skills to function in these roles as beginning practitioners. . . . Therefore, our specific goal was to help nurse practitioners, who had already developed beginning skills as clinical specialists, to become effective collaborative practitioners of mental health in all settings in which mental health can be promoted.

OTHER CLINICAL SPECIALISTS IN PSYCHIATRIC NURSING

Community mental health is not the only area in which the psychiatric nurse may specialize. The field of psychiatry is so broad that specialization in some particular content or functional area has become necessary if psychiatric nurses are to develop a level of expertise. The future development of the profession and the fulfillment of the mental health needs of the people will be dependent on the number and quality of nurses prepared to be experts in their chosen area. In the content area there are a growing number of child psychiatric nursing specialists, and nurses who specialize in working with emotionally disturbed adolescents, as well as a relatively new specialty, the geriatric nurse specialist. Other content areas include specialists in a particular method of therapy, such as crisis therapy, drug therapy, family therapy, or gestalt therapy, or with patients with a particular disorder or disability, such as the renal dialysis patient, nonverbal patients, autistic children, the mentally retarded, and the chronically ill or neurologically disabled patients with emotional problems. Functional specialists include psychiatric nurse consultants to schools, to public health agencies, and to police departments; psychotherapists and counselors in a wide variety of settings; researchers, facilitators, educators, administrators, social activists, specialists in primary prevention of mental disorders, and specialists in rehabilitation. New areas of specialization are opening up so fast that the literature cannot keep up with them. By 1970, the growing number of doctoral programs in nursing made it possible for psychiatric nurses to obtain the necessary theory and supervised clinical experience with patients which would enable them to attain to an advanced level of clinical practice and, in addition, would provide them with the opportunity to acquire much-needed research skills.

THE PSYCHIATRIC NURSE
AS AN INDEPENDENT PRACTITIONER

One of the most recent developments in the changing role of the psychiatric nurse is that of the independent practitioner—the last step in the long journey from "handmaid of the physician" to self-determination. The first forerunner of this role concept in nursing literature is found in a paper by Catherine Norris, "Direct Access to the Patient" (1970). Norris (1970, p. 1007) defines *access* as a two-way process which "includes patient access to the nurse as well as nurse access to the patient. It does not necessarily mean primary therapeutic responsibility for the nurse, *but it certainly does not negate this kind of responsibility*" (editors' italics). Independent practice takes this next step. It includes access to patients but also primary responsibility for nursing practice. It is Norris's contention (1970, p. 1008) that *"direct* access to one's patient, or client, is mandatory for a profession'' (italics those of Norris). In other words, nursing cannot consider itself truly a profession when a doctor may still write orders that prescribe what a nurse may discuss with a patient. Norris (1970, p. 1010), in speaking of the need for the nurse's commitment in direct access, states what also could serve as an excellent definition of *independent practice*, "The nurse must be committed to function professionally in meeting health needs. This means that she must lay claim to the parts of health care which she defines as nursing, and that she must take full responsibility for her own functioning and her own decisions."

Since Dr. Norris's paper appeared in 1970, several examples of the nurse functioning as a primary practitioner have been published in the nursing literature. Jordan and Shipp (1971) describe the role of a nurse specialist in the follow-up care of twenty diabetic patients and compare the results of her work over a period of one to two years with that of a comparable group of patients treated for the same period of time by physicians. The patients treated by the nurse learned more about health maintenance, had less hyperglycemia, kept clinic appointments better, and recorded urine tests more carefully than those treated by the physicians. Another example is provided by Avey (1973), who describes her work as a primary care practitioner with cerebral palsied children and their families. In her role as coordinator for the cerebral palsy clinic she was instructed to act as a primary physician and was given authority to act independently without a physician's order. She ordered laboratory tests, screened and referred patients to designated specialists, evaluated treatment plans and made necessary changes, clarified instructions of physicians for parents, consulted with a child's schoolteachers, provided health information, and gave emotional support. She writes (1973, p. 661), "My role is not that of a true specialist, but rather a generalist. When I visit a home to help a young mother learn to position her child, I act as a physical therapist; when counseling a distraught family who's just been told the diagnosis is 'cerebral palsy,' a social worker; and, when ordering physical therapy, a physician."

PRIVATE PRACTICE

A number of psychiatric nurses, to the writer's personal knowledge, have broken away from the current health delivery system and have set themselves up in private practice. Most of them have found that in psychiatry it takes considerable time to gain acceptance and build up a practice. However, an increasing number of nurses with graduate degrees in psychiatric nursing have been attracted to this type of practice. Some of the reasons for this interest can be found in a paper by Kinlein (1972, p. 22), who explains,

> Rarely did I have the time to give the kind of nursing I wanted to give because of the demands of the organized operation of the institution on the patients and on me. Even when I identified nursing needs as paramount at a given time in relation to other needs, and as I was meeting those nursing needs, I was unable to prevent the intrusion of other people and departmental routines that caused me to terminate my nursing care.

She was also frustrated by a lack of authority commensurate with the responsibility placed upon her, and she was puzzled by the fact that in spite of her professional status as a nurse so many of her judgments and actions in nursing were dependent on medical sanction. She writes (1972, p. 23), "I became convinced that the only way to identify precisely and satisfactorily the nursing needs of people was to change the setting in which I came in contact with persons in need of nursing care." So she opened her own office. In this setting she was able to see clients on an episodic or continuing basis, to make home visits, and to work with groups. When asked what she does, she responds (1972, p. 24), "In the process of meeting their [her clients'] nursing needs, I have given direct physical and psychological care, emotional support, and health counseling, in states of illness and health."

GROUP NURSING PRACTICE

A still more recent development is group nursing practice. A proposal for independent group nursing practice and a plan for operationalizing such a project were published by Murray (1972). She suggests that the time has come for the organization of groups of nursing personnel, professional and nonprofessional, working as a team, to provide care for individuals or groups of patients in a variety of health agency settings. A panel of consultants from other health professions would be available to members of the team. The team would be based in a community health center with access to nearby medical diagnostic and treatment facilities. Team members would make initial contacts with residents of the community in need of health services. The nursing team would care for patients from the first stages of illness or injury and would follow the patient throughout his entire illness and convalescence, providing necessary nursing care. The nurse-patient relationship established during the course of illness would be sustained to maintain subsequent health measures as long as the patient continued to live in the community. This plan model is but one possible model for group practice.

A group of nurse specialists in San Francisco are in the process of developing a private group practice. The members will be nurses with graduate degrees and advanced clinical practice with specialized clinical interests such as child psychiatry, cardiopulmonary problems, community mental health, crisis intervention, and family and group therapy, and a generalist who will function primarily as a consultant. They will maintain a suite with both offices and treatment rooms. The project will be financed by patient fees (Sitzman, 1973). There are still many problems to be worked out in connection with both individual and group independent nursing practice. Answers to these problems can come only from further experimentation and experience.

REFERENCES

Avey, Melodye (1973): "Primary Care for Handicapped Children," *American Journal of Nursing,* vol. 73, no. 4, pp. 658–661.

Davidites, Rose M., and Florence S. Williams (1969): "The Training Program," in Gertrude A. Stokes (ed.), *The Roles of Psychiatric Nurses in Community Mental Health Practice: A Giant Step,* Faculty Press, Inc., Brooklyn, pp. 121–130.

Fujiki, Sumiko, Bonnie C. Clayton, Nada J. Estes, Marion E. Kalkman, and Opal H. White (1967): *Defining Clinical Content Graduate Nursing Programs: Psychiatric Nursing,* Western Interstate Commission for Higher Education, Boulder, Colo.

Hall, Bernard H., et al. (1952): *Psychiatric Aide Education,* Menninger Clinic Monograph No. 9, Grune & Stratton, Inc., New York.

Jones, Maxwell (1953): *The Therapeutic Community, A New Treatment Method in Psychiatry,* Basic Books, Inc., Publishers, New York.

Jordan, Judith D., and Joseph C. Shipp (1971): "The Primary Health Care Professional Was a Nurse," *American Journal of Nursing,* vol. 71, no. 5, pp. 922–925.

Kalkman, Marion E. (1952): "What the Psychiatric Nurse Should Be Educated to Do," *The Psychiatric Quarterly Supplement,* part 1.

Kinlein, M. Lucille (1972): "Independent Nurse Practitioner," *Nursing Outlook,* vol. 20, no. 1, pp. 22–24.

Levine, Maurice (1952): "Principles of Psychiatric Treatment," in Franz Alexander and Helen Ross (eds.), *Dynamic Psychiatry,* The University of Chicago Press, Chicago, pp. 307–366.

Lewis, Garland K., Marguerite J. Holmes, and Fred E. Katz (1961): *An Approach to Education of Psychiatric Nursing Personnel, Report of Seminar Project for Teachers of Psychiatric Aides,* League Exchange 33858, National League for Nursing, 10 Columbus Circle, New York.

Lidz, Theodore (1955): "General Concepts of Psychosomatic Medicine," in Silvano Arieti (ed.), *American Handbook of Psychiatry,* Basic Books, Inc., Publishers, New York, pp. 647–658.

Menninger, Karl (1959): "The Psychiatric Aide," in Bernard Hall (ed.), *A Psychiatrist's World: The Selected Papers of Karl Menninger, M.D.,* The Viking Press, Inc., New York.

Murray, Louise (1972): "A Case for Independent Group Nursing Practice," *Nursing Outlet,* vol. 20, no. 1, pp. 60–63.

Norris, Catherine M. (1970): "Direct Access to the Patient," *American Journal of Nursing,* vol. 70, no. 5, pp. 1008–1010.

Noyes, Arthur P. (1953): *Modern Clinical Psychiatry,* 4th ed., W. B. Saunders Company, Philadelphia.

Richards, Hilda (1970): "Community Mental Health Nursing," *American Journal of Nursing,* vol. 70, no. 5, p. 1020.

Santos, Elvin, and Edward Stainbrook (1949): "A History of Psychiatric Nursing in the Nineteenth Century," *Journal of the History of Medicine and Allied Sciences,* Winter, pp. 48–74.

Seymer, Lucy R. (compiler) (1954): *Selected Writings of Florence Nightingale,* The Macmillan Company, New York.

Shryock, Richard H. (1959): *The History of Nursing,* W. B. Saunders Company, Philadelphia.

Sitzman, Judith (1973), Personal Communication.

Stokes, Gertrude A. (1969a): "The Development of the Special Training Project, the Psychiatric Nurse in Community Psychiatry, 1964–1968," in Gertrude A. Stokes (ed.), *The Roles of Psychiatric Nurses in Community Mental Health Practice: A Giant Step,* Faculty Press, Inc., Brooklyn, pp. 17–41.

———(1969b): "Sequential Development of Programs in Primary, Secondary, and Tertiary Prevention in the Community Mental Health Center," in Gertrude A. Stokes (ed.), *The Roles of Psychiatric Nurses in Community Mental Health Practice: A Giant Step,* Faculty Press, Inc., Brooklyn, pp. 43–74.

Tudor, Gwen E. (1952): "A Sociopsychiatric Nursing Approach to Intervention in a Problem of Mutual Withdrawal on a Mental Hospital Ward," *Psychiatry,* vol. 15, no. 2, pp. 193–217.

Ullman, Montague (1969): "Overview of the Evolution of the Maimonides Community Mental Health Center and the Training Project, the Psychiatric Nurse in Community Psychiatry," in Gertrude A. Stokes (ed.), *The Roles of Psychiatric Nurses in Community Mental Health Practice: A Giant Step,* Faculty Press, Inc., Brooklyn, pp. 1–16.

University of Maryland School of Nursing and National Institute of Mental Health (1967): *Work Conference in Graduate Education: Psychiatric-Mental Health Nursing,* April 24–28, Baltimore.

U.S. Department of Health, Education, and Welfare (1964): *Community Mental Health Centers Act of 1963,* Title II, Public Law 88–164, *The Federal Register,* May 6, pp. 5951–5056.

Williams, Florence S. (1969): "The Role of the Psychiatric Nurse in Secondary Prevention," in Gertrude A. Stokes, (ed.), *The Roles of Psychiatric Nurses in Community Mental Health Practice: A Giant Step,* Faculty Press, Inc., Brooklyn, pp. 53–74.

PART TWO

Mental Health
and the Life-Span

2

THE DEVELOPMENTAL MODEL

Eugenia Waechter

The developmental model as a theoretical stance toward the study of human behavior and personality dysfunctions is receiving increased emphasis within recent years. Researchers, using this model, view deviant behavior as primarily the result of deprivations, inadequacies, and distortions in the satisfactions of the individual's basic developmental needs throughout his life span. Great stress is therefore placed on the study and investigations of successive phases of development, of the tasks inherent in each developmental stage, of the variables involved in the successful mastery of such tasks, and of the processes involved in the transition from one stage to another.

Personality dysfunction, as defined by the norms of a particular society, can then be seen as an understandable, if not inevitable, result of the individual's inability to master tasks or life experiences by virtue of inadequacies in his environment, because of other concurrent life stresses, or because of emotional, social, or intellectual immaturity at the stage in which these experiences occurred. Personality distortions can be viewed primarily as variations of "normal" functioning and can be understood in the light of the normal processes of growth and human development. Plans for therapeutic intervention also place primary emphasis on the strengths and resources that the individual has acquired throughout the developmental stages.

PURPOSES OF THE STUDY OF DEVELOPMENTAL THEORY

Current developmental theory is allied to many other fields in the study of the human individual, in that its goal and purpose are to delineate broad principles which can be utilized for the accurate description, explanation, and prediction of behavior. It differs from other theoretical formulations in that it stresses continuity of behavioral patterns throughout the life cycle and is concerned with sequences of events. It also emphasizes the unitary nature of the developmental process and the constant interaction of the organism with its psychological, social, and physical environment. Whereas most disciplines stress concepts which are germane to the particular prevailing theoretical stance or mode of thinking, researchers using developmental theory strive for a wider understanding of the developmental process by scrutiny of behavior from various perspectives and by reorganization of previous knowledge.

The purposes of the study of developmental theory are threefold. The first is to illuminate the causality of behavioral characteristics in particular individuals. Through continuous study and systematic investigation, the boundaries of "normal" or "average" rates of development and behavior are being established, an achievement which contributes perspective in the evaluation of the individual. However, the ultimate goal in this field is not merely to produce a series of portraits of the child and adult at successive steps in development, but to clarify the process of change involved in such transformation. Knowledge of normal limits within stages, nevertheless, is necessary to evaluate current or past physical, intellectual, emotional, or behavioral abnormalities or any problems in one or more of the developmental stages or areas. Understanding of the factors affecting each area of development (physical, social, emotional, intellectual) in terms of the process of change also offers clues for the amelioration of problems and modification of behavior through direct therapeutic intervention, manipulation of environmental variables, or support of available internal and external strengths. The prediction of one variable from another often becomes possible within reasonable margins for error, and the scientific understanding of causality can lead to alterations and controls within the environment of the individual.

Knowledge of norms—of process and variables involved in the transformation of one phase to another—may then serve not only for diagnosis, but also in the outlining of treatment plans. The therapist who is knowledgeable regarding the elements necessary for healthy development and functioning will have a broader basis for alertness to the possible results of insufficiency or distortion in one of these areas.

However, the thesis of multiple causality must always be kept in mind. Limitations imposed by inadequate or insufficient knowledge within the discipline or incomplete understanding of the history of the individual under evaluation may result in inappropriate therapeutic intervention.

Knowledge of developmental theory also serves as a basis for a more comprehensive understanding of adult behavior. Frequently, the origin of adult behavioral dysfunctioning is to be found in early experience within the home, as was first outlined by Sigmund Freud. The importance of childhood events in adult behavior, neurosis, and psychosis is no longer in question. Adult personality, philosophy, attitudes, and feelings are known to be strongly influenced by the individual's earliest relationships. Satisfactions, needs, choice of defenses, and coping styles can usually be traced to beginning patterns in childhood. Knowledge, therefore, of the individual's early responses to both care and stress, and of his early environment, gives much useful information on which to base a sound treatment plan for problems which first become evident in adulthood.

Another important reason for the current interest in developmental processes has to do with the deeper understanding of the many social problems facing this society. Such crucial problems as racism, sexism, juvenile delinquency, crime, and international tension can often be illuminated through knowledge of the origin of attitudes and of the formation of the individual personality structure. Such knowledge can also spur social action based on research findings related to childhood influences.

Other applications of knowledge of developmental theory include the modification of childrearing practices and improvement in the education of our children. The effects of various social and cultural climates on individual development is now of intense interest to individual researchers who are investigating the effects of differing school situations on the development of self-concept and self-esteem, the influences of the group on attitude formation and attitude change, the effects of social pressure and attitude on the personality and behavior of children from minority groups, and the effect of educational practices on intellectual development of all children. Therefore, knowledge of normal development can be most germane to many applied fields and relevant for professionals from the helping disciplines who are cooperating and collaborating with other social institutions and systems.

As a summary, therefore, the study of normal developmental theory is an important end in itself; but, in addition, knowledge so derived can have important practical applications in the understanding and prediction of the behavior of particular children—and of adults and of group phenomena—in forming the basis for therapeutic plans and also in the formation of hypotheses which point the way for further investigation of variables important to developmental outcomes.

DEFINITIONS IN DEVELOPMENTAL THEORY

The field of human development as a discrete area of study and knowledge is of fairly recent origin. Traditional ways of thinking fostered a strong inclination to reify events and to fractionate wholes into discrete parts according to assumptions about the relation of variables. Such analytic methods have been immensely productive to the understanding of isolated events, but they are inadequate to explain the complexities of organisms and human institutions.

Today we are recognizing that the human organism is an open system, constantly interacting with its environment. This conception poses a challenge to the rigidities of cause-and-effect thinking and has engendered a willingness to explore new ways of thinking and studying the multidimensional and dynamic events in development. There are also compelling human needs to spur attempts to create a new discipline of human development.

The task of articulating the great array of empirical observations into an integrated, coordinated conception of human development is becoming of increasing interest and importance. Interest in problem areas has become intense in recent years, and it has resulted in vast numbers of studies on important new topics, such as constitutional differences among neonates, relationships between personality and intellectual development and between physical changes and psychological conflicts. Such research and concern are exciting in that the further information provides us with an ever clearer picture of the dynamics of human development, the complexity of interactional effects between the environment and the organism, and the hopes, motives, and rewards which underlie and maintain behavior.

Growth versus Development

Ambiguity still exists among the often interchangeably used terms *growth, maturation,* and *development.* The term *growth* has traditionally been defined as any increase in the size, weight, or power of an organism, whereas *maturation* implies the progression toward adult levels of functioning. Originally the term *development* was applied to observable increase in size or structure of an organism over a period of *time.* When taken over into the psychosocial realm, it acquired the additional consideration of progressive changes in an individual's adaptive functioning. Today, the terms are used to distinguish entirely independent dimensions of development.

Growth implies the biological and physiological substrate of behavior in the multiplication of cells which results in increments in size, and the differentiation which gives rise to tissues and organ systems. Incremental growth and differentiation enable the organism to become capable of functioning at a higher level. Dynamic process is also important in that there is continuous interchange with the environment in the absorption of food elements and in the functions of breathing and eliminating. Replacement phenomena, retention and release, and change in constituents of cells are also germane to behavior change, as, for instance, in the process of aging and in behavioral responses to puberty or menopause.

Individual variability, as well as continuity and regularity, also is demonstrable in the process of growth. Rate of increases in size and timing of continuities and discontinuities are highly idiosyncratic within broad ranges of normality. Such individual variability may often contribute directly to behavioral manifestations at all ages throughout the life cycle.

Changes in cell number, size, and differentiation also contribute to other aspects of the interaction between organism and environment. The nature, quantity, and quality of sensory inputs are often dependent on structure, whereas it has recently been demonstrated that the reverse is also true. The growth of structure is dependent on function and on environmental and sensory stimulation. For instance, it has been demonstrated that myelenation of nerves occurs more rapidly with optimum levels of sensory input and variability.

The term *maturation* has been used to refer to the change in the underlying process of a behavioral trait which occurs without the demonstrable effects of specific practice. This definition, then, implies the separation of innate factors from direct learning in the acquisition of a behavior sequence. Such a separation can be demonstrated in some instances; but in most cases it is difficult to distinguish the relative impact of genetic factors versus acquired or learned components of the behavior. This distinction, however, has formed the history of theoretical viewpoints relative to development, as will be seen in a subsequent section of this chapter.

Assumptions and Characteristics of Developmental Theory

Developmental theory encompasses all of the changes which take place during the dramatic transition from the relatively helpless state of earliest infancy to physical and emotional maturity. It is, then, legitimately concerned with genetic endowment and its relationship to observable behavior, with the effect of physical characteristics on behavior, with the neural substrates of behavior, and with learned modifications of early behavior patterns and the effects of experience.

The developmental model is particularly concerned with process as related to the product. That is, the approach is to treat development as a process which merits explanation rather than mere description or portraits of the organism through successive phases of the life cycle. Thus, it is concerned with the process of transition from one stage to another, and of identifying the variables which facilitate or impede progress. This conception is concerned with those characteristics which remain constant over the life span and is a vital ingredient in differentiating this field of knowledge from other disciplines.

The concept of development assumes that lawful continuity exists within the life cycle and that change is dynamic and basically one-directional. Therefore, although developmental theory recognizes both stability and constancy, it has a primary focus on *change over time.* This viewpoint is in contrast to the stance of many sciences, including those which study human behavior, which are primarily interested in phenomena which occur during a circumscribed interval of time, or *contemporaneous* phenomena. The primary interest of developmental theory, on the other hand, is in the function of time itself (or age) as one crucial variable in the transition and transformation of one stage to another.

The basic assumption underlying developmental theory is that each successive stage of the life cycle builds on the preceding one and that the mastery of designated developmental tasks in one stage contributes substantially to the successful traversing of succeeding phases. This conception implies a regularity in the developmental process without specifying uniformity. Conversely, failure to master designated developmental tasks in one area of development may have long-lasting effects in later functioning in that personality ingredients are inadequate to the challenge of more difficult developmental tasks.

Another basic assumption characterizing the field is that development is extremely complex, and that many areas (i.e., physical, social, emotional, and cognitive) are overlapping and undergoing change simultaneously. Thus, although frequently a particular area of development may be selected for strenuous examination, it is always recognized that such a separation is artificial, in that in actuality each area of development impinges on the other and influences change. For example, the interactional quality of cognitive growth and language growth are well recognized.

Other questions of interaction are still under debate. Questions related to the relative influence of the reciprocity of the organism and his environment, the impact of the organism on wider society, the relative emphasis which should be placed on overt observable behavior versus subjective or internal experience, etc., are still debated by developmental theorists.

Characteristics of Developmental Theory as a Science

Differences between scientific disciplines are usually a function of differences in language and concepts utilized and in methods selected to study phenomena. In the physical sciences, there is a high degree of similarity in the language used, and the experimental method of hypothesis and deduction is eminently suited to the study of phenomena in a laboratory setting.

In the study of human development, theorists differ widely in the language they use to describe personality formation and in the approaches they utilize to study behavior. Furthermore, the phenomena under investigation, those of human behavior, are also a part of their subjective experience, so that there is constant danger of observer bias in objective and accurate evaluation of the objects and phenomena under study. Interaction between experimenter and subject may influence the results of the study in many subtle ways.

There are also special problems inherent in the study of change over time that preclude study in a laboratory setting. Although many phenomena can be so studied—for example, processes involved in learning—for many others it is simply not feasible to apply experimental procedures. Developmental phenomena are generally extremely complex, involving the interaction of many variables, and are of long duration. Rigid control of variables is often difficult to achieve, and reproducing situations as they occur in real life is impossible or leads to questionable or insignificant results.

Many of the phenomena which interest developmentalists are those which preclude synthesis in an artificial setting. The acquisition of values, the process of cultural transmission, attitude formation, etc., are the result of interaction within the home, school, and wider society. Furthermore, experimental methods used in animal studies, such as deprivation, abuse, or frustration, are simply not applicable or ethically possible in the study of human situations.

For these reasons, developmental theory is largely a natural science, relying on the study of phenomena as they occur in the settings in which children and adults habitually move. This condition necessitates special considerations to avoid the pitfalls of biased observations, confusion of subjective and objective experience, and extrapolation of interpretation.

37

Interdisciplinary Nature of Developmental Theory

In contrast to many "pure" sciences, developmental theory draws heavily on such related disciplines as psychology, sociology, anthropology, genetics, psychoanalysis, biology, and physiology in the formulation of theoretical constructs and in suggesting areas of study. Each of these disciplines is also devoted to the study of human beings or of human society, and thus has much to contribute to the understanding of developmental processes. Knowledge of the physical substrate of the human individual is necessary in understanding and predicting behavior; whereas knowledge of the individual's relationship to his society and culture is imperative in the fuller elucidation of the end product of developmental processes. Individual differences can be explained only through a thorough understanding of the impact and interaction of innate and experiential factors throughout the life cycle.

Therefore, developmental theory covers a broad and interdisciplinary canvas, dealing with *all* the facets of childhood, adolescence, and adulthood. This concept distinguishes the discipline from that of psychology, which usually tends to be focused on characteristic behavior at different age levels.

Developmental Theory as a Distinct Area of Study

Despite the heavy reliance on findings from related disciplines, the field of human development claims a number of distinctive features which buttress the argument that it should become elaborated as a distinct field for theory and inquiry. First, as has been noted, developmental theory is concerned with *change* as a function of time and is focused on the variables involved with the *transition* periods in ongoing development. Secondly, developmental theory draws together many fragmentary and scattered studies into a more coherent body of knowledge. Although there is as yet no one complete theory of human development, great strides are being made in correlation of data and approaches from diverse sources, which give promise of ultimately arriving at a unified theory of human development.

HISTORICAL BACKGROUND OF INTEREST IN DEVELOPMENTAL PROCESSES

Early History—Middle Ages to the Seventeenth Century

Although writers in all periods of history have been interested in the behavior of children, childhood as an important period of life itself has not always been recognized. The "training" or education of children in order to produce desirable adult behavior was among the first topics to be explored. Plato recommended that particular training be given to the young relative to their individual talents and aptitudes. Socrates also commented on educational practices and complained about the behavior of youth toward their elders.

During the Middle Ages, many pseudoscientific writers discussed the "Ages of Life," and the symbolism of numbers and correspondences was a common theme to explain mysterious phenomena in behavior and human biology. A thirteenth-century "encyclopedia" or compilation of writings (*Le Grand Propriétaire de toutés choses, très utile et profitable pour tenir le corps en sante,* compiled by B. de Glanville, translated by Jean Corhichon, 1556) compares the ages of life to the seven planets then recognized. The period of childhood was divided into two phases characterized primarily by immaturity in all areas of functioning and was otherwise given little attention. The age of adolescence covered an age span of 20 years and was so designated because of the dawning ability to "beget children" and because in this age "the limbs are soft and able to grow and receive strength and vigour from natural heat." The period of youth, lasting until forty-five years of age, occupied the central position among the ages in that it was seen as the period of greatest responsibility, productivity, nobleness, and strength. "Senectitude," halfway between youth and old age, was characterized by an increase in "gravity of bearing and habits." "Old age" was divided into two phases: one lasting until aged seventy, and the last or "Senies" ending in death. The period of old age received little positive comment and was seen as a period of deterioration in all areas of functioning.

In France, until the seventeenth century, only the periods of childhood, youth, and old age were generally recognized, with the exact ending of the period of childhood left in severe doubt. Ambiguity between the phases of childhood, adolescence, and young adulthood was actually widespread until the last century, when "youth" became the subject of concern for many moralists and politicians.

Medieval art does not attempt to portray childhood in a realistic manner, but rather miniaturizes the characteristics of adult figures. Montaigne (1958) epitomized the thinking of the sixteenth century with the comment that children had "neither mental activities nor recognizable bodily shape." Too much investment in children was indeed hazardous, since childhood was extremely fragile and most children did not live to see adulthood.

The seventeenth century proved to be a turning point in attitudes toward children and in recognition of childhood as an important developmental phase in itself. Interest was evidenced by the recognition and adoption of childhood linguistic forms, as can still be seen in the French words *toutou* and *bonbon,* portraits of children became more numerous, and literature of the era demonstrates concern relative to the development of the young.

The education of children also became of more general and serious interest at this time, although marked by spiritual and intellectual unrest. Along with classical humanism, there now developed an interest in the natural world and man's relation to his environment. The birth of science emphasized the natural laws of the universe. Such individuals as John Comenius were forerunners of modern education methods (1592–1671) in insisting that classroom materials be adapted to the interests and abilities of the pupils, and in emphasis on the superiority of learning through sensory experiences rather than through memorizing.

Early Preformationist Approaches

This extreme position, which had roots in antiquity, was a topic of controversy in the first quarter of the seventeenth century. Residues of this approach were later to be seen in the developmental theory of Jean-Jacques Rousseau.

The preformationist thesis, in essence, averred that all human attributes, physical characteristics, character, values, and emotions were present before birth in the human embryo or even in the germ cell. A microscopic human being was thought to exist in the germ cell (the homunculus), which merely grew in size within the uterus and after birth.

A century following the invention of the microscope, this belief still dominated the thinking of the time. Constant conflict raged between the ovists and the animalculists, who differed as to whether the miniature human was in the ova or the sperm cell. Direct microscopic investigation was finally carried out to dispel the theory of complete prestructure; however, it was destined to have its impact on the psychological thinking of future generations. Roots of this extreme position could later be seen in the theory of predeterminism, which stressed the unfolding of behavioral patterns as predetermined by genetic endowment. Variations of this viewpoint are still widely believed and debated today.

Predeterministic Theory of Jean-Jacques Rousseau

A foremost proponent of predeterministic theory was Jean-Jacques Rousseau (1712–1778), a figure of conflict in his time, since his emphasis on freedom and personal choice was in direct variance to the former classical tradition of discipline and authority. Although Rousseau did not negate the importance of experience in developmental outcomes, he emphasized the regulation of development through internal factors. He felt that freedom should be given to the child to "unfold" naturally, since the child's nature was innately "good." Evil and tyranny in the world, according to Rousseau, were the result of the corruption of society and man's enslavement of his fellow man. Rousseau believed that the formal education of his day corrupted the mind of the child, and his ideas of "free activity," rather than "words, words, words," underlie some of the more progressive ideas of education to this day.

Rousseau rejected the notion of original sin, and replaced this with the theory of innate and natural goodness, postulating the thesis that development is a series of stages which are transformed, one into another, in accord with a prearranged design. Education, therefore, involved noninterference with the natural course of events. Although there are many errors and half-truths in Rousseau's *Emile* (1762) (he accepted a recapitulation theory of human development, opposed reasoning with the young, etc.), it is a classic in the history of developmental theory, and he is often given credit for the key idea of discovery of the child. Much of the work of students of intellectual development, including that of Piaget, has as its basis ideas and assumptions stemming from the thinking of Rousseau. The "stage" theory is one which is familiar to modern students of developmental theory.

Rousseau can also be said to be the first great advocate of children and of the importance of childhood as an important phase of life in its own right. His statements, "Nature wants children to be children before they are men. If we deliberately pervert this order, we shall get premature fruits which are neither ripe nor well flavoured, and which will soon decay," can be said to have shocked the world as to its ignorance of childhood (Pieper, 1951–1953, p. 79). Further, since he considered experiences during the first few years of life as vitally important to further development, he can be said to have anticipated much of today's emphasis on early experience.

Early "Tabula Rasa" Approaches

These early approaches represented the reverse extreme of the continuum in minimizing the effects of genetic endowment and placing great stress on the external environment in the determination of developmental outcomes. John Locke (1637–1704), from whom the movement stemmed, believed that reason and knowledge were derived from experience, and his concept of the mind as a blank sheet of paper at birth (the *tabula rasa*) is still seen as one of the major approaches to developmental theory. Although Locke and his followers did not negate that natural impulses do occur in children, he and his followers minimized the contributions of genetic endowment and of internal factors in behavior and stressed the predominant role played by the environment, of behavioral plasticity, and of the limitless potentialities of man under proper environmental conditions.

The human infant was conceived as amorphous, so that with proper modeling and education any desired outcome could be achieved. The natural impulses of children were not ignored, however, for both Locke and his followers advocated that children should be trained in self-discipline and self-control from "their very cradle," an idea later adopted by such psychologists as John Watson, the originator of behaviorism in the 1920s. In this era, psychologists from this school advocated specific child-rearing practices, such as impersonal handling, strictness, and the importance of habit training.

Interestingly enough, both of the extreme positions of predeterminism and *tabula rasa* approaches agreed in essence that the individual contributes very little to his own development, and that the child is really very little different from the adult. The early "humanists" stressed stern and authoritative control over children, ignored individual differences, age levels, and variations in children's abilities or capacities. Early behaviorism denied the role of subjective experience and emphasized the stimulus-response character of human behavior and learning. The era of nonpermissiveness in childrearing was a natural outgrowth of such beliefs.

Beginnings of Direct Observation

The beginning of direct observation as a method of understanding human development and behavior was first noted in the eighteenth century through a number of baby biographies.

Johann Pestalozzi (1746–1827), a Swiss, and probably the most famous teacher in the history of education, became fascinated by the emerging interests of children and of their growing motor development. Realizing the lack of objective data on child development, he carefully observed and recorded the development of his own son. He was later to become known for his use of realia in education, as in the teaching of biology and geography through the use of field trips, and for his insistence that the preparation of teachers be based on an intimate knowledge of the child and of his development.

The following century saw many such biographical observations, including those of Tiedemann, Charles Darwin, and Amos Bronson Alcott, the father of Louisa May Alcott. Although such recordings have many shortcomings in that observations are often unsystematic, biased, subjective, and based on only one subject, they were nonetheless valuable in the formation of hypotheses which could later be tested with larger groups of children and in stimulating interest in the development of children. Indeed, the observations Jean Piaget made of his own three children are still read with widespread interest today.

BEGINNINGS OF CURRENT DEVELOPMENTAL THEORY

One of the major influences of the belief in predetermined development was Charles Darwin, whose theory of natural selection of inherited variations as a basis for evolution influenced much of the zeitgeist of the time, including psychological thought.

One of Darwin's great admirers, G. Stanley Hall, president of Clark University, was one of the first to systematically study groups of children in an effort to discover the "content of their minds" (Hall, 1890, p. 139). Hall also espoused Rousseau's conception of the child as basically good. He further speculated that the child, in traversing stages of development to maturity, recapitulates the phylogenetic and cultural history of the human race. His major interest in the period of adolescence was spurred by its resemblance to the period of storm and stress in human history.

Although G. Stanley Hall wrote voluminously, his major influence was destined to be through his students, among whom can be numbered Lewis M. Terman and Arnold L. Gesell. Early concern with intelligence testing in America, and the period of normative approaches to child behavior, were greatly influenced by Hall and by the prevailing evolutionary approach to cultural anthropology.

Arnold L. Gesell

The assumption of genetically predetermined development particularly stresses aspects of unlearned behavior. According to this concept, not only physical characteristics, but also behavioral organizations, automatically unfold regardless of environmental influences. This viewpoint supported the belief in fixed intelligence and initiated the widespread normative and descriptive studies of sequences of behavior and development which were popular in the early 1930s. These norms or stages were strictly related to age and described the specific age at which various skills or characteristics normally appear.

Arnold Gesell's theory of maturation reiterated Rousseau's emphasis on the internal control of development rather than of specific practice or learning. Although he did not repudiate environmental influences entirely, he averred that "environmental factors (merely) support, inflect and modify but . . . do not generate the progressions of development" (Gesell, 1954). His thesis maintained that developmental sequences evolve inevitably in all cultures in basic uniformity through the universality of neural maturation. Undesirable behavior was conceived as stage-specific and could be best managed through a policy of noninterference. Today it is known that individual experience and cultural environment make important contributions to all developmental sequences.

Early Behaviorism

The entry of behaviorism on the scene of American child psychology can be traced to discontent with introspective analyses of mental data and to the burial of psychological work in discussion; to an active anti-instinct campaign; to the desire for separation of psychology from philosophy; and to growing insistence on placing the disciplines related to human behavior on a scientific basis. It was also influenced by Darwin's theory of evolution, by growing concern with psychometrics as introduced by Binet, by experiments in classical conditioning undertaken by Ivan Pavlov and his associates in Russia, and by the interplay between neurophysiology and psychology which influenced the direction of research toward the problems of learning and adaptation.

The interest in stimulus-response methodology was heightened by the hope and belief that this approach could offer an organized theoretical body of knowledge based on the hypothetical-deductive method. The approach also gave promise of offering a plausible solution to problems for cooperative research across disciplines to establish a cumulative and scientific effort.

John B. Watson, considered to be the father and forerunner of modern behaviorism, began his experiments in conditioning by establishing an infant laboratory in the second decade of this century. From this work flowed many of the well-known and classical manuscripts of early behaviorism, including his analysis of emotions (Watson, 1919), and his classical conditioning of Albert (Watson and Rayner, 1920).

During this time, animal studies also became popular as an indirect method for the study of human behavior and learning. The close, naturalistic observation of animals, and the vision of reinforcement as a natural selection process to select out adaptive animal behaviors, resulted in a concentrated emphasis on problems associated with learning. Animals were eminently suited for this purpose, since genetics could be controlled to some extent, and techniques could be standardized.

The stimulus-response model was slow to cross over into the field of human study in the first half of this century partly because of the antithetic gestalt, genetic, and Freudian point of view in developmental theory extant at that time. Learning theory tradition, which grew out of Watsonian behaviorism, was also delayed because of the resistance to assumptions that human behavior is learned, and that the stimulus is the cause and the response is the effect. A significant movement, however, did emerge in the mid-1950s, and behavior theory and behavior analysis became widely understood in the professional culture of American psychology.

Summary of Historical Trends

The nature-nurture controversy is no longer a matter for heated debate, since all schools of thought recognize the importance of both elements in human development. No one now seriously contends that development is on an either-or basis, or that one variable excludes the other. However, the relative influence of one or the other of the positions is still important in determining differences between theoretical stances in developmental theory. Emphasis on the predeterministic view is still viable and has contributed important concepts to current developmental theory relative to universals, such as the nature of the unconscious mind, and to stage theory, which is an important tenet of developmental theory today. Cognitive and psychoanalytic theory is also still prominent in developmental literature, and particularly the former has generated much research effort. The *tabula rasa* approach, on the other hand, with its emphasis on the role of the environment and experience in determining developmental outcomes, is becoming increasingly prominent in the form of social learning theory.

The interactionist point of view is a fairly recent one—a stance which recognizes the contributions of both heredity and environment and stresses that developmental outcomes are the result of individual experience, which is a product of both genetically determined and environmental variables. Although there is no single theory of human development extant today, this point of view gives promise of synthesis of related theory with application to the problems of practice. Such a comprehensive, theoretical base, or conceptual framework, would not only systematize knowledge and research efforts, but would enable helping professionals to better utilize theory in problem-solving activities.

CONTEMPORARY DEVELOPMENTAL THEORY

It is now increasingly recognized that diagnosis or prognosis can be attempted only when all the variables contributing to behavior are recognized. Furthermore, since most developmental research is primarily concerned with general trends, most research findings are only tangential to most practical problems of developmental or behavioral deviations. Unwarranted extrapolation must be avoided in the consideration of behavioral characteristics or therapeutic planning for an individual. Nevertheless, principles and concepts derived from current theories are indispensable in the understanding of both normal and abnormal development and in the planning for prevention or treatment of deviations.

Developmental Continuity

There is also no longer great debate as to whether development occurs through uneven forward spurts or is a gradual, even process. It is now known that in some areas of development, such as in the cognitive realm or in physical growth, there may be sudden, discontinuous changes, whereas simultaneously in other areas the changes toward maturity may be more gradual. Both types of changes are characteristic of general developmental theory. When established patterns are discarded or undergo radical revision, disequilibrium results which has been characterized as "developmental stress or crisis." Successful or unsuccessful resolution of such normative periods of crisis or stress determines the progress toward physical and psychosocial maturation. Recognition of these normal developmental crises, anticipatory guidance, and therapeutic or supportive efforts may spell the difference between successful mastery of inherent developmental tasks or failure to successfully traverse the period toward emotional maturity.

Although physical growth and changes may show sudden or seemingly abrupt changes, most psychosocial changes from one level to another are more gradual, with a great deal of overlapping of behavioral patterns, as previously stated. This constancy permits the formulation of an ordered group of concepts in studying the developmental process. Behavior which has been relinquished for the most part may reoccur sporadically in subsequent periods, and occasionally throughout life. More advanced patterns of adaptation may also occasionally appear prior to full attainment of a new phase of functioning.

Since development encompasses many differing processes, rates of change may vary between developmental areas simultaneously. Some processes may be undergoing rapid change whereas in others change may be very gradual. Growth spurts may occur during phases of gradual cognitive change, or the development of self-concept may be altered drastically during periods where physical growth is comparatively static.

Many factors operate in the relative dominance of continuity or discontinuity in developmental change. Cultural relativity may be an important contributing variable, as, for example, in the various acceptance of patterns of dependency and aggression in boys and girls. Some patterns of behavior may be sanctioned by a particular society whereas others are disapproved for a particular age or sex. Other factors may be related to parental comfort or tolerance of a particular behavioral sequence; to individual childrearing patterns; to environmental changes, pressures, or demands; or to internal conflict states.

Stage Theory and Developmental Crises

Although most developmental theorists now subscribe to the interactionist point of view of continual organism-environment interaction as a basis for behavior and developmental outcomes, they differ in the relative stress or emphasis placed on discontinuities in development—usually termed "stage theory" and "developmental crisis."

Stage theory assumes a developmental pattern within the age span studied and stresses interindividual similarities in function or behavior within stages. The criteria for stages involve the following factors:

1. Each stage involves a period of gradual formation of skill or behavioral manifestations and a period of attainment. When the individual has attained the new level, consolidation of elements subsumed in the stage occurs with progressive organization.
2. Each structure or stage contains within it at the same time the attainment of one level of functioning and the starting point of the next stage. Therefore, there is a merging of one stage with another in a continuous process.
3. The order of succession of developmental phases is invariant. Although it is assumed that individuals go through each stage in the given sequence, rates of progress vary as a function of innate factors, cultural expectations, environmental conditions, and so forth.
4. Through the process of integration, each new level of functioning contains within it preceding structures or behavior patterns of earlier stages.

The two main theories which emphasize sequential phases in development are psychoanalytic theory, epitomized by Freud's psychosexual stages, and cognitive theory, as illustrated by the intellectual stages of Piaget. Social learning theory does not place as much stress on stages of development, although some of the criteria for stages can be seen in the motivational systems of Robert Sears. Behaviorists in the Skinner tradition attack stage theory, since it implies some internal bases for development. Stage theory also assumes that development is not a complete product of learning, and is therefore more related to the predeterministic history of developmental theory rather than to the *tabula rasa* approach.

Each stage in each system is named for its immediate achievements in the emotional, cognitive, or motivational realms, respectively, and stresses qualitative *differences* in the functioning of the organism.

The transitional periods, when one phase merges into another, are of particular interest to the developmental theorist in terms of the variables associated with the process of change. Much research interest is currently devoted toward determining levels of timing and readiness, and the variables associated with changes, in order to assess whether appropriately timed environmental inputs, such as specific training, can be utilized to accelerate progress through the stages. Stage theorists therefore do recognize both genetic and environmental determinants, and also subscribe to the interactional basis of development.

The culture in which the individual lives is known to influence the developmental stages in both cognitive and personality theory. Child-rearing practices vary markedly from culture to culture, as do other environmental variables; so that the ages at which stages occur may differ from one society to another. An illustration of this is the acceleration of motor development of infants in Uganda due to maternal influences resulting in specific practice, as described by Ainsworth (1967). Personality development may also be influenced greatly by the particular family constellation which is predominant in a particular culture. Cognitive development may be markedly affected by the particular belief systems in a given society.

Other environmental factors which may influence personality and cognitive levels are related to specific educational efforts, deprivation or enrichment of general stimulation, and physical characteristics of the individual. The interrelationship of developmental areas may also influence progress in a particular realm; for example, aggressiveness and assertiveness in the personality characteristics of a child result in more rapid intellectual growth and progress through the stages of cognitive development.

The term "normative developmental crisis" is generally used to designate those transitional periods in which qualitatively new or discontinuous changes in behavior are being formulated. It is during this period that both internal and external factors, acting in concert, exert pressure toward relinquishment of former modes of functioning and speed the establishment and adoption of more mature behavior patterns. These periods do not appear abruptly, but are usually heralded by preparatory loosening of personality integration.

The factors which precipitate these periods of developmental crisis usually stem from cultural expectations or pressures for modification of behavior as mediated by the family group or wider society, or by such internal need states as physiological alterations.

The element of stress or anxiety is inherent in each transitional period, since reorganization of personality involves a disequilibrium in which former security measures and coping capacities are no longer adequate. Threats to self-esteem may also be encountered, in that the individual may experience uncertainty as to his adequacy in mastering the new developmental tasks. Former integration, which has given the individual a sense of security, must be relinquished for unknown future gratifications which may seem uncertain, difficult to acquire, and confusing. Threat of failure and the promise of increased responsibilities may engender anxiety which triggers defensive maneuvers in order to protect the individual. Change may be resisted strenuously, or regression may occur in efforts to avoid disorientation. When the transitional period is prolonged because of cultural conditions, a transitional subsociety may be established in order to provide for group identification and a lessening of anxiety. This phenomenon can be seen in the adolescent subculture in American society.

The terms *critical period* and *sensitive period* are also utilized to designate such transitional states. More specifically, however, the terms designate discrete periods of the life cycle during which environmental input may exert the greatest effect. This concept implies a general principle of behavioral organization; that is, that once a system becomes organized, it becomes progressively more difficult to reorganize the system. Modification of behavioral systems, then, is most appropriate during the period of first organization.

The concept of critical periods in development was first outlined by J. P. Scott in observations of the social development of animals. He and his collaborators found fairly distinct natural periods during which various kinds of circumstances have effects when they appear at one period but not when they occur at another. If the individual is deprived of necessary stimulation during the sensitive period when he is maximally susceptible, some degree of nonachievement in the particular sphere of development is felt to be unavoidable. Since the younger individual is in the process of organization of functioning and behavior, the concept is usually applied to certain periods of childhood. The younger individual is also felt to be more vulnerable to environmental stimulation by virtue of an inadequate experimental background to withstand frustration (Scott, 1958).

The hypothesis of critical periods, then, postulates differential sensitivities in certain affectual, intellectual, or social techniques at different developmental stages. The onset of the sensitive period is determined by "optimal readiness" and is closed when the new behavioral system is organized. This concept stipulates a certain degree of "irreversibility," i.e., learnings established during such periods may be maximally resistant to change. Such critical time-linked processes are now increasingly recognized, and possibilities for more effective exploitation of these epochs will, no doubt, be of increasing interest not only to cognitive and personality developmental theorists, but also to other disciplines. For example, it has been suggested that it is conceivable that, in the future, manipulations of maternal physiology might be used to enhance certain characteristics of faculties of the unborn fetus (Scheibel and Scheibel, 1964). Thus, it may become possible to structure the ongoing experiences of the organism, directly or indirectly, in such a manner that optimum development will be facilitated.

CURRENT THEORIES OF DEVELOPMENT

Currently the diverse viewpoints and approaches to theory in human development utilize conceptual frameworks which do consider the process of development as influenced by numerous variables, including the social matrix of the individual, cultural norms, attitudes, behaviors, and the like. Differences between them revolve around differential stress on the various components contributing to development and on particular perspectives of certain areas of total development. Each of the theories provides the professional with certain therapeutic tools and understandings which aid in assessing individual and group phenomena and in planning interventions to support or hasten development. Considered concurrently, the theories complement each other and provide the professional with an associated conceptual framework of total development.

Psychoanalytic theorists, as currently exemplified by Erik H. Erikson and David Rappaport, particularly consider the emotional development of the individual, drawing from the early formulations of Sigmund Freud. Special emphasis is given to signals from the preconscious and unconscious mind in revealing motivations for behavior, and the task of the ego is seen as maintaining a bridge of continuity as the individual passes through inevitable phases of ontogeny.

Human behavior is viewed as resulting from an interplay of two basic innate drives: (1) the drive to gratify the self and reach out, and (2) the drive to return to an earlier phase of lesser complexity in living. Erotogenic zones, and their behavioral expressions during early development, are seen as leading to future attitudes and personality expression throughout life.

Psychoanalytic theorists then emphasize sequential phases in maturation, which are seen as developmental crises culminating in individual psychosocial solution and growth. Erikson sees these phases as continuing throughout the life cycle, each building on the preceding phase. Successful resolution of the phases results in accomplishment of a sense of: (1) basic trust, (2) autonomy, (3) initiative, (4) industry, (5) identity, (6) intimacy, (7) generativity, and (8) integrity (Erikson, 1969). Further elaboration of these phases and of psychoanalytic theory will be found in the following chapters.

Researchers in social learning theories emphasize observable behavior change which is the result of a particular environmental stimulus. All behavior is conceptualized as response to external stimuli which may be strengthened or decreased by the consequences of the behavior. A *reinforcer,* immediately following the action, may be either positive or negative, and may consist of either material rewards or deprivations or social sanctions. A further tenet of social learning theory is that all behavior is learned through such antecedent-consequent linkages.

Social learning theory has continued to be a vigorous movement since its beginning in the mid-1950s. Scientists of this tradition emphasize the necessity for operational definitions, tend to engage in tightly controlled experiments, and eschew interpretations of observed behavior. For these reasons, greater reliance on instrumentation in investigation of human development has become prominent.

Cognitive theorists, as exemplified by Jean Piaget, attempt to answer such questions as: "From where do general ideas or universally held concepts derive?" "Is human knowledge something different from animal knowledge?" and "Do we acquire the general knowledge implied in intelligence in the same manner in which we learn any particular skill or fact?"

Scientists with a cognitive theoretical orientation are primarily concerned with organizational activities *within* the individual, rather than with environmental stimuli, with the genesis of the *whole* and the interrelationship of structures (structures of the whole), and with the elaboration of these mental structures from the purely reflexive to the complexities of formal logic. They view all attributes of human behavior as a consequence, primarily, of the evolving intellectual capacity of the individual to organize his experience. Thus, human affect or emotions also evolve from the same process as their intellectual counterparts, and these are interrelated. Since experience is seen as dependent on the individual's perception and conception of stimuli and events, intellectual functions form the basis and core of all human behavior.

Cognitive theory resembles psychoanalytic theory in emphasis on phases and stages of development, in utilization of empirical research as a tool to substantiate or refute facts previously established by logic, and in insistence on a cosmic unity and logical consistency of research findings.

The equilibrium of the individual is also of basic concern to cognitive theorists, but this equilibrium is viewed as a constantly changing situation and the goal of all human functions: biological, affective, and mental. Mental equilibrium is only momentarily attainable; the individual is constantly "becoming," for he is constantly striving for a new, advanced state while building on previous acquisitions. Development is seen as an inherent, evolutionary process with sequences of developmental phases remaining invariant. However, the environment is viewed as affecting growth through inputs which may accelerate or retard the rate of succession.

Cognitive theorists, along with psychoanalysts, also place great importance on the first period of human development. It is during this critical phase that the individual must receive the necessary stimulation to become an active part of his environment, to coordinate his actions, to confront an environment which makes demands, and to learn to adapt through assimilating experience and accommodating his behavior with the result of an ever-increasing repertoire of behavior.

Thus intelligent behavior is seen as problem-solving capacity based on a hierarchial organization of symbolic representations and information-processing strategies. Continuous interaction between the organism and the environment makes possible a continuous reorganizing of the structures of the mind which allows for an ever-increasing capacity to respond to stimuli remote in space and time and to an even greater ability to solve more complex problems. As the individual reaches maturity, these accomplishments permit him to operate with the sum total of possibilities rather than with merely the empirical situation.

METHODS OF STUDY IN HUMAN DEVELOPMENT

Studies in human development are often necessarily imprecise because of the nature of the phenomena under scrutiny. Much data must be gathered indirectly, resulting in problems related to the sincerity and honesty of communications. Most phenomena of development are also extremely complex and overlapping. Since the interest of researchers in development is in change over time, the possibility of transitory or extraneous factors may make for inconsistency between measurements. Consideration, then, must be given to many variables which may impinge on the area under study, and strict control is difficult in that most studies cannot be done under laboratory conditions. In addition, because of the extended nature of many studies, the maintenance of a study population can be a specific hazard.

To a great extent, the selection of a given research method is a function of the age of the subjects. With young children, the investigator is handicapped because of: (1) the necessity for rapport with the subject in order to secure his cooperation, (2) limitations in language ability, (3) limited attention spans, and (4) distractability. On the other hand, young children may be much more open in their responses and have less tendency to conceal their perceptions, attitudes, and emotions.

In spite of these difficulties, the precision of research in human development has increased remarkably in a relatively brief period of time. The problems enumerated are not unique to developmental study, and with the utilization of careful sampling and measuring techniques, it is certainly possible to satisfy the criteria for scientific data.

Approaches to Study

Since both individual characteristics and group phenomena are of interest to the developmental scientist, a number of approaches characterize developmental research. The *idiographic,* or individual, clinical approach is often utilized and is certainly of value, since greater depth of knowledge of the individual can be achieved, shedding light on the complex relationships of the individual's heredity and life experiences. However, complete understanding of the individual requires particularization of knowledge gained from large groups of subjects. Such systematic investigation of large groups of subjects utilizes a *nomothetic* approach. Both idiographic and nomothetic approaches are necessary and useful, particularly to the professional who is interested in the major factors underlying behavior of a unique individual with whom he is interacting.

The *longitudinal* approach is appropriately chosen to study change in phenomena over time and in study of continuity and discontinuities of behavioral expression. Such a research approach necessitates study of the same individuals over an extended period of time —often a decade or longer. This can obviously be of great value in the study of the stability of behavioral characteristics, in the study of long-term effects of early experience, and in the study of factors affecting fluctuations in such characteristics as intelligence and dependency. The difficulties in such an approach involve the expense of the research, the problems of maintaining the subject population over long periods of time, and the bias involved in selection of a stable and cooperative population, which may not be representative of larger segments of our society. In addition, the researchers must necessarily have a long-term commitment to the study.

In the *cross-sectional* approach, the investigator has the advantage of studying larger numbers of subjects of a particular age group. Comparisons of characteristics can then be done between age groupings. Such an approach also has the obvious advantage of being less expensive, in addition to avoiding the pitfall of loss of subjects or sample bias.

In many cases, the cross-sectional and longitudinal approaches may complement each other. For instance, the behavioral manifestations of aggressiveness may be studied cross-sectionally as a factor of age; whereas the longitudinal approach may give clues as to the individual stability of the behavior or of antecedents for behavior expression of aggression and hostility.

Manipulative experimental designs can be utilized in both longitudinal and cross-sectional research. Correlational analysis attempts to demonstrate a relationship between two variables, i.e., early experience and later intelligence. In developmental research, *age* is usually the fundamental variable, as related to a particular aspect of developmental progression. The shortcoming of this approach is that of inference; that is, a demonstrated correlation between variables does not substantiate antecedent-consequent relationships.

More complex and sophisticated manipulative designs are becoming increasingly prominent, particularly in the learning theory approach to the study of human development. Time-sampling techniques, controlled observations, and the structuring and manipulation of stimuli in laboratory conditions are now providing important insights, particularly in learning phenomena. It can be anticipated that such studies will continue to increase in light of the concern in our society related to the education of children.

CURRENT INFLUENCES IN DEVELOPMENTAL THEORY

Many of the questions toward which current research is directed center on delineating "normality" in development, and, conversely, on discriminating when deviant development becomes pathological. We still know very little about the vast number of combinations and permutations which go into the formation of what is considered mature behavior. Behavior which may be symptomatic of a pathologic condition in a mature person may be appropriate in a child at a particular stage of development.

Developmental lines are also not culture free. Only when we know for which society an immature personality is being prepared can we begin to determine the right climate for the child, the range and latitude of acceptance of deviance, and the experiences which may provide for optimum functioning in adulthood.

Some answers to these questions are currently being provided from cross-cultural research. The work of Ainsworth (1967) in Uganda, of Sprio (1965), Bettelheim (1969), and Kraft (1966) with kibbutz children, of Landy (1965) in Puerto Rico, of Coles (1964) with American black children, and of many others is giving us insight into the role of infant experiences in later development, the relative impact of parental and peer-group interaction on personality, the sources of strength and the role of struggle in unsupportive environments, and the factors which influence the capacity for survival under stress and for endurance in adverse circumstances. Current work with disadvantaged children, with ghetto families, and with the retarded is giving us new insights into the role of environmental forces in achievement of potential in all phases of development—physical, mental, and emotional. Work with ghetto children and black families also tells us a great deal about the manner in which individuals view their world and why some individuals are satisfied to make peace with what life brings to them while others struggle valiantly to change their environment. Many of these findings also give us important information regarding the coping patterns of handicapped children and suggest avenues for encouraging motivation toward change.

Although all areas of human development continue to interest researchers, work on aspects of physical growth has declined, whereas interest in mental growth has doubled or tripled in intensity. Work is also accelerating in the parameters influencing school achievement and in the role of personality factors and parent-child interaction within the family. Disturbances in personality formation and functioning have received increased attention, not only in treatment aspects, but also because of the light thus thrown on factors influencing normal development. This interest in personality disturbances has led to concern with delinquent behavior and adolescent behavior problems and to consideration of the enticing possibility of predicting such behavior. Concomitant with this growing interest in personality is the decreasing emphasis on socioeconomic factors as a cause of delinquency.

Much attention is also now being focused on the importance of the infant's perceptual experiences to later learning and socialization. Much of our knowledge about early environmental influences has come from studies of gross deprivation or trauma. Only within the past 10 years has attention been directed toward the effects of enriching or facilitating experiences in larger categories of future behavior. Such studies have linked the effect of early manipulation of environmental stimuli to later resistance to stress (Levine, 1962), to adult height and weight (Landauer, 1964), to later emotionality and exploratory behavior (Denenberg, 1969), and to later social capability (Mason, 1968).

Research investigating individual differences at birth, which is currently under way in many centers, is also of great importance to the problem of stimulus input. The inherent activity patterns of infants may well be found to interact with optimal levels of stimulation, which may be found to be different for the passive infant versus the active one. Results of this current research may give us needed clues for providing optimal environments for all infants during the first years of life.

The field of behavioral genetics has the potential for providing valuable information related to the role of inherited characteristics in intellectual and emotional behavior. Current findings giving evidence of a hereditary component of such personality traits as dominance, assertion, self-confidence, activity, and vigor and the need for achievement may greatly influence future plans for intervention in health care.

Many other lines of research in development are of significance for the delivery of health care. Among these is research on the mechanisms which affect learning and motivation in children. The role of discrepancy with previous mental structures, the role of anxiety in learning, the implications of class differences in responsiveness to teaching methods, the influence of teacher tempo and characteristics, the contingencies inherent in reward and punishment, and the role of the model are all currently under intensive investigation. The findings from such research will have great applicability to methods employed by health professionals in helping children and adults to assimilate new and better ways of coping with their environment.

REFERENCES

Ainsworth, M. (1967): *Infancy in Uganda,* The Johns Hopkins Press, Baltimore.
Bettelheim, Bruno (1969): *Children of the Dream,* The Macmillan Company, New York.
Coles, Robert (1964): *Children of Crisis,* Little, Brown and Company, Boston.

de Glanville, B. (1556): *Le Grand Propriétaire de toutes choses, très utile et profitable pour tenir le corps en santé* (translation, J. Corhichon).

Denenberg, V. H. (1967): "Stimulation in Infancy, Emotional Reactivity and Exploratory Behavior," in David C. Glass (ed.), *Neurophysiology and Emotion*, Rockefeller Foundation, New York.

Erikson, Erik (1963): *Childhood and Society,* W. W. Norton & Company, Inc., New York.

Gesell, Arnold L. (1954): "The Ontogenesis of Infant Behavior," in Leonard Carmichael (ed.), *Manual of Child Psychology*, 2d ed., John Wiley & Sons, Inc., New York.

Hall, G. Stanley (1890): "The Contents of Children's Minds," *Pediatric Seminar and Journal of Genetic Psychology,* vol. 1, p. 139.

Kraft, I. (1966): "Some Observations on Kibbutz Children," *Children,* vol. 13, p. 195.

Landauer, Thomas, and J. Whiting (1964): "Infantile Stimulation and Adult Stature of Human Males, *American Anthropologist,* vol. 66, p. 1007.

Landy, D. (1965): *Tropical Childhood,* Harper Torchbooks, Harper & Row, Publishers, Inc., New York, 1965.

Levine, S. J. (1962): "Psychophysiological Effects of Infantile Stimulation," in E. L. Bliss (ed.), *Roots of Behavior,* Paul B. Hoeber, New York.

Mason, W. (1967): "Early Social Deprivation in Non-human Primates: Implications for Human Behavior," in David C. Glass (ed.), *Neurophysiology and Emotion*, Rockefeller Foundation, New York.

Montaigne, Michele (1958): *"Essais,"* vol. 2, no. 8, in *Complete Writings,* Stanford University Press, Stanford, Calif.

Pieper, G. W. (1951–1953): "The Educational Classics," *History of Education Journal,* vols. 3–4, p. 79.

Rousseau, Jean-Jacques (1933): *Emile,* English edition, Dent Publishing Company, London.

Schiebel, M., and A. Schiebel (1964): "Some Neural Sub-strates of Postnatal Development," in M. Hoffman and L. Hoffman, *Review of Child Development Research,* vol. 1, Russell Sage Foundation, New York.

Scott, J. P. (1958): "Critical Periods in the Development of Social Behavior in Puppies," *Psychosomatic Medicine,* vol. 20, pp. 42–53.

Sprio, M. (1965): *Children of the Kibbutz,* Shocken Books, New York.

Watson, John (1919): "A Schematic Outline of the Emotions," *Psychological Review,* vol. 26, pp. 165–196.

———, and R. A. Rayner (1920): "Conditioned Emotional Reaction," *Journal of Experimental Psychology,* vol. 3, pp. 1–14.

3

DEVELOPMENTAL REACTIONS IN INFANCY AND CHILDHOOD

Patricia C. Pothier

There is a crisis in child mental health in this country today which is a challenge to all mental health workers who are interested in prevention and treatment of mental illness in children and youth.

In the United States of America today, there is a higher percentage of children and youth than at any previous time. Over half of the population is under twenty-five years of age. Of this group who are eighteen years of age and under, one-fourth live at or below the poverty level and are considered to be potentially at high risk both physically and psychologically. In the total age group under twenty-five years, there are estimated to be 10 million children needing some type of treatment. Of these, only 7 percent are receiving care (Joint Commission on Child Mental Health, 1970, pp. 147–149).

For those children labeled as in some degree of distress, the Joint Commission report (1970, p. 251) states that these children fall into the following etiological categories:

> (1) Due to faulty life experience, surface conflicts which arise from developmental tasks (80%); (2) Due to deeper conflict internalized within the self, commonly labeled as neuroses and those due to responses to physical handicaps or disorders, (10%); (3) Due to severe mental disorders such as the psychoses and severe mental retardation, (5%). This classification and relative percentages involved in each give clear indication for planning preventive strategies around developmental tasks which are aimed at prevention of mental illness in children.

The Joint Commission on Child Mental Health report concludes (Joint Commission on Child Mental Health, 1970, p. 16), "As of today, the treatment of the mentally ill child in America remains uncertain, variable, and inadequate. This is true on all levels, rich and poor, rural and urban. Only a fraction of our young people get the help they need at the time they need it." In addition to the above, the commission also points out that there is no organized and integrated program aimed at the prevention of mental illness or the promotion of mental health of children and youth.

To protect and preserve these children under twenty-five—one of our nation's most valuable human resources—the Joint Commission calls for broad planning that supports the initiation of innovative programs for both prevention and treatment. It also calls for new pools of manpower trained to perform new roles, and a continuous evaluation of these innovative programs, through research, to determine their effectiveness in preventing mental illness.

Hetznecker and Forman (1971, p. 366), in their article "Community Child Psychiatry," call for a new direction to meet the treatment needs of children. They state that psychiatry now understands how poverty and its consequences have altered therapeutic concepts and treatment interventions. Treatment approaches are needed which stress developmental aspects of cognitive, social, and vocational as well as emotional areas. They see a change in delivery of services which includes new professional and nonprofessional roles and different types of services from the traditional model. They further state that they see the following deficiencies in current mental health programs for children:

1. A paucity of community-adapted programs
2. Few mental health programs in "disadvantaged" schools
3. Lack of mental health principles integrated into school climates
4. Too much attention on psychopathology and not enough on promotion of adaptive and coping skills in poor children
5. Little inclusion of programs for children in community mental health centers
6. Failure to evaluate existing programs

The Joint Commission (1970, p. 249) also strongly recommends program planning based on the developmental model rather than on the traditional medical or clinical model.

THE ROLE OF THE NURSE IN PREVENTION AND TREATMENT OF MENTAL ILLNESS OF INFANTS AND CHILDREN

In the American Nurses' Association statement on psychiatric nursing (1966), in the section on child psychotherapy, general statements were made regarding the therapeutic role of the nurse, the nurse's role as manipulator of the environment, and his role as an agent of change in all areas of child welfare. The document further states that the clinical specialist in psychiatric nursing of children has the following functions:

1. To provide direct nursing care to children and families on either a short-term or long-range continuing basis, using a variety of treatment techniques
2. To provide immediate, on-the-spot therapeutic intervention in behavioral crises
3. To serve as a leader of parent groups, professional groups, and other interested groups in the community
4. To teach, supervise, and consult with nursing and other personnel who work with children
5. To collaborate with the members of various disciplines concerned with the health and welfare of children and to serve as liaison between these persons and disciplines
6. To act as an innovator in effecting therapeutic changes in the health and welfare of children
7. To serve as consultant to professionals by: assisting in the indentification of problems; the modification and solution of problems

Evans (1968, p. viii), in her exploration of the role of the nurse in community mental health, further states the need for psychiatric nurses to develop creative independent roles in the areas of prevention and therapeutic care. The nurse can be a key person in the whole area of prevention. Because this is a relatively new field, and at this time roles have not been clearly defined, the psychiatric nurse is in a key position to establish a role in this area. Even with the blurring of roles, Evans (1968, pp. 90–95) states that she sees the nurse being involved in activities such as identification of potential problems and helping people to cope with developmental crises by strengthening their coping skills. Bolman (1967, p. 5), in his outline of preventive psychiatric programs for children, includes the services and activities of nurses in all programs from the prenatal period through school age.

Since the focus of the developmental approach is the normal stresses in the life process, the nurse needs to have a sound foundation in normal growth and development processes. From this base the nurse can be involved in planning and implementing strategies that foster optimum development, can identify beginning signs of disturbance, and can develop strategies that help the child use his normal coping skills to deal with the stressful situation. In addition, the nurse needs clinical skills in effective intervention strategies of secondary and tertiary prevention.

The remainder of this chapter will focus on the crucial stages of personality development in infancy and childhood, some of the factors which influence the outcome of these stages, and a variety of programs aimed at primary and secondary prevention and treatment of mental illnesses in children. Nurses may not be specifically mentioned as being involved in the programs. However, based on the statements in the foregoing section, it can be inferred that nurses are being prepared to assume a variety of roles in these programs.

PREVENTION AND TREATMENT OF MENTAL ILLNESS IN INFANTS AND CHILDREN

Primary Prevention

Caplan (1961, pp. 3–5) states that primary prevention of mental disorders in children relates to reducing the rate of mental disorders in a population of children rather than focusing on an individual child. The goal is to provide preventive programs which are aimed at providing some assurance that developmental needs of infants and children will be met in order to reduce the rate of mental disorders in the total population.

Bolman and Westman (1967, p. 1058), in an overview of programs aimed at prevention of mental disorders, state that there are three types of programs: (1) those that focus on the child, (2) those focusing on the family, and (3) those focusing on society. Programs with a focus on the child include prenatal care, perinatal care, special defects, parent-child relationships, and school problems. Family programs include day care centers, preschool facilities, home helpers, planned parenthood, and assistance to families in crisis and to deprived or disorganized families. Societal programs include mental health planning, community organization, educational changes, and income and health maintenance.

To ensure that developmental needs of infants and children are met at critical periods, the Joint Commission (1970, pp. 3–5) recommends the type of broad program which will provide the following:

1. The right to be wanted
2. The right to be born healthy
3. The right to live in a healthy environment—physically and psychologically
4. The right to satisfaction of basic needs—nutrition, housing, medical, and psychiatric care
5. The right to continuous loving care
6. The right to acquire the intellectual and emotional skills necessary to achieve individual aspirations
7. The right to receive care and treatment through facilities which are appropriate to their needs and which keep them as closely as possible within their normal social setting

The Commission further recommends that where needs are obviously not being met, or in high-risk groups of infants or children where needs are most likely not to be met, early intervention take place at critical stages. At this stage the child is most vulnerable and possibly irreparable damage can be done (Joint Commission on Child Mental Health, 1970, p. 27).

As previously stated, approximately 80 percent of the children and infants labeled as being in some type of distress are exposed to inadequate life experiences, a situation which blocks achievement of developmental tasks. Therefore, interventions aimed at helping children satisfy their developmental needs could possibly prevent the occurrence of minor developmental deviations. These deviations if neglected could eventually lead to more severe difficulties and mental illness. An example of a strategy based on a program of primary prevention could be counseling or education with a group of young mothers. The focus of this intervention is to assist them in the management of their infants prior to the time when the infant enters a developmental stage. The aim of the intervention is to assure ease of transition into the next stage with a minimum amount of anxiety on the part of the infant.

Secondary Prevention of Mental Illness in Infants and Children

Basic to secondary prevention is intervention at the time of early warning signs or symptoms. For example, the nine-months-old infant's experiencing severe separation anxiety could be prevented from further handicapping of his personality development if intervention were applied to the disturbed mother-infant relationship at this stage. Although these interventions are in fact remedial in nature, their purpose is to prevent more complex or further handicapping problems from developing.

Tertiary Programs Related to Treatment of Mental Illness

The Joint Commission (1970, p. 40) defines the *emotionally disturbed child* as one whose progressive personality development is interfered with or arrested by a variety of factors so that he shows marked impairment in the capacities expected of him for his age and endowment in the following areas:

1. Reasonable, accurate perception of the world
2. Impulse control
3. Satisfying relations with others

4. Learning
5. Any combination of the above

Where the child is impaired in a severe and/or complex way, remedial or tertiary programs are initiated. Such programs are built on a model of health with a focus on developmentally appropriate behavior and a minimum amount of medical diagnostic classification. Services are provided in community-based facilities which allow the child to remain in as near normal a setting as possible. Where institutionalization is necessary, the programs should be highly individualized with a treatment and rehabilitation focus (Joint Commission, 1970, p. 27).

Child Advocacy System

One of the major problems in initiating intervention strategies at any level is that the child with the unmet need is often the child without an advocate. The most outstanding example of the need for child advocacy is the case of the battered child whose parents are the direct major and ongoing cause of the child's trauma, and without an advocate the child is at the mercy of destructive parents. Much more subtle situations arise in children at the poverty level who do not receive appropriate food, housing, or medical care and may be the victims of racial prejudice. The child needs not only an advocate for specific individual interventions but a system of advocacy that assures that needed programs and services will be available. The Joint Commission (1970, pp. 9–10) recommended to Congress and to the President the appointment of a National Advisory Council on Children as the major source for providing for and planning child advocacy at all levels—federal, state, and local. Within the Commission recommendation related to child advocacy and crucial to its implementation was the recommendation to establish child development councils throughout the country. The function of the child development councils would be (Joint Commission, 1970, p. 15):

1. To integrate existing, fragmented local services, and to ensure that each child's needs are met through advocacy and improved interagency arrangements
2. To guarantee in every community adequate diagnostic, treatment, care, special education, and social services for children with emotional, mental, behavioral, social, and physical disturbances through leadership in planning new services, reorganizing existing services, and ensuring that children in need receive the necessary care and treatment
3. To guarantee every child an adequate education
4. To involve parents in planning and supporting services in behalf of their children

The child psychiatric nurse who has a professional commitment to the mental health of all children also has a responsibility to assume leadership in child advocacy. The child psychiatric nurse can function as an advocate by being actively involved in child development counseling centers, local mental health programs, and the passage of legislature effecting child mental health.

High-Risk Population

Much of the literature on prevention suggests that activity be aimed at high-risk population. The usual connotation of the designation *high-risk persons* is: those who live at or below the poverty level. And because of the nature of our society, these people are usually racially and culturally different from the majority of the population above the poverty level. Coles (1967, p. 1972), Murphy (1962), and Garmezy (1971) raise some serious and important issues in relation to the (automatic) categorizing of poor people in high mental health-risk categories.

Coles (1967), in his extensive study of poor black people living in stressful situations, finds an amazing amount of stability and resiliency. He recognizes many of the hazards of poverty and racism. For example, often a child has to be taught to give up parts of his innate personality in order to survive. Coles also notes how often the role of adversity can also foster growth and strength (1967, p. 326). In summarizing, Coles (1967, p. 341) states that it is the "social experience of the black child that becomes a series of psychological experiences which give form and structure to life." He learns to adapt to a white world and protects himself by assuming different behaviors with different situations.

Garmezy (1971, p. 101) suggests that there is a need for basic research regarding who is "vulnerable" and how it is that some children are "invulnerable." He further recommends that research be focused on families and mothers in "high-risk" areas who do produce competent children, to find out what they do and how they do it. Related to the suggestion for study by Garmezy are the assumptions of Murphy (1962, p. 2) on coping in children. She defines *coping* as the ability to deal with new, stressful experiences where responses are not automatic. A study of vulnerabilities and invulnerabilities might focus on how families foster or hinder their children's coping skills.

Parent Education

One of the major activities which is included in prevention at all levels of development is parent education; however, as the Joint Commission points out (1970, p. 348), there is a great need for more knowledge on how to foster growth and development; how to narrow the gap between parents and children within a rapidly changing society; and in what specific areas to prepare for parenting. The report further states that educational programs usually reach only 5 percent of those in need, and that usually those parents are not the ones who are in most need of improving their parenting skills.

Brim (1961, pp. 122–124), in his discussion on methods of educating parents, states that although there are differences between education and therapy, there are also many overlaps and similarities. The main difference is that education is directed toward conscious and near-conscious aspects of the individual's personality, whereas therapy is directed more toward unconscious material. He further makes the following basic assumptions regarding parent education:

1. Choice of method depends on ends of programs.
2. Parents—mostly the mother—can effect child's mental growth.
3. Those aspects of parent behavior which influence development of mental disorders are subject to influence by education.
4. No single traumatic event, but day-by-day interactions, builds abnormal behavior patterns.
5. Parents who are involved in planning and implementing their own learning experience have more effective behavioral change.

CRUCIAL STAGES AND INFLUENCES ON PERSONALITY DEVELOPMENT IN INFANCY

Introduction to Infancy

Infancy is the period of living that starts with the birth of the individual and proceeds to the emergence of the capacity for communication through speech (approximately one and a half years). However, a consideration of the infant must of necessity include the influences of the prenatal period and of the birth process itself and their effect on the developmental tasks of infancy. Greenacre (1952, p. 3) states that the infant is dependent on prenatal organization to meet his immediate postnatal needs, and Lourie (1971, p. 34) suggests that age be measured from time of conception.

Prenatal and Birth Influence

Current research indicates that there are two major factors in prenatal development which affect the infant's personality: genetic factors and environmental factors.

In relation to genetic factors, early research by Jost and Sontag in 1944 indicated that genetic factors influence the development and functioning of the autonomic nervous system, that part of our nervous system which accounts for awareness of many emotional states. Later, in 1965, a study by Gottesman indicated a relationship between genetic composition and a tendency toward social introversion and inhibition and a tendency toward social extraversion and activity level. More recent studies by Vandenburg (1971, pp. 513–514) indicate that genetics has the following effects on human behavior:

1. Heredity influences human behavior in many of the aspects commonly measured by psychological tests.
2. Four of six factors essential to intelligence are under strong genetic control— numerical, verbal, spatial, and word fluency. Reasoning and memory are not so heavily controlled by genetics.
3. Motor skills affected by heredity include hand dexterity and ability to walk a balance beam.
4. In personality, there is a high degree of heritability for factors of activity, vigor, impulsiveness, and sociability.

Genetic irregularities are also known to be etiological factors in some birth defects and syndromes, such as Down's Syndrome.

Prenatal environmental influences also have their effect on the developmental functioning of the infant. Davison and Dobbing (1966, p. 4045), in their studies, found that poor nutrition influences the neuromuscular development if there are deficiencies which affect myelinization at this vulnerable period in brain development. Also affecting the development of the neuromuscular system are viral infections at the time of myelinization. Rubella has been identified as a specific causative agent in many birth defects. Further studies indicate that certain drugs, such as thalidomide, affect the development of the fetus, and studies are being carried out today on the influences of popularly used psychedelic drugs. Studies on the emotional state of the mother indicate that prolonged emotional strain has an enduring effect on the child (Sontag, 1944, pp. 1–5; Davids et al., 1961, pp. 74–77). The age of the mother has also been the object of an intensive study which indicates that in the mother whose age is under twenty or over forty there is a significant increase in the incidence of birth defects. The teen-aged mother has been especially studied in relation to being high-risk in prematurity, birth defects, dietary deficiency, and frequent drug usage.

The birth process itself has been the subject of much study and theorization in relation to its influence on the infant and subsequent personality development. Montague, in 1950, indicated that excessive drug usage during birth could exert permanent influences on subsequent personality development. Greenacre (1952, p. 3) states that the whole birth process exerts an influence on future psychophysiological patterns of the child, particularly in relation to distribution of energy and strength of drives. She further states that abnormal birth and poor antenatal condition produce a state of chronic tension and a susceptibility to excitation which she characterizes as a predisposition to anxiety (Greenacre, 1952, p. 7). Although anxiety as we know it exists only with a dawning ego sense, some of the individual psychological content exists in irritable responsiveness of the organism. This responsiveness is organized loosely in reflex responses and exists as somatic memory traces which later exert psychological pressures. Abnormal and painful birth adds to this store of psychological content (Greenacre, 1952, p. 8).

Individual Differences

This composite of constitutional and environmental influences both prenatally and during the birth process accounts for the wide variety of individual differences which have been studied recently in great detail (Escalona, 1962; Korner, 1967; and Chess, 1961). Lourie (1971, p. 34) draws attention to the need to begin to inventory these constitutional differences in vulnerability and to devise methods of handling to prevent poor solution to children's individual problems. Such problems as deviant arousal patterns, sleep deviations, high and low energy levels, variant sensory thresholds, and inadequate ability to protect self or summon help from the environment are examples of individual vulnerabilities that can be noted in infants. Research is needed which will categorize these differences and which will also test methods of handling these special problems and would promote optimal development through the stages. This type of research data could then be computerized and would be available through retrieval systems as a base for planning intervention strategies with infants and their parents. This type of planning and programming for effective handling of individual differences at an early stage is particularly important because of the concept of critical or optimal periods of development. Each stage has a developmental time limit in which appropriate stimulation is needed in order to foster optimal development (Barnard, 1971; Ambrose, 1963). If individual differences are not taken into account in handling the child during these optimal periods, his developmental needs will not be met for that particular period. The child whose needs are not met at one stage carries over their deficit to the next stage, thus affecting all future personality development.

Stages and Influences in Infancy

Developmental tasks and their concomitant anxiety are seen as basic personality organizers. Historically, Freud (1959, pp. 75–175) stated that the ego was the "seat of anxiety" and further stated that anxiety has a physiological base in the birth process and in infancy. Physiological responses are pressed into service to alert the organism to danger. He further states that there is a later transition of the physiological states to an emerging psychological structure where ego formation can be identified. As Greenacre (1952, p. 8) states, these physiological tensions are carried over as psychological traces that are experienced as a predisposition to anxiety.

Sander (1962, p. 165) states that adaptation between the mother and infant in a given stage involves an issue. He further identifies time segments in which these issues arise. The first phase is one of undifferentiation (0 to two and a half months), as described by Hartman et al. (1946, pp. 11–38); Spitz (1946, p. 20); and Escalona (1962, pp. 11–37). This is the first stage of imprinting socialization through the process of attachment. To ensure the life of the child and, in fact, the species itself is the process of *imprinting,* which has been defined by Gray (1958, pp. 155–166) as the "innate disposition to learn the parent."

Before the studies of Harlow (1966, pp. 244–272), it was thought that the attachment was strictly a learned response with the reward being the gratifications which the infant received by having his needs met by his mother. This learning is a part of the attachment process, but the studies of Harlow indicate that the infant is born with the capacity to emit attachment behavior toward the person caring for it. These behaviors include clinging, vocalization, smiling, scanning, and following.

Although the studies of Harlow (1966, pp. 244–272) show these innate factors leading to attachment, how well this period is handled depends on the degrees of *specific* appropriateness the mother is able to maintain in response to her baby's highly individualized cues regarding his state and needs (Sander, 1962, pp. 165–166).

The next phase is when true reciprocity in response begins to appear between the mother and infant at about five to twelve months (Spitz and Wolf, 1946, p. 59). The mother smiles and the baby, who now has the ability to fixate on the mother's face, smiles back. The attachment or symbiotic period continues until around the ninth month. The way in which the baby expresses himself and imitates social exchange at this stage is dependent upon his ability to respond and the way in which he is responded to by his mother (Bowlby, 1958, pp. 350–373).

Sometime between six and eight months, the baby develops the ability to differentiate his mother's face from those of other human beings (Bronson, 1968, pp. 350–358). Studies of infants at this stage noted a fear of novelty and an experience not pleasurable to the infant at seeing another face. This process has been stated as the ontogenetic rather than phylogenic basis of anxiety (Brody, and Axelrod, 1970, p. 34). However, this fact does not negate the phylogenic effects of the mother's ability to continue to meet the child's needs during this process of separation and the child's insistence and persistence in having his needs met. It is during this stage that Brody (1970, p. 56) sees the infant as developing anxiety preparedness, which, she states, is an adaptive reaction of the infant to penetration of his protective shield. The protective shield, although having its base in physiological paths, leads to concomitant emergence of rudimentary ego functions and the effect—anxiety. The protective shield allows for both active and passive accommodations to stimuli, which may be expressed as a tendency to appeal for help when stimuli become too excessive. Without the appropriate symbiotic imprinting of the earlier stage, the infant would not develop the ability to experience anxiety and also to develop attachment to other objects later.

The infant, without impediment from constitutional or environmental factors, continues to grow in separation from his mother and in his beginning self-identity. This growth leads quite naturally to the next stage, where the infant continues to develop autonomy (Erikson, 1959, p. 51). The issue here is how the individual style of self-assertion by the child is dealt with, especially when he is opposing his mother's wishes (Sander, 1962, p. 166).

Primary and Secondary Prevention in Infancy

Primary prevention strategies during the prenatal period itself can influence the number and quality of unusual vulnerabilities impinging on the newborn infant. Preventive programs should broadly include an environment and a society that provide for the basic needs of the pregnant mother; adequate medical care during pregnancy, the birth process, and postpartum; counseling and education in parenting; and the spacing and prevention of parenting in high-risk situations, such as those of very young and older women, and in relation to genetic factors. An example of a primary preventive strategy in this area is a school nurse who meets with young high school students to talk with them about parenthood responsibilities and the effect of parenting on very young children.

In addition to general programs of supportive health care, many parents of infants can benefit from child growth and development experiences that help them understand what to expect from their child, how to handle developmental problems, and how to identify deviations in development. An additional safeguard in assuring appropriate development during this period is systematic periodic observation of the infant's development in homes, doctors' offices, child health clinics, and day care centers, especially in areas with a high-risk population (Work and Call, 1965, p. 9). Although traumatic events do have an impact on the infant, it is the subtle day-by-day interplay of forces in the evolution of the child—the environmental interaction—that shapes the character, the unfolding, and the molding of human personality (Pavenstedt, 1962). Therefore, it is this type of daily interaction at crucial periods of development that must be observed and guided, with provisions made for intervention as needed. Nurses are often in key positions to carry out these systematic observations and/or to organize and train others in observation of parent-infant interactions.

Call (1963, pp. 451–459) describes a significant piece of primary prevention in well-child conferences. The staff of the conference observed the interactions of an infant and mother as being typical of those described in the development of early infantile autism. Following this observation, interventions were planned both at the conference and through home visits by a public health nurse. The mother was exposed to demonstration and explanation about infant care, and within a short period of time she began to interact and to relate to her infant in a manner more appropriate to the infant's developmental needs.

A number of studies indicate that different methods of childrearing have a differential effect on infant development. A study by Brody (1970) reports the results of periodic observation of and interviews with normal mothers during their prenatal periods and through the infant's first year of life. The study indicates a relationship between patterns of mothering and favorable or unfavorable development in infants.

The mothers in Brody's study were evaluated in relation to quality and consistency of empathy, control, and efficiency. The infant's development was evaluated by the Gesell Scale of Infant Development. Favorable developmental signs considered in the first year were (1) smooth physiological function, (2) superior control of ego function, (3) superior function of pleasure, and (4) ease of adaptation to stressful stimuli. The converse of these were indications of signs of disturbance.

On the basis of observable data, the mothers could be classified into seven types. The mothers whose children had the most favorable signs of development and the least signs of disturbance had the following characteristics:

1. Were cooperative in the study.
2. Gave accurate reports with appropriate affect.
3. Placed little emphasis on standards of behavior for themselves and their infants, or on their competence as mothers.
4. Were open to influence on childrearing.
5. Were interested in infant moods and activity.
6. Provided physical care which was considerate and efficient.
7. Were free to initiate social and motor activity; to communicate by glance, voice and, touch; and to respond to infants' wishes for activity and sociability.
8. Showed affection, encouragement, and praise, and seemed to enjoy mothering beyond routine care.

The other mothers were on a continuum from these most adequate mothers with the least signs of disturbance to the type of mother who had the most signs of disturbance and the least signs of favorable development. These latter mothers had the following characteristics:

1. Poor and unwilling observers and reporters about their children
2. Vague, evasive, self-centered
3. Negative and irritable
4. Tense, dissatisfied, angry or flippant, nonchalant regarding their maternal role
5. Uninterested in learning more about infant care or in increasing their competence as mothers
6. Critical of their infant's behavior and openly hostile toward it
7. Overconcerned with their own appearance and responding mechanically and as little as possible
8. Apt to carry out basic routines without observable sensitivity to the infant's feelings
9. During visible infant distress, prone to speak to the infant abusively, to complain, to ignore, or to punish it
10. At times, overaffectionate; either positive or negative involvement exaggerated, or behavior neutral and joyless
11. Lacking in maternal intimacies as between mothers and infants, when observed

Using this kind of data, it would be appropriate for nurses or child care workers trained and supervised by nurses to observe mother-infant interaction and infant development during critical stages in infancy among high-risk population, e.g., young and older mothers, mothers who fit a family or individual pattern of producing children with a high rate of disturbance, and children with marked individual differences.

The nurse or supervised child care worker with a solid foundation in infant and child development who regularly observes parent-infant interaction can provide the following services:

1. Anticipatory guidance for infant-parent interaction before the infant moves into a new developmental stage. An example is preparation of the parents for the separa-

tion stage when the infant needs gradual and gentle handling with and around strangers, and also needs more opportunity to cling to its mother.

2. Demonstration for the parents of appropriate handling of infant behavior by being a role model in her visits. She may also provide supervision and reinforcement to the parents as they interact with the infant following her demonstrations.
3. Corrective intervention when she observes disturbed infant development resulting from inappropriate parent-infant interactions.
4. Referral of families to other mental health facilities for counseling when the above measures are not effective in reducing infant developmental disturbances.
5. Advocacy for the infant where parents are not able to use available resources to reduce abnormal deviation of their infants.

Throughout the country, preventive infant programs are developing and expanding. The following are a few examples of this type of program.

In New York, through the Child Development Center of the Jewish Board of Guardians (Lilleskov et al., 1970, p. 281), a full- and part-time infant care unit was set up in a high-risk community housing project to provide consistent alternative care when mothers of infants needed to go to work or school or were simply unprepared for or overwhelmed by their mothering role. The program also offered emergency care in the home at times of crisis, postnatal assistance in the home, and counseling and education in childrearing for parents or groups, or on an individual basis.

Hunt (1971, pp. 13–35) describes parent and child centers in which the aim of intervention is to teach mothers of poverty greater skills in childrearing so that they can experience success and increase their competence. The parent and child centers provide nontraditional educational opportunities that include demonstrations; imitation and modeling; explanation of childrearing practices; and concern for mothers. In addition, the center provides leadership in the formation of day care facilities which incorporate developmental educational components for infants, toddlers, and preschoolers.

A similar program is described by Badger (1971, p. 168) in which there was a concerted effort to reach the apathetic mother who usually did not attend educational experiences. Through involvement in an educational process that valued them and their ability to be con-tributors, mothers who had seemingly hopeless and helpless attitudes were able to change. Part of the program was mother-centered, with an opportunity for her to be involved in a group experience, and the other part was child-centered, with the mother being taught and supervised in how to play, interact with, and teach her infant and young child.

Tertiary Programs

In situations where there are numerous signs of disturbance, where there are severe physical defects, or where the mother cannot assume an appropriate mothering role, the demonstrations and developmental guidance of child care workers may not be sufficient to decrease the signs of disturbance and foster optimal development. The infant with severe physical and/or mental deficits will need the help of other specialized health care workers such as physical therapists, nurses, psychologists, or psychiatrists trained in child psychiatry. Mothers may also need counseling and/or therapy in order to work through their emotional response to producing a defective infant and/or the grief of loss of the expected normal infant. An example of preventive intervention in the possible abnormal development of a child with a physical defect is that of a cerebral palsied infant who stiffened his body and turned away when his mother picked him up. The mother assumed that the infant was rejecting her, was quite depressed, and in fact now rejected the infant. However, when she was helped to understand that her infant's response was due to reflexes, and when she was taught how to handle her infant in a way that avoided stimulating the reflex patterns, she was able to develop a closer attachment to the infant and hence to meet his normal developmental needs.

In the case of the child who has severe emotional deficits, or suffers physical abuse as the result of poor parenting, it is appropriate for the parents to be involved in an intensive psychotherapeutic program. However, since personality change leading to ability to assume a parenting role may take considerable time, it is important to plan for alternate parenting experiences for infants during this most crucial period of development. Alternate types of parenting could be full- or part-time day care, and foster home care. The infant with behavior described as infantile autism may also fall into this category. In the mental health field there is great controversy regarding the etiology and treatment of infantile autism; however, the fact remains that, regardless of professional controversy, the parents often cannot cope with the autistic infant's behavior in a way that fosters development. There may be a need to provide the parents and infant with respite care, day care, or foster home care alternatives in addition to the prescribed treatment program.

The last type of intervention leads to a major philosophical change in the thinking and approach of professionals and nonprofessionals who deal with children. In the past we have often functioned with the assumption that *all* families can meet *all* needs of their children;

however, it is now more readily accepted that they cannot, and that infants need protection at crucial early stages of their development. It may be the role of the community child advocacy system to intervene in situations where infants are in danger of being permanently damaged, by arranging with the families for out-of-home care and/or placement until the parents are able to assume more therapeutic parenting roles or until the child has passed through crucial vulnerable stages of development. Often the nurse who is in contact with the family in homes and clinics must take this most important step as the infant's advocate.

DEVELOPMENTAL STAGES AND INFLUENCE IN CHILDHOOD

Introduction to Childhood

At the end of the period when the infant's separation from the mother has been relatively smooth and he begins to assume a separate identity, there develops a solid foundation for his continued and broader socialization. The main purpose of the parents' attempts to socialize their child is to guide the child in acquiring personality characteristics, behavior, values, and motives which the culture considers appropriate.

For the child, this is the period of beginning communication through speech and separation, individuation having been well established; the child then begins to expand his relationships to a larger world. He begins to form relationships with people of his own age level who share his attitudes toward authority and activities. Throughout the childhood period he continues to expand his association with compeers, and the period ends when the satisfaction and security of another person become as significant as his own.

Variables in Personality Development in Childhood

Kagan and Moss (1962, pp. 13–16), in a longitudinal study of development during childhood, were able to identify four child behavior variables related to personality development: (1) motive behaviors aimed at attaining cultural goals, (2) sources of anxiety and conflict, (3) defensive responses to anxiety situations, and (4) modes of interpersonal interaction.

Motive behavior refers to overt goal-related behavior which has been learned by the child to attain specific goals. The common goals are social recognition, task mastery, nurturance, appropriate sex interest and gratification, affiliation with peers, and perception of injury or anxiety in others. The sources of anxiety in the preschool child are around fear of loss of parental love as he moves away from them toward more independence, anticipation of physical injury, and expression of aggressive, sexual, and dependent behavior. In the school-age child the main sources of anxiety are fear of failure to master socially valued skills, intellectual incompetence, personal inadequacy, and deviations from sex-role standards. As in infancy, the intensity of the anxiety in the child is a function of the child's basic constitution and environmental interaction. The previously stated anxiety sources in the child are motives for defensive behavior. These are learned behaviors which are aimed at the specific goal of amelioration of unpleasant states. The major defensive behaviors of childhood are regression, denial, projection, repression, and withdrawal.

Other factors in child personality development are the mode of social interaction, the quality of interpersonal interactions, the approach-avoidance pattern, the amount of spontaneity or tension, and the amount of domination or submission.

Murphy, in *The Widening World of Childhood* (1962), looks at the way children cope with new normal and abnormal stresses of life. It is through experiences in coping that the child develops a patterned way of dealing with newness (Murphy, 1962, p. 2). New and strong situations have different meanings for different children and cause different reactions based on the child's individual differences and his infantile experiences to newness and the mother's ability to meet his specific needs in relation to newness (Murphy, 1962, p. 57). The child develops a repertoire of coping strategies that allow him to control the direction of his attention and interest; control of anxiety; management of stress so that negative or anxiety reactions are balanced with positive gratification (Murphy, 1962, p. 280).

The longitudinal study at the Fels Institute described by Kagan and Moss (1962, p. 272) was able to identify that those behavioral tendencies which have their foundations in infancy become "crystallized" during the childhood period and continue on through adulthood.

Preschool Stages and Influences

During the first year of life the parents, particularly the mother, are usually seen by the infant as supporting persons who gratify the infant's needs as soon as these are identified. In the second year the parents, recognizing the need and readiness of the child, begin the process of socialization and inhibit undesirable behavior which the infant finds pleasurable. The child is expected to delay or curb gratification. This process is the first normal source of friction between the parent and the child. There are little solid research data on the best way to socialize a child, but the major goal is to minimize the friction and conflict that arise naturally.

Part of the child's readiness to participate in the socialization process is dependent on the socialization aspects of infant development. Normally the infant learns to please the parents, thus ensuring affection and protection and avoiding unpleasant feelings generated by punishment and rejection. If the infant has not experienced gratification from his parents and the desire to please them, the next stage of development in which he is expected to delay or curb gratification will be more difficult. He may have the physiological readiness but not the psychological readiness to give up pleasurable behaviors.

To develop a sense of autonomy, the child must have a feeling of confidence in his ability to deal effectively with his environment (Mussen et al., 1969, p. 261). He needs to be able to develop mastery over bodily function and skill in manipulation, and in this process he must face the reality that there are rules connected with these functions. For example, in developing a sense of autonomy, the child needs to gain control over his bowels and bladder, but at the same time he finds there are rules regarding elimination that are imposed on him by his parents. The child's response to the rules or limits is negative behavior that usually takes the form of aggression toward parents.

Behaviors Associated with Conflict and Anxiety

Aggression in childhood is universal, and the tendency or capacity has some innate components (Lorenz, 1966). However aggression is expressed, its nature, form, and control are learned (Bandura and Walters, 1965, p. 101). The child learns that he can get what he wants through aggressive behavior and may become skilled in using this method of controlling others (Sears, 1953, pp. 135–234). The child also learns from his parents that some types of aggression are rewarded and some are punished. Bandura and Walters (1965, p. 105) indicate that parents, beyond being differential reinforcers of aggressive behavior, also serve as models for learning acceptable and unacceptable aggressive behavior. The research of Kagan and Moss (1962, p. 201) at the Fels Institute documents the importance of sex typing in relation to the form of expression of aggressive behavior in children.

Frustration is also seen as a major factor in the expression of aggression in preschool children. When the child is blocked or curbed in goal-seeking behavior, he experiences a threat to his self-esteem. He may be blocked by external barriers, internal conflicts, or feelings of inadequacy or anxiety that inhibit goal-seeking behavior. There is a wide range of individual differences at this age in how much or how little frustration can be tolerated; also, there is a difference in the expression of response to frustration. For some children, the major response to frustration is regression to a level of more comfort rather than overt acts of aggression to gain control and reduce the anxiety of their inability to control the environment (Barker et al., 1943, pp. 441–458). The amount of conflict and anxiety related to the expression of normal aggression in the preschool child is related to the way parents accept and support the child in this developmental response.

In the preschool years, the major sex-related behaviors are masturbation and sexual curiosity. The major methods of dealing with these behaviors in American families is to restrict sex-related actions, e.g., not allowing or punishing masturbation or exposure of genitals in public, and nonlabeling or redirecting of sexual activity. Both of these actions quite possibly lead to anxiety regarding sexual activity. Less anxiety develops if parents handle sexual curiosity and behavior realistically without embarrassment or punishment. They should also answer children's sexual questions with content that is appropriate to their level of understanding (Mussen et al., 1969, pp. 328–329). There is evidence in studies by Gagnon (1965, pp. 212–228) that sex-connected experiences in early life have lasting influences on the way sex is conducted in later life.

The dependency motive is the wish to be nurtured and to be comforted, to be close emotionally, and to be accepted. This motive is still very strong in the early preschool period (three to four years) and may be expressed in a variety of individual ways. Where dependent needs are met in the early preschool years, the child develops a security and is then able to move into more independent behavior in the four- to five-year-old and on into the later childhood years (Mussen et al., 1969, p. 343). Where the mother is inconsistent in relating to dependent behavior—sometimes rewarding and at other times punishing—reward for dependent behavior tends to increase dependent behavior and decrease the development of independent behavior (Sears, 1957, pp. 173–174).

INFLUENCE OF PLAY ON PERSONALITY DEVELOPMENT

Throughout childhood, play is the natural medium of self-expression in the child. It is the method he uses for self-mastery, coordination, and mastery over objects. From his play the child is able to form images and patterns of relatedness which form a whole out of parts.

Play activity is recognized as a complex assortment of the child's conscious and unconscious expressions (Erikson, 1963, p. 32). Through play, the child is able to act out areas of concern that he is unable to verbalize. Play is the language and work of the child in which he often uses objects to act out his conflicts. Play also may have the effect of catharsis that speech has for the adult. The child who, as the result of external or internal motivation, is unable to engage in active play, limits his ability to use a tool that fosters mastery of developmental tasks.

Role Identification in Personality Development

Identification is the process which leads the child to incorporate the characteristics of another person within his own personality. It is not a conscious process, nor the result of training (Mussen et al., 1969, pp. 356–357). In the development of identification with another person, there must be motivation to be like the model and the presence of some characteristics in the child which are similar to those of the model. The child sees his parents as having abilities he would like to possess, such as control or power over others, mastery over the environment, and the ability to give or withhold love, and he identifies with these.

An interrelated concept is that of identification and sex typing. In the ideal situation, appropriate sex typing occurs through identification with the parent of the same sex.

This parent is seen as nurturing and has desirable characteristics. Ideally, both parents consistently reward sex-appropriate behavior and discourage sex-inappropriate behavior (Mussen and Rutherford, 1963, pp. 586–607). In the process the child is able to adopt the behavior, values, attitudes, and interests of his own sex. Kagan and Moss (1962, p. 271) state that sex-role identification is central to selective adaptation and maintenance of behavior. The expressions of aggression, competition, passivity, dependency, and sexuality are in part determined by the child's assessment of the congruence of the behavior with cultural sex-role standards. Children are motivated to behave in many ways congruent with hypothetical ego-ideals and models of masculine or feminine qualities. In addition, most humans need to act and behave in ways that are congruent with standards which reflect their ideal. Any behavior or belief that increases the discrepancy between the child's evaluation of himself and his idealized model provokes anxiety and is avoided, whereas any behavior that decreases the discrepancy between the self-evaluation and the model of the self is rewarded and repeated.

Development of Conscience

There is evidence of beginning conscience formation in the preschool years. The child develops a set of standards of acceptable behavior and acts according to these standards. He feels guilty if he violates them. The process of conscience development at this stage is closely related to identification with the parents (Murphy, 1947, p. 543). Anxiety about punishment or loss of love may be the major motivation to acquire the standards that please the parents. Becker (1964, p. 183) states that optimum superego development is closely related to the parents' ability to arouse unpleasant feelings in the child about his misbehavior. These feelings are independent of threats and encourage the child to take responsibility for his actions. Defects in beginning superego development may be seen as inadequate identification with significant others. This inability to identify may be based on the fact that the child does not experience his parent or parents as being nurturant or having enough positive similarities to identify with.

Extra-Family Influences on Preschool Personality Development

As the child grows older and begins to move away from the family, new socialization agents compete with those of the parents. The most important new socialization agents to preschoolers are peers and teachers in nursery schools.

The nursery school program has been the focus of many studies regarding the effect of attendance on preschool children. Hattrick (1967, pp. 180–190) reports that the nursery school child makes rapid gains in social participation compared with nonattending peers. He is less inhibited, more spontaneous, independent, self-assertive, self-reliant, curious, and interested in his environment. Individual attention by nursery school teachers may reduce a child's maladaptive behavior and strengthen adaptive behavior. In this process, there is an increase in the child's self-confidence, frustration tolerance, and ability to persist in a task (Allen et al., 1964, pp. 511–518).

Peers also act as reinforcers for behavior in preschool children. They become new models for imitation and identification. In the peer group, the models are the most popular persons. These popular models are the most friendly, often engage in cooperative play, tend to reinforce others, and are least dependent on adults (Charlesworth, 1967, pp. 993–1002).

So as the child emerges from the preschool years to school age, his world expands from the close one-to-one relationship with his mother to interrelations with the family, and then to small-group relationships away from the family structure.

Primary and Secondary Prevention in Preschool Children

The programs of health maintenance, parent education, and observations should continue on to this age period. Observation and intervention programs could be carried out in homes, well-child conferences, day care centers, and preschools, with services being provided by nurses and child care workers similar to those described for the infant-parent relationship.

Day Care

One of the most important current issues in primary prevention in the preschool child is the need for developmental day care programs for mothers who work or who are unable to provide for the developmental needs of their children. Keyserling (1971, p. 434) in "Day Care Challenge" states that a survey by the U.S. Labor Department and the Children's Bureau in 1965 found that over one-third of the mothers with children under six years of age are working. The study indicated the following regarding arrangements made for the child when the mother was unable to care for him:

1. *Own Home Care*: Mostly inadequate, depending on siblings or fathers to care for the children.
2. *On Their Own*: A conservative estimate of 18,000 children under six years are "latchkey children."
3. *Other Home:* A variety of quality—from very good to poor custodial.
4. *Group Centers:* Quality spotty.

Zigler (1972) describes developmental day care as a major step beyond custodial day care for young children. Developmental day care provides opportunities for emotional, social, intellectual, and physical development under the direction of trained child caretakers. This type of care is based on planned programs which include nutritious meals, medical and dental examinations, and parent participation. To staff these centers, Zigler describes the new profession of child development associates, who will be trained at the associate degree level through the Office of Child Development. The goals of the developmental day care program are to:

1. Enhance the child's self-image
2. Foster trust in, and enjoyment of, other people, as well as respect for the rights of others
3. Develop problem-solving ability
4. Develop motivation, achievement, and competence in learning
5. Provide children opportunities to develop and refine their intellectual, physical, and social skills
6. Encourage expression of ideas and feelings through effective use of language
7. Provide materials that encourage creative play and learning with a minimum of frustration and a maximum of challenge (Klein, 1972, p. 5)

In addition to day care programs, Warren, (1972, pp. 28–29) describes night care centers. These centers provide safe, consistent care for children whose parents work at night. Another preventive aspect of the program is to offer a place for children to go for activity in the evening when family tensions are often highest, and when the potential for emotional or physical injury or trauma to children may be greatest.

The child psychiatric nurse has an excellent opportunity to participate in the developmental day care programs. First, the nurse has the opportunity to provide indirect services through education and training of new categories of child caretakers. The child psychiatric nurse is also prepared to offer consultation to child care staff in the area of normal growth and development needs of the children, management of behavior problems, recognition of physical problems and defects, and referral to appropriate treatment sources.

The child psychiatrist nurse can provide direct services, such as individual and group counseling with children who are experiencing behavior problems, parent education, and parent counseling.

Tertiary Programs

Preschool children who have been identified as severely disabled developmentally with emotional, intellectual, or social defects, or any combination of these, need intensive treatment. Treatment is essential at this malleable age to prevent the disabilities from becoming crystallized and to prevent further handicapping. The preferred treatment is to keep the child in as near as normal a setting as possible and to involve the child and his family in a treatment program. There are a growing number of community day treatment centers and psychoeducational day schools that provide services for such children and their families; however, community support of these sorely needed agencies is still quite inadequate. An example of an outstanding agency which is supported by a federal grant is the Julia Ann Singer Pre-School Psychiatric Center in Southern California (Williams, 1971, p. 319). The goals of the center are to modify the child's maladaptive social behavior and to interrupt inappropriate familial training that perpetuates learning difficulties and emotional disturbance.

The agency expands its treatment potential by using a maximum number of indigenous workers from the community. Parents, teachers, students, and volunteers are trained by mental health professionals in the agency to serve as primary therapeutic agents for emotionally disturbed preschoolers. These therapists are trained in techniques of behavior modification, sensorimotor stimulation, and family demonstration.

When the child's behavior has improved significantly, the agency arranges for transfer to a normal school setting. However, before the child is placed, the prospective teacher is released from her regular classroom assignment to receive training at the center. This training focuses on the management of the child to be placed in the teacher's class. This part of the program makes use of the progress made during the preschool years and allows the child to continue his "normalization" in a regular classroom setting.

Where there are no appropriate facilities available for preschoolers with developmental disabilities, or when his own home cannot meet the child's developmental needs, it may be necessary to consider out-of-the-home placement. Pratt (1971, p. 269) reports on "assembled foster families," which is an intervention model aimed at interrupting the cycle of poor or inadequate parenting. Young children who are abandoned, or who have parents who cannot meet their specific developmental needs, are placed in family settings of from one to five children with stable, well-adjusted couples who are committed to long-term family care. Extensive support is offered by mental health specialists through home visits, group education, and counseling with the groups of foster parents involved in the project. Foster care is also seen as an important link—as an extension of in-patient programs for children. Here, again, there is a great need for the provision of mental health support services (Rice and Semmelroth, 1968, p. 539). All too often the child who learns to function well in a treatment setting is placed in a foster home with little support for the child or the parents. The end result may be that the child is returned to the in-patient setting. Both child and foster parents suffer from this situation. In most cases this problem could be avoided by organized systematic visits by child psychiatric nurses or other mental health workers prepared to deal with the mental health needs of disturbed children.

Stages in Personality Development in the School-Age Child and Influences on Them

Five major developmental tasks have been identified for the school-age child to accomplish:

1. The development of intellectual and academic skills and the motivation to master them
2. The crystallization of sex-role identification
3. Increased autonomy and independence
4. The development of moral standards and conscience
5. Learning to deal appropriately with anxiety and conflict (Mussen et al., 1969, p. 545)

Whether the school-age child is able to accomplish these developmental tasks depends on his prior and present life experiences. If his earlier developmental needs have been met, he will be able to expend his energy in working on age-appropriate developmental tasks. He will have ego development that allows him to be in control of his aggressive, sexual, and dependency impulses. The child with prior faulty life experiences in which his developmental needs have not been met may have poor control over his impulses. This child may not have the full amount of energy to pursue and accomplish developmental tasks of his age group.

School Adjustment and School Influence on the Child

Aside from the initial separation from his mother, the next major influence on the child's life is his entrance into school. This entrance into the larger world forces the child to deal with a number of tasks at the same time:

1. Separation from his mother for most of the day and consequent reduction of dependent ties
2. Contact with a new adult, the teacher, who makes many demands on the child and may not be seen as rewarding
3. The development of intensive, meaningful relationships with peers (Mussen et al., 1969, pp. 546–647)

An important factor in initial school adjustment is the personality of the teacher. Mussen, Conger, and Kagan (1969, p. 554) summarize their research on the relation of teacher personality and teacher effectiveness:

Most children seem to do best under well-trained democratic teachers who know their subject matter, are interested in their pupils, and are not overly concerned with their own problems. Such teachers encourage the students to actively participate in the learning process while maintaining leadership, direction, and, when necessary, reasonable discipline. In contrast, optimal academic and personal growth will not be stimulated in most students by the teacher who is either rigidly authoritarian, hostile, or unresponsive to students' needs; or by the teacher who is indecisive, uncertain, poorly trained, or too occupied with her own anxieties and personal problems.

Although these statements are true in general, there are differences in the way a child perceives the teacher (Cheong 1966, pp. 446–449). There is some evidence that students might be able to function more effectively with teachers who have similar personality patterns and with similar social, economic, and cultural and racial background as the child (Mussen et al., 1969. p. 555).

An area of current special interest in which the fit between teacher and child is discrepant and which influences the achievement of the child is that of the "culturally disadvantaged" or "culturally different" student. The child may enter school with developmental deficits resulting from cultural influences of his family, or from a generally poor social milieu which conflicts with school expectations, which may affect his ability to achieve in academic tasks (Coleman, 1966, p. 10). Since the educational needs of these children are greater, there should be more assistance and better-prepared teachers for these children. All too often these children attend schools in which the environment does not provide motivation to learn and in which the staff are poorly prepared to meet their unique problems (Conant, 1961, p. 12). Although federal legislation has been enacted to improve this situation, there are still too many ghetto schools that are victims of racial and cultural discrimination. For these children there is a need to look for different kinds of approaches to education that will stimulate the child to use and value the qualities, attitudes, and differences that stem from his cultural background. Along with curriculum changes there is also a need for preparing teachers who can understand and meet specific needs of children with a cultural background different from that of the white middle class (Museen et al., 1969, pp. 566–567).

Another influence on the child's ability to achieve relates to his level of anxiety in the classroom, particularly in situations which involve testing. Studies indicate that children with high levels of anxiety have impaired academic achievement (Feldhusen, 1962, pp. 403–409; Frost, 1965, pp. 167–175; Keller, 1962, pp. 19–22; and Sarason et al., 1960, p. 12). Sarason et al. (1960, pp. 13–16) hypothesize that the anxious reaction of children to classroom tests or test-type situations is a reflection of the child's experiences at home before formal schooling begins. The test-anxious child often has had earlier unmet dependency needs which caused the child to experience great hostility toward his parents. This hostility could not be expressed because of the child's need for approval and the fear of loss of parental love. The teacher who is aware of the child's level of anxiety may be able to structure the teaching style so that support is offered to the anxious child. Such structuring allows the child to reduce his anxiety level and increases his ability to function at a level that is nearer his capacity.

Influence of Peers on Personality Development in Childhood

In addition to the educational process and the personality of the teacher herself, another important influence on the school-age child is his peer relationships. Whether a child adapts significant peer-group relations depends a great deal on whether the child is able to gain or want acceptance by his peers and can identify with them. Where the values of peers, teachers, and parents are somewhat related, there are fewer conflicts; but often the behavior that the peer group demands is in conflict with that required by teachers and parents. In this situation the child then has to decide whether adult or peer approval is more important to him (Mussen et al., 1969).

The peer group becomes a major socializing agent for the child in teaching him how to interact and how to handle conflicts and anxiety regarding aggressive and sexual activities; and it also provides an opportunity for him to develop a realistic concept of who he is in relation to others his own age. During middle childhood, children often form into small, informal groups—"the neighborhood gang." The activities and interests of these groupings are usually strongly sex-typed.

PRIMARY AND SECONDARY PREVENTION OF MENTAL ILLNESS IN SCHOOL-AGE CHILDREN

Mental Health in the Schools

Although there is some difference of opinion as to whether or not schools have any responsibility for the mental health of students (Dingman and Boettscher, 1971, p. 328), there is a growing acceptance of the school as an appropriate setting to provide a number of mental health services for school children (Leuchter, 1968; Allinsmith and Goethels, 1962; and Stickney, 1968). Leuchter (1968, p. 575) and Stickney (1968, p. 1407) point out that the schools have been assigned by law the task of educating and caring for most of the communities' disturbed children and at the same time have been granted no funds and no trained personnel or insufficiently trained personnel for this crucial assignment. In addition, teachers have not been adequately prepared for the responsibility of educating disturbed children.

Role of the Mental Health Specialist in the School Setting

Stickney (1968) and Allinsmith (1962) see the major role of the mental health specialist as providing indirect services through consultation to and education of school personnel to help them with the following tasks:

1. Incorporation of mental health principles in teaching
2. Early identification of problems
3. Classroom management of children with problems
4. Crisis intervention with children and families

In addition, the child psychiatric nurse and other health specialists may provide direct services through individual and group counseling to those children who have been identified as having problems (Michne, 1971, pp. 18–25; Pazdur, 1969, pp. 349–457).

Primary Prevention—Mental Health in the School Curriculum

Redl (1959, p. 40 and p. 127) sees the mental health role of the school in primary prevention as being able to provide a healthy framework for child development by gearing the school curriculum to growth needs and also to individual differences which are based on past experiences. He sees the core of school activities as being a guide for children in learning activities so that they can master their environment and gain self-confidence (Redl, 1959, p. 228). Minuchin et al. (1969, xii) adds to these statements that mental health is not an appendage to the school, but a vital part, and that there should be an infusion of mental health principles into the educational process at all levels. Allinsmith and Goethels (1962, pp. 92–124) states that the school has the following specific opportunities to practice primary prevention by:

1. Reducing the incidence of traumatic events
2. Minimizing undesirable reactions to traumatic events when they do occur
3. Preparing children for entrance to school
4. Providing a mentally healthy classroom environment
   a. Activities to express tension
   b. Human relations and human behavior classes
   c. Teacher's use of human behavioral dynamics to promote understanding in all subjects

Further curriculum implications for fostering mental health are stated by Lowenfeld and Brittain (1970, pp. 5–13). They state that since man learns through his senses, a curriculum that promotes greater awareness of all the senses and not just a focus on cognitive development will promote more learning. They also state that children need to have an active part in their learning process and to be able to identify with what they do with self and others.

An example of incorporating behavioral understanding in the classroom is described by Doyal (1971, p. 311) in an elementary school project. The goal of the project was to help children understand that aggression is a normal form of behavior that should be understood, accepted, and modified or controlled. Using an experimental design, the project demonstrated that classroom discussions and experiences around the area of aggression did modify the way children handled and reacted to hostile behavior.

A different kind of program is described by Schiff (1971, p. 322) in a 6-year program in Chicago ghetto schools. Large-group discussions were conducted in classrooms and involved children, their parents, and their teachers. The purpose of the discussions was for all concerned to explore what school is all about, to raise the self-image, and to bring out feelings of worth and responsibility for all concerned. The program was evaluated in relation to the child's adaptation to the student role as judged by teachers' reports on the child and on his reading and arithmetic test scores. The findings supported the fact that this approach fostered growth in academic learning.

Most teachers are not prepared by their previous education to incorporate and implement mental health strategies in the classroom setting. Some schools are beginning to recognize that mental health skills are essential in teacher education; however, the teachers also will need the help of mental health specialists for consultation and up-to-date in-service education. Specifically, teachers need training in group dynamics, normal growth and development, and mental health principles, as well as motivation to achieve greater self-maturity (Allinsmith and Goethels, 1962, pp. 102–124).

Secondary Prevention—Early Identification

Bower (1961, p. 353) states that the schools are in a strategic position to identify beginning problems in school-age children and to plan appropriate preventive interventions. He believes that teachers can be trained to be valid observers and "suspecticians" (Bower, 1960, p. 28).

The emotionally handicapped child can be identified as a child with any, or a combination, of the following characteristics which are apparent to a marked degree over a period of time and cannot be accounted for by low intelligence or other defects:

1. Inability to learn, or to master skills
2. Inability to build or maintain satisfactory interpersonal relations with peers or teachers
3. Inappropriate types of behavior or feelings under normal conditions
4. General mood of depression or unhappiness
5. Tendency to develop psychosomatic symptoms associated with learning situations, e.g., headaches, stomachaches (Bower, 1960, p. 9)

Sarason et al. (1960, p. 263) cite the need to identify at an early age the child who has an abnormal degree of anxiety related to school functioning. In their study they determined that the conventional measures of assessment of the child often do not pick up anxious children, such as the "bright-anxious" child. They suggest the use of testing procedures that indicate patterns of strength and weakness, problem-solving ability and the child's attitude toward himself (Sarason et al., 1960, p. 270).

Van Fleet (1970, p. 320) and Wyatt (1970, p. 319) describe community-initiated programs aimed at early identification of and intervention in "high-risk" groups of young children as they entered the school setting. In addition to the initial identification of children with developmental lags as they entered kindergarten, the programs provided special comprehensive services to the child, the parents, and the teachers in an attempt to prevent further deviation, or, as Deutsch (1964, p. 172) terms it, the "cumulative deficit" of the "disadvantaged child."

Intervention Strategies

After recognition that a child has some type of learning problem related to school, appropriate assessment of the specific learning abilities and disabilities of the child is in order to plan a psychoeducational program based on the assessment (Valett, 1969, p. 2). The child is evaluated on his abilities and disabilities in the following areas:

1. Gross motor functioning
2. Sensorimotor integration
3. Perceptual motor skills
4. Language ability
5. Conceptualization
6. Social-emotional functioning

The child with learning disabilities has specific difficulty in acquiring and using information or skills that are necessary for problem solving and needs special education based on the identified strengths and deficits (Valett, 1969, p. 3).

In order to provide as normal a learning situation as possible within the child's specific disabilities, it is preferable that the psychoeducational program be carried out in the normal classroom, or with the child spending only part of his day in special-class experiences. In all his classes he is involved in specific kinds of remedial experiences with teachers or other specialists who are prepared to help him with his specific disabilities. Such experiences might include such activities as perceptual-motor therapy, remedial reading, language instruction, and group or individual counseling.

For children whose disabilities are such that normal-class experience is not beneficial either to the child or to the other children in the class, "contained" classes may be necessary.

Marrone and Anderson (1970, pp. 694–701) describe a type of innovative public school programming for emotionally disturbed children. In a separate or contained class setting, the children are able to explore and express their feelings about themselves and school, to work through some of their blocks to learning, and perhaps to experience success for the first time in the school. Teachers for these children need special training and continuous support from mental health specialists in order to provide continuing therapeutic experiences for the children, as well as to maintain their own mental health in the face of the daily demands and crises that arise in these classrooms. Child psychiatric nurses in school settings can provide milieu interventions in the classroom besides consultation and support to these teachers who must meet the large demands of their children daily.

TREATMENT PROGRAMS FOR EMOTIONALLY ILL CHILDREN

In many school districts there are no programs for disturbed children within the school setting. There are also children who are too disturbed to benefit from the special classes, even if they were offered. For the latter there are very few treatment facilities available. Frequently the only alternative is admission to a state hospital, often located at some distance from the child's home and usually providing only custodial care rather than therapy.

An exception to this situation is found in Hobbs (1970, p. 310), "Project Re-Ed: New Ways of Helping Emotionally Disturbed Children." This innovative program is an example of a federally funded project that meets the needs of severely emotionally disturbed children. The goal of Project Re-Ed is to return the child as quickly as possible to a normal life setting by around-the-clock reeducation in all areas of the child's life, and by intensive work with the parents.

Within the program for these severely disturbed children, the children are not labeled with diagnoses. The only requirement is that the child have normal intelligence, get in serious difficulty in the school setting, and be unable to remain in school. The staff is composed of teacher-counselors who are selected on the basis of their willingness and capacity to relate to these disturbed children. The focus of their psychoeducational approach is to help the children cope with the here-and-now problems of everyday living.

Hobbs's philosophy is that the emotional disturbance of the child is a manifestation of a breakdown in an ecological system, composed of the child, his family, his neighborhood, the school, and the community. The focus of treatment is on a high expectation of the child for normal behavior with an emphasis on self-fulfillment rather than pathology. The average stay of the children is 7 months; the cost, $25 a day or a total average cost of $5,000. The follow-up studies of these children have shown remarkable improvement. The comparison of those children who spend most of their lives in traditional institutions with the treatment results of these children is appalling, not only in terms of human wastage, but also in financial expenditure. Hertha Riese (1962) in *Heal the Hurt Child* depicts the plight of the severely damaged black child who is given an opportunity for a new life through an intensive humanistic, educational therapy approach.

Such programs as Hobbs's and Riese's are the exceptions; and although there are increasing numbers of day treatment programs and private psychoeducational schools for severely disturbed children, unfortunately the communities where these children live and which contribute to the ecological breakdown which has trapped the child have not assumed or are not able to assume responsibility for providing appropriate treatment services to these children. Many nurses have been prepared to assume responsibilities in child mental health programs. They have a deep commitment to improving mental health services for children. However, because child mental health services have been so poorly supported by communities, these highly trained specialists are often not able to contribute where they are most needed.

REFERENCES

Allen, K. Eileen, et al. (1964): "Effects of Social Reinforcement on Isolated Behavior of a Nursery School Child," *Child Development,* vol. 35, no. 2, pp. 511–518.

Allinsmith, William, and Carl W. Goethels (1962): *The Role of Schools in Mental Health,* Basic Books, Inc., Publishers, New York.

Ambrose, J. A. (1963): "The Concept of a Critical Period for the Development of Social Responsiveness in Early Human Infancy," in Brian M. Foss (ed.), *Determinants of Infant Behavior,* vol. 2, John Wiley & Sons, Inc., New York, pp. 201–226.

American Nurses' Association (1966): *Conference Group on Psychiatric Nursing Practice,* The American Nurses' Association, New York.

Badger, Earladeen G. (1971): "A Mothers' Training Program," *Children,* vol. 18, pp. 168–169.

Bandura, Albert, and Richard H. Walters (1965): *Social Learning and Personality Development,* Holt, Rinehart and Winston, Inc., New York.

Barker, Roger G., T. Dembo, and K. Levin (1943): "Frustration and Regression," in R. G. Barber, J. S. Kounin, and H. F. Wright (eds.), *Child Behavior and Development,* McGraw-Hill Book Company, New York, pp. 441–458.

Barnard, Kathryn (1971): "What Are the Effects of Early Stimulation on Later Development?" Unpublished manuscript, University of Washington, Seattle, Wash.

Becker, Wesley C. (1964): "Consequences of Different Kinds of Parental Discipline," in Martin Hoffman and Lois Hoffman (eds.), *Review of Child Development Research,* Russell Sage Foundation, New York, pp. 169-208.

———and J. C. Westman (1967): "Prevention of Mental Disorders: An Overview of Current Programs," *American Journal of Psychiatry,* vol. 123, no. 9, pp. 1058–1068.

Bolman, William M. (1967): "An Outline of Preventive Psychiatric Programs for Children," *Archives of General Psychiatry,* vol. 17, no. 1, pp. 5–7.

Bower, Eli M. (1960): "Early Identification of Emotionally Handicapped Children in School," Charles C Thomas, Publisher, Springfield, Ill.

———(1961): "Prevention in a School Setting," in Gerald Caplan (ed.), *Prevention of Mental Disorders in Children,* Basic Books, Inc., Publishers, New York, pp. 353–359.

Bowlby, John (1958): "The Nature of the Child's Tie to His Mother," *International Journal of Psychoanalysis,* vol. 39, pp. 350–373.

Brim, Orville (1961): "Methods of Educating Parents and Their Evaluation," in Gerald Caplan (ed.), *Prevention of Mental Disorders in Children,* Basic Books, Inc., Publishers, New York, pp. 122–141.

Brody, Sylvia, and Sidney Axelrod (1970): *Anxiety and Ego Formation in Infancy,* International Universities Press, Inc., New York.

Bronson, Gordon W. (1968): "The Fear of Novelty, *Psychological Bulletin,* vol. 69, pp. 350–358.

Call, Justin (1963): "Prevention of Autism in a Young Infant in a Well Child Conference," *Journal of American Academy of Child Psychiatry,* vol. 2, pp. 451–459.

Caplan, Gerald (1961): *Prevention of Mental Disorders in Children,* Basic Books, Inc., Publishers, New York.

Charlesworth, Rosalind, and Willard W. Hartup (1967): "Positive Social Reinforcement in the Nursery School Peer Group," *Child Development,* vol. 38, pp. 993–1002.

Cheong, G., and M. V. DeVault (1966): "Pupils' Perceptions of Teachers," *Journal of Educational Research,* vol. 59, pp. 444–449.

Chess, Stella (1961): "Temperament in the Normal Infant," in Jerome Hellmuth (ed.), *Exceptional Infant,* Brunner Mazel Inc., New York, pp. 143–150.

Coleman, James S. (1966): *Equality of Education,* U.S. Government Printing Office, Washington, D.C.

Coles, Robert (1972): "Breaking the American Stereotypes," *Time,* vol. 99, no. 7, pp. 36–42.

———(1967): *Children of Crisis,* Little, Brown and Company, Boston.

Conant, James B. (1961): *Social Dynamite in Our Large Cities,* Commission on Children and Youth, Washington, D.C.

Davids, Anthony, Spencer Devault, and Max Talmadge (1961): "Anxiety, Pregnancy and Childbirth Abnormalities," *Journal of Consulting Psychology,* vol. 25, pp. 74–77.

Davison, A. N., and J. Dobbing (1966): "Myelinization as a Vulnerable Period in Brain Development," *British Medical Bulletin,* vol. 22, pp. 40–45.

Deutsch, Martin P. (1964): "The Disadvantaged Child and the Learning Process," in Frank Reissman, Jerome Cohen, and Arthur Pearl (ed.), *Mental Health of the Poor,* The Free Press of Glencoe, New York, pp. 172–187.

Dingman, Paul, and William Boettscher (1971): "Interlocking Responsibilities: A Critical Issue for the Mental Well-Being of School Children," *American Journal of Orthopsychiatry,* vol. 41, no. 2, pp. 328–332.

Doyal, Guy T., John Ferguson, and Ida Rockwood (1971): "Group Method for Modifying Inappropriate Aggressive Behavior in the Elementary School," *American Journal of Orthopsychiatry,* vol. 41, no. 2, pp. 311–312.

Erikson, Erik (1963): *Childhood and Society,* W. W. Norton & Company, Inc., New York.

———(1959): "Growth and Crisis in Normal Personality," *Psychological Issues,* vol. 1, pp. 50–100.

Escalona, Sybil L. (1962): "The Study of Individual Differences and the Problem of State," *Journal of American Academy of Child Psychiatry,* vol. 11, pp. 11–37.

Evans, Frances M. C. (1968): *The Role of the Nurse in Community Mental Health,* The Macmillan Company, New York.

Fabian, Alice, and Herman Tanner (1971): "Role of Psychiatric Consultant to Day Care Centers in Ghetto Communities," *American Journal of Orthopsychiatry,* vol. 40, no. 2, p. 280.

Feldhusen, John F., and Herbert J. Klausmeier (1962): "Anxiety, Intelligence and Achievement in Children of Low, Average, and High Intelligence," *Child Development,* vol. 33, pp. 403–409.

Freud, Sigmund (1959): *Inhibition, Symptom, and Anxiety,* Standard Edition, Hogarth Press, London.

Frost, B. P. (1965): "Intelligence, Manifest Anxiety, and Scholastic Achievement," *Alberta Journal of Educational Research,* vol. 2, pp. 167–175.

Gagnon, John H. (1965): "Sexuality and Sexual Learning in the Child," *Psychiatry,* vol. 28, no. 3, pp. 212–228.

Garmezy, Norman (1970): "Vulnerability Research and the Issue of Primary Prevention," *American Journal of Orthopsychiatry,* vol. 40, no. 2, pp. 217–221.

Gottesman, Irving I. (1968): "Personality and Natural Selection," in Steven G. Vandenburg (ed.), *Methods and Goals in Human Behavior Genetics,* The Johns Hopkins Press, Baltimore, pp. 63–74.

Gray, Paul H. (1958): "Theory and Evidence in Imprinting in Human Infants," *Journal of Psychology,* vol. 46, pp. 155–166.

Greenacre, Phyllis (1952): *Trauma, Growth and Personality,* W. W. Norton & Company, Inc., New York.

Harlow, Harry, and Margaret H. Harlow (1966): "Learning to Love," *American Scientist,* vol. 54, no. 3, pp. 244–272.

Hartman, Heinz, Ernst Kris, and Rudolph M. Lowenstein (1946): "Comments on the Formation of Psychic Structure," *The Psychoanalytic Study of the Child,* vol. 2, pp. 11–38.

Hattrick, B. W. (1967): "The Influence of Nursery School Attendance on the Behavior and Personality of the Pre-School Child," *Journal of Experimental Education,* vol. 5, pp. 180–190.

Hetznecker, William, and Marc A. Forman (1971): "Community Child Psychiatry," *American Journal of Orthopsychiatry,* vol. 41, no. 3, pp. 350–370.

Hobbs, Nicholas (1970): "Project Re-Ed: New Ways of Helping Emotionally Disturbed Children," in Joint Commission on Mental Health of Children, *Crisis in Child Mental Health: Challenge for the 70's,* Harper & Row, Publishers, Inc., pp. 310–312.

Hunt, James McV. (1971): "Parent and Child Centers: Their Bases in Behavior and Educational Sciences," *American Journal of Orthopsychiatry,* vol. 41, no. 1, pp. 13–21.

Joint Commission on Mental Health of Children (1970): *Crisis in Child Mental Health: Challenge for the 70's,* Harper & Row, Publishers, Inc., New York.

Jost, H., and Lester W. Sontag (1944): "The Genetic Factors in Autonomic Nervous System Functioning," *Psychosomatic Medicine,* vol. 6, pp. 308–310.

Kagan, Jerome, and Howard A. Moss (1962): *Birth to Maturity, A Study in Psychological Development,* John Wiley & Sons, Inc., New York.

Keller, E. O., and V. Rowley (1962): "Anxiety, Intelligence, and Scholastic Achievement in Elementary School Children," *Psychological Reports,* vol. 11, pp. 19–22.

Keyserling, Mary D. (1971): "Day Care Challenge," *Child Welfare,* vol. 8, p. 434.

Klein, Jenny W. (1972): "Educational Components of Day Care," *Children Today,* vol. 1, no. 1, pp. 5–7.

Korner, Anneliese F. (1967): "Some Hypotheses Regarding the Significance of Individual Differences at Birth for Later Development," in Jerome Hellmuth (ed.), *Exceptional Infant,* Brunner Mazel, Inc., New York, pp. 191–205.

Leuchter, H. J. (1968): "Are Schools to Be or Not to Be Community Health Centers?" *American Journal of Psychiatry,* vol. 125, pp. 575–576.

Lilleskov, Roy K., Martha L. Gilbert, Thelma Mikelov, and Clara Barksdale (1970): "Planning an Infant Care Unit with Communtiy Participation," *American Journal of Orthopsychiatry,* vol. 40, pp. 281–283.

Long, Nicholas J., William C. Morse, and Ruth G. Newman (1966): *Conflict in the Classroom: The Education of Emotionally Disturbed Children,* Wadsworth Publishing Company, Inc., Belmont, Calif.

Lorenz, Konrad (1966): *On Aggression,* Harcourt Brace Jovanovich, Inc., New York.

Lourie, Reginald (1971): "The First Three Years of Life: An Overview of a New Frontier Psychiatry," *American Journal of Psychiatry,* vol. 127, no. 11, pp. 33–39.

Lowenfeld, Victor, and W. Lambert Brittain (1970): *Creative and Mental Growth,* The Macmillan Company, New York.

Marrone, R. Thomas, and Nancy Anderson (1970): "Innovative Public School Programming for Emotionally Disturbed Children," *American Journal of Orthopsychiatry,* vol. 40, no. 4, pp. 694–701.

Michne, J. (1971): "Group Therapy in an Elementary School," *Social Casework,* vol. 52, no. 1, pp. 18–25.

Minuchin, Paul, Barbara Biber, E. Sherino, and H. Zimiles (1969): *The Psychological Impact of School Experience,* Basic Books, Inc., Publishers, New York.

Montague, M. (1950): "Constitutional and Pre-Natal Factors in Infant and Child Health," in Milton Senn (ed.), *Symposium on the Healthy Personality,* J. H. Macy Foundation, New York, pp. 148–175.

Murphy, Gardner (1947): *Personality,* Harper & Row, Publishers, Inc., New York.

Murphy, Lois B. (1961): "Prevention Implications of Development in the Pre-School Years," in Gerald Caplan (ed.), *Prevention of Mental Disorders in Children,* Basic Books, Inc., Publishers, New York.

———(1962): *The Widening World of Childhood,* Basic Books, Inc., Publishers, New York.

Mussen, Paul H., John J. Conger, and Jerome Kagan (1969): *Child Development and Personality,* Harper & Row, Publishers, Inc., New York.

———and E. Rutherford (1963): "Parent-Child Relations and Parental Personality in Relation to Young Children's Sex-Role Performance," *Child Development,* vol. 34, pp. 586–607.

Pavenstedt, Ernest (1962): "Opening Comments," *Journal of American Academy of Child Psychiatry,* vol. 1, p. 140.

Pazdur, Helen (1969): "Innovation: The School Nurse as a Mental Health Specialist," *Journal of School Health,* vol. 39, no. 7. pp. 449–457.

Pratt, Catherine, and Laurence A. Cove (1971): "Assembled Foster Families: A Practical Experiment," *American Journal of Orthopsychiatry,* vol. 41, no. 2, pp. 269–271.

Redl, Fritz, and William W. Wattenburg (1959): *Mental Hygiene in Teaching,* Harcourt, Brace Jovanovich, Inc., New York.

Rice, Dale L., and Sara Semmelroth (1968): "Foster Care for Emotionally Disturbed Children," *American Journal of Orthopsychiatry,* vol. 38, no. 3, pp. 539–542.

Riese, Hertha (1966): "Educational Therapy: A Methodical Approach to the Problem of the Untreatable Child," in Nicholas J. Long, William C. Morse, and Ruth G. Newman (eds.), *Conflict in the Classroom,* Wadsworth Publishing Company, Inc., Belmont, Calif., pp. 321–332.

———(1962): *Heal the Hurt Child,* University of Chicago Press, Chicago.

Sander, Louis W. (1962): "Issues in Early Mother-Child Interaction," *Journal of American Academy of Child Psychiatry,* vol. 1, pp. 141–166.

Sarason, Seymour B., Kenneth S. Davidson, Frederick F. Lighthall, Richard B. Waite, and Britton D. Ruesbush (1960): *Anxiety in Elementary School Children,* John Wiley & Sons, Inc., New York.

Schiff, Sheldon K. (1971): "New Look at Children's Potential: Results of a Six-Year Community Wide Mental Health Program for over 10,000 Children," *American Journal of Orthopsychiatry,* vol. 41, no. 2, pp. 322–323.

Sears, Robert R., et al. (1953): "Some Child Rearing Antecedents of Aggression and Dependency in Young Children," *Genetic Psychological Monographs,* vol. 4, pp. 135–234.

Sears, Robert R., Eleanor E. Maccoby, and H. Levin (1957): *Patterns of Child Rearing,* Harper & Row, Publishers, New York.

Sontag, Lester W. (1944): "War and Fetal Maternal Relationships," *Marriage and Family Living,* pp. 1–5.

Spitz, Rene (1946): *The Ontogenesis of Human Communication,* International Universities Press, Inc., New York.

———and Katherine M. Wolf (1946): "The Smiling Response," *Genetic Psychology Monograph,* vol. 34, pp. 57–125.

Stickney, Stonewall B. (1968): "Schools Are Our Mental Health Centers," *American Journal of Psychiatry,* vol. 124, pp. 1407–1414.

Valett, Robert E. (1969): *Programming Learning Disabilities,* Fearon Press, Palo Alto.

Vandenburg, Steven G. (1971): "Genetics of Human Behavior," in Julius Segal (ed.), *The Mental Health of the Child,* National Institute of Mental Health, Washington, D.C., pp. 513–514.

Van Fleet, Phyllis P., and Robert Brownbridge (1970): "Young Children at Risk: A Three Year Research and Demonstration Project Concerned with Early Intervention and Prevention of Learning and Behavior Problems," *American Journal of Orthopsychiatry,* vol. 40, no. 2, pp. 320–322.

Warren, Virginia L. (1972): "Night Care Center," *Children Today,* vol. 1, no. 1, pp. 28–29.

Watt, N. F., R. D. Stolorow, Amy W. Lutensky, and D. C. McClelland (1970): "School

Adjustment and Behavior of Children Hospitalized for Schizophrenia as Adults," *American Journal of Orthopsychiatry,* vol. 40, no. 4, pp. 637–657.

Williams, Frank S. (1971): "The Effectiveness of Community Mental Health Treatment and Prevention Programs for Children," *American Journal of Orthopsychiatry,* vol. 41, no. 2, pp. 319–321.

Work, Henry H., and Justin D. Call (1965): *A Guide to Preventive Child Psychiatry,* McGraw-Hill Book Company, New York.

Wyatt, Gertrude L., Elaine F. Loomis, and Lois L. Scott (1970): "Early Identification and Training of So-Called High Risk Children," *American Journal of Orthopsychiatry,* vol. 40, no. 2, pp. 319–320.

Zigler, Edward (1972): "Focus on Day Care," *Children Today,* vol. 1, no. 1, front cover piece.

4

DEVELOPMENTAL REACTIONS IN ADOLESCENCE

Helen Pazdur Monea

Our adolescents now seem to love luxury. They have bad manners and contempt for authority. They show disrespect for adults and spend their time hanging around places gossiping with one another. . . . They are ready to contradict their parents, monopolize the conversation in company, eat gluttonously, and tyrannize their teachers.

Socrates (470 B.C.–399 B.C.)

This particular day was one of joy, happiness, sorrow, sadness, and anger. To feel all of these emotions is quite strange. For on this day, I left home to live on my own.

Clark Burnside (1971)

For centuries societies have struggled through the crisis of adolescent development. In Socrates' day, youth was a time of conflicts and turbulent feelings, as it is in contemporary society. In studies in the behavioral sciences of psychology and sociology increased effort has gone into the understanding of why young people behave as they do. In the United States today we are particularly conscious of youth because we have the largest adolescent population in our history. There are 93 million young people under the age of twenty-five, and 38 percent of today's young people range in age from ten to nineteen (Joint Commission, 1970). A nation with such a wealth of children and youth has great potential and responsibility for expanding the growth of these youngsters into mentally and physically healthy adults.

A tragedy lies in the fact that we, as a nation, often neglect our children and youth, particularly in regard to mental health (Joint Commission, 1970). The Commission reports that "at least 1,400,000 of our youngsters under eighteen need psychiatric care." Eight to 10 percent have emotional problems and are in need of specialized services; 2 to 3 percent are severely disturbed; and $^6/_{10}$ percent are psychotic. Only a fraction of these young people receive the help they need at the time they need it. The major unmet need of adolescents is for improved institutional care. The majority who pass through the state institutions each year are not being helped but are, indeed, often worse for the experience. Mental health community facilities are even more deficient in services to adolescents.

THE CONCEPT OF PREVENTION AND THE ROLE OF THE ADOLESCENT PSYCHIATRIC NURSE

Caplan defines *primary prevention* as an effort made through various programs toward lowering the risk of mental disorders in a community and increasing its capacity to resist such influences. If a person does not have the resources to cope successfully with the difficulties he faces, he may seek unhealthy means of problem solving which lead to increased vulnerability or directly to mental disorder (Caplan, 1964). Caplan emphasizes the importance of beginning primary prevention by placing special emphasis on prenatal care and suggests the prerequisites for subsequent healthy mental development. These include both the physical and the psychosocial needs of nurturing, which can be considered to be love and affection, support of need to grow away from dependence and toward independence, opportunity for identity development through socialization process, opportunity for development of consistent relationships in which to develop trust and self-confidence, and opportunity for learning to problem-solve and cope with unexpected crisis (Caplan, 1964, pp. 288–289).

In the normal process of growth and development, there are maturational crises such as the transition from childhood to adolescence (Williams, 1971). Adolescence in particular seems to accelerate the growth of problems both numerically and in terms of severity. The stress of rapid body change is compounded by increasing physical-genital maturity and the concomitant psychological adjustment to these changes and to the expectations of society. Higher standards are held for adolescents than for younger children, and, since adolescents are capable of embroiling themselves in greater difficulties than younger children, their deviant behavior is considered more serious (Joint Commission, 1970). In striving for independence, for identity, and for peer approval, children, as they grow, experience conflicts; and many, as adolescents, refight crises unresolved in earlier years (Anthony, 1969).

Caplan defines a *crisis* as an interruption of the balance of an individual's ability to problem-solve. Anxiety occurs, followed by an extended period of emotional upset. The outcome is governed by the kind of interaction which takes place between the individual and the key figures in his emotional milieu throughout the crisis period (Caplan, 1951). Appropriate intervention offers the opportunity for regaining equilibrium or restoring to full function that which existed before the crisis. In addition, the process of crisis and intervention ideally provides the individual with an opportunity for personality growth.

ROLE OF THE NURSE IN PREVENTION OF MENTAL ILLNESS

Evans states that primary prevention will be a major focus of mental health nursing when community mental health programs become established. The nurse's role in the community will be geared toward helping people to cope with problems and to deal with stress (Evans, 1968). There are psychiatric nurses prepared by their education and training to deal with distress in children and adolescents (Boston University, 1968). Their expertise in counseling parents, teachers, and youth workers can be utilized in a variety of settings, such as prenatal clinics, child care centers, and schools. Counseling by psychiatric nurses with children, adolescents, and families is utilized in schools as well as in homes (Pazdur, 1969; Pothier, 1968). They can also function as consultants to professionals and nonprofessionals concerned with the general welfare of the community (Boston University, 1968).

Secondary prevention deals with early recognition and intervention to prevent further mental disorder and to end the disorder as soon as possible (Evans, 1968). Since the psychiatric nurse is also knowledgeable in the area of growth and development, he can recognize and assess adolescents' problems and plan appropriate interventions.

Tertiary prevention is related to remedial programs. The Joint Commission envisions remedial programs built more on the model of health than of illness. They recommend that future programs provide a new and broader range of services to seriously disturbed adolescents, juvenile delinquents, mentally retarded, and their families. An increase in the development of community-based facilities would permit adolescents to be treated as much as possible in their normal settings, as well as provide highly personalized treatment and rehabilitation services in institutions for those adolescents unable to remain in the community.

The psychiatric nurse-clinical specialist prepared to work with adolescents can function as a therapist in individual and group work, as a milieu therapist, as a counselor, or as a teacher of parents of emotionally disturbed or mentally retarded. He should be able to function as a collaborator with other mental health and psychiatric professionals and consult with professional and nonprofessional individuals and groups in regard to care, education, and welfare of children and adolescents. Further, he functions as a consumer and participant in research, as an educator of other nurses and child care personnel in a variety of settings, and as a change agent for providing for the needs of children, families, and community (Boston University, 1968).

These roles may expand and change to meet the demand of changing needs of delivery systems and the nurse's increasing responsibilities for promoting change through the introduction of new ways of caring for and about children. The need for innovative programs to alter the gap in quality and quantity of services to youngsters is pointed out by the Joint Commission on Mental Health of Children.

BECOMING AN ADVOCATE FOR YOUTH

"We proclaim that we are a nation devoted to its young" (Joint Commission, 1970, p. 1). The evidence from the Commission's report reveals that we have failed to take adequate care of our adolescents and that adolescents have been treated as second-class citizens (Work, 1971). One problem holding up the delivery of services to minors is the fact that many agencies hesitate to provide treatment for adolescents without parental permission. In a New York City hospital, a fifteen-year-old boy with a badly cut hand was accompanied by parents to the emergency room, where the cut was stitched. He returned alone a week later for removal of the stitches and the hospital refused to treat him because his parents were not there. In a Midwestern city, a sixteen-year-old girl sought contraceptive advice from a private gynecologist and was refused because she had no business "doing things like that," and the doctor was unwilling to examine her without parental consent (Brody, 1972, p. 1). Similar incidents occur when adolescents seek respite from destructive parents where there has been psychological or physical harm. Adolescents may need protective guardians of their rights as human beings.

One recommendation of the Commission is that there be established a national advisory council on children and youth, to be responsible for studying and gathering information on the problems of children and youth in the United States. A state child development agency would be responsible for developing a state plan in conjunction with federal guidelines to meet the needs of children and youth. On the local level, the plan would call for local child development authorities' child development councils. The councils would act as direct advocates for children and youth and be imbued with the responsibility of arranging complete services from preventive to diagnostic and treatment services (Joint Commission, 1970).

Social action is another approach to primary prevention (Evans, 1968). Eisenberg points to the role of the mental health professionals which encompasses both the professional and the citizen. Professionals have a heightened moral responsibility for social action because of their specialized knowledge (Eisenberg, 1966). Professionals alone and in collaboration with others are becoming increasingly active. A national organization entitled Common Cause consists of professionals and laymen working to give the community a voice in bringing about change to meet the needs of people. Dr. Bertram Brown, Director of NIMH (National Institute of Mental Health), has presented a description of projects that would prepare citizens to serve as child advocates (Ramshorn, 1971). Graduate students in the Child Psychiatric Nursing Program at the University of California, San Francisco, are given the opportunity to prepare themselves for the advocacy role through seminar and clinical experiences. The child psychiatric nurse has a responsibility for being involved in the community in protecting and improving the mental health of children, as well as in informing the community of societal conditions which are adversely affecting the mental health of children (Boston University, 1968).

The rationale for advocacy is based on democratic principles; therefore the health professionals interested in becoming advocates should consider all manner of individuals, children as well as adults, poor as well as middle-class, minority groups as well as dominant majority. In general, groups with power develop services to meet their own needs while the needs of less powerful groups are neglected. The advocate attempts to intervene in this process by making public planning less one-sided through special help to groups that are usually ignored (Guskin and Ross, 1971). Studies seem to support the observation that middle-class Americans scorn and patronize the poor and racial minorities (Coles, 1972).

More and more health professionals are becoming advocates. Some results of the work of advocacy are evident; for example, legislation has been enacted abolishing the requirement of parental consent for minors seeking medical treatment in some states. The American Medical Association has endorsed the right of teen-aged girls to receive contraceptive advice on their own consent (Brody, 1972). Child psychiatric nursing students who have been active in promoting preventive mental health services for children and youth in San Francisco have been included as part of a district mental health team; this example indicates one way which nurses can expand mental health delivery services (Finley et al., 1972).

DEVELOPMENTAL APPROACH IN UNDERSTANDING ADOLESCENT BEHAVIOR

Aristotle (384–322 B.C.) introduced a concept of human development which remained dominant within European philosophy for 1,500 years (Groffman, 1970). He divided the developmental period of the human being into three stages of 7 years each: infancy, boyhood, and young manhood. These three stages were accepted throughout the Middle Ages and reoccur in some modern psychological theories of development in the German literature (Muus, 1966).

The Industrial Revolution exercised a tremendous effect upon the place of the child and the adolescent within the societal group. In the late nineteenth century, the developmental needs of children and adolescents were not considered. Leaders such as Rousseau and Pestalozzi, through their revolutionary theories of education, were responsible for recognition of individual differences (Crow and Crow, 1965). Another prominent leader was G. Stanley Hall, who is credited as father of the scientific psychology of adolescence (Muus, 1966).

Generally, there is consensus that adolescence is divided into two stages, early and late, with no clearly marked division between the two. In early adolescence the young person is concerned with emancipation, independence, and freedom from the family; during late adolescence, there is concern with one's place in the wider world and the developing of a capacity for intimacy with the opposite sex (Joint Commission, 1970).

The age span devoted to adolescent development will vary in different cultures as well as in definition. Over the past 50 years, within Western cultures, the adolescence period has increasingly lengthened (Offer, 1971). The Joint Commission on Mental Health of Children studied young people up to twenty-five years of age in considering programs for children and youth. The boundary was extended as far as twenty-five because society today often demands of adolescents long periods of educational and vocational preparation prior to their assuming adult responsibilities. In the United States, adolescents are grouped according to school enrollment. Junior high schools have adolescents in age ranges from twelve to fourteen years old; high schools carry the fourteen- to eighteen-year-olds. The eighteen-year-old to twenty-one-year-old may either begin work or continue education (Offer, 1971). This chapter will focus mainly on the age range of twelve through eighteen years.

Adolescent Developmental Model

The developmental model considers the normal process of growth and development, including critical physical and emotional changes which occur during adolescence, and is based on the theory that "optimal development in adolescence depends on successful accomplishment of the developmental tasks in infancy and children" (Eisenberg, 1969). According to Erikson, the adolescent is faced with the task of overcoming a sense of identity diffusion as well as of achieving a sense of identity. This task will be hampered or delayed if the adolescent is unable to achieve successfully a sense of trust in infancy, a sense of autonomy in childhood, a sense of initiative in the play age, and a sense of industry in school age (Erikson, 1959).

A developmental stage is "the time when a capacity first appears or at that period when it is so well established and integrated that the next step in development can safely be initiated" (Erikson, 1959). Each stage has a critical alternative with a potential crisis. Variables that affect the phases include irreversible biological processes, cultural influences which affect the desirable rate of development, and the idiosyncratic response of the individual (Maier, 1969). The sequence of stages thus represents a successive development of the component parts of the psychological personality. At the end of adolescence, the adolescent must find a certain integration as a relatively conflict-free psychosocial arrangement—or remain defective and conflict-laden (Erikson, 1959). Eisenberg notes that clinical experience has shown that adolescence will be an unusually stormy, prolonged, and poorly resolved experience if it follows a childhood marked by severe deficits (Eisenberg, 1969).

Another function of adolescent development is expansion of the cognitive process. Piaget characterizes the growth and development of cognition through phases and stages. The adolescent enters the phase of formal operations in which he acquires the capacity to think and to reason beyond his own realistic world. He finds pleasure in manipulating ideas without any commitment on his part. His main interest centers on reevaluating different social points of view (Maier, 1969). The idealism of adolescents is based on their dissatisfaction with the world that adults have created and leads them to challenge basic premises (Eisenberg, 1969; Erikson, 1970).

Acting Out: An Adolescent Phenomenon

Theoretically, acting out is recognized as an expected phenomenon in adolescence and as a normal psychological phase (Blos, 1966; Erikson, 1970). Because the adolescent uses mostly action and fantasy in synthesizing his world, his impulses find expression in action rather than in symbolic thinking.

The term *acting out* has been used inappropriately to label behavior that is not acting out but acting upon an impulse. Acting upon an impulse differs from acting out in that in the latter case there is no awareness of the reason underlying the action. Since the adolescent's ego is not developed sufficiently to integrate experiences, the acting upon an impulse is a measure of mastery through trial and error (Josselyn, 1965). Further misuse of the term "acting out" is seen in its application to a patient's behavior on moral grounds or because it is considered nonconforming as measured against the therapist's culture or socioeconomic class background (Robertiello, 1965).

In understanding the concept of acting out, there are three aspects to consider: a predisposition to acting out; the manifestation of behavior in acting out; and the function of the acting-out mechanism (Blos, 1966). All three aspects are not necessarily interrelated. Acting-out behavior can occur without evidence of predisposition, can be stimulated by an acute circumstance such as a maturational event (puberty, adolescence), or can be due to a structural characteristic of the ego (Blos, 1966).

Fenichel explains the predisposition arising from intense narcissistic needs and intolerance of tension (Fenichel, 1945). Greenacre refers to predisposing factors that include a visual sensitization producing an inclination for dramatization, a distorted relationship between thought, speech, and action, and an unconscious belief in the magic of action (Greenacre, 1950; Blos, 1966).

Carroll states that, since the sense of reality in the acting-out individual is weak, the disposition to a rich fantasy life allows no compromise with reality. Adolescents with this disposition state that their fantasies are more real than the outer world. They turn away from the outer world as soon as their gratification need ceases. The young drug user is an extreme example of an adolescent choosing the "reality" of his fantasies as opposed to reality of the outer world

(Carroll, 1954; Blos, 1966). Erikson views the adolescent excursions into fantasy as an appropriate method of handling identity diffusion. "In the healthy adolescent, a great capacity for fantasy is matched by ego mechanisms that permit him to go far into dangerous regions of phantasy or social experiment and to catch himself at the last moment . . ." (Maier, 1969, p. 64).

In the process of gaining independence, the adolescent develops a sense of helplessness and has a need to deny it through actions which exaggerate his independence, thereby denying his dependence on reality. He develops the attitude of "Nobody can tell me" (Blos, 1966, p. 122). Typical adolescent acting-out behavior is usually transient and can serve the cause of progressive development through the experimentation it allows (Blos, 1966).

A word of caution is noted by Dr. Lidz in pointing out the differences in symptomatology between acting-out boys and girls; for example, a sociopathic girl usually has a primary problem of promiscuity while the sociopathic boy's problems are related to stealing and aggressiveness (Rexford, 1966).

The similarity between action and acting out in the adolescent is not always clearly differentiated in clinical work. There are several adolescent characteristics which blur the concept of acting out, such as: the adolescent's flux between regressive and progressive movements; ego detachment from parental figures; the ego impoverishment that is experienced; reaching toward the outside world to compensate for ego impoverishment; and the efforts of ego synthesis (Blos, 1966). Blos suggests that the standard concept of acting out may be too narrow for explaining adolescent phenomena and that reconsideration should be explored to enhance its clinical usefulness.

In discussing Blos's concept of acting out, Wermer points to the fact that the significance of acting out will vary by cultures and society; behavior regarded as pathological acting out in one culture may be ego synthesis in a different milieu. Therapists, parents, and teachers are cautioned to keep an open mind about what is pathological acting out and what is ego synthesis through action. Wermer (1966, p. 14) strongly suggests that unless therapists, caseworkers, and teachers are prepared to be the patient's external reality and be willing to be acted upon, they retreat to another area of practice which does not deal with adolescents.

Developmental Reactions in Adolescence: Normal Versus Abnormal

It is as difficult to differentiate the acting-out process from typical adolescent traits as it is to define what constitutes normal adolescent behavior. The definitions of normality vary among the disciplines that use the concept of normality. Erikson emphasizes the importance of successful mastery of the various stages in the normal development of the identity process in which the ego faces disruption in each stage; the normal, mature person is considered to have successfully overcome the disruptions in each stage of his development (Offer, 1971).

Definitions of normality are difficult to formulate, particularly in the field of adolescent research, since the emotional conflicts seen as normal adolescent turmoil by one investigator may be viewed as pathological by another (Offer, 1966). Offer and Sabshin completed a study of high school boys in an attempt to define criteria that would describe the modal adolescent. These criteria included good object relationships with adults, ability to resolve conflicts, and almost complete absence of gross psychopathology and severe physical defects (Offer and Sabshin, 1966). Future studies of adolescents need to include girls in order to determine any differences between the sexes.

Some clinicians view normal adolescent turmoil as resembling borderline psychopathology. Weiner states that although this notion persists in the thinking of many clinicians, recent data reviewed by Offer indicate that adolescent turmoil reflects psychopathology rather than normal development, that turmoil is an infrequent phenomenon, and that most adolescents achieve their personal identity gradually without any major disruptions (Offer, 1969).

Developmental Arrests

There is a large group of adolescent psychiatric patients of normal intelligence and average physical capability who have a stable self-concept and awareness of basic reality, yet act in such inappropriate ways that they appear "crazy" (Easson, 1969). They are not psychotic but have a severe developmental arrest. The concept of developmental arrest is somewhat novel as a psychopathological entity with no description or theory (Fleming and Altshul, 1963; Gedo, 1966). Gedo developed a tentative definition from Fleming and Altschul: ". . . A striking picture of immaturity in self-image and in the development of ego ideal and super-ego structures is apparent. Reality-testing, impulse control, object need, and self-object awareness are not adequate for adult functioning" (Gedo, 1966, p. 25).

Easson states that it is essential to differentiate the adolescent with developmental arrest from the psychotic adolescent because the treatment is different (Easson, 1969). In diagnosing the adolescent, it is important that the relationship capability be carefully evaluated so as to show that the youngster is not psychotic but has instead a stunting of ego growth and severe developmental arrest in relationship ability. Many adolescents show immature behavior in terms of childlike behavior patterns. The temporary regression may be due to excessive stress or emotional strain. The adolescent is embarrassed to maintain such childlike behavior, but certain disturbed adolescents do not feel silly about the behavior. The behavior is part of their behavioral repertoire, and they have not progressed beyond the infantile pattern of relating (Easson, 1969).

Many parents of this teen-age group do not have the parenting ability of giving love and control, for they themselves have not experienced being mothered or loved. Some parents have found pleasure in the infantile demands of their adolescent children, while others have been unable to control or direct their youngsters so as to give them the external support needed for learning self-control and self-growth. Other youngsters have such strong drives and energy that even an optimal home environment may not help them gain control (Easson, 1969).

Families of all these teen-age patients have developed fears of mutual destructiveness early in the life of the child. Easson in his book *The Severely Disturbed Adolescent* (Easson, 1969, p. 177) quotes a fifteen-year-old:

> I never knew what to depend on with my folks. They always say what they think I want and then they do something different behind my back. They make me so mad, I could smash them. I told my old man that—and now he always does what he thinks I want. He is a stupid chicken shit. I won't ever hit them—I don't need to. They always do what they think I want and then they pretend they do it because they decided that way anyhow. Who do they think they are fooling? They do it because I say so and I hate their guts for doing it.

The adolescent quoted above controlled his environment through his childish threats. Because the behavior made the parents feel weak, they responded with poorly concealed hatred in letting him have his way. The result was that they stood by and watched their son destroy himself. The vicious circle continues as the youngster who needs control and stability continues to confront and attack the adults who fail to control him (Easson, 1969).

Easson believes that many adolescents who suffer developmental arrests have the potential of emotional growth in becoming socially acceptable human beings. During treatment, as with all other adolescents, it is essential that his environment include staff who are not intimidated by the teen-ager's threats and who can help him take the responsibility for his own behavior. Easson states that when "these teen-agers start to gain pleasure from mastery and ego growth, they may show rapid emotional maturation and development" (Easson, 1969, p. 181). When they learn to trust themselves and others, they may increase their relationship ability. As they begin to appreciate their growth, they react by mourning the pleasures they have never had and may feel bitter over the loss. They need help in facing the sadness and anger of the loss and in moving on to accepting adult responsibilities (Easson, 1969).

ADOLESCENT SUICIDE AND DEPRESSION

Suicide, suicidal threats, and attempts of suicide are considered severe forms of acting out (Glaser, 1965). The death rate by suicide rises during adolescence. Suicide is virtually nonexistent at five to fourteen years of age; there is increasing frequency between fifteen and nineteen; and it more than doubles again in the twenty to twenty-four-year age group (Joint Commission, 1970).

Exact figures on suicide among adolescents are not known because the aura of stigma attached to suicide hampers accurate data collection. Also related is the failure of some researchers to distinguish between various categories of attempted and committed suicides (Seiden, 1969). Mintz conducted a study of prevalence of suicide attempters, and the results indicated that the attempters were younger (age range fourteen to twenty-four) than the completed suicides. Further data revealed that the sex ratio for attempts by females was three to one in comparison with males; the reverse was true in the completed suicides. More accurate knowledge regarding the attempters as opposed to the committers will bring about effective remedial action (Seiden, 1969; Mintz, 1964).

The problem of suicide attempts is significant in adolescents because they outnumber the completed suicides by a ratio of fifty to one (Jacobziner, 1960; Seiden, 1969). Twelve percent of all suicide attempts in this nation have been made by adolescents, of which 90 percent were adolescent girls (Balser and Masterson, 1959; Seiden, 1969).

The suicidal behavior of adolescents may be a "cry for help" in dealing with problems of sexual identification and related impulses (Schneer et al., 1961; Seiden, 1969). A crisis in sexual identity can develop from a failure to achieve masculine or feminine identity or from concerns over homosexual tendencies which may lead to suicidal attempts (Bigras et al., 1966; Seiden, 1969). For some adolescents sexual identification is adequate, but the increase in sexual impulses of adolescence may lead to anxiety, guilt, and frustration (Seiden, 1969). Seiden reports studies of suicidal attempts in adolescent girls that show that their guilt over sexual acting out was a major factor that precipitated their act (Seiden, 1969).

The role of depression has usually been linked to suicidal potential. A study by Lourie suggests that the clinical picture of depression does not appear until late adolescence as a factor, while contrary results were found in studies where the characteristic of depression was identified in half of the young people (Lourie, 1966; Seiden, 1969). Symptoms of depression vary widely according to age. Toolan describes crying and eating and sleeping disturbances as evidence of depression in infants; temper tantrums and accident proneness as displaced depressive feelings in latency-aged children; boredom, restlessness, and fatigue as "depressive equivalents" in adolescents (Toolan, 1969; Seiden, 1969). He states that depression is a reaction to loss, whether it is real or fantasied, and that the developmental stage at which the loss occurs has profound significance for personality development.

Teicher and Jacobs studied adolescents who had a high rate of parental loss in childhood. One group attempted suicide; another did not. The study revealed that it was not just parental loss in childhood which predisposed some subjects to depression and suicide later in life, but the loss of love at a particular time (Teicher and Jacobs, 1966; Seiden, 1969). The loss of a love object occurring during adolescence does not prevent further object-relationship because the critical years for development have passed; however, the adolescent may develop hatred for the former love object. Adolescent girls who attempt suicide show a history of loss of a father and may be particularly vulnerable because of the deprivation of a paternal figure (Zimbaca, 1965; Seiden, 1969).

Impulsiveness is often considered a factor in suicide threats and attempts. Jacobziner related the high incidence of suicide attempts in adolescent girls to "the greater impulsivity of the young female" to react suddenly to stress (Jacobziner, 1960; Seiden, 1969). On the other hand, Teicher and Jacobs argue that suicide attempts are not impulsive decisions when a longitudinal view of the total life history of a person is considered; the act is a rational decision in ending a long history of problems in life adjustment (Teicher and Jacobs, 1966; Seiden, 1969).

Another link to suicide is drugs. There is limited evidence as to the direct causal connection between adolescent drug use and suicide. Even where there doesn't seem to be any underlying depression, the drug may be a catalyst in touching off underlying emotional conflicts to the point of increasing the adolescent's self-destructive tendencies (Seiden, 1969).

One important factor in suicide among adolescents is their attitude toward death. Studies have concluded that youth live in the present and have little concern for the future (Kastenbaum, 1959; Seiden, 1969). They handle death by denial or displacement. Studies have shown that suicidal adolescents feared death less than nonsuicidal peers (Seiden, 1969).

Family and Cultural Factors

A relationship between suicide and broken homes has been noted in the United States and throughout the world. Seiden points to the fact that there seems to be a correlation between youth who commit or attempt suicide and broken homes (Seiden, 1969). Jacobs and Teicher, however, stress the need to consider the history of broken homes in the context of the total life of the adolescent. In studying adolescent suicide attempts, they found that the nonsuicidal group had had a stable home life in the preceding five years and the suicide attempters had not (Jacobs and Teicher, 1967; Seiden, 1969).

Grollman postulates the concept of the suicidogenic family in which a family member, very often an adolescent, unconsciously becomes the object of aggression of family members and acts out the covert antisocial impulses present in other members of the family (Grollman, 1971).

Cultures influence the suicide rate in three ways: (1) by producing psychological stresses within their members, (2) by the acceptability of suicide, and (3) by alternative behaviors provided (Seiden, 1969). In countries where attitudes toward suicide are tolerant, such as Austria and Germany, there is higher incidence of self-destruction than in countries where suicide is looked upon as cowardly or a sign of mental disturbance, as in England and the United States (Bakwin, 1964; Seiden, 1969).

A mass of adolescent suicide attempts in Northern Cheyenne Indians occurred when there was no culturally approved way of expressing aggression, such as a buffalo hunt or intertribal warfare. There were no alternatives by which they could deal with the deprivation of the expression of deep tribal emotions; thus they developed an attitude of hopelessness and helplessness (Dizmang, 1967; Seiden, 1969). The Indian adolescent has a double identity crisis: he experiences not only the identity crisis of adolescence, but also carries the additional burden of his particular culture's identity crisis. He has difficulty identifying with his Indian heritage, which leads to loss of pride. Further, because he is not accepted by the dominant culture, he is unable to identify with it (Resnik and Dizmang, 1971). One coping mechanism he uses is suicide. Resnik and Dizmang believe that this double bind applies to other minority-group children as well (Resnik and Dizmang, 1971).

Prevention of Suicide in Adolescents

Many health professional writers recommend educating parents, children and youth, and the community at large regarding suicidal behavior. Jacobziner recommends that parents learn the psychodynamics and needs of adolescents (Jacobziner, 1965; Seiden, 1969). Jan-Tausch suggests that preventive efforts be expanded in the school setting by encouraging more personalized teacher-pupil relationships and participation in extracurricular activities to combat withdrawal. Each school counselor should be encouraged to assist students in the process of acquiring at least one friend (Jan-Tausch, 1963; Seiden, 1969). The nurse-counselor in particular often has the opportunity for early detection of suicidal clues in adolescents and can offer support to the students and, if necessary, refer them for further therapy. He can also help to educate the school community about suicidal behavior and interventions via parent-teacher meetings, in-service education for teaching staff, and adult evening classes and as guest speaker in high school classrooms.

Of particular importance in dealing with suicide-prone adolescents, in either the community or the treatment setting, is the psychiatric nurse's skill in helping people in the adolescent's milieu cope with their anxieties by facilitating their expression of feeling as well as by offering guidelines for a protective environment, i.e., removing possibly destructive instruments, providing appropriate supervision and activities, and watching for significant changes in mood, affect, or physical activity which could indicate a decision to terminate life.

During the period in which suicidal tendencies are overt, hospitalization may be necessary as a precautionary measure. Glaser indicates that unless the suicidal threat or absence of resource persons makes hospitalization imperative, remaining outside the institutional setting is the desired course for the patient, since the hospitalization experience will often increase feelings of isolation and helplessness (Glaser, 1965; Seiden, 1969).

Recent research has been done which deals with the parents of adolescents who committed suicide. The parent group disclosed feelings ranging from grief and bewilderment to hostility, denial, and subsequently guilt and depression (Seiden, 1969). The investigators recommended early contact with families after a suicide of an adolescent and follow-up interviews, which have therapeutic and cathartic value (Herzog and Resnik, 1968). Health professionals are not immune to similar grief reactions of anger, guilt, or depression after losing an adolescent client through suicide. They may need assistance from colleagues in order to express their own reactions to the death as well as any self-destructive fantasies of their own.

DRUGS AND THE ADOLESCENT

The increasing attention focused on drug use and abuse by children and youth in the United States stems partly from the spread of drugs from the lower socioeconomic groups to include the middle and upper classes as well. Drugs are not new to the ghettos of metropolitan areas or crowded tenements of our inner cities. "They are a way of life, as common as the Mister Softie truck is in white suburbia" (Anderson, 1971, p. 392). However, with the entrance of widespread drug use on the middle-class scene, the problem has recently come to be a major focus of middle-class concern (Anderson, 1971).

There are many social as well as personal factors that contribute to the "psychological readiness to experiment with or start taking drugs" (Cameron, 1968, p. 1270). The teen-age population varies remarkably; it comprises multiple subcultures, racial groupings, and ethnicities. Consider the values and behavior of the black adolescent in Harlem, the 4-H clubbers in rural Kansas, and the adolescent Chicanos in Southern California. Their backgrounds vary by ethnic background and socioeconomic class (Weiner, 1972). It is necessary to consider these important variables in order to compile reliable data from which to plan preventive and remedial programs.

Findings of a research study of high school students in a rural community reflected the differences in the sociocultural milieu of white and black students. The incidence of drug use among white, middle-class students increased with the students' socioeconomic status. Among black students, drug use decreased with increased socioeconomic levels; they used marijuana more than white students; and religion was a factor in discouraging drug use. White students, on the other hand, were significantly influenced by their families where a strong family identification existed; however, the black students were not as significantly influenced by family ties. The investigators concluded that although the incidence of drug use was high, the total amount consumed was not; that is, almost one-half of the students had used drugs only once out of curiosity. The latter phenomenon can be seen as a function of the natural risk-taking behavior and curiosity of adolescents (Globetti and Brigance, 1971).

Auster also discusses the differences in drug use pattern among varying social groups. The lower-class ghetto individual has often used opiates and cannabis, while these drugs are fairly new to the middle- and upper-class youth (Auster, 1969). In the middle- and upper-class population, Auster classifies adolescent drug users into three categories. The first group is composed of these adolescents who could be readily recognized as psychologically disturbed with or without the use of drugs. Their problems, including disturbed family relationships, preceded the escape to drugs. Drug termination for them is unlikely until their underlying difficulties are altered. They use drugs for stimulation and so that they won't feel so "dead" internally. The second group is made up of adolescents who need group acceptance. They will take nearly any drug to go along with the crowd. Group pressure is a primary reinforcer with this type of adolescent, and the "high" that is obtained is a secondary gain. Their psychological handicap is their inability to make their own decisions as opposed to following the wishes of the group. They have little sense of "self," mistrust relationships, and turn inward for relief. Curiosity is the incentive to the use of drugs for the third group; after brief periods of experimentation, they continue to use drugs intermittently for coping with personal problems. They do not depend upon the drugs to resolve developmental challenges of adolescence, but as a facilitator to the process instead (Auster, 1969).

Weiner takes issue with the incidence of drug abuse. He reports recent studies that demonstrate a lower rate of teen-age drug use than has been previously recorded (Weiner, 1972). He points out that inadequate sampling in the survey as well as the highly publicized nature of adolescent deaths due to overdosage have given us an exaggerated view of the prevalence of drug abuse in youth. Weiner goes on to cite another study suggesting that well-adjusted youngsters do not turn to drugs, but that the minority of teen-agers who do so are those students who are not doing well in school either academically or in extracurricular activities. He refers to these studies not to minimize the presence of or seriousness of the drug problems, but to bring into perspective the fact that groups of young people approach their developmental tasks in different ways and that drug abuse is not a normal pattern of adolescent behavior.

Contemporary Society and the Adolescent

"Today's young people live in a world of splendid potential and of terrifying threat" (Joint Commission, 1970, p. 141). A crisis exists in our society because of the necessity to adapt to overwhelming changes.

Toffler refers to the greatly accelerated rate of change in our society as "future shock" (Toffler, 1970). He suggests that young people are the first to experience the symptoms of future shock. Youth is reacting to these rapid changes by massing a social movement toward a society of identity seeking (Glasser, 1972). They reject the "corporate state" and the value of the establishment, and many perceive them as a generation that will revitalize our humanity, freedom, and a sense of community (Reich, 1970). On the other hand, the silent majority thinks otherwise. A change in values is not necessarily operating, but rather a change in their application. Youth's disinterest in achievement may be interpreted as rejection; however, they are not rejecting achievement per se, but are questioning its expense (Auster, 1969). There is evidence that changes produced by the youth movement are already apparent in terms of greater tolerance toward differences in individual appearance and attitudes and in the realization that emotion is the equal of reason and intellect (Dalrymple, 1972).

"There is little evidence to support the widespread impression that most teen-agers are in revolt against the values of their family and society" (Weiner, 1972, p. 21). Only 10 percent of today's adolescents are motivated to renounce societal norms, according to Lipsett and Raab (Weiner, 1972). Weiner distinguishes three different categories of dissident youth: (1) college or college-bound students whose parents have liberal political attitudes; (2) youth from the working class and lower middle class whose families are interested in preserving societal norms and resist the liberal attitudes and activities; (3) a group of dissatisfied youth, mainly black and often culturally disadvantaged, who want the system as it is but also equal social, educational, and occupational opportunities for themselves within it (Weiner, 1972).

American society is moving into a "role-dominated society," in which self-identity, self-expression, and cooperation are the human concerns (Glasser, 1972). The phenomenon that is visible in contemporary society in terms of a search for self-understanding is an effort to escape the prevalent sense of alienation and uncertainty. Middle- and upper-class adolescents are involved in the same process—the search for self-understanding (Auster, 1969). Their search is qualitatively different from that of older generations. Their developmental experiences have been very much different. Today, the adolescent lives in a world where technology has changed the significance of living. The search, then, is for intensifying internal experiences to bring about more awareness that may help him to assess and adapt to new life situations. Drugs have been a way of heightening internal perceptions; group experiences are another more socially acceptable way; Eastern meditation forms still another way, although more difficult for most adolescents to achieve (Auster, 1969).

Drug Prevention Programs

Auster proposes that schools have the greatest potential for preventive programs because they have the most contact with children and youth. For both the adolescents searching for self-understanding and those seeking improved "sense of self," relevant, innovative, and sound educational programs can help establish pathways alternative to the use of drugs. Educating the teacher and the administrator in understanding the experiences of youth which draw them to drugs is imperative. This understanding can best be achieved through experiential education programs wherein the curriculum would afford the students the opportunity to "experience directness and immediacy and their emotional concomitants, with the areas under study, with each other, and with the teacher. This is the real challenge" (Auster, 1969, p. 286).

Dambacher and Hellwig suggest nursing strategies for the young adolescent drug user who is in remedial care on a ward (Dambacher and Hellwig, 1971). They approach their plan from the premise that normal human functioning depends upon a variety of external stimuli as well as upon continuous meaningful contact with the outside world. They speculate that the young drug users rely on internal stimulation from the drug and, therefore, respond minimally to the external world. Drugs sabotage these needs, disturb the perception of the user, and reduce his external contacts. To alter this situation, Dambacher and Hellwig manipulate the drug user's environment to increase external stimuli, both in the hospital unit and through outside physical settings, such as beaches, stores, and rock music. Another strategy used is perception correction, which utilizes feedback therapeutically in order to correct the patient's perceptions of his behavior and to help him make alternate plans for managing his world.

The above strategies can be useful in working with adolescent drug users in any setting: schools, youth guidance centers, community clubs, or directly in the home environment. A consultant such as a child psychiatric nurse specialist could help staff, teachers, parents, and youth leaders develop and implement a plan based on the principles described. He could also be a significant person in the planning and implementation of a drug prevention program through experiential education.

SEXUAL IDENTITY CRISIS IN ADOLESCENTS

She took my hand and I suddenly felt alive and living as I had never felt before. My heart jumped up and screamed, "What the hell is going on?" My mind said, "I don't know, but whatever it is I am digging it."

Clark Burnside (1971)

The stirring of heterosexual feelings in adolescence, as vividly described above, indicates that the process of biological and emotional development is evolving toward the developmental task of sexual identity. "Biological development and emotional readiness for heterosexual relationships do not proceed at the same pace" (Offer and Offer, 1971, p. 31). Although the sexual impulses are present with increasing strength, there may be psychosocial hindrances that delay expression of these urges. Studies of high school male and female adolescents found a difference of several years between the time adolescents were biologically ready for reproduction and the time that they engaged in intense heterosexual relationships. The results of these studies and others seem to show that "adolescent sexuality remained an emotional taboo as well as an environmental one" (Offer and Offer, 1971, p. 32; Douvan and Adelson, 1966). Therefore, the claim that there is increased sexual experience among today's adolescents because of the movement toward change in sexual practices is not supported; however, the change seems to be in more open discussions of sex (Offer and Offer, 1971).

Erikson contends that "sexual experimentation will provide a necessary part of identity formation, but sexual pleasure need be preceded by a sense of one's own identity" (Offer and Offer, 1971, p. 34; Erikson, 1968). A crucial aspect of sexual identity is learning role-appropriate behavior. Comparative studies indicate that learning appropriate sexual behavior is less dependent upon hormones than upon conditioning. The development of sexual behavior is influenced by cultural and psychosocial experiences. In learning the appropriate role of one's sex, an individual becomes aware of the element that one is either female or male (Roessler, 1971).

Maier describes Erikson's view of the polarization continuum of sexual identity versus bisexual diffusion in terms of the adolescent's need to resolve bisexual conflicts and to feel identified with his own sex role. It is difficult for the adolescent to conceive of himself as a bit of both. The period of adolescence furnishes situations and attitudes for a young person which provide continued experimentation that can contribute toward a sense of identity with adults of his sex (Maier, 1969, p. 63).

Learning one's sex role begins in childhood with emulation of the like-sexed parent, inculcation of cultural patterns, and experience with peer interaction. The child learns through the process of feedback, positive and negative, as to what are the expected and appropriate behaviors (Eisenberg, 1965). Margaret Mead has described the universal role of the female as being more certain than that of the male in that she begins with the simple identification with her mother. The male's role, however, is less certain; in the male's earliest experience of self, he is forced to conceive of himself as essentially different from his mother (Mead, 1949). Keniston points to the fact that the American family complicates masculine sexual identification for a boy. Since the mother controls most of the things he wants (love, approval, security), and because the father is absent during the work day, the boy establishes an early bond with his mother (Keniston, 1965, p. 305).

The current feminist movement also has implications for future roles and identification experiences for children, adolescents, and adults. Many women are in search of a new, independent role that is less confining than the "triangle of children, kitchen, church" (*Time,* 1972, p. 26). Since the process of increased feminine autonomy is complicated, only a few implications are noted here.

Confusion of roles as well as clarity of identification for both sexes may develop. Parents who are pioneering the reverse roles of mother working and father responsible for home duties have to be secure in their own identities in order not to cause confusion in their children. Parents who share equal responsibility and contact with their children provide more opportunity for sexual identification.

Implications related to increased sexual autonomy as opposed to the double standard may alter girls' learning sex roles, and, thereby, categories of promiscuity and delinquency for girls may need to be changed. Basic concepts about what constitutes mental health in men and women may also need to be altered as the issue of increased feminine autonomy is pursued.

Homosexuality

When the adolescent has been unable to identify with the same-sexed parent, a situation for predisposition to homosexuality may develop (Coons, 1971, p. 261). Kirkendall found that one out of every five boys (sixteen to twenty-four years of age) had been or were concerned about homosexuality (Kirkendall, 1968). Society increases anxiety regarding homosexuality in adolescent girls and boys by signaling to young people that they would be considered a heterosexual or homosexual by the age of sixteen or seventeen. Many adolescents are distressed by the common assumption that if one is not heterosexual, one must then be homosexual (Coons, 1971). Coons reports that this inference often produces a homosexual panic in college freshmen. Their anxieties are usually alleviated when they explore their behavior and fantasies and become aware that they have confused heterosexual retardation with homosexuality (Coons, 1971).

The etiology of homosexuality is complex, and research has failed to verify genetic, constitutional, or hormonal factors as direct causes (Bowers, 1972; Eisenberg, 1965; Rubin, 1970; Semmens and Krantz, 1970). There are many factors that may produce the complicated phenomenon, such as inappropriate identification with opposite-sexed parent or role reversal of parents, too high cultural expectations, as well as rigid male and female social roles and easier access to sexual gratification from one's own sex during adolescence (Hooker, 1961). Psychiatric theory relates the phenomenon to disturbed family relationships. Beiber states that both female and male homosexuality originate from a "continuity of pathologic parent-child relationships" (Beiber, 1969, p. 2640). He offers hope that the gender identity formed in childhood is not irreversibly set. Children who enter adolescence as potential homosexuals can be helped to achieve their heterosexual potentials in order to offset homosexual development. It is important that early identification be implemented before the continuation of the homosexual experiences becomes fixated.

Sexual Promiscuity

Berman has found that adolescents deeply disturbed about their identity express their need to be themselves through sexual promiscuity (Berman, 1969). They perceive the sexual activity as freeing them from an inhibiting society. Upon closer examination, Berman found that the activity was mainly for physiological release as opposed to a need for interpersonal needs. Adolescent girls involved in unrestrained sexual activity have difficulty in establishing relationships and seem unconcerned about pregnancy. Berman defined the recurring theme of the personal freedom struggle in patients as an attempt against being involved (Berman, 1969).

Since there is confusion in the concept of promiscuity, some factors to be considered in assessing an adolescent would include a definition (such as excessive sexual acting out) in terms of the adolescent's total background, any differences between girls' and boys' behavior, and the therapist's own subjective attitude about promiscuity which could influence the assessment.

The detachment of sex from interpersonal contact can clearly be seen in the schizophrenic. Although the schizophrenic is highly threatened by closeness, he is capable of physical and sexual intimacy without being very disturbed by it. His sexual participation may diminish anxiety for him but it frequently shows perverted behavior (Frank, 1969).

The Pregnant Teen-ager

The pregnant teen-ager is a high risk medically. The high incidence of premature births and other complications suggests that female reproductive organs may not be functioning in the same manner in the early and middle adolescence that they would in a later stage of life. In addition, many teen-age pregnancies occur out of wedlock, and subsequently pressure of incurring negative social sanction is experienced along with emotional and economic problems (Osofsky, 1968).

The number of out-of-wedlock pregnancies has been increasing both in the United States and abroad. Teen-agers contribute a high percentage of illegitimate births, with the greatest number occurring among fifteen- to nineteen-year-olds (Osofsky, 1968). In some cases teen-age girls are eager to become mothers as the result of anxiety related to the turmoil of adolescence; they hope to escape to the "less turbulent state of adulthood" (Harris, 1971). However, teen-age motherhood carries with it its own difficulties. Since problems of emotional maturation are not resolved, some young mothers treat their infants either as toys or as rival siblings. Harris notes that the emotional immaturity of adolescent parents is a contributing factor in the battered infant syndrome (Harris, 1971).

In reviewing the research related to the problem of illegitimacy, Osofsky reports that during the 1940s and 1950s, psychological and psychiatric studies defined teen-age, out-of-wedlock pregnancy as a symptom of an underlying emotional difficulty. In the 1950s and 1960s studies began to include environmental factors as well. All services for the pregnant teen-ager, married or not, are inadequate, particularly for the poor and nonwhite women, who usually constitute the highest-risk group. A basic problem of the pregnant teen-ager is that she is denied control of her own body through the paucity of available sex education, the lack of contraceptive information, the difficulties in obtaining an abortion, and the powerful social sanctions against providing these services (Osofsky, 1968).

Nursing Strategies and Sexual Identity of Adolescents

The psychiatric nurse working with adolescents has a responsibility for assisting the young person in his developmental task of searching for sexual identity, through direct and indirect methods such as teaching, counseling, consulting, and acting as an advocate, by providing him with appropriate and sufficient resources regarding sex information, and with medical and psychological support. The psychiatric nurse works with adolescents through youth groups, planned parenthood clinics, classrooms, and other community agencies. He has a responsibility for helping staff, parents, and youth leaders to understand and relate to the adolescent in his search for a healthy sexual identity.

Giggling and laughter which often accompany sex discussion in teen-age groups are related to anxiety, and the understanding nurse can intervene appropriately to reduce the anxiety so the adolescent can utilize the learning experience to clarify and validate his perceptions and feelings about his sexual development (Pazdur, 1969). Through this process, he can develop a healthy attitude about sex as he learns about the biological growth toward heterosexual relationships. The nurse also understands that the dating process for the adolescent is a source of great interest as well as of anxiety about intimacy; that some adolescents are anxious about being or becoming homosexual; and that some adolescents act out their anxieties through multiple sexual activities.

The nurse is in a strategic position to assist in the prevention of unhealthy sexual identity as well as to help those teen-agers who have differing sexual identification. In his contacts with small children and their families through nursery schools, home visits, or community agencies, the nurse can assess maladaptive behavior at an early age that may indicate a beginning sex-role confusion. The nurse can refer the family to an appropriate agency or be himself the primary therapeutic agent. The nurse can make a significant contribution to healthy adolescent development by advocating the rights of youth to services related to sex information, counseling, and medical care.

ADOLESCENT DELINQUENCY

The adolescent who acts out in an antisocial way is called a *delinquent*. The term is used in several ways. The legal concept of delinquency postulates a type of behavior that is forbidden by law; the cultural concept indicates behavior that is not congruent with the value demands of the dominant culture; and the clinical concept of delinquency refers to the psychological conflicts that are causing the behavior (Redl and Wineman, 1951).

The major offenses of the delinquent adolescent include stealing, truancy, fire setting, vandalism, and cruelty ranging on a continuum to murder (Johnson, 1959). Delinquency rates rise from age eleven, are five times higher among boys than among girls, and are higher in the poverty areas of large cities than in rural or suburban areas. There is an estimate that 11 percent of all children in the United States will reach a juvenile court by the age of nineteen. In 1965, individuals eighteen years or younger were charged with 61 percent of all auto thefts, 45 percent of the larceny charges, 52 percent of all burglary, and 24 percent of charges of forcible rape (Joint Commission, 1970).

The concept of delinquency is wider in scope because of the number of factors involved and the difficulties encountered in defining with certainty the nature and extent of the problem (Short, 1966). Two categories suggested as causative of antisocial behavior are (1) delinquents from "normal" families driven by unconscious conflicts, and (2) the delinquent gang or sociologic group which operates at any socioeconomic level (Johnson, 1959).

Although gang delinquency is not limited to the working class, it is less common among the middle and upper classes. There are psychological factors that indicate differences between delinquent and nondelinquent boys. Delinquent boys generally have great concern for status because of their feelings of inferiority; show very poor social and interpersonal skills; and are highly anxious and extremely self-centered. The group spirit of the delinquent gang, contrary to a gang of "nondelinquent" boys, has little warmth or trust, and the bravado is a cover-up for feelings of dependency. Frequently, the group members have received little love or discipline, and many of their homes lacked a father (Joint Commission, 1970).

The Joint Commission on Mental Health of Children reports that we continue to fail our children in providing them with needed services, and this failure is nowhere more evident than in the area of delinquency. Most delinquents are dealt with harshly instead of receiving the remedial services that they need. Delinquents from disadvantaged minority and poverty groups are more often committed to correctional institutions than to treatment facilities and are more likely to be treated brutally by police than are middle-class adolescents. Psychiatric or counseling assistance through the juvenile corrective facilities is also lacking (Joint Commission, 1970).

The rapid increase in delinquency, especially among the poor, makes the preventive approach a necessary requirement. A recommendation of the Commission is that noninstitutional, community-based programs be established in which youth participation is encouraged. Further research is needed to clarify the many factors that contribute to developing an antisocial personality. Above all, an immediate effort by the community to plan and implement these recommendations is needed, as well as greater consideration of the rights and needs of children and of adolescents, who are "yesterday's neglected children" (Joint Commission, 1970, p. 376).

PSYCHOSIS IN ADOLESCENCE

"There is no symptom of the disturbed adolescent that does not in one way or another fit into the category of normal adolescence" (Joint Commission, 1970, p. 372). In adolescence certain behaviors resembling psychosis such as schizophrenia may occur. Corboz points to the similarities between a beginning schizophrenic psychosis and a crisis of puberty. The adolescent at puberty becomes more seclusive, has mood swings oscillating between depression and exhilaration, loses himself in fantasy at times, is aggressive toward siblings, and is impertinent to his parents (Corboz, 1969). The degree of rigidity of these symptoms and the extent to which they cripple are the criteria for measuring the young person's behavior against that of a normal adolescent (Joint Commission, 1970). The healthy adolescent will maintain contact with reality although he may show behavior that seems pathological in certain environments while behaving normally elsewhere. On the other hand, the schizophrenic's strange behavior is not altered by changes in his environment (Corboz, 1969). Corboz states that when hallucinations and delusions appear, there is little doubt that the adolescent is suffering from a schizophrenic illness.

In distinguishing between normal and abnormal mental disturbances, consideration should be given to the similarity of psychosis to behavior in drug-induced states. Early phases of acute psychosis many times cannot be differentiated from drug experience (Redlich and Freedman, 1966; Freedman, 1971). The similarities are heightened sensitivity, euphoria, tension, narcissism, and feelings of body change. There are indications that schizophrenia in adolescence is less frequent than previously believed. With improvements in treatment, there is evidence that many adolescents were misdiagnosed as schizophrenic. An adolescent, overburdened with demands made upon him, may suffer a psychotic breakdown and upon recovery not show any schizoid characteristics. Such an illness should not be confused with schizophrenia (Joint Commission, 1970). "The essential criterion for diagnosing adolescent psychosis is complete recovery" (Krevelen, 1971, p. 382).

When considering the possibility of an adolescent schizophrenic disturbance, one should determine whether the illness is in its initial stages or began in a previous stage of personality development (Corboz, 1969). There are two types of adolescent schizophrenia: one marked by adolescent onset, the other with its roots in an earlier period (Krevelen, 1971). Corboz cites studies that report that only 1 percent of all schizophrenics manifest their illness before the age of ten and 4 percent before the age of fourteen.

Easson describes two types of disturbed adolescents: (1) the reactive psychotic and (2) the process psychotic or nuclear schizophrenic (Easson, 1969). In the former disturbance, the adolescent has experienced early trauma in his interpersonal relationships and may not have had sufficient ego strength to deal with continued anxiety-arousing relationships as well as with the burdens of the emancipation task of adolescent years. He copes by retreating into an autistic world. In the latter disturbance, Easson includes the symbiotic or schizophrenic children who have carried their illness into adolescence and are relatively "comfortable" within that personality state (Easson, 1969).

Thoughts on Prevention of Mental Illness

Schonfeld states that mental health specialists interested in prevention should consider the "individual at a stage in his life cycle when previous identifications are up for review, new ones are being formed and prior to continuing the reproductive stage and transmitting maladaptive patterns to the next generation" (Schonfeld, 1971, p. 504). He suggests a comprehensive view of planning community programs for adolescents which to be most effective would include a multidisciplinary approach, provisions for prevention, diagnosis, treatment, and rehabilitation. These services would offer care at the appropriate time and place and would be responsive to the adolescent's needs. In dealing with the needs of the adolescent, three levels of services are explored: the schools, the general community, and community mental health services.

In the school setting, Schonfeld recommends that teachers learn about the categories of adolescent disturbances and how to cope with them in the classroom. Buckle (1966), in his discussion of prevention, recommends that schools be primarily oriented toward undertaking preventive milieu therapy and that teachers primarily learn to be milieu therapists and secondarily instructors, in order to help students take initiative in learning. Reorientation of educational philosophy as well as great change in the attitude of the community toward the role of the schools would obviously be required. Buckle's suggestion of preventive milieu therapy in the classroom may be futuristic and would undoubtedly raise the issue among educators and parents as to the school's function and responsibility for nonacademic endeavors. However, such innovative planning is an urgent need today if we are to provide adolescents the maximum opportunity for developing into healthy adults.

This writer recommends the development of a pilot program that would support several multidisciplinary mental health teams in satellite stations located within the school community for the purpose of prevention. The services would be specifically designed to assist adolescents to achieve and maintain a healthy growth process both psychologically and physically. The team could offer teacher training in milieu therapy; classroom work with teachers and students in learning about growth and development in relation to their bodies; counseling and seminars with topics related to the adolescents' needs, such as sex education, drugs, and parent-teacher conflicts; parent-teacher-student communication group seminars to facilitate further understanding between adults and adolescents. A free drop-in atmosphere within the satellite system would be necessary so that students, staff, and parents would feel less inhibited about seeking out the available resources. Similarly, it would be equally incumbent upon school personnel to maintain an open-door policy toward the health team involved in the school setting.

Adolescents are difficult to work with, for they can be treated neither as children nor as adults. If they are treated as children, the process prevents maturation; and if they are treated as adults, the process may burden their egos (Schonfeld, 1971). The psychiatric nurse who is professionally prepared to work with this age group would thus be a logical person from the satellite team to function as a mental health trainer for teachers learning to become milieu teacher-therapists. Clerical and custodial staff in the school many times develop a rapport with the student and can relate to him according to his needs. They might possibly be included in a training program. A problem which may arise by including auxiliary staff could be union objections to extra services not included in the job specifications. Another problem to consider would be an anti-mental health attitude of the auxiliary staff.

In teaching and consulting with the school community, the psychiatric nurse would help students and adults in the process of predicting and becoming aware of emotional distress, as in the case of moving into a new neighborhood, an addition to the family, or a severe illness of a family member. The nurse could also assist staff and students in coping with major crisis resulting from a death, divorce, or severe accident.

Today the psychiatric nurse who is prepared for working with adolescents focuses his attention on prevention. He functions as a counselor, family therapist, and parent-group leader, as well as consultant, educator, and researcher, in helping adolescents and all those involved with youth toward a better understanding of an adaptation to the ever-changing developmental process of adolescence.

Schonfeld recommends that treatment services be part of the school setting and include psychotherapy and special education for disturbed adolescents. Within the community at large, he recommends effective recreational and social programs as functions of primary prevention, as well as a range of treatment modalities. Foster homes, group homes, emergency services, and specialized adolescent clinics are a few of the treatment services suggested. For further discussion of treatment services and innovative programs, the reader is referred to Schonfeld (1971) and the Joint Commission on Mental Health for Children (1970).

REFERENCES

Anderson, Clarence C. (1971): "Drugs—America's Current Visible Hysteria," *Journal of Drug Education,* vol. 1, no. 4, pp. 391–399.

Anthony, James (1969): "The Reactions of Adults to Adolescents and Their Behavior," in Gerald Caplan and Serge Lebovici (eds.), *Adolescence: Psychosocial Perspectives,* Basic Books, Inc., Publishers, New York, pp. 54–78.

Auster, Simon L. (1969): "Some Observations on Adolescent Drug Use," *Educational Leadership,* vol. 27, no. 3, pp. 281–286.

Bakwin, Harry (1964): "Suicide in Children and Adolescents," *Journal of Pediatrics,* vol. 50, pp. 749–769.

Balser, Benjamin H., and James F. Masterson (1959): "Suicide in Adolescence," *American Journal of Psychiatry,* vol. 116, pp. 400–404.

Beiber, Irving (1969): "Homosexuality," *American Journal of Nursing,* vol. 69, no. 12, pp. 2637–2641.

Berman, Leo H. (1969): "Freedom and Sexuality," *Disease of the Nervous System,* vol. 30, no. 11, pp. 731–786.

Bigras, Julian Y., Yvon Gauthier, Collette Bouchard, and Yolande Tasse (1966): "Suicidal Attempts in Adolescent Girls: a Preliminary Study," *Canadian Psychiatric Journal,* Supplement, pp. 275–283.

Blos, Peter (1966): "The Concept of Acting Out in Relation to the Adolescent Process," in Eveoleen N. Rexford (ed.), *A Developmental Approach to Acting Out,* Monographs of the Journal of American Academy of Child Psychiatry, International Universities Press, Inc., New York, pp. 118–143.

Boston University School of Nursing (1968): *Nursing in Child Psychiatry: Work Conference,* Programs in Mental Health-Psychiatric Nursing, NIMH.

Bowers, Faubion (1972): Homosex: Living the Life, *Saturday Review, Feb. 12, pp. 23–28.*

Brody, Jane E. (1972): "New Laws Help Minors Obtain Own Health Care," in *New York Times,* Mar. 5, pp. 47.

Buckle, Donald (1966): "Children and Schools: A Reaction," in Henry P. David, *International Trends in Mental Health,* McGraw-Hill Book Company, New York, pp. 223–228.

Burnside, Clark (1971): *Personal Journal,* Unpublished paper, Diablo Valley Junior College.

Cameron, Dale C. (1968): "Youth and Drugs," *Journal of American Medical Association,* vol. 206, no. 6, pp. 1267–1271.

Caplan, Gerald (1951): "A Public Health Approach to Child Psychiatry," *Mental Hygiene,* vol. 35, pp. 235–249.

———(1964): "The Role of Pediatricians in Community Mental Health (with Particular Reference to the Primary Prevention of Mental Disorders in Children)," in Leopold Bellak's *Handbook of Community Psychiatry and Community Mental Health,* Grune & Stratton, Inc., New York, pp. 287–299.

Carroll, Edward J. (1954): "Acting Out and Ego Development," *Psychoanalytic Quarterly,* vol. 23, pp. 521–528.

Coles, Robert (1972): "Breaking the American Stereotypes," in *Time,* Feb. 14, pp. 36–48.

Coons, Frederick W. (1971): "The Developmental Tasks of the College Student," in Sherman C. Feinstein, Peter L. Giovacchini, and A. A. Miller (eds.), *Adolescent Psychiatry,* vol. 1, Basic Books, Inc., Publishers, New York, pp. 256–274.

Corboz, Robert (1969): "Endogenous Psychoses of the Adolescent," in Gerald Caplan and Serge Lebovici (eds.), *Adolescence: Psychosocial Perspectives,* Basic Books, Inc., Publishers, New York, pp. 275–279.

Crow, L. D., and Alice Crow (1965): *Adolescent Development and Adjustment,* McGraw-Hill Book Company, New York.

Dalrymple, Willard, (1972): "The Youth Revolution: It Is Over and It Has Won," in *Intellectual Digest,* vol. 2, no. 11, pp. 80–81.

Dambacher, Betty, and Karen Hellwig (1971): "Nursing Strategies for Young Drug Users," in *Perspectives in Psychiatric Care,* vol. 9, no. 5, pp. 200–205.

Dizmang, Larry H. (1967): "Suicide among the Cheyenne Indians," *Bulletin of Suicidology,* July, pp. 8–11.

Douvan, Elizabeth, and Joseph Adelson (1966): *The Adolescent Experience,* John Wiley & Sons, Inc., New York.

Easson, William (1969): *The Severely Disturbed Adolescent,* International Universities Press, Inc., New York.

Eisenberg, Leon (1965): "A Developmental Approach to Adolescence," in *Children,* vol. 12, no. 4, pp. 131–135.

———(1969): "A Developmental Approach to Adolescence," in Dorothy Rogers (ed.), *Issues in Adolescent Psychology,* Appleton-Century-Crofts, Meredith Corporation, New York, pp.21–30.

———(1966): "Preventive Psychiatry: If Not Now, When?" in Henry P. David (ed.), *International Trends in Mental Health,* McGraw-Hill Book Company, New York, pp. 63–77.

Erikson, Erik H. (1959): *Identity and the Life Cycle,* International Universities Press, Inc., New York.

———(1968): *Identity: Youth and Crisis,* W. W. Norton & Company, Inc., New York.

———(1970): "Reflections on the Dissent of Contemporary Youth," *International Journal of Psychoanalysis,* vol. 51, pp. 11–22.

Evans, Frances Monet Carter (1968): *The Role of the Nurse in Community Mental Health,* The MacMillan Company, New York.

Fenichel, Otto (1945): *Psychoanalytic Theory of Neurosis,* W. W. Norton & Company, Inc., New York.

Finley, Brooke, Elizabeth Jordan, Ann McCue, Marcia McLain, Lloyd Miller, and Mary Wierda (1972): *The Position of Child Psychiatric Nursing in the Delivery of Mental Health Services to Children in the City and County of San Francisco,* Unpublished paper, June.

Fleming, Joan, and Sol Altshul (1963): "Activation of Mourning and Growth by Psychoanalysis," *International Journal of Psychoanalysis,* vol. 44, pp. 419–431.

Frank, Leonard (1969): "Humanizing and Dehumanizing Aspects of Human Sexuality," *Disease of the Nervous System,* vol. 30, no. 11, pp. 781-786.

Freedman, Daniel E. (1971): "On the Use and Abuse of LSD," in Sherman C. Feinstein, Peter Giovacchini, and A. A. Miller, *Adolescent Psychiatry,* vol. 1, Basic Books, Inc., Publishers, New York, pp. 75–107.

Gedo, John E. (1966): "The Psychotherapy of Developmental Arrest," *British Journal of Medical Psychology,* March, vol. 39, part 1, pp. 25–33.

Glaser, Kurt (1965): "Suicide in Children and Adolescents," in Lawrence Edwin Abt and Stuart L. Weissman (ed.), *Acting Out,* Grune & Stratton, Inc., New York, pp. 87–99.

Glasser, William (1972): "The Civilized Identity Society," *Saturday Review,* Feb. 19, pp. 26–31.

Globetti, Gerald, and Roy S. Brigance (1971): "The Use and Non-use of Drugs among High School Students in a Small Rural Community," *Journal of Drug Education,* vol. I, no. 4, pp. 317–322.

Greenacre, Phyllis (1950): "General Problems of Acting Out," *Psychoanalytic Quarterly,* vol. 19, pp. 455–467.

Groffman, Karl J. (1970): "Life-Span Developmental Psychology in Europe: Past and Present," in L. R. Goulet and Paul B. Baltes (eds.), *Life Span Developmental Psychology: Research and Theory,* Academic Press, Inc., New York, pp. 54–68.

Grollman, Early A. (1971): *Suicide: Prevention, Intervention, Postvention,* Beacon Press, Boston.

Guskin, Alan E., and Robert Ross (1971): "Advocacy and Democracy: The Long View," in *American Journal of Orthopsychiatry,* vol. 41, no. 1, pp. 43–57.

Harris, Herbert X. (1971): "The Range of Psychosomatic Disorders in Adolescence," in John G. Howells (ed.), *Modern Perspectives in Adolescent Psychiatry,* Brunner Mazel, Inc., New York, pp. 237–253.

Herzog, A., and H. P. Resnik, (1968): "A Clinical Study of Parental Response to Adolescent Death by Suicide with Recommendation for Approaching Survivors," *Proceedings Fourth International Conference for Suicide Prevention,* N. L. Farberow (ed.), Los Angeles International Association for Suicide Prevention, pp. 381–390.

Hooker, Evelyn, (1961): "Homosexuality—Summary of Studies," in Evelyn Ruth M. Duvall, *Sex Ways in Fact and Faith,* Association Press, New York.

Jacobs, Jerry, and Joseph D. Teicher (1967): "Broken Homes and Social Isolation in Attempted Suicide of Adolescents," *International Journal of Social Psychiatry,* vol. 13, no. 2, pp. 139–149.

Jacobziner, Harold (1965): "Attempted Suicides in Adolescents by Poisoning: Statistical Report," *American Journal of Psychotherapy,* vol. 19, no. 2, pp. 247–252.

———(1960): "Attempted Suicides in Children," *Journal of Pediatrics,* vol. 56, no. 4, pp. 519–525.

Jan-Tausch, J. (1963): *Suicide of Children 1960–63: New Jersey Public School Students,* State of New Jersey Department of Education, Trenton, N.J.

Johnson, Adelaide (1959): "Juvenile Delinquency," in Silvano Arieti (ed.), *American*

Handbook of Psychiatry, vol. 2, Basic Books, Inc., Publishers, New York, pp. 840–856.

Joint Commission on Mental Health of Children (1970): *Crisis in Child Mental Health: Challenge for the 1970's,* Harper & Row, Publishers, Inc., New York.

Josselyn, Irene (1965): "The Acting Out Adolescent," in Lawrence E. Abt and Stuart L. Weissman, *Acting Out,* Grune & Stratton, Inc., New York, pp. 68–75.

Kastenbaum, Robert (1959): "Time and Death in Adolescence," in Herman Feifel (ed.), *The Meaning of Death,* McGraw-Hill Book Company, New York, pp. 99–113.

Keniston, Kenneth (1965): *The Uncommitted,* Dell Publishing Company, New York.

Kirkendall, Lester A. (1968): "Adolescent Homosexual Fears," in Lester A. Kirkendall and Isadore Rubin (eds.), *Sex in the Adolescent Years: New Directions in Guiding and Teaching Youth,* Association Press, New York.

Lourie, R. S. (1966): "Clinical Studies of Attempted Suicide in Childhood," *Clinical Proceedings of Children's Hospital of the District of Columbia,* vol. 22, no. 6, pp. 163–173.

Maier, Henry W. (1969): *Three Theories of Child Development,* Harper & Row, Publishers, Inc., New York.

Mead, Margaret (1949): *Male and Female,* William Morrow & Company, Inc., New York.

Mintz, R. S. (1964): *A Pilot Study of the Prevalence of Persons in the City of Los Angeles Who Have Attempted Suicide,* Unpublished manuscript (presented at American Psychiatric Association Meetings, Los Angeles, May), UCLA Neuropsychiatric Institute.

Muus, Rolf E. (1966): "Theories of Adolescent Development—Their Philosophical and Historical Root," in *Adolescence,* vol. I, no. 1, pp. 22–44.

Offer, Daniel (1969): *The Psychological World of the Teenager,* Basic Books, Inc., Publishers, New York.

———and Judith Offer (1971): "Four Issues in the Developmental Psychology of Adolescents," in John G. Howell (ed.), *Modern Perspectives in Adolescent Psychiatry,* Brunner Mazel, Inc., New York, pp. 28–44.

———and Melvin Sabshin (1966): *Normality: Theoretical and Clinical Concepts of Mental Health,* Basic Books, Inc., Publishers, New York.

Osofsky, Howard J. (1968): *The Pregnant Teen-ager,* Charles C Thomas, Publishers, Springfield, Ill.

Pazdur, Helen C. (1969): "Innovation: The School Nurse as a Mental Health Specialist," *The Journal of School Health,* vol. 39, no. 7, pp. 449–457.

Pothier, Pat (1968): "A Thing Called Hope," *Journal of Psychiatric Nursing,* vol. 6, no. 1, pp. 15–19.

Ramshorn, Mark T. (1971): "The Major Thrust in American Psychiatry: Past, Present and Future," *Perspectives in Psychiatric Care,* vol. 9, no. 4, pp. 144–155.

Redl, Fritz, and David Wineman (1951): *Children Who Hate,* The Free Press, New York.

Redlich, Fredrick C., and Daniel X. Freedman (1966): *The Theory and Practice of Psychiatry,* Basic Books, Inc., Publishers, New York.

Reich, Charles A. (1970): *The Greening of America,* Random House, Inc., New York.

Resnick, H. C. P., and Larry H. Dizmang (1971): "Observations on Suicidal Behavior among American Indians," *American Journal of Psychiatry,* vol. 127, no. 7, pp. 882–887.

Rexford, Eveoleen N. (1966): "A Developmental Concept of Acting Out," in Eveoleen N. Rexford (ed.), *A Developmental Approach to Problems of Acting Out,* International Universities Press, Inc., New York, pp. 6–21.

Robertiello, Richard C. (1965): "Acting Out or Working Through," in Lawrence Edwin Abt and Stuart L. Weissman, *Acting Out,* Grune & Stratton, Inc., New York, pp. 40–45.

Roessler, Richard T. (1971): "Sexuality and Identity: Masculine Differentiation and Feminine Constancy," *Adolescence,* vol. 6, no. 22, pp. 187–196.

Rubin, Isadore (1970): "Coping with Homosexual Fear," in James P. Semmens and Kermit E. Krantz, *The Adolescent Experience,* The Macmillan Company, New York, pp. 98–114.

Schneer, Henry I., Paul Kay, and Morris Brozovsky (1961): "Events and Conscious Ideation Leading to Suicidal Behavior in Adolescence," *Psychiatric Quarterly,* vol. 35, no. 3, pp. 507–515.

Schonfeld, William A. (1971): "Comprehensive Community Programs for the Investigation and Treatment of Adolescence," in John G. Howell (ed.), *Modern Perspectives in Psychiatry,* Brunner Mazel, Inc., New York, pp. 483–511.

Seiden, Richard H. (1969): *Suicide among the Young, A Supplement to the Bulletin of Suicidology,* National Clearinghouse for Mental Health Information.

Semmens, James P., and Kermit Krantz (eds.) (1970): *The Adolescent Experience,* The Macmillan Company, New York.

Short, James F. Jr. (1966): "Juvenile Delinquency: The Socio-cultural Context," in Lis Wladis Hoffman and Martin L. Hoffman (eds.), *Review of Child Development Research,* vol. 2, Russell Sage Foundation, pp. 423–468.

Socrates, in Anthony James (1969): "The Reactions of Adults to Adolescents and Their Behavior," in Gerald Caplan and Serge Lebovici (eds.), *Adolescence: Psychosocial Perspectives,* Basic Books, Inc., Publishers, New York, p. 77.

Teicher, Joseph D., and Jerry Jacobs (1966): "Adolescents Who Attempt Suicides: Preliminary Findings," *American Journal of Psychiatry,* vol. 122, no. 11, pp. 1248–1257.

Time (1972): *The American Woman,* Special Issue, March 20, pp. 25–104.

Toffler, Alvin (1970): *Future Shock,* Random House, Inc., New York.

Toolan, James M. (1969): "Depression in Children and Adolescents," in Gerald Caplan and Serge Lebovici (eds.), *Adolescence: Psychosocial Perspectives,* Basic Books, Inc., Publishers, New York, pp. 264–274.

————(1962): "Suicide and Suicidal Attempts in Children and Adolescents," *The American Journal of Psychiatry,* February, vol. 118, pp. 719–724.

van Krevelen, D. Arn (1971): "Psychoses in Adolescence," in John G. Howells (ed.), *Modern Perspectives in Adolescent Psychiatry,* Brunner Mazel, Inc., New York, pp. 381–403.

Weiner, Irving B. (1972): "Perspectives on the Modern Adolescent," *Psychiatry,* vol. 35, no. 1, pp. 20–31.

Wermer, Henry (1966): "Discussion, Peter Blos, The Concept of Acting Out in Relation to the Adolescent Process," in Eveoleen N. Rexford (ed.), *A Developmental Approach to Acting Out,* Monograph of the Journal of American Academy of Child Psychiatry, International Universities Press, Inc., New York, pp. 137–143.

Williams, Florence (1971): "Intervention in Maturational Crisis," *Perspectives in Psychiatric Care,* vol. 9, no. 6, pp. 240–246.

Work, Henry (1971): "Advocacy for Children: Challenge for the 1970's," *Children,* vol. 18, no. 18, pp. 31–32.

Zimbaca, Nicole (1965): "Suicide in Adolescents," *Concours Medical,* vol. 87, pp. 4991–4997.

5

DEVELOPMENTAL REACTIONS IN YOUNG ADULTHOOD

Paula J. LeVeck

Although the young adult years can range from the age of seventeen to fifty, depending on one's theoretical orientation, in the division of the life span into phases, usually early or young adulthood is thought to encompass the early twenties through the late thirties. Within this relatively brief period, given total life expectancy, man must make decisions which have momentous, if not governing, impact on the rest of his life. That fact, coupled with the knowledge that young adults are prone to illness and have a high rate of hospitalization, is cause for alarm and study by all persons involved in the preservation and promotion of health and the prevention of mental illness.

Most of the studies of human development have focused on the first quarter of life; that is, infancy, childhood, and adolescence. Consequently, there is great need for extensive longitudinal studies of the maturing and aging processes beyond the first 18 years. Even the simple delineation of the life cycle represents widely disparate views. Bromley (1966) gives ages twenty-one to twenty-five as early adulthood and twenty-five to forty as middle adulthood. Other systems suggest that early maturity is from seventeen to twenty-five and maturity from twenty-five to fifty (Birren, 1964). This reflects, it seems to the writer, the greater problem which should be mentioned at the outset, which is that although there are useful age-specific theories to describe and explain human development, at present there are no comprehensive theories for the entire life cycle. Not only is there absence of agreement about phases in adult development, but maturity, which is the prime achievement of adulthood, remains a nebulous concept badly in need of continued research. After an extensive review of the theoretical and developmental literature on maturity, Heath concluded that the maturing person becomes stably organized, integrated, allocentric, and autonomous and more of his internal and external experiences become symbolized and available to awareness (Heath, 1965). These characteristics need further study and refinement to provide useful information on what comprises maturity.

For Erikson, adulthood develops from the resolution of the problem of intimacy versus isolation (Erikson, 1968). Bischof suggests that adulthood is the period when we are fulfilled (Bischof, 1969). To Maslow, adulthood and maturity involve the continuous process of becoming and are apparently achieved by the self-actualized person, whom he describes with a long list of attributes (Maslow, 1970). For Freud, maturity is purportedly, the ability to love and to work (*lieben und arbeiten*) (Erikson, 1968). Empirical studies of maturity suffer from absence of comparable measures in selection and assessment of population, dubious reliability of judgment procedures, and lack of cross-validation of studies. Difficulties in studying maturity also arise out of the fact that criteria for maturity may focus on anatomical, physiological, psychological, or social growth, rather than on the complex interplay among all the individual's systems. Coupled with these drawbacks is an observation by Margaret Mead, relevant to the understanding of young adulthood in the 1970s: "The people who have grown up since World War II have been bombarded by all the fragmented things in the world, and have never experienced a whole culture. They are overcome by it too early so that they never learn to sense the holistic quality, the pattern within the diversity of a social system" (Mead, 1970, p. 61). That the bombardment of the immediate past, present, and anticipated future will explode into the young adult's psyche and his private and public life is obvious. The nature of this bombardment and its effect on adulthood and maturity are speculatory.

Studies from the fifties and sixties provide information on some dimensions of the transition from adolescence to adulthood, and there are others which focus on adaptation to adulthood, with its accompanying stresses and responsibilities. In 1940–41, Perceival Symonds and others studied forty junior and senior high school boys and girls through a variant of the apperception test (T.A.T.) method, using a special set of pictures designed to tap adolescent fantasy (Symonds et al., 1949). In 1953–1954, Symonds, Silverman, and Wexler conducted a follow-up study of twenty-eight of the original forty subjects, using projective tests and interviews (Symonds, 1961). In general, the subjects represented the lower middle class.

One general conclusion of the Symonds study was that there was a marked persistence of themes in fantasy over the 13-year interval between the first study and its predecessor—enough to make it possible to identify the narrator and to match the stories told 13 years apart when they were mingled indiscriminately with the stories of other narrators (Symonds, 1961, p. 209). However, there were some general changes in themes. The increase in depression over the previous study was frequently referred to as a clear-cut finding of this study. The researchers conclude that this finding may represent the natural outcome of adolescent fantasy and may also explain what has happened to hostility and aggression formerly present in adolescence. "If young adults have lost the aggressive content of their fantasies, some of it may have been directed into work, but some of it otherwise unexpended, may have been turned inward to appear in the form of regret, discouragement, and surrender." Other general impressions and findings of this study included the following: "Becoming an adult does not mean shedding one personality for another, but rather using the personality that one has to meet the emergencies of adult years" (Symonds, 1961, p. 196). This finding supports the view that basic changes in personality do not occur in young adults.

A more recent study, rich in findings, is that by Rachel Dunaway Cox (Cox, 1970). Sixty-three undergraduate students, all student council members and believed to be good examples of positive mental health, were studied while in college and again 10 years later. *Normal* in this study was defined as the capacity to function passably in all roles on a day-to-day basis, reality-oriented, out of hospitals, and contributing appropriately to their family and community. The researchers' expectations that a group of normal people would still be normal 10 years after college was fulfilled. Over 95 percent of the sixty-three had become financially self-supporting and all were functioning in their selected roles. What is pertinent to note is that these subjects, considered "normal" if not above normal, had, in their accounts of the 10-year interval, evidenced that: "At least ten had gone through periods of profound disheartenment, in four of these cases the discouragement probably verged on a mild depression. One subject experienced an anxiety state. One had attempted suicide. Two others had briefly considered it. Serious problems in their marriages had distressed thirteen" (Cox, 1970, p. 45).

The important thing to the researchers was the subjects' ability to carry on even though they had encountered stress and experienced difficulties. Six specific areas of their life during the 10-year period were investigated, namely: further education, work, marriage, parenthood, relation to one's parents, and management of money, since these were seen as major dimensions through which adult life moves forward. Reported stresses in all spheres were discussed and also categorized as unidirectional or reciprocal. Some stresses, such as occupation-rated stress, were considered endemic to young adulthood. Stresses were definitely experienced by most members of the group, but in general, as well-functioning people, the typical disappointments that occur in young adulthood did not have debilitating effects.

The report of the Joint Commission on Mental Illness and Health is another study using self-reported data. Their findings did not support the definitions of mental health and maturity widely used and accepted among professionals. For example, it was found that money and its related advantages, as well as children, marriage, and family, were a major source of happiness, and that the greatest cause of worry was economic and materialistic. Other findings which related particularly to young adult Americans are the following:

1. "Younger and better educated people are happier but worry more than those who are older or less educated" (Gurin et al., 1960, p. xiv).
2. Women reported a greater experience of distress in all areas of adjustment. This raised questions, which were acknowledged by the researchers, whether women really are subjected to greater stress, less able to manage difficulties, more attuned to interpersonal relationships, or less protective of felt inadequacies than males.
3. Nearly one in four adult Americans says that sometime in life he has felt sufficiently troubled to need help. One in seven sought it (p. xx).
4. Among those who sought help, 42 percent reported their problems centered around their marriages, 18 percent reported personal adjustment difficulties, and 12 percent designated troubles involving their children (p. xx).

In regard to occupation, men in clerical positions and wives of unskilled workers stood out as reporting the greatest sense of unhappiness and discontent. In general, women, younger persons, and the better-educated sought assistance for problems most frequently. Sex, age, and education stood out as the factors most relevant to successful adjustment. The better-educated were capable of experiencing not only greater introspection than other members of the group, but also enhanced well-being and satisfaction and awareness of the scope of interpersonal frustrations and gratifications. The younger subjects had, on the whole, more concerns and doubts than the older population. This may indicate more involvement and greater demands among the younger people rather than reflect a decreased functioning when compared with the less active older subjects.

DEVELOPMENTAL THEORIES

Freud's contribution to knowledge about healthy adults is contained in his conception of the genital character—an individual who had successfully completed the preceding stages of libido development, including liberation from the oedipal situation. Erikson added social and cultural dimensions to psychoanalytic theory when he evolved his epigenetic, phase-specific theory covering the entire life span of man. His sixth stage—intimacy versus isolation—describes the tasks of young adulthood. According to Erikson, following the resolution of the identity crisis during adolescence, man's next developmental task is to resolve the crisis of intimacy versus isolation. Intimacy is not limited to sexual patterning but also includes psychosocial relatedness, to share with and care about another without loss of one's own autonomy. Indeed, it may not even involve sexuality, for example, as in close friendships and comradeship. Early adulthood is the period when one hopefully overcomes tendencies to distance self from others—a carryover from adolescence—and instead establishes his genitality in sexual mutuality and develops the capacity to love. "Love as mutual devotion, however, overcomes the antagonisms inherent in sexual and functional polarization and is the vital strength of young adulthood" (Erikson, 1968, p. 137).

Harry Stack Sullivan's developmental approach ends with late adolescence, which "extends from the patterning of preferred genital activity through unnumbered educative steps to the establishment of a fully human or mature repertory of interpersonal relations, as permitted by available opportunity, personal and cultural" (Sullivan, 1953, p. 237). What he includes in late adolescence frequently gets realized in young adulthood in this society. However, Patrick Mullahy in *Psychoanalysis and Interpersonal Psychiatry* makes it clear that Sullivan's personality theory ends with adulthood, which is "a total situation including another person (or conceivably two other persons) in a total activity, prevailingly sexual in character, the resolution of which is complete in the sense that it does not proceed into disturbing situations, which in turn would require resolution." The important criterion which determines that one is an adult is when "he can establish a durably satisfying relationship with another person—a relationship in which the sexual drive or desire is the conspicuously effective integrating motive" (Mullahy, 1970, p. 126). Inextricably connected with sexual integration is the capacity for collaboration with one or more others. One can glean from Sullivan's writings that he thought our particular culture rendered the accomplishment of mature adulthood difficult because of its exaggeration of sexual differences and obstacles resulting from social and legal controls on marriage and parenthood. Sullivan was clear in his view that marriage ideally facilitated the commingling of sexual and intimacy needs, but that this union often fell woefully short of achieving that blend.

Jurgen Ruesch suggests that salient features of development are related to age-level and age-specific interference with communicative behavior. In young adulthood, from nineteen to approximately the late twenties, one masters complex and diverse communication roles and rules, and in work situations learns subservience. In middle adulthood, from thirty to middle forties approximately, he learns communication with age inferiors and children and switches to a position of greater responsibility in communication transmission (Ruesch, 1964, p. 34). During a brief two decades, the gamut of interactional expertise, it would seem, is presented for mastery, in increasingly accountable situations.

In terms of ego development, adulthood means that the individual exercises greater control, giving priority to long-term benefits rather than immediate satisfactions. A mature ego has the capacity to endure anxieties and frustration without the loss of foresight or problem-solving ability, and to resort only infrequently to escapist behaviors. The individual must also come to terms with his own identity, especially as it is expressed through vocational choice and commitment to a meaningful, intimate relationship with another person. Decisions in these two realms of adult life have far-reaching and long-lasting effects and may be the most important decisions of one's lifetime. Prerequisites ideally include liberation from dependency needs; establishment of an identity separate from one's family; and capacity for enjoying closeness without fear of annihilation. Solomon, discussing adulthood somewhat differently, but still within the framework of ego psychology, writes that ego integration in a mature adult produces a balanced sense of values. Through the acquisition of high levels of concept formation, one assesses, compares, and determines purposeful action. But there is also a capacity for disintegration when confronted with inexorable conflicts. These conflicts could conceivably be in home life or parenting, in occupational life, or in social and recreational spheres. "What we can consider as a real maturity involves the efficient organization and integration of experience with all of the problems that are inherent in all the areas in which man operates" (Solomon, 1954, p. 215).

OCCUPATION

According to Peter Drucker, a well-known management consultant, "The probability that the first job choice you make is right for you is roughly one in a million. If you decide your first choice is the right one, chances are you are just plain lazy" (Hall, 1968, p. 22). That is an extremely cogent remark, especially in light of the widely held view that when a young adult enters into an occupation he is also donning a community status, establishing social parameters, and perhaps even patterning marriage and family. Indeed, work choice is often the predominant determinant of one's entire style of life as an adult. For many people this decision is often whimsically or mistakenly made in that the information, experience, and self-knowledge which would enable them to make a wise decision are not yet acquired.

For most men, and some women, in our society, the chief developmental activities in young adulthood relate to job adjustment. Often the major education for an individual seeking an occupation is the knowledge and skills necessary for a particular line of work. Frequently preparation has already begun in high school or college, especially when students could identify interest areas while still in adolescence. When there are job-related difficulties which point to inadequate preparation or inappropriate vocation selection, the question arises whether high school and college vocational counselors and programs are imperceptive or whether decisions regarding life occupations are made prematurely before men and women have sufficient psychological knowledge about themselves.

It has been suggested that some college graduates realize, when seeking employment, that they are essentially postadolescents with self-identity and authority conflicts yet to be resolved. Others have received excellent, technical education but are lacking in instruction in interpersonal skills, so desperately needed in most work situations (Schein, 1968). Schein found that 50 percent of the 1964 graduates of Massachusetts' Institute of Technology Sloan School of Management left their jobs, as did 67 percent of the 1963 graduates and 73 percent of the 1962 graduates. Some of the latter group were working in their third or fourth job. Other graduates say that their formal education, although ostensibly job-related, was largely not relevant to actual job requirements.

The choice of occupation is often an overdetermined one in that a variety of motives operate simultaneously. In this culture desires for challenge and growth, enjoyment and satisfaction, and economic security or power are usually the strongest ones. The orientation toward achievement and upward mobility by which success or failure is measured often plays a major role. Through the selection of an occupation one begins to utilize particular potentialities of himself— technical, interpersonal, intellectual, creative, etc. As he moves into an increasingly stable position, other systems also may become involved, such as friendship, social, and community networks. Sometimes the presentation of one's self is almost completely linked with occupation, so that an individual is known and judged by what he does rather than by what he is.

Problems of vocational choice are more significant to men than to women at present, in that marriage and children still take priority over career development for many women. However, women who do not aspire to a place in the world of work are sometimes inextricably bound to their husband's career choice, which may bring them to either the peak of satisfaction or the depths of despair. For other women, entry or reentry into an occupation after perhaps 10 to 20 years of mothering may create tremendous stress. Their occupation-related talents and skills frequently have been understimulated and unchallenged. With great effort these women strive for an economic position which allows them to express their needs for independent achievement after a 15-year moratorium.

Our culture offers few unambiguous guidelines for adolescents and young adults to assist them in preparing for the occupation of their choice, with the exception of certain highly specialized careers which have clear-cut steps which must be completed before admission to that career is granted. Nonetheless, by the late teens and early twenties, unless military service has interrupted vocational advancement, young adults are expected to attain full adult status through commitment to a suitable occupation or profession. From a developmental point of view, when the selection congruent with the individual's overall physical and psychological maturity has not been premature and has evolved gradually occupational choice will be made without undue stress. But if such a choice stems from unresolved conflicts from the past, severe ramifications may eventually emerge. The decision to pursue achievement in one area versus another may stem from the need to be more financially secure than one's parents were. If the family of origin was economically stable, then the need may be to maintain a comparable status. Pressure from family members, notably parents, may interfere with the young adult's choice of occupation. When career advancement is slow or dubious, especially for upward-striving persons, frustration and mild depression may ensue. Perhaps the most devastating discovery is that one has not made the right choice. Many adults now are forced into untimely or unexpected confrontation between self needs and employment needs, especially in such fields as electronics and aerospace. It is an occupational hazard that one's employment may be terminated in one's thirties and forties. For some persons this has provided the incentive to embark on other, more productive endeavors. For others it has meant agonizing reappraisals of life's values which often precipitate depressions and withdrawal responses. Another built-in hazard, for those adults who are not "mobicentric men," is the movement from one place to another depending on business or corporation needs (Jennings, 1970). Mobicentric men value change (prime examples are the business executive and the hippie); for others, the repeated uprootings may result in individual or family crises.

MARRIAGE

"The monogamous marriage not only has positive social impact, but also allows for the greatest personal intimacy and involvement in a continuing collaborative endeavor. In addition, it goes a long way toward simplifying a person's existence by establishing efficient and dependable routines of living" (Rosenbaum and Alger, 1968, p. x). This statement reflects the mainstream beliefs associated with the state of marriage. Although there is often an extended period between high school or college completion and marriage, the expectation and advantages of eventual marriage have been clear. In all societies, structured relationships of some kind are established between adults of both sexes.

In the United States, marriage has undoubtedly been the relationship which is most highly rated. The married pair, preferably wth children, has constituted the basic social unit through which culture has been transmitted. But now the divorce rate has increased about three times what it was a half-century ago. According to Weiss (1970):

Although we have only imperfect statistics on divorce, and hardly any statistics on separation and desertion, it would appear that the chances of a marriage ending for some reason other than the death of one of the spouses is better than one in four, and perhaps approaches one in two.

This should lead us to consider whether there are facets of marriage in this society which make the promise of marriage difficult for some and impossible for others to realize. The fact of impermanence of the marital state has already so shattered adolescents' and young adults' romantic idealism regarding marriage that many alternatives to this previously highly desirable state are now sought after. Perhaps part of the difficulty relates to the nature of marriage in contrast to other extended intimate adult relationships, in that it becomes a very public matter, carrying social status and legal responsibilities. Community interest in marriage never wanes; couples are ceaselessly reminded that they are under surveillance, with duties in regard to the way they fulfill their roles as spouses and/or parents.

According to many marriage counselors, a major prerequisite for a successful marriage is the requirement that the persons involved have achieved independence from their own families, that is, independence sufficient to allow for intimacy with another adult as well as the ability to further one's own integration as a separate and autonomous but interdependent being.

Sexual desires and the desire for children are strong motives propelling one toward marriage. The rigid delineation of behaviors into sex-linked roles has also weighed heavily on the desire of many persons to marry. For persons raised in families where activities and functions were clearly dichotomized into male and female categories, the sense of incompleteness and need for a counterpart is often especially strong. Another impetus stems from the universal incest taboo. One's generic family usually frustrates the expression of sexual feelings within the family system. The resolution of the oedipal triangle encourages gradual emotional independence from the family. A new union is then sought with a person of the opposite sex.

The process of selecting a mate is fraught with conscious and unconscious elements and contingent upon a host of developmental and current experiences. Successful ego development is possible, in part, through the resolution of a series of ambivalent object relationships to an outcome which enables one to move toward satisfying future relationships. If early family relationships were predominately "good," the chances for gratifying, mature adult relationships are far greater than in families with poor relationships. If the parents were preponderantly frustrating or hostile, the person will experience persistent unfulfilled needs relating to his parents which he will most likely attempt to meet through his spouse. If the spouse is unprepared, or unable, to fulfill his expectations, resentment, disillusionment, and frustration occur and, finally, marital conflicts. These dynamics operate not only unconsciously, but also ambivalently. The mate selected is expected to help resolve one's conflicts, but at the same time there is also the hope that he will help maintain the status quo. The stronger the unconscious determinants, the less possible "free" marital choice becomes.

Dicks has written, "Marriage is the nearest adult equivalent to the original parent-child relationship. Thus its success must revolve around the freedom to regress" (Dicks, 1963, p. 129). From his point of view, the expression of parent-child residue becomes a condition of growth and is what we all seek in the ideal mate (Dicks, 1963, p. 129):

> To be able to regress to mutual childlike dependence, in flexible role exchanges, without censure or loss of dignity, in the security of knowing that the partner accepts because he or she projectively identify with, or tolerate as a good parent this "little needy ego" when it peeps out—this is the promise people seek when they search for the one person who will be unconditionally loving, permissive, and strong—who will enable one to fuse all past object relations into a meaningful whole and be enhanced by it.

When young adults, struggling with their identity in a number of spheres, fail to fulfill certain dimensions of marriage, especially when expectations are not openly communicated, the basis for mental disharmony and perhaps divorce is set.

Sexual expression during courtship or dating, honeymoon, and early stages of marriage is usually experienced by couples as irresistible and overwhelming. Sexual attraction is probably perceived to be the major characteristic endearing one person to the other. In addition to the overpowering nature of sexual drives, man and woman must experiment with sexual behavior in order to learn what feels most pleasurable to self and the beloved one. Patterning and pacing of affectionate gestures and sexual intercourse may undergo several changes, until the spouses establish the height of mutuality. Working out sexual preferences and differences simply parallels the effort which must be made in other areas of marriage—role relationships and functions, whether complementary or symmetrical.

Sexual problems which emerge may reflect temporary adjustment difficulties of indicate more deep-seated difficulties. Interpretations of male impotence, for example, range from fear of engulfment and/or destruction by a woman while having intercourse, to less pathological explanations such as anxieties due to inexperience, or lack of knowledge about his wife and her wants. Frigidity in the woman may be a clue to her fear of intimacy or fear of "letting go" or lack of preparation through foreplay. Her husband may show a subtle or obvious lack of concern about her readiness which produces feelings of resentment and inability to enjoy mutuality. Sexual stalemates between spouses frequently mirror power struggles which originated from other issues, such as distribution of labor within the home and economic decisions related not only to expenditures but also to the determination of who shall have the right to gainful employment. In a healthy marriage, in time, sex becomes more integrated and predictable, but sought after nonetheless, because it continues to be quite pleasurable and rewarding.

In light of strong criticism now being leveled at marriage as an institution, it is interesting to note that a book has come out in favor of this arrangement, but with some reformation. George and Nena O'Neill, authors of *Open Marriage,* think that marriage need not be abandoned but that it needs to be reshaped as a relationship which is mutually fulfilling because it allows for growth of both persons within and outside of marriage. Marriage can be salvaged if the role enactment required by the legal nature of marriage does not preclude development of individuality within the two-person union.

PARENTHOOD

Parenthood is a developmental crisis in that, from the moment birth occurs, marriage is irreversibly altered. Homeostasis is shattered, and when equilibrium is reestablished, which may require months, it is accompanied by profound changes. The fact of birth renders some familiar patterns of interacting for the parents obsolete. Birth necessitates development of schedules, communication, and interpersonal behaviors which incorporate and stimulate the new infant. Ideally, parenting should occur at the height of one's physical, emotional, and intellectual development, and within a marriage, but actual situations rarely approximate perfection. However, it is remarkable that spouses who have varying, if not opposing, backgrounds and attitudes regarding child care and inadequate self views respond to untimely babies with responsible and growth-facilitating behavior.

Pregnancy is an anticipatory period when an offspring is known to exist but at the same time is not visible and is an unknown entity to the prospective parents. And the change in family dynamics may even begin during these nine months in that fantasies and anxieties about the unborn baby begin to emerge and influence the relationship between the husband and wife. The actual preparation for the baby which occurs also points to potential and significant changes. According to Rainwater, attitudes and behavior regarding family planning are influenced by two social class factors: the role expectations of the spouses in their marital relationship and the behavior and values expected of men and women outside the family (Rainwater, 1965). Dyer found when he interviewed urban middle-class parents whose first child was under two, that 53 percent of the couples had a "moderate" or "severe" crisis with the birth of their first child. Couples who were rated as having good marital adjustment and some who had been married for three or more years reported less crises (Dyer, 1963). Christensen's research indicated that perhaps 20 percent of all first births in our society were conceived before marriage (Christensen, 1966). That means at least one-fifth of American couples are denied a sufficient experience with marriage before embarking on parenthood. It does not seem surprising that the parental role produces severe reactions in that couples are suddenly faced with a totally dependent infant who requires relentless 24-hour care. The transition from a marriage to a family is sudden and abrupt. The adjustment is further accented because there are few guidelines to successful parenthood, and because through their own growth and development spouses have not been adequately or systematically prepared to assume this adult role. It must also be recognized that conception, in contrast to engagement or marriage, even in the age of contraception, may not have been voluntary. As Rossi states, "It [conception] may be the unintended consequence of a sexual act that was recreative in intent rather than procreative" (Rossi, 1968, p. 31).

The symbolic meanings of pregnancy are legend. They include fulfillment of one's biological destiny; opportunity to nurture and mold a new person; a visible expression of a love relationship between husband and wife; evidence of marital consummation, fertility, and virility; proof of equality with one's own parents; and achievement of status, especially in our child-minded society.

On the other hand, pregnancy can signify grave dangers to some potential mothers. Those who are uncertain of their own identity and autonomy, who seriously doubt their capacity for mothering, or who have simultaneous desires for career development may experience severe conflict. For others it means continued competition with mother, exacerbation of unmet dependency needs, fear of pain or mutilation during childbirth, or anxiety or depression during pregnancy. For any one of these reasons or a combination of them, a woman's ability to mother may be temporarily hampered or totally impaired. If there are intrapsychic conflicts or external attenuating circumstances regarding childbearing, the capacity to meet the infant's continuous need for mothering is crucially interfered with.

Unplanned pregnancies, especially the conception premaritally, are known to be associated with greater friction in marriages and higher divorce rates (Arasteh, 1971). Of all the white couples interviewed in a large national sample, 17 percent said that their most recent conception was unwanted and 31 percent of nonwhite couples admitted this

(Whelpton et al., 1966). Postpartum psychoses are also associated with unplanned pregnancies among women who already have a history of nervous complaints (Nilsson et al., 1967). All of this is rather alarming in view of the widespread availability, supposedly, of contraceptive pills and devices. From the medical and technical viewpoint, the problem of controlling numbers of human population has been solved. Obviously the same cannot be said for the individual and social psychological aspects of contraception. Contraception could be so helpful in that it permits the timing of offspring. Adults can now plan deliberately whether or not to have children, when, and how many. But the issues around conception are many and complex, and the need to produce offspring, even out of wedlock, remains a strong and frequently gratified desire.

In this society, part of the difficulty for women and men with natural and strong desires for generativity and creativity who are eager to parent is the absence of parent substitutes such as existed when extended families were more prevalent. Particularly in urban areas the individual parent's responsibility is increased in that neighborhoods consist of small, separate, nuclear families who are often strangers to their neighbors. What is seen as the problem of modern mothers may be society's failure to establish substitutes for the relatives who used to participate in caring for babies and children. Also, "it may be that the role requirements of maternity in the American family system extract too high a price of deprivation for young, adult women reared with highly diversified interests and social expectations concerning adult life" (Rossi, 1968, p. 27). Rossi even suggests, "The possibility must be faced, and at some point researched, that women lose ground in personality development and self-esteem during the early and middle years of adulthood whereas men gain ground in these respects during the same years" (Rossi, 1968, p. 34). The increasing acceptance of women, including wives and mothers, into the labor markets points to the need for child care centers staffed by competent parental surrogates and child care professionals.

Also worthy of serious consideration is the impact of what is called *sex-role blurring* as men and women move away from traditional sex-linked behaviors, such as the masculine instrumental role and the feminine integrative one (Parsons and Bales, 1955). If our society liberates itself from the rigid male-female role concepts, the resulting behavioral freedom may develop more spontaneous and integrated parents—which may have profound implications for the next generations.

As children grow older, the interplay between them and their parents may lead to problems and conflicts—difficulties which seem to stem from the inevitable confrontation between the youngster, who is striving for identity, and his parents, who think they have found theirs. But within the parents may occur the reactivation of residual unresolved areas of conflict from their own family of origin, as they parallel events in the family they have sired. Adolescent turmoil in particular creates havoc in American families when the parents' past is rekindled by their teen-agers' activities, values, and conflicts. At another level parents must cope with their constantly changing roles depending on the phase of their child's development, on the needs specific to that phase, and on society's dictates and pressures.

Parental failures are usually more newsworthy than their successes, as any perusal of the mass media will show. Parents are answerable to many professionals should anything happen to their child. Yet, with few exceptions, parents are amateurs in childrearing. The prevalence of Freudian theory, with it's emphasis on the irrevocable programming which occurs during the first five years of life, has further frightened parents. Also injurious and unjust to parents, according to Brim, is the view that many parent educators may have been unconsciously presenting their middle-class values for all parents to emulate, rather than presenting information, guidelines, and problem-solving techniques. Such information should be free of value judgments and derived from the variety of subcultural groupings which influence childrearing patterns (Brim, 1959). It is well known that social class patterns vary widely, but this fact has often been seemingly overlooked in books and advice for parents raising children.

Even Norbert Wiener, the genius behind the development of the modern computer, wrote, "Thus, like all families, we had our problems to consider and our decisions to make. I am neither certain of the correctness of the policies I have adopted nor ashamed of any mistakes I might have made. One has only one life to live, and there is not time enough in which to master the art of being a parent" (Weiner, 1956, p. 224).

TRENDS IN YOUNG ADULT LIFE

A major issue confronting the world of young adults in the 1970s is that of differentiating between behavioral symptoms induced by society's inequities and malfunctioning and those created by the individual's intrapersonal, neurotic conflicts. A serious student of human development and psychopathology can no longer confine his interest to the intricate interplay between individual men and women and between children and parents. Society's role in forced injustices, stereotyping, exploitation of minority groups, and sexual typecasting must be included as central to the struggle for the attainment of maturity, etiology of crisis, and behavioral reactions, and to the development of frustrations in young adult life.

The Hippie Movement and Communes

When one uses a systems approach to the study of the adult developmental stage, group reactions rather than strictly individual ones become the focus of interest. In the United States, perhaps the most visible trend was the hippie movement, or the counter-culture. As an adult developmental reaction, this revolution involved rejection of the larger society, including many of its customary practices in work, marriage, childbearing, and childrearing. In terms of collective action, the movement lacked strength, but its effect on traditional values has been enormous, since the new norms were frequently in total opposition to the established ones.

The "hip scene" originated among the flower people, who were mostly teen-agers, during the summer of 1966 in the Haight-Ashbury district of San Francisco. But those who went on to become "genuine hippies," in that they considered themselves free from society's constrictions and hypocrisies, and truly espoused love, brotherhood, and nonviolence, were well into their twenties but "under thirty." Johnson, in discussing the beatnik movement of the fifties headed by Kerouac and the hippie movement of the late sixties was struck by the large numbers in the eighteen-to-thirty age range. It was his contention that they were passing through delayed adolescence experiencing a prolonged period of attempting to resolve their adolescent ambivalence and conflicts into the usually productive adult years. He pointed to the importance of the peer group, the reaction against authority and established mores, and the rigid standards akin to the rebellion seen in earlier phases of development (Johnson, 1969).

This older hippie's removal of himself from the establishment often occurred after deliberate and agonizing confrontation between individual and societal values. His rejection was not impulsive, and it was total, and he often physically isolated himself within a commune (of which there are now probably several hundred). According to Kanter, (1970, p. 53)

Communes have been started by political radicals, return to the land homesteaders, intellectuals, pacifists, hippies and dropouts, ex-drug addicts, behavioral psychologists following B. F. Skinners' *Walden Two,* humanistic psychologists interested in environments for self-actualization, Quakers in South America, ex-monks in New Hampshire, and Hassidic Jews in Boston.

Generally the communal population strives to create a healthy family system in that they incorporate some characteristics of extended families, such as collective and shared childrearing, interpersonal warmth, and closeness of relationships. Some communes place greater emphasis on changing traditional roles between men and women, especially the monogamatic arrangement; although pairing may occur in some circles, generally several adults are sexually and emotionally accessible to each other.

Sexual Behavior

The advent of contraception and legitimate abortion have been instrumental in freeing sexual behavior, but the emergence of new ways of thinking about adult relationships have also found expression in the area of sex. Some of these new ways of thinking about adult relationships include: (1) the question of whether or not marriage has become outmoded as a basic requirement for family life in Western culture; (2) people seeking to change attitudes in regard to sexual behavior as well as increasing their options for a variety of marriage arrangements; (3) the possible failures of marriages to fulfill personal and social purposes, which increasing numbers of divorces would indicate, and (4) the question frequently raised by divorce of whether it is an inept attempt to resolve a problem or a step which facilitates the process of maturation in both partners.

Many young adults engage in sexual intercourse without reference to procreation or marriage. Many choose to live together without formal marriage, bound by affection and love rather than by legal or religious sanction.

For growing numbers of those already married, the liberalization of views regarding extramarital sex and the interest in group marriages or partner switches, although scarcely a mass movement, represent very appealing alternatives to monogamous marriage. Charles and Rebecca Palson made an 18-month participant observation study of 136 swingers. Instead of finding that swinging created jealousy or mental problems or splits among the couples, they concluded that this activity in some instances had quite positive effects on the marriage. According to the researchers, "It does this by re-romanticizing marriage, thereby making it tolerable, even enjoyable to be married. In a very important way, then, swinging is a conservative institution" (Palson and Palson, 1972, p. 37). It has been predicted that swinging will become part of marriage for from 15 to 25 percent of couples (Palson and Palson, 1972).

Psychology Today's research questionnaire on sexual attitudes and practices received more than 20,000 responses. Certainly the findings cannot be applied to the general young American public, but they do reflect the attitudes of the politically liberal, young, well-educated adults of relatively high socioeconomic status (Athanasiou et al., 1970).

Examples of findings are that less than one in ten recommend virginity until marriage. Forty percent of the married men and 36 percent of the married women engage in extramarital sex. Although group marriage is approved of by twice as many men as women, 9 percent altogether favor this arrangement. And less than 50 percent actually disapprove. Forty percent of the men, compared with 25 percent of the women, said that "having children had an entirely positive effect on marriage. Women tend to say that . . . the effect was negative, or both positive and negative." Regarding abortion, two-thirds were in favor of the availability of legal abortion on demand.

The sexual revolution has by no means stabilized at this moment in history; but as new attitudes and behaviors become incorporated and accepted into American life, we can expect important changes with accompanying stresses in young adult life styles.

Women's Liberation Movement

A movement with great impetus and numbers is women's liberation, or the new feminism. If, as the result of this movement, the basic status of women does change, it is certain then that family, childrearing, and society at large will also undergo marked changes. According to Shulamith Firestone, "The heart of woman's oppression is her child-bearing and childrearing roles" (Firestone, 1970, p. 72).

Germaine Greer maintains that: "The 'normal' sex roles that we learn to play from our infancy are no more natural than the antics of a transvestite" (Greer, 1971, p. 21). Although these pronouncements may sound radical and overly rhetorical, they are challenging traditional beliefs—such as the privacy of the nuclear family with its sex-linked role models, or the idea that the mother-child relationship is crucial to a child's optimal development.

The maternal instinct is being attacked as a myth perpetrated by, and comfortable to, males. And Margaret Mead maintains that the accentuation of the continuing mother-child relationship, with the view that separation is injurious if not irreversibly traumatic, is one devastating form of antifeminism committed by males. She says, "On the contrary, cross-cultural studies suggest that adjustment is most facilitated if the child is cared for by many warm people" (Mead, 1971, p. 477).

The attacks on obvious inequities between men and women in

relation to employment and educational opportunities are being taken quite seriously. Suggestions for change in our most basic of social structures, the family, are far less warmly received. Yet who can look at the family pattern of the dominant mother and ineffectual father, which purportedly produced so much pathology in offspring, without wondering whether there is not some connection between that sick system and the external social and sexual inequalities. In the privacy of the home the battleground was erected and the battles culminated in psychological and sometimes physical damage to the children as well as to the spouses (Miller and Mothner, 1971).

Chesler, a New York psychologist, entitles an article of hers "Men Drive Women Crazy." Her explanation of the fact that more women seek psychotherapy than men is that women are permitted and encouraged to do so, and therapy, like marriage, is an approved institution of social control. In writing about woman's unhappiness, she states: "Most women are unhappy because they have been trained to be passive and dependent in a world that values activity and strength" (Chesler, 1971, p. 97). As major upheavals do occur as a result of woman's changing self-view and consequent behavior, the nature of interaction between women and men, and between women and children, will also undergo monumental change.

Gay Liberation

Bisexuality and/or homosexuality are prevalent responses which often have their onset during the young adult years. Prior to the 1960s, homosexuals were categorized as sexual perverts, undesirable citizens, and malignant influences in need of psychotherapy and/or hospitalization. In recent years, especially in certain urban areas, homosexuals have become a recognized and articulate minority group. The old stereotype of the homosexual which kept homosexuals on the lunatic fringe of society is now giving way to the view that homosexual acts are natural responses of affection felt for members of the same sex.

Many writers now cease to represent homosexuals as tragic, guilt-ridden people; instead they represent them as individuals who have selected an alternative style to the heterosexual way of life. Homosexuals themselves are exposing their oppression and are confronting the vast majority of adults who condemn their homosexual choice. The stigma of homosexuality has by no means disappeared. But homosexuals have managed increasingly to assert themselves with pride and anger despite their lack of genuine acceptance by the rest of society.

It has been estimated that one in twenty adults is homosexual

(Magee, 1966). It is only a small percentage of that one in twenty who seek therapy, because many have made a satisfactory adaptation to a homosexual way of life. Nonetheless, "There are very few who do not feel, at least in part, the need to live a double life" (Altman, 1971, p. 29). They still experience persecution, discrimination, and intolerance, as well as religious views that they are sinful. Freud did not consider homosexuality an illness, but many modern psychiatrists do. Treatment has ranged from intensive, long-term analysis to aversion therapy. Goals of treatment have ranged from optimum adjustment to a homosexual way of life to complete conversion to heterosexual behavior. One can expect that the traditional clinical interpretations of sexual "deviancy" will be submitted for serious reappraisal. If the social and psychodynamic interpretations of homosexuality change, attitudes and therapeutic programs will also undergo important modifications.

PSYCHIATRIC NURSING IN RELATION TO YOUNG ADULT DEVELOPMENTAL REACTIONS

The psychiatric nurse's major task, prior to actual intervention with young adults, is to identify his own attitudes and opinions regarding this stage of development. There is a need to recognize, analyze, and eliminate the biases, stereotypes, and misinformation which abound in the media and in the helping professions and to understand adults— their behavior, values, problems, role conflicts, and adaptation patterns in the process of maturing. The psychiatric nurse, who is often a member of the young adult category, also has the task of separating his own "growing pains" from those observed in others. It is mandatory that the multiple and complex influences which determine behaviors in each of us be properly appreciated and clearly defined so that one can perceive a situation from the client's perspective rather than from one's own. Authentic and therapeutic encounters can proceed only when this prerequisite is met.

As potential adult stresses are enumerated and defined, it becomes obvious that preparation for adult living is woefully inadequate at the high school and college levels. In addition to the concentration on the knowledge clusters and technical aspects of job preparation (which, as it exists, is insufficient), courses are needed at these levels which focus on all facets of adult living. Sex education, recently introduced, is a breakthrough, but equal time needs to be allotted to other dimensions of individual expression and interpersonal relationships as well as to other aspects of adulthood, such as marriage (including alternatives to marriage), parenting, and childrearing.

In terms of primary prevention, if psychiatric nurses want to be instrumental in decreasing harmful psychosocial influences and increasing health-facilitating influences, they must get involved with institutions preparing people at the high school and college levels. Nurses could be originators, coordinators, and/or teachers of courses which focus on the adult and his needs in a changing society. For example, a nurse with an understanding of human behavior, family dynamics, and child psychology is quite capable of teaching courses which relate to crises in adult and family relationships, as well as of teaching courses in normal growth and development. In relation to specific crisis events—both developmental and accidental—courses can be designed which include information and discussion on the nature of the risks, possible outcomes, alternate ways of dealing with stress, and professional and community resources, all richly interwoven with actual examples from life experiences.

Psychiatric nurses, in their efforts toward primary prevention of mental illness, are often able to initiate contact with high-risk populations. This category would include persons generally found in physicians' offices, prenatal clinics, unemployment offices, prisons, divorce courts, and centers for unmarried mothers, as well as new community residents, the poor, welfare recipients, and parents of premature, deformed, or mentally retarded infants and children. A nurse could establish individual, group, or family conferences with both educative and therapeutic aims. For example, prospective parents undergo a tremendous psychological upheaval as they move from traditional male-female sex roles to an individualistic, egalitarian approach to parenting. The role diffusion which results leads in some instances to temporary disorganization and disintegration of the family unit. Dissemination of health information, accompanied by frank and open seminar discussions led by a psychiatric nurse or other mental health professional, could prevent unnecessary symptomatology and loss of functioning in many young adults. Another relevant topic for exploration is that of childless marriages, which are becoming increasingly popular and respectable as a result of the current problem of overpopulation. Spouses can be happy and fulfilled without children, especially if their attitudes toward children are not hostile or ambivalent and if the absence of children is not contrary to their personal and cultural concepts of the good life.

Sometimes the nurse may prefer to act as a consultant to other professionals or paraprofessionals who are already engaged with client groups rather than to be the discussion leader, or he may prefer to evaluate the results of programs already in operation or to launch experimental programs for specific populations as a researcher.

Many researchers have found that young adults experience symptomatic reactions and incapacitating illnesses. Eisler and Polak assessed the social and situational events preceding the psychiatric hospital admission of 1,500 patients and collected specific data on the relative frequency of these stressors for 172 patients in four major psychiatric diagnostic groups (schizophrenia personality disorder, depression, and transient situational reaction). They identified fifteen social system stressors: marriage, work, migration (relocation), illness, financial, problems, separation, death, sex, pregnancy, legal difficulties, school, family, childhood, adolescence, aging, and interpersonal relationships. The average age of the males was 31.77 and of the females, 30.96. Findings showed an average of three stressors in the two-year period preceding admission. Nearly one-half were marital and/or family stress, one-third were actual or threat of separation, and one-half, in the males, were work stresses (Eisler and Polak, 1971).

Paykel and others interviewed 185 depressed patients and 938 community residents regarding stressful life events. They found that the depressed patients reported almost three times as many such events as the controls in the six months prior to the depressive episode. The prevalent events cited were marital difficulties, deaths, illnesses, and work change. It would appear from these studies that a series of developmental and accidental crises do act as precipitants to behavioral reactions and classical symptomatology in young adults, with due appreciation, of course, for the role played by community resources, family and social systems, and personality characteristics of the person experiencing the event (Paykel et al., 1969).

Statistics from the federal government for the year 1968 show alarming facts. The statistics came from the following four categories: first admissions to public mental hospitals, first admissions to private mental hospitals, discharges from general hospitals with psychiatric services, and terminations from outpatient psychiatric clinics. The age groups ranging from twenty to forty-four years accounted for from 44 to 47 percent of the total patient population, although they represent less than one-third of the total life span (United States Department of Health, Eucation, and Welfare, 1968).

The psychiatric nurse becomes an agent of secondary prevention, that is, treatment, when the responses to stress and crises have already occurred. With knowledge of early signs and symptoms of anxiety and conflict, the nurse can combine observational and interviewing skills to assess the clients for whom he will provide nursing care. This includes participation in early diagnoses and referrals and the identification of problematic or ineffectual reactions. The nurse may also suggest treatment techniques of choice on the basis of familiarity with the client and his experiences. He may also engage, individually or in collaboration with other mental health professionals, in a variety of treatment modalities. Intensive one-to-one therapy with the goal of significant personality change for the client may be used. Group therapy for a variety of purposes may be the preferred mode of treatment when several young adults are available for sessions. For groups of mothers, impoverished intellectually by constant and isolated care of young children, major treatment goals may be environmental manipulation and utilization of community resources rather than character shifts or uncovering of marital problems. Suburban housewives, who develop feelings of estrangement and depression, often with concomitant problems of alcohol and drug addiction as the result of trying to keep up with competitive, successful, commuting husbands, may need intensive group therapy to develop a sense of autonomy, self-worth, and personal identity separate from that derived from their husbands' careers. Family therapy may be indicated for conflicts between parents and children, and marital therapy for tensions residing primarily in the marital relationship.

The competent nurse clinician, prepared at the graduate level, can be active at all levels and through every phase of young adult care. Treatment modalities, which require an understanding of their theoretic bases, working principles, and supervised experience, include short- and long-term individual, group, and family therapy and crisis intervention. Treatment may often be provided within the community through community mental health centers, private clinics, and general or psychiatric hospitals, as well as in non-health agencies and in the patient's home.

Nurses mainly involved in rehabilitation or tertiary prevention must have frequent communication with their hospitalized patients, as well as their families or friends outside the institution. It is also necessary to ensure that patients maintain the social contacts on their own to prevent social alienation and withdrawal. Creating a therapeutic environment (interpersonal and physical) which is stimulating and which permits patients to function at their optimum can also be very helpful.

Often persons in their twenties and thirties with diagnoses of manic depressive psychoses and schizophrenic reactions, especially the paranoid type are admitted to mental hospitals. If their response to drugs and/or psychotherapy is not immediately evident, and it sometimes is not, the full-treatment regimen is often discontinued and the beginning stages of chronicity and inadequate social function appear.

Whether the regressive course is inevitable or contributed to by our current lack of knowledge and skills to reverse certain human processes, it is essential that the quality of life be upheld by psychiatric nurses and that these nurses relentlessly pursue treatment and research efforts to guarantee use of clients' maximum potential.

REFERENCES

Allen, James R., and Louis, J. West (1968): "Flight from Violence: Hippies and the Green Rebellion," *American Journal of Psychiatry,* vol. 125, no. 3, pp. 120–126.

Altman, Dennis (1971): *Homosexual,* Outerbridge and Dienstfrey, New York.

Anthony, James, and Therese Benedek (eds.) (1970): *Parenthood,* Little, Brown and Company, Boston.

Arasteh, J. D. (1971): "Parenthood: Some Antecedents and Consequences: A Preliminary Survey of the Mental Health Literature," *Journal of Genetic Psychology,* June pp. 79–202.

Athanasiou, Robert, Philip Shaver, and Carol Tavris (1970): "Sex," *Psychology Today,* July, pp. 39–52.

Bardwick, Judith M. (1971): *Psychology of Women,* Harper & Row, Publishers, Inc., New York.

Bernard, Jessie S. (1956): *Remarriage: A Study of Marriage,* Holt, Rinehart and Winston, Inc., New York.

Birren, James E. (1964): *The Psychology of Aging,* Prentice-Hall, Inc., Englewood Cliffs, N.J.

Bischof, Ledford (1969): *Adult Psychology,* Harper & Row, Publishers, Inc., New York.

Brim, Orville G. (1959): *Education for Child Rearing,* Russell Sage Foundation, New York.

Bromley, Dennis B. (1966): *The Psychology of Human Aging,* Penguin Books, Inc., Baltimore.

Caplan, Gerald (1964): *Principles of Preventive Psychiatry,* Basic Books, Inc., Publishers, New York.

Chesler, Phyllis (1971): "Men Drive Women Crazy," *Psychology Today,* July, pp. 18, 22, 26–27, 97–98.

Christensen, Harold T. (1950): *Marriage Analysis,* The Ronald Press Company, New York.

———(1966): "Scandinavian and American Sex Norms: Some Comparisons with Sociological Implications," *Journal of Social Issues,* vol. 22, pp. 60–75.

Cox, Rachel Dunaway (1970: *Youth into Maturity,* Mental Health Materials Center, New York.

Dicks, H. V. (1967): *Marital Tensions: Clinical Studies towards a Psychological Theory of Interaction,* Basic Books, Inc., Publishers, New York.

———(1963): "Object Relations Theory and Mental Studies," *British Journal of Medical Psychology,* vol. 36, pp. 125–129.

Duvall, Evelyn Mills, and Renton Hill (1953): *When You Marry,* D. C. Heath and Co., Boston.

Dyer, E. (1963): "Parenthood as a Crisis: A Restudy," *Marriage and Family Living,* vol. 25, pp. 96–201.

Eisler, R., and P. Polak (1971): "Social Stress and Psychiatric Disorder," *The Journal of Nervous and Mental Disease,* October, pp. 227–233.

Erikson, Erik H. (1959): *Identity and the Life Cycle,* International Universities Press, Inc., New York.

————(1968): *Identity: Youth and Crisis,* W. W. Norton & Company, Inc., New York.

Firestone, Shulamith (1970): *The Dialectic of Sex,* Bantam Books, Inc., New York.

Goode, William J. (1956): *After Divorce,* The Free Press, New York.

Goulet, L. R., and Paul B. Baltes (1970): *Life Span Developmental Psychology Research and Theory,* Academic Press, Inc., New York.

Greer, Germaine (1971): *The Female Eunuch,* McGraw-Hill Book Company, New York.

Gurin, G., J. Veroff, and S. Feld (1960): *Americans View Their Mental Health,* A Nationwide Survey, Joint Commission on Mental Illness and Health, Basic Books, Inc., Publishers, New York.

Hall, Mary T. (1968): "A Conversation with Peter Drucker on the Psychology of Management," *Psychology Today,* March, pp. 21–25, 70–72.

Heath, Douglas H. (1965): *Explorations of Maturity Studies of Mature and Immature College Men,* Appleton-Century-Crofts, Inc., New York.

Henry, W. E. (1971): "The Role of Work in Structuring the Life Cycle," *Human Development,* vol. 14, no. 2, pp. 125–131.

Jennings, Eugene (1970): "Mobicentric Man," *Psychology Today,* July, pp. 34–35, 70–72.

Johnson, James (1969): "The Hippy as a Developmental Task," *Adolescence,* Spring, pp. 35–42.

Kagan, J., and H. A. Moss (1962): *Birth to Maturity,* John Wiley & Sons, Inc., New York.

Kanter, Rosabeth Moss (1970): "Communes," *Psychology Today,* July, pp. 53–57, 78.

Kelly, E. Lowell (1955): "Consistency of the Adult Personality," *The American Psychologist,* vol. 10, pp. 659–681.

Klerman, Gerald (1971): "Clinical Research in Depression," *Archives of General Psychiatry,* April, pp. 305–319.

LeMasters, E. E., (1970): *Parents in Modern America,* Dorsey Press, Homewood, Ill.

Magee, Bryan (1966): *One in Twenty, A Study of Homosexuality in Men and Women,* Secker and Warburg, London.

Maslow, A. H. (1970): *Motivation and Personality,* 2d ed., Harper & Row, Publishers, Inc., New York.

Mead, Margaret (1970): "A Conversation with Margaret Mead and T. George Harris on the Anthropological Age," *Psychology Today,* July, pp. 59–64, 74–76.

————(1971): "Some Theoretical Considerations on the Problem of Mother-Child Separation," *American Journal of Orthopsychiatry,* October, pp. 471–483.

Miller, Jean B., and Ira Mothner (1971): "Psychological Consequences of Sexual Inequality," *American Journal of Orthopsychiatry,* October, pp. 767–775.

Millet, Kate (1970): *Sexual Politics,* Doubleday & Company, Inc., Garden City, N.Y.

Montagu, Ashley (1968): *The Natural Superiority of Women,* The Macmillan Company, New York.

Mullahy, Patrick (1970): *Psychoanalysis and Interpersonal Psychiatry,* Science House, New York.

Nilsson, A., L. Kay, and L. Jacobsen (1967): "Postpartum Mental Disorders in an Unselected Sample. The Importance of the Unplanned Pregnancy," *Journal of Psychosomatic Research,* vol. 10, pp. 341–347.

Nye, F. Ivan, and Lois W. Hoffman (1963): *The Employed Mother in America,* Rand McNally and Company, Chicago.

O'Neill, George, and Nena O'Neill (1972): *Open Marriage,* M. Evans & Company, Inc., New York.

Palson, Charles, and Rebecca Palson (1972): "Swinging in Wedlock," *Trans-Action,* vol. 9, no. 4.

Parsons, T., and R. Bales (1955): *Family Socialization, an Interaction Process,* Free Press of Glencoe, Ill.

Paykel, Eugene, et al. (1969): "Life Events and Depression," *Archives of General Psychiatry,* December, pp. 753–760.

Rahe, R. H., and T. H. Holmes (1967): "The Social Readjustment Rating Scale," *Journal Psychosomatic Research,* August, pp. 213–218.

Rainwater, L. (1965): *Family Design, Marital Sexuality, Family Size, and Contraception,* Aldine Publishing Company, Chicago.

Rosenbaum, Salo, and Ian Alger (eds.) (1968): *The Marriage Relationship: Psychoanalysis Perspective,* Basic Books, Inc., Publishers, New York.

Rossi, Alice S. (1968): "Transition to Parenthood," *Journal Marriage and the Family,* February.

Ruesch, Jurgen (1964): *Psychiatric Care,* Grune & Stratton, Inc., New York.

Schein, Edgar H. (1968): "The First Job Dilemma," *Psychology Today,* March, pp. 27–37.

Solomon, Joseph C. (1954): *A Synthesis of Human Behavior,* Grune & Statton, Inc., New York.

Sullivan, H. S. (1953): *The Interpersonal Theory of Psychiatry,* W. W. Norton & Company, Inc., New York.

Symonds, P. M. (1961): *From Adolescent to Adult,* Columbia University Press, New York.

——S. Silverman, and M. Wexler (1949): *Adolescent Fantasy,* Columbia University Press, New York.

Theodore, Athena (1971): *The Professional Woman,* Schenkman Publishing Company, Cambridge, Mass.

Trice, Harrison (1966): *Alcoholism in America,* McGraw-Hill Book Company, New York.

U.S. Department of Health, Education, and Welfare, Public Health Service (1968): *Reference Tables on Patients in Mental Health Facilities, Age, Sex, and Diagnosis.*

Vincent, Clark (1961): *Unmarried Mothers,* The Free Press of Glencoe, New York.

Warner, W. Lloyd (1953): *American Life: Dream and Reality,* The University of Chicago Press, Chicago.

Weiss, Robert (1970): "Marriage and the Family in the Near Future," in K. Elliott (ed.), *The Family and Its Future,* J. and A. Churchill, London, pp. 51–61.

Whelpton, P. K., A. A. Campbell, and J. Patterson (1966): *Fertility and Family Planning in the United States,* Princeton University Press, Princeton, N.J.

Wiener, Norbert (1956): *I Am a Mathematician,* Doubleday & Company, Inc., Garden City, N.Y.

6

DEVELOPMENTAL REACTIONS IN THE MIDDLE YEARS

Judith A. Moore

Of all the barbarous middle ages, that which is most barbarous is the middle age of man!

Lord Byron

The transition from young adult life to middle life is difficult because youth is so highly valued in American culture. It is impossible to be unaware of this glorification of youth, for it is stressed in fashion, in films, and in advertisements on billboards, radio, and television. An individual becoming middle-aged must identify with an age group that is not a particularly highly regarded one. The transition to mature adulthood is "equal in difficulty to any other period of transition in the growth and development of people" (Klemme, 1970, p. 21). It brings an awareness that the wonderful years of youth are passing and that one's body has begun its slow decline. But this aging process varies from one person to another; for example, a man of fifty may possess the general physical health of a forty-year-old man but have the hearing of a man of eighty. During this developmental period an individual might be best described in terms of many ages.

What age period sould be included in *middle age?* White (1962, p. 45) wrote that it should be considered as that period of time between adolescence and before old age. The middle-age bracket set by the American Medical Association begins at twenty-five and ends at sixty-five. Young adulthood is an unrecognized era (McCormack, 1973, p. 3). While studying the working class and the middle class, Neugarten (1968, p. 144) found that both social classes viewed the beginning of middle age differently; that is, unskilled workers considered forty as middle-aged and the middle class regarded fifty as middle-aged. Stockwell (1972, pp. 5–6) included ages thirty to sixty-four in his discussion of the middle-aged and reported that there has been an increase in the number of aged and forty to sixty-four in the last 10 years. Clearly, there is no consensus about what constitutes the middle period of life. For the purposes of this chapter, middle age will encompass the years from thirty-five to sixty-five because this would seem to reflect a compromise based on the various age categories mentioned in the literature reviewed by the writer.

The literature reveals that individuals at mid-life have not received much rigorous study. Most research of this age bracket has been "incidental to studies of development or involution or to attempts to plot data over the life span" (Soddy and Kidson, 1967, p. 61). However, recent interest in middle-aged people has sparked more researchers to undertake such study, and some of their findings will be discussed in this chapter, including the male and female climacteric, the empty-nest phenomenon, and the postparental period. Other topics to be covered include problems related to middle-age parenthood, divorce and other marital problems, employment problems of both men and women, unmarried life, and grandparenting.

THEORETICAL PERSPECTIVES

Man in mid-life has been viewed and studied from a variety of perspectives. In Erikson's (1963) work about the eight psychosocial and psychosexual stages of man, he labeled the seventh as one of "generativity versus stagnation." *Generativity* meant concern for creating and guiding the following generation. Individuals who failed to achieve this stage became personally impoverished and stagnated. While this theory of generativity can be easily applied to numerous couples who have achieved it, it fails to take into account current developments such as population explosion, ecological space, and freedom for abortion, which offer alternative goals for many other middle-aged couples. Couples who have chosen not to rear children would not consider themselves as stagnating in time. A study based on the self-image of childless couples might serve to shed further light on the applicability of Erikson's seventh stage to current mid-life developments.

Neugarten (1970) wrote that just as an individual passes through a biological cycle, he passes through a socially defined time cycle that orders major life events. There is a normative pattern that people adhere to generally; that is, there is a time when one is expected to marry, a time to raise a family, and a time to retire. "From this perspective, time is, at least, a three-dimensional phenomenon charting the course of the life cycle, with historical time, life time (or chronological age), and social time all intricately intertwined" (Neugarten, 1970, p. 72). While interviewing 100 middle-aged university graduates about the characteristics of middle adulthood, it was found that the respondents structured their life in terms of time left to live and clocked themselves according to body changes, career changes, and family changes rather than to chronological age. Neugarten speculated that it is not until adulthood that individuals developed their sense of a life cycle with inescapable turning points. From such a point of view, expected life events could not constitute crises, for parenthood, occupational achievement, menopause, and grandparenthood are normal turning points. These events are mere markers in the life cycle that precipitate new adaptations for most people rather than traumatic events leading to mental illness (Neugarten, 1970, pp. 78–79). Such a view of middle adulthood has merit, for it focuses on normal events rather than on negative, psychopathological ones. However, it may be argued that it fails to take into account individual resistance to change and such defense mechanisms as denial, projection, and distortion, which may be used in the service of the psychosocial needs in the personality structure of the individual rather than with respect to the needs of the culture. To discard the notion of crisis seems simplistic, for, as clinicians can attest, clearly many middle-aged individuals lack the personal, interpersonal, and material resources to cope with the developmental reactions encountered.

Gutmann (1967) wrote of his developmental hypothesis concerning the ego psychology of the aging process in adulthood. During the first phase (alloplastic mastery) the individual seeks to master the affairs of the outer world both for the purpose of achievement and for acquisition of independence. "To a statistically significant degree, [more] younger American men (aged 40–54) are characterized by alloplastic mastery" (Gutmann, 1967, p. 28) than are older men. He called the second stage "autoplastic mastery," in which changing the self is emphasized and men become thoughtful and philosophical rather than bent on achievement. Older men (fifty to seventy) display this type of mastery.

As a result of 8 years of intensive interviewing and projective testing of men from diverse ethnic and cultural groups, such as urban middle-class white Americans, Navajo Indians, and Mayan Indians of Yucatán, he acquired empirical evidence that there are universal patterns of age difference. His findings indicated that the human life cycle was an independent event that had fixed psychological implications. There seem to be "internal, mandatory programs of change that will shape thought, imagery and behavior in predictable ways, across a wide variety of cultures" (Gutmann, 1972, p. 418). Men and their patterns of aggression seem to illustrate his point. Young men can use aggression constructively or destructively; they channel it toward productivity, for apparently the experience of marriage and fatherhood provides the incentive needed to deploy productively their potentially combative energies. On the other hand, men of late middle age universally phase out their aggressive energies and tend toward passivity as they replace their aggression with tender, affiliative sentiments. Young men may see a field of corn and see money growing, while older men speak of the lush, green leaves and the plump, ripe kernels. Old men are sensual about the corn while young men merely love what they have produced. The study concluded that younger men repress their sensuality and delay gratification, and that older men are less likely to impose such restraints on themselves. Such a conclusion is supported by Freudian theory, which holds that younger men relegate their sensuality to the genital zones and that parenthood reinforces such a repressive process. If a man is to fulfill his family role as the breadwinner and status winner, he must not be distracted by his sensuality (Gutmann, 1972, pp. 419–422, 446). Klemme (1970, p. 21) made a similar point when he wrote that a man in his productive years must spend his energies on his work task and a man in retirement can afford to redirect his energies.

While the developmental phases outlined by Gutmann may be normal, some men are unable to negotiate a particular stage. They may fixate at one level or regress to an earlier one. In a newspaper article entitled "Stormy Day of 'Mid-Life' Crisis" (San Francisco Chronicle, July 12, 1971, p. 4), an example by Klemme is cited. "A man in his late 30's may resume extramarital dating behavior more characteristic of his earlier 20's and enjoy the relative comfort of behavior already learned, perhaps to avoid the pain of advancing to another developmental level."

Gutmann's work offers an interesting base for understanding men and their stages of adulthood. Empirical evidence supports these phases. But where do women fit into this schema, or do they even fit into such phases? The writer was unable to find in the literature a single comprehensive theoretical framework which had been adequately researched and that encompassed both men and women during mid-life. This work remains to be done and will be a complex study to complete. The conception of a theoretical framework that incorporates biological changes in both sexes, sociohistorical changes, and psychosocial phenomena spanning some 30 years will be a monumental task.

THE EARLY MID-LIFE CRISES

Why have some creative and hard-working persons like Ben Jonson, the playwright, burned out their creativity in their thirties or forties and others, such as Bach, begun to flower then? Jacques (1965) was curious about this and randomly sampled more than 300 men of the arts, music, literature, and science. As a result of his study he wrote that he believed that a mid-life crisis manifests itself in some form in all individuals. The crisis expressed itself in any one of three different ways: (1) the creative career came to an end as in actual death; (2) the capacity for creativity became observable for the first time; or (3) a particular change in the quality or the content of the creativeness occurred. When persons can become constructively resigned to man's imperfections and their own shortcomings related to work, then serenity of work and life can ensue. Moreover, to survive the mid-life crisis and to achieve mature adulthood, one must recognize that death is inevitable and that all men possess hateful feelings and destructive impulses (Jacques, 1965).

People experiencing a mid-life crisis may make compulsive attempts to remain young. To do so in the face of advancing age is the result of a complex personality phenomenon. "Tension between processes of aging and pressures to remain young may contribute to the motivation to maintain the *status quo* which many people show during the middle period of life" (Soddy and Kidson, 1967, p. 105). Other races against time include overconcern with health, increased religious fervor, and the emergence of sexual promiscuity. But new starts are coming to an end. Many early hopes and ambitions must be discarded or be relegated to far corners of the mind and destined to a kind of oblivion. As Jacques so poignantly wrote, "And because the route forward has become a cul-de-sac, attention begins its Proustian process of turning to the past, working it over consciously in the present, and weaving it into the concretely limited future" (Jacques, 1965, p. 513). Those who survive this critical transition best are frequently the ones who use their heads rather than their hands in self-evaluation and in solving life problems (Peck, 1968, p. 89).

WOMEN IN MIDDLE AGE

Two of the four basic anchors that we usually share are an intact body and body image and a meaningful identity and purpose in life (Cath, 1965, p. 174). Women in their forties frequently struggle to hang onto both simultaneously. A woman's life goals are closely related to her body; her self-concept and self-esteem are linked to the appearance and function of her body. Therefore, when a woman has a hysterectomy or a mastectomy, the anchor related to her intact body and body image is lost. Such a loss may be temporary if preoperative and postoperative teaching and counseling by nurses are made available to all women at such times. As youth, beauty, and sexual attractiveness fade, a woman in her forties may want to gratify some of her needs before the opportunity to do so is seemingly lost forever.

Kinsey's studies revealed that by the age of forty, one-fourth of all wives had engaged in at least one extramarital coitus (Packard, 1968, p. 289). The urge to engage in an affair may arise from the wish to recapture the passions of adolescence and early young adulthood. During such a love affair three things may be affirmed—namely, one's lovability, one's youthfulness, and one's desirability as a sexual being. To put it another way, it can be said (Bardwick, 1971, p. 215):

> I love and am alive.
> I am alive and therefore I love.
> I am lovable; I can love; I am a woman.
> I am not yet middle-aged.

Therein lay the ingredients for many successful soap operas, films, and novels. But to make light of all this is to miss the point that women as well as men frequently struggle to avoid their decline.

The female climacteric "refers to the involution or recognition or regression of the ovaries and includes menopause, the cessation of menstruation" (Bardwick, 1971, p. 37). The average age for a woman to experience menopause is forty-seven, an age when her vitality still remains to help her cope with it (Szalita, 1966, pp. 67, 72). Physiologically speaking, the climacteric can create such somatic symptoms as breast pain, hot flashes, and dizzy spells. The latter two are caused by vasomotor disturbances. The menstrual flow may gradually slow down or come to a quick halt. Psychosomatic symptoms include headaches, dizzy spells, transient palpitations of the heart, and mild abdominal and muscular cramps. According to Masserman (1966, p. 48), some women search endlessly for a doctor who will prescribe pills or other medications to delay the "change of life."

Psychological symptoms attributed to the climacteric include irritability, crying spells, depression, confusion, inability to concentrate, anxiety, and hypochondriasis (Bardwick, 1971, pp. 37–38). As her reproductivity declines, the mother is frequently confronted with a daughter's budding sexuality. This observation may leave the mother both anxious and depressed. Additionally, she must come to grips with the fact that her reproductive abilities have come to an end. Many women, though they can never give birth again, reportedly experience an urge to become pregnant again and reexperience the process.

The depression of women during this period is attributed to several different factors: the manner in which prior losses were handled, the depressive problems of earlier life, the lack of important roles, and the subsequent loss of self-esteem. If her major orientation and invest-ment were in the family, then the menopause may be harder on her (Szalita, 1966, p. 18), for she can no longer be a "servant of the species" (Deutsch, 1945, p. 459). When women seek psychiatric treatment during this period, they should first have a physical examination, for not all complaints of middle-aged women can be attributed to psycho-logic or psychosomatic causes.

For some women, the menopausal milestone is one to be celebrat-ed. Freedom from unwanted pregnancy is cause for rejoicing. The capacity for sexual performance and the sexual drive are not blunted, and many women develop a renewed interest in their husbands; they have "a second honeymoon" (Masters and Johnson, 1968, pp. 271–273).

In point of fact the menopause may not be the important event in understanding the psychology of middle-aged women that biologists or psychoanalysts have presumed it to be. Neugarten (1970) conducted interviewing and projective testing on 100 normal women between the ages of forty-three and fifty-three from working-class and middle-class backgrounds. All the women were married, living with their children, and had at least one child, and none had had a hysterectomy. As a group, the interviewees tended to minimize the importance of the menopause and thought it unlikely to produce stress and anxiety. More than half stated that losing their husband was their greatest concern. Two other related research studies were conducted about menopausal symptoms, and Neugarten concluded "that there was little evidence in these data to support a 'crisis' view of the climacter-ium and that the crisis theory in the literature probably reflects basic differences between clinical samples and a community sample" (Neu-garten, 1970, p. 82). Recently the magazine *Ms.* has been proclaiming that "menopause is not a traumatic experience for most women—less than half even consult their doctors about it" (Solomon, 1972, p. 16). It may be that Neugarten has empirically exploded a myth, or it may be that the women interviewed were not being altogether honest about their intensely personal experiences of menopause. Nurses are in a particularly good position to gather more data about women's percep-tions of their menopause. There is opportunity for nursing research to be done. For example, do women who have had a hysterectomy view their climacteric as a crisis? Are they worried about losing their husbands, too? And what about the women who have never married? What is their greatest concern during the climacteric? Neugarten has only touched the surface.

Whether or not the period of the climacteric creates anxiety and depressive episodes for the woman, emphasis needs to be placed on her need to learn to live with the faculties, resources, and adaptability she has, rather than those which she once had. Further, she will need to accept and be less guilty about her emerging aggressive and egocentric impulses.

WOMEN AND WORK

The changes occurring to middle-aged women necessitate that they reflect on the image they have of themselves and the one they present to the world. Such changing imagery may require a developmental adjustment or two. Bardwick believes that "the female's need to establish herself in a loving, intimate relationship, to love and be loved, is dominant" (Bardwick, 1971, p. 158). Further, she adds, maternal needs are paramount, and gratification of these needs at home or work (e.g., nursing or teaching) are motives which are dominant in women (Bardwick, 1971, p. 159). For some women, the closer they are to the reality of entering or reentering a profession, the faster their interest declines and "accidental" pregnancies occur.

Nevertheless, women in middle age are seeking and obtaining jobs. They may reinstate themselves in the kind of work they had prior to marriage and motherhood, begin a new career, or devote themselves full-time to a prior part-time job. Over 40 percent of the women aged thirty-five to forty-four are members of the labor force (Neugarten, 1970, p. 74) and 42 percent of all women between forty-five and sixty-four are working women (Simon, 1968, p. 73). These figures overlap but clearly depict an unmistakable trend, namely, that women tend to return to work when childrearing is finished. They also provide striking evidence in support of research findings that women in the thirty-five to thirty-nine age bracket have high motivation to achieve, and that women fifty-five and older have decreased achievement motivation (Bardwick, 1971, p. 193). In many families children and adolescents grow up in homes in which both mother and grandmother work. The status accorded women for their work roles helps offset the unequal or low status of women in the home. For many women, a well-paying job is not their goal; they throw themselves vigorously into PTA work, volunteer work, or some church or philanthropic ventures.

In payment, they receive necessary boosts to their self-esteem, feel needed, extend their circle of acquaintances, and acquire a rewarding way in which to expend their energies.

In our contemporary society a small minority of families could be called a "dual-career family." Rapaport and Rapaport studied sixteen such families through tape-recorded interviews and found that "the essence of the *dual-career* family as a variety of the partnership family is that there is a division of labor in relation to family functions that is distributed between the partners on an equal-status basis" (Rapaport and Rapaport, 1969, p. 7). Several areas of stress were mentioned in these families. First, there was the overload dilemma. In order to manage both career and home, these couples needed to delegate domestic chores and to deliberately set aside time for leisure activities. Secondly, stress arose as the result of the discrepancy between their personal norms and the social norms of others. Parents were constantly reviewing their own personal norms and values. A third dilemma involved the wives' problems. Women used their occupational world as the place to develop their distinct personal identities. In order to cope with the problem of split identities, most of the women compartmentalized their work role from their wife role or made conscious efforts to minimize their work role to themselves (Rapaport and Rapaport, 1969).

Even though the Rapaports' sample (sixteen families) was small, it represents some guidelines for the prevention or alleviation of stress in dual-career families. Namely, such couples could be counseled about predicted stresses and helped to engage in some problem solving prior to being caught in the middle of some of the dilemmas identified by the researchers. In the face of an ever increasing number of women actively working, we can see that a whole new arena has opened for behavioral and social science study.

MEN AND THEIR INVOLUTION

Cartoons and jokes abound regarding men and middle age. An example: "You have reached middle age when your wife tells you to pull in your stomach and you already have." This is the time for the emergence of so-called "beer bellies," and many a wife busily lets out seams of trousers or buys a larger belt for her husband. Added girth may not be all that's noted in men.

Do men experience an involution, a climacteric, or an "andropause"? The literature reflects little consensus on this question. Soddy and Kidson write that the "male has no counterpart to the visible effects of the cessation of ovulation" (Soddy and Kidson, 1967, p. 95). They point out that we know little about the cessation of spermatogenesis and believe that the only indication of male involution may be a gradual decrease in the level of functions and a lowering of aspirations of the male (Soddy and Kidson, 1967, pp. 95, 361). In contrast Szalita thinks that involution in men is inevitable. "The climacteric in the male has the same biological foundation as the menopause in the female, viz., gonadal insufficiency with concomitant atrophy of the genital apparatus, disturbances in the neuroendocrine balance and emotional reactions of varying degree" (Szalita, 1966, p. 69). More research seems indicated in this area.

Other aspects of men's middle-aging have been studied and continue to be researched. Six researchers at Yale University have completed 3 years of a 4-year study on men aged thirty-five to forty-five. Forty men (executives, blue- and white-collar workers, writers, and biologists) were interviewed. The participants reported that they experienced a turning point, a "male crisis," in their late thirties. This was precipitated by the necessity of facing obvious and indisputable signs of aging; further, they had to assess realistically the fantasies and illusions they had about themselves and their potentials (Scarf, 1972, pp. 76, 120).

The Yale findings are compatible with the studies and writings of Rümke, who reviewed what numerous psychologists and others had written about the variation in human personality. As reported by Soddy and Kidson (1967, p. 139), Rümke identified a period of "productive disintegration" in men around forty years of age. At this time men reassess their lives, note their declining physical and mental capacities, and take stock of their changing body image and the onset of such diseases as circulatory disorders, arthritis, and diabetes. Men may experience difficulty if there are discrepancies between the real and imagined body-image (the concept of body held in the mind) and self-image (the concept of the total self, feelings, body, history, and self-evaluation). It is not uncommon for a man's body-image to be incongruent with his objective physical state. He may function at a minimal and cautious level or drive himself unrealistically (Soddy and Kidson, 1967, pp. 140–141). What nurse has not seen middle-aged man with a coronary thrombosis? Can it be that these men commit "coronary suicide," as Bartemeier suggests? He hypothesized that those men experiencing coronaries may have a self-image unrelated to reality, and a body that they overtax. Premature death is often the outcome. Clinical specialists working in coronary care units are in a unique position to assess middle-aged men and assist them to acquire a more realistic self-image.

The manifestations of anxiety in middle-aged men are numerous. They arise from such things as loss of reproductive capacity, concern about acquiring cancer, worries over job status and finances, and retirement. Is it any wonder that many struggle to keep some form of status quo? Maintenance of the status quo is a way to offset declining powers, as well as a way to provide the constancy of attitude and behavior that the young and society seem to depend upon (Soddy and Kidson, 1967, pp. 143–149).

The current "hippie generation" notwithstanding, most men grow up with the belief that they will work for most of their life. Work is what a man prepares to do and what he does unless unforeseen circumstances intervene. Despite some men who change their careers at mid-life and the growing unemployment figures, the majority seem to prepare for a particular occupation and pursue it, or forms of it, for much of their lives.

There are various occupational difficulties to surmount. In reassessing themselves, some men decide that what they have achieved was not worth the emotional sacrifice involved; they acquire a new freedom from external pressure and decide to spend even more time finding out who they are and what they want (Scarf, 1972, p. 120). Others experience threats to their self-esteem and security upon the realization that they have failed to achieve as much status or earning power as they had hoped, and they give up their starry-eyed ambitions and struggle just to keep their job in the face of all their young competitors (Masserman, 1966, p. 49). Still others pass their days feeling satisfied about prior accomplishments and sense no need to continually prove themselves. The ambitious-executive types may engage in further striving as they seek to climax their careers by further amassed wealth, prestige, and power. Some who receive promotion become depressed, for despite the recognition of a man's capabilities, promotion may mean that he has surpassed his own father's accomplishments and acquired more responsibility and work to boot (Lidz, 1968, pp. 461–462). All this stress occurs at a time when his capacities to deal with stress are diminishing.

Competition may not be relegated solely to the job scene. Narcissistic and immature fathers compete at home with their sons. Benedek (1970, p. 318) cited an example in which a father tried to outdo his son in ten athletic events. He was rushed to the hospital for treatment of a coronary attack after the eighth event. (A better-adjusted father who had come to grips with his own crises would have retired gracefully from such competition.) Middle-aged fathers may be seductive to or be seduced by their adolescent daughters. One middle-aged man seen in family therapy by the writer had been found by his wife fondling and holding his young adult daughter in his arms. It is thought that father-daughter incest is probably more prevalent than has been commonly thought. Those fathers who do not succumb to overt incest may nevertheless be quite attracted to and proud of their daughters, find opportunities to take them out, and be hostile or disgruntled toward their dates. One newly married young man said jokingly that he would tie his as yet unborn daughters "to the bedrails" to prevent them from running off with young men when they were about ready to "leave the nest." Surely he was predicting some of his own middle-aged behavior.

Some men experience great concern over their decline of sexual prowess and physical attractiveness. Fulfillment is sought from women outside the marriage by many middle-aged men. After the age of fifty the incidence of sexual inadequacy takes a sharp rise and secondary impotence increases. Masters and Johnson (1968, pp. 275–278) have enumerated several factors related to the male's altered sexual responsiveness. First, the male's own sexual relationship with his wife may be monotonous. His wife is predictable and he is taken for granted; therefore, the prospect of a new, unfamiliar woman seems most attractive. Secondly, some men are so engrossed in their economic pursuits that they are less responsive sexually. Mental or physical fatigue or infirmity and overindulgence in food or drink are additional factors in the development of impotence. Finally, there is the fear of failure. "Once impotent under any circumstance, many males withdraw voluntarily from any coital activity rather than face the ego-shattering experience of repeated episodes of sexual inadequacy" (Masters and Johnson, 1968, p. 278). Men can be trained out of their secondary impotence. Sexual counselors and therapists have aided many men in regaining their sense of sexual adequacy and ability to perform.

Fathers whose ability to work has not diminished may grow mellow in their attitudes toward their wives and children. They may function as negotiators or peacemakers at home (Benedek, 1970, p. 199). They also become more receptive to the idea that it is all right to become more supportive to their families. Such men find the time to enjoy their occupation, family, wives, and leisure-time activities.

THE UNMARRIED

The literature does not abound with studies of the way in which unmarried heterosexual or homosexual men and women experience middle age. It can be assumed they experience many of the same developmental reactions as the married. Unmarried women may have to confront the fact that being childless has some significance to them. If they have lived with parents, they may easily become the ones designated to care for the parents in their old age. Unmarried men and women may have become so set in their ways that the thought of the task of adapting to married life precludes anything more than simply contemplating marriage. Lacking offspring, they may become very attached to pets. Despite this, many middle-aged single persons do marry widows or widowers, as the desire for companionship outweighs the motivation to stay single.

Lesbians and male homosexuals arrive at the conclusion that their sexual lives will be different from those of others. Despite the contemporary abortive and successful attempts made to marry by both groups, the number of actual marriages of a lesbian to a lesbian and a male homosexual to another male homosexual is small indeed. They support themselves, may or may not come "out of the closet" and declare their lack of heterosexual inclinations, and may or may not find warm and loving relationships with partners of their choice.

It remains a fact that at the present time not all individuals experience the enthusiasm for marriage that their parents and grandparents had. For the unmarried, Lidz concluded that "the realization that the turn toward the end of life has been rounded awakens anxiety and despair in proportion to feelings that one has never lived and loved" (Lidz, 1968, p. 473). The same might be said of all middle-aged people, married or unmarried, homosexual, heterosexual, or asexual.

PARENTHOOD AND MARRIAGE

Concurrently with the physical and emotional changes that occur in middle-aged individuals, they must cope with their family and marital relationships. As middle-aged parents, everything they do seems to be wrong. The law enforcement agencies tell them they lack control over their children. "Otherwise, why would he be on drugs and stealing bikes?" Adolescent children test them to the hilt and complain if they are weak. If parents are strong and intolerant of their children's fluctuating value system, health professionals condemn them for providing too rigid a home environment and for lack of ability to communicate with their children. The emotional crises of their adolescent children generally coincide with their own middle-age crises (Scherz, 1967). So many things influence young people and their attitudes that parents should not receive all the blame. A good majority of parents have done commendable jobs of childrearing.

As for the parents' marriage, it may be "happy, just tolerable, or a cauldron of explosive emotions," as Benedek (1970, p. 196) so aptly describes it. Those happily married become increasingly dependent on each other for companionship and caring. Conceivably, such couples would have many of the traits identified by Packard (1968, pp. 483–489) that seem likely to enhance marital enjoyment. The seven traits are as follows:

1. A large capacity for affection
2. Emotional maturity
3. A capacity to communicate effectively and appealingly to each others' their thoughts and feelings
4. A zest for life
5. The capacity to handle tensions constructively
6. A playful approach to sex
7. The capacity to accept fully the other person with full knowledge of his shortcomings

"Wife-swapping" and "swinging" are two new phenomena for which there have been reported positive as well as adverse effects on middle-aged individuals and couples. Some couples exchange marriage partners for weekends. The marriages may disintegrate rapidly or be healed. The couples' experiences of infidelity may make their lives richer and their companionship closer. Ackerman (1965, p. 156), reports

> In one such case, the wife reacted to the shocking discovery of her husband's romance with an attractive Negro actress with the prompt disappearance of her sexual frigidity. This change delighted her husband and impelled him to characterize his Negro *amour* as the best psychotherapist he and his wife could have had.

"Swinging" in wedlock has been studied. The term "swinging" usually refers to couples in a monogamous marriage who seek a series of sexual encounters with different partners (Constantine and Constantine, 1971, p. 163). One couple spent 18 months in a participant-observation study of 136 swingers. Couples were reached through swinger magazines, personal networks, and contact with the researchers during their lecture tours. Informants came from eight different states; the West, East Coast, South, and Midwest were all represented. Most couples were from the middle class; they were interviewed informally, after which the researchers made field notes. As such a study provided sampling problems, statistics were useless and the sample was not considered representative (Palson and Palson, 1972, p. 29).

Some of the findings of the Palsons' study bear scrutiny. To begin with, they found several couples who had developed emotional involvement and friendships with other swingers. The couples seemed to avoid jealousy by developing their "individuation." The meaning of this term was difficult to decipher from the article, but *individuation* seemed to refer to the fact that each partner recognized his counterpart to be a distinct human being and not merely a person who fulfilled a variety of roles. Another finding was that women were more likely to participate in homosexuality while few men participated in it. Some couples entered swinging as a way to achieve something new. Others entered as a way to experience a part of living they thought they had missed out on because of early marriage and responsibilities. Still other couples engaged in swinging to avoid feeling "trapped." Several couples declared that swinging had led to better communication and even led to a re-creation of romantic feelings that they had had for each other earlier in their marriage. The Palsons concluded that the extramarital activity in swinging often succeeds in solidifying a marriage (Palson and Palson, 1972). Two other writers have concluded that "the most positive contribution of the group sex phenomenon to the non-swinging world is as a preview of things to come" (Margolis and Rubenstein, 1972, p. 345). Herein, both sexes are changing their sexual identities; namely, men are less visibly threatened about their masculinity and women do not demolish the family unit in pursuit of their needs (Margolis and Rubenstein, 1972, p. 345).

But what of the marriage characterized as being a "cauldron of explosive emotion"? The later years can be ones of disenchantment, where marital conflict and unhappiness abound (Pineo, 1963, p. 393). After twenty-plus years of marriage, either partner may consider the other "not good enough for me." "In a society where people are told many times a week about the delights of model-changing, it is easier for a person to wonder why his or her attachment to a used spouse should be any more enduring than that to a used station wagon" (Packard, 1968, p. 287). While it is obviously too simplistic an explanation for divorce, Packard's revealing comment serves the function of bringing to mind a cultural influence on couples. Can they help but be affected by the communication media?

As the children grow older, they may not fulfill the scapegoat role—one that serves the purpose of avoidance of conflict between the spouses. Faced with the loss of the children who provided so much diversion and activity and the fact that they have not kept their marriage relationship in good repair, a couple may conclude that divorce is the only viable alternative. Couples who have kept up "social appearances for the sake of the children" may head for a lawyer when the children go to college or marry. Those with some hope of resolving their differences may seek religious guidance or assistance from mental health professionals. The divorces rate is high. The newly divorced must cope with social pressures and stigma, role changes, the single life, the reactions of children, friends, and relatives, and a lowered or increased sense of self-esteem. Some of those divorced will have matured sufficiently, as a result of the divorce, to select a new mate by using better judgment (Lidz, 1968, p. 469). Still others tend to select a new mate with "hang-ups" similar to those of their former spouse. If individuals weather all this, they remain middle-aged and have further obstacles to surmount happily and successfully or unhappily and unsuccessfully.

THE EMPTY NEST

An event experienced by couples in their forties and fifties is that of the children growing up and leaving the home for college, work, adventure, or marriage. Some mothers experience what is known as the "empty-nest syndrome." It is defined as "the temporal association of clinical depression with the cessation of child rearing" (Deykin et al., 1966, p. 1422). The shift from active childrearing to emotional divorce from the children is a difficult adjustment for some mothers. If such mothers have difficulty dealing with object losses, their problems are magnified. In one Boston study, researchers collected data (narrative case summaries, detailed histories, physicians' and nurses' notes, and social work interviews with families) on sixteen depressed mothers who no longer had childrearing functions. The mothers met the criteria for one of three categories as judged by two of the researchers. The categories were as follows: (1) overt conflict between patient and children at time of hospitalization; (2) latent conflict between mother and child noted by staff but not identified by family members; and (3) no conflict reported by staff or family. Seven women each were categorized as in overt or latent conflict. Those overtly conflicted were foreign-born or first-generation Americans, married as teen-agers, and socially withdrawn; few had ever worked (Deykin et al., 1966). The inference was that the depression of these women could be related to conflicts with children.

Some writers (Bardwick, 1971, pp. 215–216; Benedek, 1970, p. 199) have indicated that the empty-nest period is a crucial period of adjustment, and while their points seem well taken, three empirical studies seem to destroy this belief and relegate it to the status of a myth. Deutscher conducted a door-to-door survey in one upper-class and one lower middle-class socioeconomic area of Kansas City, Missouri. The sample consisted of thirty-one couples who lived alone, were between forty and sixty-five years of age, and had "launched" one to four children. They were asked to what extent they viewed the postparental period favorably or unfavorably. The researchers concluded that the sample provided little support for those observers who hold that postparental life in one of great difficulty (Deutscher, 1968, pp. 263–264).

A second study was one made by Sussman, who attempted to determine "if relationships between generational families were consistently related to behaving in particular social roles in middle-aged couples" (Sussman, 1960, p. 71). Fifty-seven couples between forty-five and sixty comprised the sample. Spouse rules changed significantly in postparental couples of the middle class or in low-continuity families (this term was poorly defined). Upper-class families indicated that changes in their roles had begun while their children were in the early adolescent stage of development. Parents experienced changes as users of leisure time, and most postparental males intensified their work activity. He concluded that radical changes in the lives of parents do not occur immediately after the children leave the home (Sussman, 1960).

Neugarten reports research findings of a study of the presumed "crisis" of the empty nest. "Rather than being a stressful period for women, the empty nest or postparental stage in the life cycle was associated with a somewhat *higher* level of life satisfaction than is found among other women" (Neugarten, 1970, p. 83). Statements made by an actress, Evelyn Keyes, in a newspaper article (quoted in Drewes, 1971, p. 6) seem to characterize such satisfaction.

I am a middle-aged woman, and this is the best period of my life. I feel a peace I never achieved when I was young. I was always twirling, dashing, afraid I suppose of living with myself. Now I enjoy my company very much.

Benedek believes that postparental parents have the developmental task of including the daughter's husband or the son's wife in their own family as well as in their own psychic system as an object worthy of their love. This is accomplished through identification with and separation from their own child. If successful, they become more objective with both child and in-law and less ambivalent toward the new family member (Benedek, 1970, pp. 196–197). Additionally, both parents need to have resolved their questions about their own identity before they become grandparents.

Fortunately, the only place grandmothers get swallowed by wolves is in fairy tales! Grandparents can bring much delight and joy to grandchildren, and vice versa. It is true that the arrival of the first grandchild may evoke both shock ("the third generation") and strange feelings. Where do we learn how to be grandparents? Where can we go to learn about the "psychology of grandparenthood"? Nurses in doctoral study searching for a dissertation topic might well pursue this area, for little is written about grandparenting. Perhaps one of the first clinicians to describe grandmothers was Helene Deutsch. She cited three types: (1) one who continues her own motherhood through her grandparent role, (2) one who enjoys being a grandmother but does not experience it as a continuation of her motherhood, and (3) the "grandmother par excellence" who neither identifies with nor competes with the mother (Deutsch, 1945, pp. 483–486).

Younger grandparents (under sixty-five) tend to be funseekers. They relate informally and playfully with the grandchildren and act like playmates. Leisure time is spent in such a way that authority is unimportant and mutual satisfaction is emphasized (Neugarten, 1970, p. 74). Still, it is hard to escape parenting, for when the young deposit the children with the grandparents with the goal of getting away for a day or an evening, they are asking for that nice dependable-parent image (Simon, 1968, p. 211).

LATE MIDDLE AGE

Basically, America has not had the time or the inclination to sort out late middle age from aging. But during the latter half of middle age (fifty to sixty-five), individuals prize wisdom rather than physical prowess. Socializing rather than sexualizing in human relationships becomes paramount. People are valued as distinct personalities rather than sex objects. The person of late middle age probably has the widest range of contacts with others that he will ever experience. Some grow less flexible in their ways and thinking (Peck, 1968, pp. 88–90). Research studies suggest that there is a decline in future-oriented thinking with age in adulthood, and that present-centered thinking increases with age (Cameron, 1972, p. 118).

"The instinct is to stay away from a future which has the smell of death about it" (Simon, 1968, p. 22). But this new, vivid encounter with death is a task that cannot be put off unless denial operates at a high level. Death looms ahead as a given, an inevitable occurence. One is faced with the reality that he cannot turn to his parents for much, if any, parenting. In late middle age one parents both his own children and his own parents as the latter's existence wanes and they regress. And then his parents are gone and perhaps some of his friends. Now, if never before, he faces the finitude of death. He is crossing the bridge to the last stage of his life.

In regard to the work role, blue- and white-collar workers become concerned with keeping the jobs they have. Future security takes precedence as they gradually approach retirement age. Some persons should retire for health reasons at fifty to fifty-five (Buckley, 1967, p. 35), since heart attacks are less fatal in later life and psychologically disorganizing illnesses become less common. By late middle age, the personality is integrated and ego identity has been established. However, depression increases in late middle age. Such depressive reactions are often related to anger toward the self for life's failures and to a general displeasure with the way life has gone (Lidz, 1968, p. 460).

A fascinating consequence of mid-life evolution is that "the sexes move closer together, psychologically, each partner becoming what the other used to be, and there is ushered in the unisex of later life" (Gutmann, 1972, p. 424). Gutmann sheds further light on this phenomenon by suggesting that the revolution in sex roles that the women's liberation movement wants eventually occurs to most women as the direct result of life-cycle sequences. He states that men and women are distinguished by the temporal staging of masculine and feminine traits. Men are the sex which is masculine *before* exhibiting those relationship capacities and sentiments known as feminine, and women are the sex for whom the sequence is the reverse (Gutmann, 1972, p. 243).

ADAPTIVE OUTCOMES IN MIDDLE AGE

The variations of middle-aging are infinite. The attributes of those who are most successful in coping with this phase of life have been identified in a 10-year study of some 700 citizens participating in the Kansas City Studies of Adult Life. To be a success at mid-life and adapt to the developmental changes, a person needs the following characteristics (Peck and Berkowitz, 1964, pp. 16–20):

1. Cathectic flexibility—the capacity to shift emotional investment from one person to another
2. Mental flexibility—the capacity to use prior learning as a guide for new problem solving rather than being closed-minded and inflexible
3. Ego differentiation—the capacity to enjoy a number of roles and value oneself for a variety of attributes
4. Body transcendence—the capacity to feel whole and happy because of one's social and mental powers and activities despite poor health

5. Ego transcendence—the capacity to be concerned with others' well-being, to find satisfaction in meeting their needs rather than being preoccupied with private desires for the self
6. Body satisfaction—the capacity to experience contentment and satisfaction with one's body
7. Sexual integration—the capacity to integrate sexual desires with other aspects of life in a harmonious way

On the other hand, who are some of the failures of adjustment to middle age? The aging Don Juan? The businessman who commits suicide? The "wino" sitting in the alley, surrounded by trash and guzzling "rot-gut"? The quiet, withdrawn housewife with the cirrhotic liver and the gin hidden in the flour canister? The professional woman who never can get to sleep without two sedative pills? Yes, these persons have failed somehow and have probably experienced developmental defeat. Retreats into alcoholism, sedative addiction, hypochondria, suicide, divorce, or obesity are not uncommon (McCormack, 1973; Soddy and Kidson, 1967, pp. 157–159; and Scarf, 1972, p. 122). Defeated, and more often than not lonely, they move toward old age, a time for which they are ill equipped because they never adapted successfully to mid-life.

Some middle-aged persons seek help from mental health professionals. Psychiatric nurses who are engaged in various forms of therapy, such as crisis intervention, family therapy, and brief therapy, and who are familiar with the tasks to be accomplished during mid-life, have excellent opportunities to assess and intervene with those who are failing to adjust to the pressures of middle-aging.

CONCLUDING REMARKS

Our modern industrial society is dependent on the stability of social institutions. Middle-aged persons generally control, dominate, and operate these institutions. "Thus, in addition to the pressures . . . to 'settle down' in middle age, it may be equally argued that society is dependent for its continuity and stability on the capacity of middle-aged people to assume an unvarying role, in the continuity of which the society can feel confidence and in which it will tend to confine the people concerned" (Soddy and Kidson, 1967, p. 108).

What does the future hold for the middle-aged and our knowledgeability of this developmental era? Packard suggested that we need to provide persons approaching later middle life with the opportunity to gradually "taper-off" their working days rather than have ever-earlier retirement dates. The latter assaults a person's sense of worth.

He also wrote that it was probably that women demonstrating outstanding "mothering" abilities and capacities would have opportunities to have the profession of "mother-imprinter." Such women would assist a child's natural mother to "mother" her children (Packard, 1968, pp. 365–366, 383).

Researchers and clinicians seem to be becoming more interested in the formerly neglected era of middle life. Therefore, this writer predicts that research studies and articles about the middle-aged will begin to proliferate in the professional literature. Hopefully, many psychiatric nurses will use their observations to generate some grounded theory about middle-aging or choose dissertation subjects related to some aspect of mid-life. We know little and have much to learn about the developmental reactions in the middle years.

REFERENCES

Ackerman, Nathan W. (1965): "The Family Approach to Marital Disorders," in Bernard L. Greene (ed.), *The Psychotherapies of Marital Disharmony,* The Free Press, New York, pp. 153–167.

Bardwick, Judith M. (1971): *The Psychology of Women,* Harper & Row, Publishers, Inc., New York.

Benedek, Therese (1970): "Parenthood during the Life Cycle," in E. James Anthony and Therese Benedek (eds.), *Parenthood: Its Psychology and Psychopathology,* Little, Brown and Company, Boston, pp. 185–206.

Buckley, Joseph C. (1967): *The Retirement Handbook,* Harper & Row, Publishers, Inc., New York.

Cameron, Paul (1972): "The Generation Gap: Time Orientation," part I, *The Gerontologist,* Summer, pp. 117–119.

Cath, Stanley (1965): "Some Dynamics of the Middle and Later Years," in Howard J. Parad (ed.), *Crisis Intervention: Selected Readings,* Family Service Association of America, New York, pp. 174–190.

Constantine, Larry L. and Joan M. (1971): "Group and Multilateral Marriage: Definitional Notes, Glossary and Annotated Bibliography," *Family Process,* vol. 10, no. 2, pp. 157–176.

Deutsch, Helene (1945): *The Psychology of Women,* vol. 2, Grune & Stratton, Inc., New York.

Deutscher, Irwin (1968): "The Quality of Postparental Life," in Bernice L. Neugarten (ed.), *Middle Age and Aging,* University of Chicago Press, Chicago, pp. 263–268.

Deykin, Eva, Shirley Jacobson, Gerald Klerman, and Maida Solomon (1966): "The Empty Nest: Psychosocial Aspects of Conflicts between Depressed Women and Their Grown Children," *American Journal of Psychiatry,* vol. 122, pp. 1422–1426.

Drewes, Caroline (1971): "Her Life's a Billboard," *San Francisco Sunday Examiner and Chronicle,* December 19, p. 6.

Erikson, Erik H. (1963): *Childhood and Society,* 2d ed., W. W. Norton & Company, Inc., New York.

Gutmann, David (1967): "Aging among the Highland Maya: A Comparative Study," *Journal of Personality and Social Psychology,* vol. 7, pp. 28–35.

———(1972): "The Premature Gerontocracy: Themes of Aging and Death in the Youth Culture," *Social Research,* vol. 39, no. 3, pp. 416–448.

Jacques, Elliott (1965): "Death and the Mid-Life Crisis," *International Journal of Psychoanalysis,* vol. 46, pp. 502–514.

Klemme, Herbert (1970): "Flame-out after 35," *The Rotarian,* September, pp. 21–23.

Lidz, Theodore (1968): *The Person,* Basic Books, Inc., Publishers, New York.

Margolis, Herbert F., and Paul M. Rubenstein (1972): *The Group Sex Tapes,* Paperback Library, New York.

Masserman, Jules (1966): *Modern Therapy of Personality Disorder,* William C. Brown Co., Publishers, Dubuque, Iowa.

Masters, William, and Virginia E. Johnson (1968): "Human Sexual Response: The Aging Female and the Aging Male," in Bernice L. Neugarten (ed.), *Middle Age and Aging,* University of Chicago, Chicago, pp. 269–279.

McCormack, Patricia (1973): "25 to 65? You're Neglected," *San Francisco Sunday Examiner and Chronicle,* Mar. 4, p. 3.

Neugarten, Bernice L. (1968): "Adult Personality: Toward a Psychology of the Life Cycle," in Bernice L. Neugarten (ed.), *Middle Age and Aging,* University of Chicago Press, Chicago, pp. 137–147.

———(1970): "Dynamics of Transition of Middle Age to Old Age: Adaptation and Life Cycle," *Journal of Geriatric Psychiatry,* vol. 4, no. 1, pp. 71–87.

Packard, Vance (1968): *The Sexual Wilderness,* David McKay Company, Inc., New York.

Palson, Charles and Rebecca (1972): "Swinging in Wedlock," *Society,* February, pp. 28–37.

Peck, Robert F. (1968): "Psychological Development in the Second Half of Life," in Bernice L. Neugarten (ed.), *Middle Age and Aging,* University of Chicago Press, Chicago, pp. 88–98.

———and Howard Berkowitz (1964): "Personality and Adjustment in Middle Age," in Bernice Levin Neugarten (ed.), *Personality in Middle and Late Life: Empirical Studies,* Atherton Press, Inc., New York, pp. 15–43.

Pineo, Peter C. (1963): "Disenchantment in the Later Years of Marriage," in Marvin B. Sussman (ed.), *Sourcebook in Marriage and the Family,* Houghton Mifflin Company, Boston.

Rapaport, Rhona and Robert F. (1969): "The Dual Career Family: A Variant Pattern and Social Change," *Human Relations,* vol. 22, no. 1, pp. 3–30.

San Francisco Chronicle (1971): "Stormy Days of Mid-Life Crises," July 12, p. 4.

Scarf, Maggie (1972): "Husbands in Crisis," *McCall's,* June, pp. 76–77, 120–125.

Scherz, Frances H. (1967): "The Crisis of Adolescence in Family Life," *Social Casework,* no. 4, pp. 209–215.

Simon, Anne W. (1968): *The New Years,* Alfred A. Knopf, Inc., New York.

Soddy, Kenneth, and Mary C. Kidson (1967): *Men in Middle Life,* J. B. Lippincott Company, Philadelphia.

Solomon, Joan (1972): "Woman's Body, Woman's Mind: Menopause: A Rite of Passage," *Ms.,* December, pp. 16–18.

Stockwell, Edward G. (1972): "The Changing Age Compositon of the American Population," *Social Biology,* vol. 19, no. 1, pp. 1–9.

Sussman, Marvin B. (1960): "Intergenerational Family Relationships and Social Role Changes in Middle Age," *Journal of Gerontology,* vol. 15, no. 1, pp. 71–75.

Szalita, Alberta B. (1966): "Psychodynamics of Disorders of the Involutional Age," in Silvano Arieti (ed.), *American Handbook of Psychiatry,* vol. 3, Basic Books, Inc., Publishers, New York, pp. 69–74.

White, Paul Dudley (1962): "Middle Age Fitness," *Arizona Medicine,* vol. 19, no. 3, pp. 43–48.

7

DEVELOPMENTAL REACTIONS IN OLD AGE

Irene Mortenson Burnside

Because the human being is an organism which develops and moves forward in time and is comprised of physiological, psychological, and social elements (Birren, 1964), it is necessary to consider all three in developmental reactions of the aged. In this chapter, although greatest emphasis will be on the psychological changes in the aged, the physiological changes must be considered also, because the physiological, psychological, and social problems of the aged are so interrelated. Knowledgeable psychiatric nurses intervene in all three of these areas; however, only two developmental aspects of the aged, the physiological and psychological, will be discussed in this chapter. The content of socioeconomic aspects of aging is so broad that space will not permit discussion of the important aspects of this particular area.

The first section of the chapter deals with the physiology of aging, and particularly with the structural changes. This section is followed by psychological reactions to aging. The third section deals with psychiatric problems of the aged. Each section of the chapter ends with implications for nursing. For the purposes of this particular book, the writers have taken the age of sixty-five as the arbitrary cutoff point for the onset of old age, also known as *senescence*. The term *senility* is sometimes used interchangeably with *senescence;* this is an incorrect use of the term, although it is true that senility and senescence can develop concomitantly. The word *senility* should be reserved for the psychopathological condition which may occur for some individuals in their later years.

DEFINITION OF AGING

Aging has been frequently defined. In a symposium entitled "Control of Human Aging," held in Zurich, Switzerland, Doctor Comfort described aging as "a process of increasing instability in time" (Comfort, 1971). Verwoerdt (1969a, p. 55) states, "Aging may be viewed as a process leading to increased vulnerability to stresses, such as disease, accident, widowhood, economic deprivation, or loss of status." Handler (1960, p. 200), a biologist, gives a more comprehensive definition: "Aging is the deterioration of a mature organism, resulting from time dependent, essentially irreversible changes, intrinsic to all members of a species such that with the passage of time, they become increasingly unable to cope with the stresses of the environment, thereby increasing the probability of death."

Birren (1970) states, "The term aging refers to the regularities or transformations that occur over the life span in members of a species and result in differences between young and old organisms in both structure and function." The same author distinguishes between the biological age, or the likely number of years a person will live; the psychological age, or the adaptive capacities of a person; and the social age, or the roles and social habits of an individual in regard to his culture or society.

It does not seem appropriate in this chapter to include a definition of geriatric services. The World Health Organization defines the purpose of geriatric services, which on the first reading sounds deceptively simple: "to keep the elderly in good health and happiness in their own homes for as long as this is possible" (Thomas, 1971). With the tremendous increase in the construction of new nursing homes and extended care facilities in the United States, one wonders if this is the prevailing philosophy of placement of the aged in this country.

PHYSIOLOGICAL CHANGES IN THE AGING PROCESS

There is a gradual decline in the ability of many of the organ systems to function in the aged person. The pattern of decrements and the decrease of function begins about the fifth decade (Chinn, 1970). "There is a decrease in cardiac and pulmonary reserve, decrease in voluntary muscle strength, reduction in renal function and decline in mental acuity" (Chinn, 1970). It is also generally agreed that there is a loss of neurones in the aged (Chinn, 1970; Bromley, 1966).

Some of the evidence of changes related to the physiologic determinants includes declines in: (1) speed of conduction of nerve impulse, (2) renal blood flow and filtration rate, (3) cardiac output, (4) basal metabolism, (5) vital capacity, (6) maximum breathing capacity, (7) urinary steroid excretion, (8) adrenal response to ACTH, (9) gonadal endocrine secretion, and (10) muscular strength and speed of motion. There are increases in the following: (1) cerebro-vascular resistance, (2) blood pressure, (3) peripheral vascular resistance, and (4) residual lung volume resistance. Nearly all the body systems are affected by the aging process; the two which are least affected are the gastrointestinal and the hematological system (Chinn, 1970).

Shock and White have suggested that aging is accompanied by a lack of homeostasis in the internal environment, and this lack increases gradually (Shock, 1960; White, 1960). Kohn feels that there is a lowered efficiency in the homeostatic mechanism of the older person, and this lessened efficiency is one of the most characteristic features of aging (Kohn, 1963). If the homeostasis is precariously balanced, and the aged person's equilibrium is upset, it is likely to take more time to return to previous values than it would in the case of younger persons. Several examples include the pH of the blood, the body temperature, and the blood sugar level. Diabetes is one example which illustrates the problem in attempting to distinguish between biological aging, pathological aging, and the disease itself. Old persons, who may have a glucose tolerance test which would indicate diabetes, show no evidence of the disease at the time they are clinically examined.

If the aged person is subjected to stress in the form of unusual heat or cold, he may not readily adapt to the drastic temperature changes in his environment. The writer recalls two victims of such decreased adaptation: two elderly women wandered away from extended care facilities in the Bay Area of California during the relatively mild California winter months. Both the elderly women perished in the exposure to the outdoors. Another example recalled by the writer is the rise of deaths in the aged noted during two years of group work with aged patients in a convalescent hospital. The extreme heat of the summers took its toll; one man in the group had had severe heat exhaustion during a scorching spell when the air conditioner did not work. Another ninety-year-old man in the group died during the same heat spell.

Multiple problems and multiple diagnoses are common in many of the elderly of our society. Age does not influence all of the organ systems to quite the same extent, and age does not even have a uniform effect on different organ systems even in the same individual. Therefore, it is important that health workers assess and intervene with the aged as individuals and not solely as members of an age group since there is much less homogeneity in a group of old people of the same chronological age than in a similar group of young people.

The age-related changes in the various organs and systems of the body will be reviewed briefly as they relate to the aging process. When there are structural changes in these systems, there will also be a change in the function of the system.

Dermal System

Changes in the skin are due to the aging process: loss of elasticity and pigmentary changes. Changes in the skin are a factor in the increased difficulty on the part of the aged in maintaining normal temperature of the body. There is also a tendency for the skin to bruise easily and to develop skin sores.

Muscular and Skeletal System

One of the most visible manifestations of the aging process, says Chinn (1970), is the decline in muscular function despite the infrequency of specific disease states of the skeletal muscles. A common clinical condition in the aged is the demineralization which occurs in the skeletal system, so that the loss of calcium in osteoporosis may be seen as a direct accompaniment of the aging process. The stiffening of joints and changes in bone structure may cause a reduction in height and also a stooped posture. There also may be limitation of mobility.

Cardiovascular System

The blood vessels and the heart suffer from a degenerative process. The state of the heart and peripheral vessels plays a prominent role in the health picture of the aged individual. Generalized or localized arteriosclerosis is one very important condition of the aged, and it is extremely common in persons of advanced years.

Respiratory System

In most older people, the pulmonary function is as good as that of the young under conditions of extreme stress (Richards, 1956). It seems that older persons have reduced maximum breathing capacity, reduced vital capacity, an increase in residual volume, an increase in functional capacity, and a decrease in respiratory reserve (Norris, 1956;

Agostini, 1962). "Many of the abnormalities in pulmonary function must be due in part to reduced power of the accessory muscles of respiration, in part to increased rigidity of the chest wall, and in part to the intrapulmonary changes" (Chinn, 1970). One may therefore expect to find barrel chests in elderly men and shortness of breath on exertion. Chinn discusses a "senile emphysema" which is based primarily on the loss of pulmonary elasticity (Chinn, 1970).

Gastrointestinal System

The cells which make up the lining of the gall bladder, the intestines, and the stomach, and those of the liver and pancreas are able to reproduce themselves. Therefore, it is thought that these tissues do not age as do those in the central nervous system and muscular system. It is at this time believed that these "organs remain free of significant time-related structural abnormalities" (Chinn, 1970). The reduction of hydrochloric acid starts to diminish progressively during the middle years; achlorhydria is quite common in the aged. Two clinical conditions frequently seen in the aged are constipation and diverticulosis of the large intestine.

Genitourinary System

Chinn (1970) states that there is much evidence to substantiate the belief that the kidney in the aging individual undergoes physiological change. The two most common diseases of the kidneys in the elderly are pyelonephritis and the changes concomitant with diabetes and hypertensive vascular disease.

One of the very great problems in care of the aged is the problem of incontinence. This condition also creates social problems for many aged individuals, for example, in their placement. Brocklehurst (1964) reported 25 to 50 percent of a chronic hospital patient population as being incontinent. Organic brain damage is believed to be the cause of incontinence in more than 80 percent of such individuals.

Implications for Nursing Care

Although the entire area of physiology of the aged is a challenging one for nursing research, there are some very specific areas germane to nursing. One area is that of skin care; nurses are constantly faced with the responsibility of prevention of decubiti, or healing already existing ones. The nurse also has responsibility for incontinent patients. At this writing, few studies by nurses about incontinence have been published; yet the incontinent patient is the bane of nursing practice in whatever setting the patient may be living.

The stroke patient, especially the aphasic stroke patient, is common in the case loads of most nurses, both in the acute and chronic care setting. The psychological problems directly related to the cardiovascular accident offer a field for study by nurses. The ill effects of extreme heat and cold on the aged individual have been discussed. A more sensitive assessment of the heating of the environments of the aged would increase the comfort of the aged.

Both positive and adverse drug reactions need to be investigated by nurses. In extended care facilities nurses must cope with the overdoses and the symptoms of overdosage, and often they do not have a doctor on the premises or readily accessible for consultation. Gunby, (1971) says, "Pharmacotherapy in geronto-psychiatry is still an art." Anxiety and insomnia are frequent problems in the aged; often medication is used rather than attempting to get at the cause of the distress itself, or trying alternate methods of treatment.

The physiological changes of the aging process need to be included in the curriculum of all nursing students, at whatever the level of preparation of student. Much of the major responsibility of the care of the aged lies with the nursing profession, especially in the case of aged persons in extended care facilities. The nursing profession presently lags far behind other disciplines in research and literature published about the aged.

PSYCHOLOGICAL CHANGES IN AGING

A person has more opportunity to be damaged, physically, psychologically, and socially, as he lives longer. "We must distinguish trauma and damage from normal processes" (Carp, 1969). The sensory changes and/or decrements have great impact on the lives of the aged individuals.

Sensory Loss

There is usually a sensory loss in increasing age. "Man's capacity for complex skills and even his ability to survive depend upon the reception and integration of information from specialized nerve endings, such as those in the eye, ear, skin, and muscles. However, there is not necessarily a direct relation between the sensitivity of sensory receptors and the adequacy of behavior" (Birren, 1964). The same author reminds us that we must keep in mind the principle that acuity should be interpreted in each individual, as well as how he personally adapts. This statement is important to nurses who assess aged individuals and design nursing care plans.

Vision

Vision is considered to be one of the most important of the senses. Visual acuity (that is, the smallest object that can be discriminated) declines slightly from the twenties to the fifties, and there is an accelerated rate of decline after the fifties (Birren, 1964). Studies have shown that cataracts, blindness, and impaired vision are high in the aged beyond sixty-five (Kornzweig, 1957; U.S. National Health Survey, 1959).

Audition

For some time it has been known that older persons have poorer hearing of high tones than do younger persons. There is also a greater tendency for men than for women to have impaired hearing, although there is no clear-cut reason for this. Some speculate that men in their occupational lives may have been exposed more often to high noise levels than women. If that is true, one cannot help but wonder what rock and roll listening will do to the hearing of the present young generation when they become elderly. Birren (1964) suggests that above the age of forty, individuals will begin to show some loss of high tone perception. The hearing condition due to aging is known as *presbycusis.* One hearing difficulty the aged may have is mistaking one word for another word, which often creates difficulties in communication. One of the functional evidences of presbycusis is a deterioration in the ability to understand speech. Older people who are seen by audiologists and otologists complain that speech that is still heard is no longer clear (Bergman, 1971).

The number of persons over age seventy-five with hearing impairment is five times greater than that for the age bracket of forty-five to sixty-four (U.S. Health Survey, 1959). Hearing loss may be more handicapping to some individuals than to others; some persons, because they are intelligent, seem to better interpret the sounds, even though they may be a bit deafer than other individuals around them. The severe effects of hearing loss can be seen in the social withdrawal of a hard-of-hearing person; some may also develop a suspicious nature. Many elderly persons who willingly wear eyeglasses balk at wearing a hearing aid.

Rigidity, a trait common in the aged, may be due in part to the decrements in sensation and perception. The finding of a more rigid, i.e., overcontrolled, underactive, approach to the world is more common in aged persons with impaired hearing than in the normal-hearing aged (Eisdorfer, 1960).

Gustation

There have been a number of studies done for the measurement of intensity of taste for sweet, salt, bitter, and sour substances (Cooper et al., 1959). The studies do not reveal much change in taste thresholds up to age fifty, but after the late fifties a decline was noted. Birren suggests that large changes in the sensitivity of taste probably would be a relatively late phenomenon in life occurring after age seventy (Birren, 1964). The writer is reminded of a seventy-six-year-old man's description of the food in the extended care facility: "The mashed potatoes taste like apple sauce and the apple sauce tastes like mashed potatoes." Perhaps his aging had as much to do with the taste of food as the institutional preparation of the food. The study of taste sensitivity in relation to the aging process reveals conflicting results.

Olfaction

Because of the difficulties involved in the study of the sense of smell quantitatively, there is little evidence to suggest how the sense of smell does change with age.

Pain

There has not been much success in the attempt to verify the clinical impression that there is a decrease in sensitivity to pain in old people. Pain is unlike the other sensory receptors, because the sense of pain has a high component of subjectivity. Pain serves also to warn and alert the body.

Touch

Touch has been studied by using a technique of calibrated hairs, and has been determined on these areas of the body: the cornea of the eye, limbus of the eye, lower and upper limbi, and tip of the nose. Generally, says Birren, sensitivity remains unchanged until about age fifty to fifty-five (Birren, 1964).

There can be little doubt that sensory and perceptual changes during the aging process have important and sometimes drastic consequences for the aged individual as he attempts to function in his environment or cope with his losses and problems. For many of the sensory systems, it would seem that seventy is the age at which the sensory processes are very frequently a cause of the behavior of an individual (Birren, 1964).

Psychomotor Skills

Welford (1958) has demonstrated, and there is agreement among several studies, that the maximum strength, highest in the twenties, decreases with age. Older people are often characterized by their deficits in strength, reaction time, and sensorimotor coordination.

Intelligence

There have been many studies done in an attempt to relate age and intelligence. The problems in the study lie in ferreting out age changes in intelligence from other age-related changes, for example, in general health or in societal trends, say, in the field of education. Large-scale, long-term, longitudinal studies are needed.

Implications for Nursing Care

The multitude of losses an aged individual may experience offers fertile grounds for studies, investigations, and in-depth case studies. Each of the sensory losses is important in the nursing care of an individual, and with the sensory decrements come the accoutrements of aging, such as magnifying glasses, eyeglasses, and hearing aids (Burnside, 1972). The nurse assumes much responsibility in maintaining these devices and helping the aged individual adjust to and/or accept them. The psychological impact of a new device can be great. The importance of these aspects of nursing care are nowhere spelled out more clearly than they are in the Geriatric Standards of the American Nurses' Association (1970). These standards should be available as guidelines to all nursing personnel who care for elderly clients. The ability to distinguish disease and trauma from the normal processes in aging is important for a nursing staff.

Vision Aged persons have difficulty driving at night because the aging eyes adapt more slowly and less effectively to the dark. Nursing personnel need to be sensitive to this because many elderly persons drive in the late years of their lives; some are embarrassed and handicapped by being unable to drive at night. Care of eyeglasses looms as an important nursing problem. Luminescent and enlarged phone dial numbers are helpful to the elderly person who lives at home (Burnside, 1972). Periodic eye examinations will have to be encouraged in order to have necessary lens changes made.

The loss of vision can create serious problems for those who become totally blind. These persons should be observed for hallucinations, loneliness, and withdrawal. Knowles (1968) once described to the writer a blind, hallucinating nursing home patient: "The blind patient often sees other people with her and I was very much upset that a mental institution was the only recourse for this particular patient." In-service classes need to be developed in extended care facilities which will zero in on the many problems which may be created for the aged by blindness or impaired vision.

Audition The hard-of-hearing elderly create increased communication problems in nursing care. Garbled and inaccurate communications occur persistently among an aged population (Burnside, 1973). Part of the problem lies in that often when we communicate with the aged, we do not check out whether or not they heard or understood what we have said. Consequently, many instructions are not followed at all, or they are carried out incorrectly—and sometimes unsafely. Since men have a greater tendency toward impaired hearing than women, nurses might anticipate this problem in working with aged men. The entire area of presbycusis also could be researched by nurses. We know the effectiveness of touch with both the blind and the hard-of-hearing, but what kind of touch, where, how much, how often, when? As nurses we use touch intuitively and we know its effectiveness; however, scientific studies of touch might increase our therapeutic effectiveness with the elderly.

Rigidity in the aged is often written off as stubborness for cantankerousness. Perhaps it is time to study both the rigidity in ourselves and the rigidity we see, or think we see, in the aged client. The latter observation came from reading student papers and listening to them in conferences; it became clear that sometimes the student's rigidity equalled (and occasionally surpassed) that of the aged client he or she was describing.

ADAPTATION IN OLD AGE

One of the adaptations of the aged person is to maintain his own identity and to realize that he has entered the last portion of his life. Such identity is difficult to maintain in the face of negative attitudes about the aged in our society. Also, his role as parent—as a worker—may have been taken from him; he must adjust to steady, sometimes serious, losses. Loss of spouse is particularly difficult for aged persons who have been married for many years. It is also difficult for some to find a satisfying home arrangement. The individual or couple may be forced to adjust to a drastically reduced income. Elderly persons are often found to be caring for individuals much older than they are. The author recalls a seventy-six-year-old woman who had to hospitalize her ninety-six-year-old mother with a colostomy because she could no longer care for her at home.

It is clear, then, that survival in later life means adjustment and adaptation. Those who survive are an elite group; they need to be studied over time. Perhaps we would then better understand the coping mechanisms and adaptation techniques which could be shared with other aging individuals who are in similar situations.

This has been a cursory glance at the normative reaction to aging. Now for a look at some of the problems and also the functional psychiatric disorders that are seen in the aged population.

Psychiatric Problems in the Aged

Thomas (1971) uses the term *psychogeriatric* to describe "a group of patients who may or may not have physical illness, but who do have a psychiatric condition and who, as a consequence, require care and attention, and applies to the age 60-plus." In his writings, Verwoerdt uses the term *geropsychiatry* (Verwoerdt, 1969b; Verwoerdt and Eisdorfer, 1967).

The increased life span means an increase in psychiatric problems for aged persons. Comfort quoted an unidentified psychiatrist who said that he felt most people could live with their problems 70 years, but he was not sure if there would not be more mental illness if another 10 years were added to their life span (Comfort, 1971).

Loss and Loneliness

Although there are losses throughout all phases of life, there are special losses during middle age, such as children leaving home, the end of the work period for either a man or a woman, plus the decline in physical vigor, which has been described in the section on physiological aging in this chapter. Aged persons also may experience sharp declines in their incomes, and, in fact, may have to give up a style of living to which they may have been accustomed—for example, moving into a smaller home, or giving up a home for an apartment. Such moves may create other losses.

It is difficult for the aged to compensate for the loved ones they lose, and this seems especially true when they lose a spouse. It is not uncommon for nurses to be working with a spouse who has been recently widowed after 40 or 50 years of marriage. Busse has described this loss as "the most grievous assault of all." Loneliness frequently follows the loss.

The loneliness of the aged person or client is well known to the practicing nurse, and most particularly to the public health nurse with a case load predominantly of elderly people, many of whom reside alone. Institutionalized elderly will also often complain of loneliness in spite of their communal living arrangements. Busse distinguishes between being alone and loneliness. He defines loneliness as ". . . the awareness of an absence of meaningful integration with other individuals or groups of individuals, a consciousness of being excluded from the system of opportunities and rewards in which other people participate" (Busse, 1969).

There are few research studies which have studied a problem of loneliness (Busse, 1969). Shanas and associates (1968) conducted a cross-national survey to examine the experience of subjective loneliness and the social isolation in the aged. Moustakas (1960) wrote a sensitive and poignant article about the loneliness and the psychotherapy of an elderly client. Clark formulated logical steps for defining the concept of loneliness. She states there are themes or threads which are important for nurses to understand. Although she was not addressing herself to loneliness in the aged per se, the themes do have relevance for gerontological nursing. One theme is that loneliness is a part of man's humanity. This theme is also found in Thomas Wolfe's masterful writings. Another one is that being related to others can relieve loneliness. Still another theme suggests that there are defenses used to help protect the individual from loneliness; loneliness can be experienced in varying degrees; the suggestion is made that the inability to love may be related to the degree of loneliness felt. Another theme is the indication that there is some hope for relief of that loneliness in order to be able to relate to others (Clark, 1968).

Toffler, in his book, *Future Shock,* describes the plight of many elderly Americans: "Thus, despite extraordinary achievements in art, science, intellectual, moral, and political life, the United States is a nation in which tens of thousands of young people flee reality by opting for drug-induced lassitude . . . a nation in which legions of elderly old vegetate and die in loneliness" (Toffler, 1970).

Anxiety in the Aged

Generally anxiety is considered to be important in most of the theoretical systems in psychiatry (Engle, 1962; Fenichel, 1945; Sullivan, 1947). Peplau's contributions to psychiatric nursing on the subject are well known (Peplau, 1952). Busse summarizes work done by Eisdorfer, Powell, and Shmavonian, by saying, "It appears that response to an anxiety-producing stimulus in the elderly is often delayed and may be increased or decreased, depending on which manifestation of anxiety is being measured. Furthermore, the same stimuli which produce anxiety in younger persons may not produce the same reaction in the elderly, and vice-versa" (Busse, 1969; Shmavonian et al., 1963).

Burnside feels that many aged institutionalized patients do not reveal their anxiety (Burnside, 1971a). The same writer wrote about patients in a group who used somatic complaints to mask their anxiety (Burnside, 1971b). "Classical anxiety reaction (with 'free floating' anxiety) appears to be rather uncommon in the aged. Instead, anxiety is frequently manifested by symptoms of somatic distress" (Verwoerdt and Eisdorfer, 1967).

Anxiety is not uncommon in the aged. If a specific cause or problem can be delineated, then clarification of the problem at hand may be enough to assist in reduction of the anxiety. At other times arrangements need to be made with other disciplines or the family to be certain that the aged person receives concrete help. But it is well to remember that anxiety may not arise out of a special problem alone, but could well be related to the overall problem of the aging process itself. Busse points out the helplessness which many aging persons are apt to experience regarding their life situations, and especially the dependency on others which can give rise to a gamut of emotions in the aged. The writers say, "Dependency can be tolerated more easily if the individual can be sure that the support upon which he is relying will not be withdrawn at any moment" (Busse, 1969). This writer saw the impact of loss of nursing staff members upon a group of aged persons during group therapy. As one after another of their favorite nurses resigned, the group expressed sadness and felt that no one else would take care of them as well. One man was particularly upset because a nurse who had spent much time with him when he had suffered heat exhaustion left. He truly felt this nurse had saved his life.

Because anxiety is a state which prepares one to act in emergency situations, it constantly fluctuates. But if the cause of the anxiety is not resolved, other mechanisms go into effect to reduce that anxiety, and one must deal with such defense mechanisms. Therefore, it is important to treat heightened anxiety; the treatment may be preventive psychiatric nursing that can prevent the development of other symptomatology. In this connection one constantly has to keep in mind the problems of overuse of drugs in the aged, since drugs are often given to reduce anxiety.

Insomnia in the Aged

Sleep is a normal physiological function in the individual, and for some persons it is a means of escape and withdrawal from the problems of life. "Chronic insomnia, on the other hand, can most commonly be attributed to unsolved emotional conflict involving feelings of guilt and hostility with fear of retaliation" (Busse, 1969). The pattern of sleeping changes in some important ways in the elderly. Deep sleep in the elderly virtually disappears. Older people also require a longer period of time to fall asleep (Kahn et al., 1969; Kales et al., 1968). The sleep of the aged person is lighter and he awakens more frequently. These changes are even more pronounced in individuals who have significant organic brain disease (Feinberg et al., 1968).

Hypochondriasis

It is only recently that hypochondriasis has been considered a distinct disease entity rather than syndrome. The second edition of the *Diagnostic and Statistical Manual of Mental Disorders* of the American Psychiatric Association has listed hypochondriacal neurosis as a separate neurotic condition (American Psychiatric Association, 1968). Among elderly women patients hypochondriasis is frequent (Early et al., 1969). Busse (1969) states:

> [There are] three psychological mechanisms which play a major role in the dynamics of hypochondrias: a withdrawal of psychic interest from other persons or objects and a centering of this interest upon oneself, one's own body, and its functioning; (2) a shift of anxiety from a specific psychic area to a less threatening concern with bodily disease; and (3) use of physical symptoms as a means of self-punishment and atonement for unacceptable hostile or vengeful feelings toward persons close to the individual.

The same writer explains that it is easy to see why an older worker whose only interest was work could shift his interest onto normal body functions. Also, old persons who may be anxious over losses such as social prestige or finances may shift their anxiety to concerns about their bodies.

Depression

Depression is a common psychiatric problem seen in the elderly. The high suicide rate seen in elderly men gives one some indication of the severity of the depression many of the aged experience in the later years of life.

The psychotic depressive reaction seen in the aged is comparable in symptoms and psychodynamics to depressions found in any age. Verwoerdt (1969a) says that "the psychodynamic background usually involved the experience of a loss, either real or imagined, which is not primarily age-specific (death of a parent, loss of a spouse, a disappointment in vocational aspirations, etc.)"

Levin sees two general ways in which the depressed patient might be viewed; one is "the carrier of a powerful anger in search of an outlet," and another is that of "the carrier of a powerful libido in search of gratification." He classifies problems of external factors which disturb the libido equilibrium of depression into four main categories: (1) loss, (2) attack, (3) restraint, and (4) threats. Although these factors occur in different combinations and may be present at all ages, they are seen by this psychiatrist as occurring more commonly in old age, and he states, "Since their impact is often unconscious, they frequently remain unrecognized not only by the patient but also by others" (Levin, 1965).

Although there are many psychiatric aspects of aging important to nursing, only the most common ones are discussed here. One other important problem in geropsychiatry is the patient with the diagnosis of chronic brain syndrome. Nurses are constantly requesting help and information in working with these elderly patients. The condition of chronic brain syndrome has been previously discussed in another chapter in the book.

Senility

"If the ability to reach affectionate others decays with senility, and this deterioration of the communication bridges in turn narrows the traffic which provides for the integrity of the inner world, it is equally true that the withdrawal of affection by others is a main force that pushes the aging into senility" (Etzioni, 1971).

Butler (1971) emphatically states, "Senility is a waste basket term and not acceptable in medicine. We have no measurable indicators for it." He states that the following possibilities must be considered when there are symptoms indicative of senility: (1) a beginning depression, which may be revealed by confusion, (2) the beginning of a reversible brain disorder, (3) chronic brain disorder, which could either be stable or be progressive at various rates. There are four early symptoms to watch for: (1) change in the attention span, (2) memory changes, (3) altered intellectual grasp, and (4) a lowered responsiveness in the patient. The cause of senile psychosis is not known (Butler, 1971).

Noyes and Kolb feel that the psychodynamics of senile dementia "may be understood as a series of ontogenetically related ego regressions. Thus, as the patient becomes aware of the gradual impairment of his capacities, there is at first an intensification of already existing character defenses—'he grows more like himself.'" If the usual defenses do not reduce anxiety, then symptoms such as depression, persecution, and hypochondriasis emerge. These symptoms serve to protect the individual against death fears and also the possible losses he faces. A senile patient moving into a long phase of deterioration will not be likely to manifest depression; he is more prone to use projection and also to make paranoid accusations (Noyes and Kolb, 1968). Weinberg has also discussed these defense mechanisms used by the aged. He gave the example of an elderly woman accusing people of stealing from her; it was her way of coping with her loss of mastery (Weinberg, 1970).

Although this discussion is about senile dementia, one should also consider aspects of normal aging. An unidentified writer once stated that an aged person is the way he always was, only more so, which is still another way of stating that he "grows more like himself." Although in normal aging the person may become forgetful, less responsive, and less active because of sensory changes, one cannot glibly label an aged person as senile; unfortunately, this is frequently done. However, it is true that the traits seen in younger years may become pronounced in late years of life. For example, stubborn persons become even more stubborn in old age. Frugal persons sometimes become misers. These are negative qualities, but positive qualities remain also in old age.

One point that Noyes and Kolb (1968) make about the ego regression of senile dementia is that the regression is not specific for senile dementia, for it may be seen in schizophrenics who are deteriorating also.

The signs of senility are often conspicuous, for the skin is thin and wrinkled. The special senses lose acuity. There may be a weight loss. Muscles waste away, and the person's gait is not steady; he may shuffle. The speech is slow and the voice harsh. The handwriting is shaky and there may be tremors of head and hands. There may be amnesia, and there is a tendency to reminisce about personal events.

An increasing amount of study is being done on reminiscing. Noyes and Kolb (1968) write,

> This retention of memory for remote events and loss for recent ones seems reasonable in view of the theory that the hypothetical neuronal circuit patterns responsible for memories become more strongly established with time. The longer, then, the pattern has been established, the more strongly does memory resist degenerative states such as those of senility.

Orientation is defective. Senile persons often wander off and are lost. Policemen in communities are often quite familiar with these people, since they return them to their homes or convalescent hospitals frequently. Old people may become forgetful and, not remembering where they placed things, may accuse others of stealing. They often hoard articles either on their person or in some secret hiding place. Restlessness at night is common, and sometimes there is destructive behavior that relatives cannot cope with. Obstreperous and destructive aged patients create real problems in long-term case facilities.

Noyes and Kolb (1968) feel that the nocturnal delirium may be due to the problems the aged have with vision at night. They say that aged persons "with senile states become disoriented within an hour when placed in darkened rooms due to failure to retain their spatial location; they then become anxious and more confused." Daytime sleeping is common among senile persons.

Implications for Nursing

The implications for nursing in the care of the client with senile psychosis are many.

1. Close observation of clients is necessary to pick up the symptoms described above by Butler that indicate approaching senility. Butler (1971) has also given clinical differentiations of psychosis with cerebral arteriosclerosis as distinguished from senile psychosis.
2. Nurses working with senile psychosis need to be able to intervene in depression, agitation, and paranoid states. It would be helpful if nurses could teach the staff some of the psychodynamics of the behavior. Destructive behavior in aged patients often frightens newly trained ancillary help, as well as the other residents in a facility. A nurse's aide once came to the writer frantically saying, "The man in Room 4 has had a coronary." A newly admitted old man who had carcinoma of the brain was standing up in his bed swinging at anyone who came close to him. He was almost blind, hard of hearing, and very frightened. Reduction of anxiety is another fruitful area for nurses to study. Little has been written about the anxiety of the aged.
3. A better understanding of the value and use of reminiscing in aged patients would be

useful in nursing care of the aged. There is beginning work and experimentation in this special area by interested practitioners.

4. Special in-service classes should be geared to night personnel, who have different problems in institutions from those that daytime and evening shifts face. There should be soft night lights in the patient's room, and a minimum of shifting the patient about. Schwartz has written about one deplorable condition nurses could change, and that is the tremendous use of drugs used for sleep rather than considering nursing interventions that could be therapeutic (Schwartz, 1971). She suggests that the way the patient is put to bed at night is important, and among contented patients there is less disorientation at night.

5. Nurses could also teach relatives who are caring for patients in their homes about some of the problems and how to solve them. Visiting nurses play a tremendous role here. Follow-up visits by hospital staff when a patient is discharged would be useful. When patients are transferred from one institution, a "patient advocate" or a liaison nurse is useful in disseminating information about the patient and in making the transition easier for staff, patient, and relatives (Conti, 1973).

6. Nursing educators will have to take more responsibility for upgrading their own knowledge about gerontology and geriatrics, and to begin to integrate increased gerontological content into existing programs. Educators need to consider ways to increase the motivation of students to work with the aged. Students have frequently described negative attitudes of faculty members about geriatrics and the aged.

7. Nurses themselves are going to have to demand classes and information about gerontology, and about care of special problems which arise in the aged. As nurses assert themselves and express an interest in and need for the classes and workshops, there is greater impetus for knowledgeable professionals to teach and share their information.

8. Publishers of nursing journals will have to make increased efforts to solicit articles about care of the aged. Journals provide recent, easily available material to educators, practitioners, and students. However, there continues to be a paucity of articles about the aged client and his care at this writing.

9. Adequate nutrition, management of health, and early detection of illness are also in the domain of the nurse caring for any aged patient or client, but particularly the senile person.

10. Increased knowledge about psychosocial aspects of nursing care of the senile patient is important. The aged individual needs to maintain his dignity and also to feel emotionally secure, and this is true of the senile person, too. Care for the aged senile patient also means caring about him.

SUCCESSFUL AGING

It is difficult to describe successful aging, and yet the term is used rather frequently. *Successful aging* is individualistic, and one needs some criteria to describe, or as a baseline to determine, what is successful aging. The tasks given by Clark and Anderson (1967), as they describe the process of aging adaptation, comprise one such criterion:

1. Perception of aging and definition of instrumental limitations
2. Redefinition of physical and social life space

3. Substitution of alternative sources of need satisfaction
4. Reassessment of criteria for evaluation of the self
5. Reintegration of values and life goals

The same writers also give a detailed description in the research study of one subject, whom they considered to have aged successfully. The above guidelines could be useful for nursing students, particularly in designing nursing care plans and assessing strengths and limitations of the client. Also, students need to be encouraged to search for more positive adjustments to and aspects of the aging process. There is still much emphasis on the disease-oriented, medical model. We need to remember that old age itself is not an illness.

Erikson's developmental model of the eight stages of man is also useful in studying normal aging. He uses the terms *integrity* and *despair* to describe the eighth stage of man. Although guidelines are not spelled out as definitely in this theory, students can still assess an individual by carefully studying Erikson's model (Erikson, 1968). For example, Bancroft (1973) has written about her application of the concepts of integrity versus despair in two aged clients in her public health nursing.

The concepts of adult personality development by Neugarten may also be useful in understanding normal growth and development (Neugarten, 1964). Gunther has described course content developed for a nursing class, "to provide knowledge of aging as a normal developmental process, of the problems of the aged, and of the community resources available, and from this knowledge to derive implications for the nursing of the aged" (Gunther, 1969).

More literature by the aged themselves also would help change the pervasive negative views of old age. Florida Scott-Maxwell has beautifully described old age in her diary, *The Measure of My Days.* Coleman McCarthy, writing in *The Washington Post,* aptly described the book, "The testimony of someone who has lived nearly a century, and whose house of memories is not crammed with useless antiques, is crucial" (McCarthy, 1972).

Butler (1971) has suggested we need an archive to preserve some of the wisdom, knowledge, and expertise of our present aged. Nurses are in a position not only to listen to old people's reminiscing and "life reviews," but to encourage them to record them.

Old people in other cultures have been viewed as sages. A young man from Nigeria who lived in the home of the writer stated that they did not need psychiatrists in Nigeria because "our old people are our psychiatrists." The wisdom of our aged people in the United States is seldom tapped. A retired dean of a school of nursing deplored the fact that in the world of nursing the expertise of many retired deans was so seldom sought (Nahm, 1972).

There are admirable qualities seen in the elderly which one tends to overlook. They have a direct manner about them. Since they have so little to lose, often they say and do exactly as they feel. There is a congruency about them—what they say matches how they say it. What they believe matches the way they behave. Patience, time, and less need to hurry are attributes of the aged which contribute to their roles as grandparents.

Many old people appear to know very well who they are, where they have been, and where they are going. They have lived a long while and know their faults and virtues. Florida Scott-Maxwell (1969) described it,

> Age only defines one's boundaries. Life has changed me greatly, it has improved me greatly, but it has also left me practically the same. I cannot spell, I am over critical, egocentric and vulnerable. I cannot be simple. In my effort to become clear I become complicated. I know my faults so well that I pay them small heed. They are stronger than I am. They are me.

One should encourage the individuality seen in elderly persons. In institutions for the aged and long-term care facilities, this is often neglected. The model patient is expected to be "good," subdued, and not make excessive or unusual demands. Yet Guillerme reminds us, "There can be no doubt that man is most likely to endure by becoming more and more individualized; freedom to think and act as an individual is still one of the best ways of postponing the onset of incurable senility."

Nursing Implications

By the time an aged patient reaches a nursing care facility or is seen by a public health nurse, his behavior is generally such that the family, friends, or relatives can no longer tolerate it. The importance of preventive care is paramount in the aged. Nurses have absorbed many of society's negative views toward the aged and the aging process. Student nurses still prefer to select young patients for one-to-one relationship therapy. It is encouraging to note that group work with the aged by nurses is increasing (Gillin, 1973; Morrison, 1973; Blake, 1973; Holtzen, 1973; Stange, 1973; Holland, 1973; Burnside, 1973). Family therapy with aged families is, as yet, not commonly practiced by nurses. The aged family may consist of a variety of constellations, such as elderly siblings living together; or widowed mother and daughter; or a widower and his widowed daughter. The paucity of literature on family therapy with the aged is indicative of the lack of interest in this mode of therapy for the elderly. At this writing no nurse-written articles were found in the literature.

Nurses could be effective and made considerable changes in such areas as one-to-one relationship therapy, group work, and family therapy with the aged. Nurses could begin to build a body of geriatric nursing knowledge which will be increasingly necessary for practice as our population continues to age. Wheeler (1970) has predicted an age-centered culture, and describes the change as "the rise of the elders."

Nursing students will have to be motivated by enthusiastic, knowledgeable teachers who can serve as role models. More gerontology will have to be included in curricula at all levels. Clinical specialists in geriatric nursing are needed now. Research by nurses in the care of the aged is desperately needed. The importance of nurses working with multidisciplines cannot be overstressed, since aged patients often have complex multiple problems. Butler (1971) points out some areas that this writer considers areas for nursing intervention and research at this point of time:

Old age is a period of multiple, rapid, and profound losses, including the loss of choice. Medical and psychiatric efforts must be directed toward making restitution where possible, and promoting realistic acceptance where fundamental change is impossible. . . . The resources of the community must be exploited. Home care is the probable therapeutic trend of the future.

Riesman's provacative words, written some years ago, are still appropriate to conclude a chapter on developmental reactions in aging (Riesman, 1954):

Many of the suggestions currently made for improving the adjustment of the elderly seem aimed simply at finding ersatz preservatives, not at any inner transformations that would permit self-renewal. . . . Too quick an effort to assure a smooth adjustment results in this merely substitutive activity, whereas allowing a person to be confronted for a time with nothingness might save him—or destroy him—depending on what inner resources he could muster to the challenge.

REFERENCES

Agostini, E., and R. Margaria (1962): "Aspects of Respiratory Physiology in the Aged," in H. T. Blumthal (ed.), *Aging around the World*, vol. 4, *Medical and Clinical Aspects of Aging*, Columbia University Press, New York, pp. 133–154.

American Nurses' Association (1970): "Standards for Geriatric Nursing Practice," *American Journal of Nursing*, vol. 70, no. 9, pp. 1894–1897.

American Psychiatric Association (1968): *Diagnostic and Statistical Manual of Mental Disorders*, 2d ed., Washington, D.C.

Bancroft, Ann V. (1973): "Integrity and Despair: A Contrast of Two Lives," in Irene M. Burnside (ed.), *Psychosocial Nursing Care of the Aged,* McGraw-Hill Book Company, New York.

Bergman, Moe (1971): "Changes in Hearing with Age," *The Gerontologist,* vol. 2, no. 2, part 1.

Birren, James E. (1970): "An Introduction to Contemporary Gerontology," in James E. Birren (ed.): *Contemporary Gerontology: Issues and Concepts,* Gerontology Center, University of Southern California, Los Angeles.

———(1964): *The Psychology of Aging,* Prentice-Hall, Inc., Englewood Cliffs, N.J.

Blake, Dorothy R. (1973): "Group Work with the Institutionalized Elderly," in Irene M. Burnside (ed.), *Psychosocial Nursing Care of the Aged,* McGraw-Hill Book Company, New York.

Brocklehurst, J. C. (1964): "The Etiology of Urinary Incontinence in the Elderly," in W. F. Anderson and B. Isaacs (eds.), *Current Achievements in Geriatrics,* Cassel and Co., Ltd., London, pp. 115–121.

Bromley, D. B. (1966): *The Psychology of Human Aging,* Penguin Books, Baltimore, p. 58.

Burnside, Irene M. (1971a): "Loss: A Constant Theme in Group Work with the Aged," *Hospital and Community Psychiatry,* vol. 21, no. 6, pp. 173–177.

———(1971b): "Gerontion: A Case Study," *Perspectives in Psychiatric Nursing Care,* vol. 9, no. 3, p. 103.

———(1971c): "Long Term Group Work with Hospitalized Aged," *The Gerontologist,* vol. 2, no. 3, part 1, p. 217.

———(1972): "Accoutrements of Aging," in Lois N. Knowles (ed.), *Nursing Clinics of North America,* W. B. Saunders Company, Philadelphia, p. 295.

———(ed.) (1973): *Psychosocial Nursing Care of the Aged,* McGraw-Hill Book Company, New York, pp. 3–14.

Busse, Ewald W., and Eric Pfeiffer (1969): "Functional Disorders in Old Age," in Ewald W. Busse and Eric Pfeiffer (eds.), *Behavior and Adaptation in Late Life,* Little, Brown and Company, Boston.

Butler, Robert (1971): "Clinical Psychiatry in Late Life," in Isadore Rossman (ed.), *Clinical Geriatrics,* J. B. Lippincott Company, Philadelphia.

Carp, Frances (1969): "The Psychology of Aging," in Rosamonde Boyd and Charles G. Oakes (eds.), *Foundations of Practical Gerontology,* University of South Carolina Press, Columbia, S.C.

Chinn, A. B. (1970): "Physiology of Human Aging," in James E. Birren (ed.), *Contemporary Gerontology: Issues and Concepts,* Gerontology Center, University of Southern Califronia, Los Angeles.

Clark, Eloise (1968): "Aspects of Loneliness: Toward a Framework of Nursing Intervention," in Loretta Zderad and Helen Belcher (eds.), *Developmental Concepts in Nursing,* Southern Regional Educational Board, Atlanta, pp. 33–40.

Clark, Margaret, and Barbara G. Anderson (1967): *Culture and Aging,* Charles C Thomas, Springfield, Ill.

Comfort, Alex (1971): Speech presented at Control of Human Aging Conference, Zurich, September 2.

Conti, Mary L. (1973): "Continuity of Care for Elderly Discharged Hospitalized Patients," in Irene M. Burnside (ed.), *Psychosocial Nursing Care of the Aged,* McGraw-Hill Book Company, New York.

Cooper, R. M., I. Bilash, and J. P. Zubeck (1959): "The Effect of Age on Taste Sensitivity," *Journal of Gerontology,* vol. 14, pp. 56–58.

Early, L. W., and Otto von Mering (1969): "Growing Old in the Out-Patient Way," *American Journal of Psychiatry,* vol. 125, pp. 963–967.

Eisdorfer, Carl (1960): "Rorschach Rigidity and Sensory Decrement in a Senescent Population," *Journal of Gerontology,* vol. 15, pp. 188–190.

Engel, George (1962): "Anxiety and Depression Withdrawal: The Primary Affects of Unpleasure," *International Journal of Psychoanalysis,* vol. 43, parts 2 and 3, pp. 89–97.

Erikson, Erik (1968): *Identity, Youth, and Crisis,* W. W. Norton & Company, Inc., New York.

Etzioni, Amitai (1971): "Home—A Buberian Play," *Psychotherapy and Social Science Review,* vol. 5, no. 10, p. 27.

Feinberg, E., M. Braun, and E. Shulman (1968): "E.E.G. Sleep Pattern in Mental Retardation," in *E.E.G. and Clinical Neurophysiology; Diagnostic and Statistical Manual of Mental Disorders,* 2d ed., American Psychiatric Association, Washington, D.C.

Fenichel, Otto (1945): *The Psychoanalytic Theory of the Neuroses,* W. W. Norton & Company, Inc., New York.

Gillin, Lee B. (1973): "Factors Affecting Process and Content in Older Adult Groups," in Irene M. Burnside (ed.), *Psychosocial Nursing Care of the Aged,* McGraw-Hill Book Company, New York.

Guillerme, Jacques (1963): *Longevity* (translated by Mark Holloway), Walker and Company, New York, pp. 129–130.

Gunby, Bjorn (1971): *Psychopharmacy in Old Age,* Paper presented at the Sixth European Congress of Clinical Gerontology, Berne, Switzerland, September.

Gunther, Laurie M. (1969): "A New Look at the Older Patient in the Community through the Eyes of Nursing Students," *Nursing Forum,* vol. 8, no. 1.

Handler, P. (1960): "Radiation and Aging," in N. W. Shock (ed.), *Aging, Some Social and Biological Aspects,* publication no. 65, American Association for the Advancement of Science, Washington, D.C., The Horn-Shafer Company, Baltimore, p. 200.

Holland, Diana L. (1973): "Co-Leadership with a Group of Stroke Patients," in Irene M. Burnside (ed.), *Psychosocial Nursing Care of the Aged,* McGraw-Hill Book Company, New York.

Holtzen, Verna L. (1973): "Group Work in a Rehabilitation Hospital," in Irene M. Burnside (ed.), *Psychosocial Nursing Care of the Aged,* McGraw-Hill Book Company, New York.

Kahn, E., and C. Fisher (1969): "The Sleep Characteristics of the Normal Aged Male," *Journal of Nervous and Mental Diseases,* vol. 148, pp. 477–494.

Kales, A., et al. (1968): "Sleep and Dreams—Recent Research on the Clinical Aspects," *Annals of Internal Medicine,* vol. 68, pp. 1078–1099.

Knowles, Lois R. (1968): Personal communication.

Kohn, R. R. (1963): "Human Aging and Disease," *Journal of Chronic Disease,* vol. 16, pp. 5–21.

Kornzweig, A. L., M. Feldstein, and J. Schneider (1957): "The Eye in Old Age," *American Journal of Ophthalmology,* vol. 44, pp. 29–37.

Levin, Sidney (1965): "Some Comments on the Distribution of Narcissistic and Object Libido in the Aged," in Martin A. Berezi and Stanley H. Cath (eds.), *Geriatric Psychiatry: Grief, Loss, and Emotional Disorders in the Aging Process,* International Universities Press, Inc., New York. Also published in International Journal of Psychoanalysis, vol. 48, pp. 200–208.

McCarthy, Coleman (1972): *Opinion,* vol. 8, no. 4, p. 6.

Morrison, Julianne M. (1973): "Group Therapy for High Utilizers of Chronic Facilities," in Irene M. Burnside (ed.), *Psychosocial Nursing Care of the Aged,* McGraw-Hill Book Company, New York.

Moustakas, Clark (1960): "Communal Loneliness," *Psychologica,* vol. 3, pp. 188–190.

Nahm, Helen (1972): Personal communication.

Neugarten, Bernice L. (1964): "A Developmental View of Adult Personality," in James E. Birren (ed.), *Relations of Development and Aging,* Charles C Thomas, Springfield, Ill.

Norris, A. H., N. W. Shock, M. Lansdown, and J. H. Falzone (1956): "Pulmonary Function Studies: Age Differences in Lung Volume and Bellows Function," *Journal of Gerontology,* vol. 2, pp. 379–387.

Noyes, Arthur P., and Lawrence C. Kolb (1968): *Modern Clinical Psychiatry,* 7th ed., pp. 250–258.

Peplau, Hildegard E. (1952): *Interpersonal Relations in Nursing,* G. P. Putnam's Sons, New York.

Richards, D. W. (1956): "The Aging Lung," *Bulletin New York Academy of Medicine,* vol. 32, pp. 407–417.

Riesman, David (1954): "Some Clinical and Cultural Aspects of Aging," *American Journal of Sociology,* vol. 59, pp. 379–383.

Schwartz, Doris (1971): "Nursing Care of the Aged," in Isadore Rossman (ed.), *Clinical Geriatrics,* J. B. Lippincott Company, Philadelphia.

Scott-Maxwell, Florida (1969): *The Measure of My Days,* Alfred A. Knopf, Inc., New York.

Shanas, Ethel, et al. (1968): *Old People in Three Industrial Societies,* Atherton Press, Inc., New York, pp. 258–287.

Shmavonian, B. M., and E. W. Busse (1963): "Psychophysiological Techniques in the Study of the Aged," in C. Williams et al. (eds.), *Processes of Aging,* vol. 1, Atherton Press, Inc., New York, pp. 168–183.

Shock, N. W. (1960): "Some of the Facts of Aging," in N. W. Shock (ed.), *Aging, Some Social and Biological Aspects,* publication no. 65, American Association for the Advancement of Science, Washington, D.C., The Horn-Shafer Company, Baltimore, pp. 241–260.

Stange, Astrid Z. (1973): "Around the Kitchen Table: Group Work on a Back Ward," in Irene M. Burnside (ed.), *Psychosocial Nursing Care of the Aged,* McGraw-Hill Book Company, New York.

Sullivan, H. S. (1947): *Conceptions of Modern Psychiatry,* William A. White Foundation, Washington, D.C.

Thomas, R. Glyn (1971): *Psychogeriatrics in the Community,* W.H.O. Regional Office, Copenhagen.

Toffler, Alvin (1970): *Future Shock,* Random House, Inc., New York.

United States National Health Survey (1959): *Health Statistics,* Series B, no. 9, p. 9.

Verwoerdt, Adriaan (1969a): "Biological Characteristics of the Elderly," in Rosamond R. Boyd and Charles G. Oakes (eds.), *Foundations of Practical Gerontology,* University of South Carolina Press, Columbia, S. C., p. 55.

————(1969b): "Training in Geropsychiatry," in Ewald Busse and Eric Pfeiffer (eds.), *Behavior and Adaptation in Late Life,* Little, Brown and Company, Boston.

————and Carl Eisdorfer (1967): "Geropsychiatry: The Psychiatry of Senescence," *Geriatrics,* vol. 22, pp. 139–149.

Weinberg, Jack (1970): Lecture, University of Southern California, Los Angeles, July.

Welford, A. T. (1958): *Aging and Human Skill,* Oxford University Press, London.

Wheeler, Harvey (1970): "The Rise of the Elders," *Saturday Review,* December 5.

White, A. (1960): "Some Biochemical Aspects of Aging," in N. W. Shock (ed.), *Aging, Some Social and Biological Aspects,* publication no. 5, American Association for the Advancement of Science, Washington, D.C., The Horn-Shafer Company, Baltimore, pp. 137–145.

8

DEVELOPMENTAL REACTIONS IN THE DYING PERSON

Janice E. Hitchcock and Irene Mortenson Burnside

This chapter describes the developmental reactions which occur in the dying process. The first part of the chapter reviews the literature, and although not an exhaustive review, it does reflect the work and thinking of professionals who represent a variety of health disciplines. The current, frequently used theories are described in greater detail than some of the other theories presented.

The second part of the chapter focuses on death and dying occurring in the later years of life. With the sharp increase in the aged population, the health professions, particularly the nursing profession, face problems peculiar to the dying aged. At the present time, few patients die at home, since death generally occurs in a hospital setting or a nursing home. The aged themselves view nursing homes as places to die or as halfway houses to the mortuary. A growing amount of research and literature from many disciplines reveals increasing interest and concern about the dying aged person; however, the paucity of research and literature by nurses about the dying aged is striking. The chapter ends with implications for the nursing profession.

Death may come to us at any time throughout life. However, for the aged person, death and the process of dying are the imminent and final act of life (Worcester, 1961; Schneidman, 1970). His response to the prospect of death and the dying process will be determined by his reactions to other developmental tasks. Although for some aged people death comes quickly, for others death may approach slowly and the dying process may take weeks and months, and often chronic illness, increased dependency, and suffering accompany the process. Many aged people express more concern about these aspects of dying, and the accompanying sense of hopelessness, helplessness, and isolation, than about actual death itself (Kübler-Ross, 1970).

Since death and dying are subjects which many people consider taboo while many others merely prefer to avoid them, the aged person frequently comes to the end of his life having little preparation for this final task; the process of dying is one which the individual has seldom faced, and death is a total unknown. Until recent years, most theoreticians and clinicians alike avoided the process of dying and death as topics for study and research. The expression of emotions and thoughts regarding the concept of death and dying had been left to theologians, artists, writers, and poets.

Although some people may not allow themselves to think specifically about the end of their life, they still have some concept about what death means to them which will inevitably affect their reactions to their own death. One's particular conceptualization of death usually relates to the culture in which he has been socialized. Members of religious groups, who believe in a life after death, have markedly different concerns from persons who believe that death is an individual's final termination. Whatever one's belief, the inevitability of death allows no rational alternatives and impels people to resort to magic and irrationality on a greater scale than in any other area of human experience (Wahl, 1959). Thus, the frightening and unknown quality of death is perpetuated.

Jung describes a life-death continuum. He views life as a "parabola of a project which, disturbed from its initial state of rest, rises and then returns to a state of repose" (Jung, 1959). He believes that the psychological curve of life refuses to conform. Sometimes the curve lags behind the biological ascent because we try to perpetuate childhood. When we finally do reach the peak of life, we try to stay on top rather than allowing ourselves to gradually slide down the other side to death. Just as fear originally prevented us from living, when death approaches, fear again stands in the way. Jung believes that from middle life onward an individual remains vitally alive only when he is ready to accept his ending.

Tillich speaks of the "eternal now." If we think of ourselves as living in a temporal "now" which is only part of eternity, then death as we know it is really our "being-no-more." The future beyond our "now" we cannot comprehend, but it is inextricably bound to our "being-not-yet," which has to do with the "unimaginable billions of years in which we did not exist" (Tillich, 1959). All this makes up eternity, of which our present existence, the "eternal now," is one part. One's own death is a private and lonely task. We can only observe the process of dying and death in others. Hopefully we can extrapolate some theories which can be helpful when the time comes to cope with our own dying. Death continues to be a subject which needs further investigation.

THEORIES RELATED TO DEATH AND DYING

There has been much written on the various factors related to death and dying which takes into account both intrapsychic and interpersonal aspects. Pattison considers death as a crisis; the stressful event poses a problem which is insoluble in the immediate future. One's psychological resources are taxed beyond one's traditional problem-solving mechanisms, and death is often perceived as a threat or danger to life goals. This state is characterized by a tension which mounts to a peak and then subsides. Unresolved key problems are awakened from both the near and distant past, such as dependency, inadequacy, and identity. During such a crisis, although the health professional cannot deal with the ultimate problem of death, he can help the individual to cope with the various aspects of the dying process: (1) fear of the unknown, (2) loneliness, (3) loss of family and friends, (4) loss of vital parts of the self-image, (5) loss of self-control, (6) loss of identity and of regression (Pattison, 1967). Pain, physical suffering, helplessness, and dependency also increase the anxiety of the dying.

The dying process is described by a number of authorities. Kalish indicates that a number of decisions influence the process (Kalish, 1965). One of the most important is the patient's right to know. From Kalish's experience and that of others, few patients need to be told they are near death; they are soon aware of it. What most dying people would like is the opportunity to discuss their feelings (Quint, 1969a; Worcester, 1961; Kübler-Ross, 1970; Strauss and Glaser, 1965). Another factor to be considered is the social value of the dying person (Glaser and Strauss, 1964). In our society, certain values are highly esteemed, such as: (1) youth, (2) beauty, (3) integrity, (4) talent, (5) parental responsibility, (6) marital responsibility, and (7) earning ability. How one is viewed in terms of his actual potential loss to society or family will influence the reactions of others to him. If the dying person is aged, the chances are great that his social loss will be perceived by those caring for him as being less than that of a younger person. The way in which his family, friends, physician, and nurses respond to the dying individual will in part determine how he copes with his interpersonal relationships as he moves through the dying process.

Social Loss

The idea of social loss is pertinent to the theory of Jourard (Jourard, 1970). He suggests that death occurs because the person is invited to die. When a person no longer has a role, as is true with the elderly in our culture, he is expected to die. "Natural death from old age can be referred to at the same time, both murder and suicide; an invitation to die, extended by others, that has been accepted by the victim" (Jourard, 1970).

Another aspect of social loss is social death. Elderly people are often treated as half-dead while they are still physically and psychologically alive (Kastenbaum, 1969). Limiting our contact and conversation with the dying person and talking at him, rather than with him, are examples of how we also contribute to this approach of handling the dying.

Worcester warns against the danger of socially and psychologically killing a patient. He emphasizes the importance of maintaining close affective contact with the patient until death. Discomfort and pain, often present in the first stages of dying, usually cease when impending death is close (Worcester, 1961). Usually, there is a gradual loss of consciousness, but often a person is conscious long after it has become physically impossible for him to communicate to others; sometimes he is conscious until the final moment of death. This fact is important for those attending the dying person to remember.

Kübler-Ross

Kübler-Ross, in her book, *On Death and Dying,* identified stages of dying that support the above statements of Worcester and others. She also pointed out some of the differences between dying in today's world and dying some years ago (Kübler-Ross, 1970). Formerly people died in their own homes surrounded by relatives, friends, and a familiar environment. Now they usually are sent to a hospital which has much life-saving equipment but offers little that is familiar or supportive and much that is anxiety-provoking. As a result, dying can be a lonely, and sometimes a needlessly long-drawn-out, process which is "impersonalized, dehumanized and mechanized" (Kübler-Ross, 1971). Death is no longer recognized as a natural part of the life process, but rather something to be avoided as long as possible. Hospitalization of the dying person tends to strengthen current taboos associated with death and dying. Death is seen by many health professionals as a failure to cure. Guilt makes them overprotective of the dying patient. Relatives are kept at a distance and may find many obstacles in their way as they try to maintain closeness to their dying loved one. Emotional expressions are usually not encouraged because it might be disturbing to others in the milieu. Opportunity for hospital personnel to learn about death and become comfortable with the experience is curtailed, if not actually prohibited, in most hospital environments.

Kübler-Ross discovered, when she was looking for dying patients as subjects for a study in a large general hospital, that the professional staff denied that there were dying patients on the ward. When she talked to patients, she learned that many knew they were dying and wanted to discuss what they were experiencing. They welcomed the opportunity to talk about themselves. In her study, Dr. Kübler-Ross described specific sequential stages that dying people experience. They may experience several stages at once, or may move back and forth from one stage to another; the progression is not necessarily an orderly one proceeding through one stage at a time.

Generally, the first response of a person hearing that he has a serious illness is shock and denial. However, most people do not continue to maintain these attitudes, unless they are with others who do not allow them an alternative. If such a patient is encouraged to accept the diagnosis, he usually is soon able to talk about his predicament. Anger follows denial, and is often expressed by the question, "Why me?" During the stage of anger the individual is usually irritable and difficult to please. He often is resentful because others are healthy, and may experience feelings of rage, impotence, and frustration.

The next stage is a stage of bargaining. The person has accepted the fact that he will die, but he wants a temporary reprieve in order to do some specific thing. Usually a bargain is made with God and may take the form of bargaining for time to attend a son's wedding or for completing some important project that has been planned.

In the next stage there comes full acknowledgment of impending death, and the dying person becomes very depressed. This stage includes such behavior as: (1) not wanting visitors, (2) crying, and (3) withdrawal from interpersonal contact. There is the acute realization that he is losing everyone; such feelings make grieving very acute and necessary. In the process of working through his feelings at this stage, he begins to decathect and separate himself from his relationships. It is necessary to pass through a stage in which the individual integrates dying into his self-concept. The outcome is acceptance and readiness to die. He may want only one close person to be near him at this time, and has said goodbye to all the others. Acceptance is different from resignation, because it is not a bitter kind of giving up or a defeat, but rather a good feeling.

This gradual disengagement does not contradict the previous statements regarding the avoidance of social death. *It is important that the decathecting begin with the dying patient. He should be the one to decide with whom he wishes to maintain contact. The degree of decathecting will vary from individual to individual.* There is also grief for loss of self.

Throughout all the stages, hope is an important element. Even when death is accepted, there is still the hope that a cure might be found or that there is meaning to this situation in which the dying person finds himself. It is important to support such hope, but not reinforce ideas that are truly unrealistic. It has been Dr. Kübler-Ross's observation that when the dying person no longer hopes, death occurs within 24 hours.

The above-described stages are necessary for the dying person to go through so that he can come to terms with death; however, how well he can complete these tasks depends a great deal on those around him. If he is surrounded by people who are unable to be candid, he may lack the necessary support to proceed beyond denial and anger. Unfortunately, many studies have shown that most of us are loath to talk about death, or we are at a different stage in the grief process than is the patient. Dr. Kübler-Ross describes how difficult it is for a patient to face death when the family is not ready to let him go or is not able to discuss his impending death with him (Kübler-Ross, 1971).

Jaeger and Simmons (1970), in their study, indicate that the majority of professional staff in nursing homes did not think that it was wise to let a patient know that he was dying. Most of the staff felt that the most therapeutic approach was to be evasive or to deny the probability of death; many also denied that they had any responsibility to support the relatives in their grief. Nurses in this study reported that they did not feel that either their patients or the relatives showed enough concern about the dying process to warrant a response from the nurses. Others have reported on the general lack of knowledge about the dying process and grief responses of patients and/or inability to deal with the issue, except to use evasiveness and denial (Quint, 1969b; Duff et al., 1968; Mervyn, 1971; Strauss and Glaser, 1965).

There continues to be gigantic gap between the needs of the patient, who is dealing with the task of dying, and the responses available to him by the significant people in his life. Our current attitudes toward death and dying actually appear to complicate, rather than facilitate, the task of dying.

INFLUENCING FACTORS IN TASK OF DYING

In addition to the attitudes of those surrounding the dying person, there are a number of factors which influence the determination of how one faces the task of dying. How the person has dealt with previous developmental tasks in his life will be a factor. For instance, if most of the conflicts in life have been handled by the use of denial and evasion, then it is likely to be difficult to proceed to an acceptance of death. If, on the other hand, many conflicts in the past were confronted directly, and the coping mechanisms were effective, then there is a good chance that there will be sufficient resources to face this final ultimate task.

Strauss and Glaser (1965) speak of four "awareness contexts": (1) closed awareness, (2) suspicious awareness, (3) mutual pretense, and (4) open awareness. Certain conditions exist to maintain each one. In closed awareness, (1) the patient doesn't recognize signs of impending death, (2) the physician doesn't tell the patient he is dying, (3) the family guards the secret, (4) medical information is withheld from the patient, and (5) the patient has no allies who help him find out about his impending death.

"Suspicious awareness" occurs if any of the above five conditions are not met and the patient suspects that he is dying. If he shows his suspicion either explicitly or by gesture, then it is open suspicious awareness, as contrasted to a closed suspicious awareness, in which he does not reveal his concern; in the latter instance, staff and family do not know of his suspicions.

Mutual pretense exists when both patient and staff or the family are aware that the patient is dying, but at least one interactant wishes to pretend this is not so and other members agree to the pretense. There are certain rules that must be followed: (1) dangerous topics should be avoided, but are permissible as long as no one breaks down, (2) the focus should be on appropriately safe topics, (3) if something happens that leads to exposure of the fiction, then each must pretend that nothing has gone wrong. Finally, an open awareness context emerges when the mutual pretense can no longer be sustained. This awareness usually occurs where physical debilitation or suffering makes the situation impossible to cling to or the patient can no longer face death alone.

In addition to the awareness context in death, it is theorized that one has a certain intention about his own death (Schneidman, 1970). Human deaths can be divided into: (1) intentioned, or (2) subintentioned. Each of these includes a number of subcategories. An intentioned death is one in which the individual plays a direct and conscious role. He may do this as:

1. A death-seeker, one who intends to end his life in a manner that makes rescue unlikely or impossible. These people usually do not stay in this category for long, because with help, they can regain their will to live.
2. Death-initiator, one who believes that he will die soon and wishes to do it for himself.
3. Death-ignorer, one who believes that physical death does not bring psychological death and takes his life in that belief.
4. Death-darer, one who bets his life on low probability of survival.

Unintentional death is a death in which the individual played no part. However, this group of persons can be subcategorized:

1. Death-welcomer—welcomes death although he did not hasten it.
2. Death-accepter—has accepted and is resigned to his fate.
3. Death-postponer—wishes that death would not occur for as long as possible.
4. Death-disdainer—is above involvement.
5. Death-fearer—fears death to the point of phobia and fights it.
6. Death-feigner—simulates self-directed movement toward death, usually for the purpose of activating others into a relationship with him.

Schneidman considered the subintentioned the most important death category, in which the individual plays an unconscious role in his demise:

1. Death-chancer—takes an action that has a limited but realistic risk of dying.
2. Death-hastener—unconsciously increases his chances for death through life style, as in alcoholism or deliberately disregarding prescribed remedial procedures.
3. Death-capitulator—through a strong emotion, effects his death, as in voodoo.
4. Death-experimenter—lives on the brink of death.

Schneidman also comments on the two-person aspect of death, and that the survivor's burden is a heavy one.

ATTITUDES OF THE AGED TOWARD DEATH

Although the process of dying can be identified, the aged person confronted with the situation will face it in his own individualistic way, which will be highly dependent on his specific resources and personality.

Feifel believes that "types of reactions to impending death are a function of interweaving factors" (Feifel, 1959). These factors include the psychologic makeup, the maturity of the person, the coping techniques available, the variables of religious orientation, the socioeconomic status, the severity of the organic process, and the attitudes of the physician and other significant persons in the patient's world.

The attitude of the individual toward death will vary according to its meaning to that individual. For those in severe emotional or physical pain, death may be a release. For others it may be an acceptable and accepted outcome of life or the anticipated beginning of another life. Others may consider death to be totally unacceptable.

Regardless of the particular attitude toward death or one's specific coping ability, there are some practical tasks which must be carried out by the dying person. Such tasks are sometimes difficult to begin if one is still ambivalent about one's dying status or not in the open-awareness context. Only those people who are told of their status and given support as they begin to cope will be able to complete their necessary objectives.

Kalish has described the tasks of the dying person which, when accomplished, have dealt with the practical components of both the physical and the emotional aspects of dying (Kalish, 1970). First, there are usually personal affairs to complete. These may have to do with final considerations about a will, business affairs to adjust, or messages to various people in one's life. If the dying can handle these considerations, he will most likely be able to approach the next task, that of dealing with the loss, both of survivors and of his own life, with courage and hope. This task will include much grief work on the part of the dying person and would account for the depression Kübler-Ross described. The next tasks have to do with participation in the planning for the dying process. The dying individual can help to arrange for medical and other care needs, such as nursing home versus family home. He can allocate his energy and financial resources for the remaining time, and anticipate the occurrence of any physical debilitation or pain. Often it is the fear of loss of performance, rather than death itself, that is the overriding concern. If the person can be helped to plan for this aspect of his life—possible loss of performance—his fear and anxiety can be greatly reduced.

When these tasks are accomplished, or at least under way, the person can begin to look to his own death encounter. Besides contending with his feeling of loss, he must deal with the unknown aspect of death and the possibility of permanent extinction or immortality. The next task concerns his decision to speed up or slow down the dying process. He may indicate whether he wants extraordinary measures taken to keep him alive, or merely whether he will or will not follow doctors' orders regarding such things as diet, exercise, or activity. To some extent, what he decides in such matters can have an effect on how long he can live.

The final task is his adjustment to the dying role and dealing with the psychosocial problems that arise. Such problems include: (1) dependency on others, (2) threat to self-concept by his condition, (3) financial care, (4) housing, (5) emotional support, and (6) lack of productivity in his environment.

Death in the Aged Individual

For the aged, dying means being faced with the history, consequences, and meaning of one's life. What is one to make of one's life if it is about to end? Erikson describes the eighth stage of man as one of either integrity or despair. He says this about the crisis between integrity and despair (Erikson, 1959):

> It is the acceptance of one's own and only life cycle and of the people who have become significant to it as something that had to be and that, by necessity, permitted of no substitutions. It thus means a new different love of one's parents, free of the wish that they should have been different, and an acceptance of the fact that one's life is one's own responsibility. It is a sense of comradeship with men and women of distant times and of different pursuits, that have created orders and objects and sayings conveying human dignity and love. Although aware of the relativity of all the various life styles which have given meaning to human striving, the possessor of integrity is ready to defend the dignity of his own life style against all physical and economic threats. For he knows that an individual life is the accidental coincidence of but one life cycle with but one segment of history; and that for him all human integrity stands and falls with the one style of integrity of which he partakes.

The poet Auden writes succinctly and beautifully of moving toward the ultimate silence of death when he says, "Saying 'Alas' to less and less." As previously stated in this chapter, aged patients, more than persons in other age groups, have come to terms with their own deaths.

One study found that people with a fundamentalist religious background were forward-looking toward death, while those with little religious activity were more likely to be evasive or avoid talking about the subject. It was also found that those in homes for the aged tended to look forward to death while those living alone or with a spouse evaded the issue. The more educated person tended to prepare for his own death more fully. Persons in good health were more likely to evade the consideration of death (Swenson, 1965).

These findings are in contrast to Wolff's study, who found that although fear of death was denied in initial interviews, subjects were open to expressing their concern in subsequent discussions. Wolff found that fear is commonly seen as a part of one's emotional response to death, and is often manifested by restlessness and insomnia in the aged. A study of 240 subjects, who were psychiatric patients over sixty-four, indicated that many fear falling asleep or being alone because "something might happen" (Wolff, 1967). Our society down-grades the status of the aged—which only adds to their fear of death and dying. Our culture tends to view aged death as abnormal rather than emphasizing the natural process of this final life event. As a result, many people fear and avoid the idea and are thus kept from dealing directly with the process.

Pattison has these suggestions for intervention with the dying person which could be used for nursing staff who design nursing care plans and assess the elderly patient (Pattison, 1967):

1. Share responsibility of this crisis so that the patient has help in dealing with the first impact of anxiety and bewilderment.
2. Make continued human contact for the patient not only available to him, but rewarding.
3. Help him in separating and with the grief over the losses of family, body-image, and self-control.
4. Take over the needed body and ego functions for him without making him feel shame; maintain respect for the person and also help him maintain his self-respect.
5. Help him to work out an acceptance of his life situation with dignity.

Defense Mechanisms

Jeffers and Verwoerdt (1969) review several different types of coping that they and others have observed when death is faced. Denial is used to avoid the painful threat from coming into full awareness; denial is considered to be one of the major defenses used to handle the fear of death. For the aged, however, it is somewhat too difficult to maintain a steady pattern of denial, simply because of the events occurring around him. For instance, there is the steady loss of close friends and associates, and even loved pets, through the years. There is an increasing slowing down because of physical disability and/or illness.

Other defenses which an aged person may use to avoid the clear awareness of death would include: suppression, rationalization, and externalization. The same authors state that these defense mechanisms may occur in clusters rather than singly; this is important for nurses to remember so that they observe for more than one coping mechanism.

Another group of defenses is discussed by Jeffers and Verwoerdt (1969). Those are the defenses which are used not so much to exclude the painful threat from the aged individual's conscious awareness as to enable him to retreat from the source of his anxiety. Such mechanisms are: regression, withdrawal, "disengagement," and what these au-thors have termed "surrender," for example, in suicide.

It is known that the actual suicide rate does increase markedly with advancing age, and especially among men. There have been few efforts toward preventing suicide in this particular age group (Breed, 1967). Rachlis (1969) reviews some of the losses involved in the adjustment to aging and makes some suggestions for creative approaches to prevention of suicide in the high-risk older male:

1. Using senior citizens as a resource to identify the suicidal older person.
2. More research to discover the link that might exist between "retirement shock" and suicide.
3. A simple index to predict who is high-risk in the aged population.

The effectiveness that suicide prevention centers have with the elderly population remains to be studied. In one follow-up study of users of a suburban suicide prevention service the authors found that out of sixty-five calls studied, only four callers were above the age of sixty-one, and only one of those four were in the age range seventy-one to eighty years (Carden and Burnside, 1969).

Besides the drastic, lethal suicides committed by the aged, Jeffers and Verwoerdt (1969) describe "occult or slow" suicides in old age. Such occult suicides may be due to depression, loss of appetite, or lowered vitality. Although there may not be any readily available statistics on such behavior, nurses who care for the elderly are quite familiar with the patient who has lost his will to live. One of the writers was once a private-duty nurse; she cared for an elderly woman who absolutely refused to eat. The patient's children were adamant about her eating and were perturbed because the nurses did not feed her more. The old woman very firmly clamped her jaws during any attempt to feed her or give her medications. "Just let me die," she would say to all. Such behavior by the patient often increases both the staff's and the relatives' determination to get food into the person.

If the elderly person is depressed, the nurses and relatives' often try to draw him out into a more active role, unaware that the withdrawal pattern may be one means of cushioning the loss of significant others which the dying person experiences. The social isolation, although often openly requested by the patient, is often ignored by staff and relatives alike. Many patients feign sleep in order to be left alone more when they are nearing death.

Less socially acceptable ways of mastering the fear of death is to withdraw by the use of alcohol and drugs. Another coping behavior described by Jeffers and Verwoerdt (1969) is that of resolution and mastery. The defense mechanisms used in these instances include: (1) intellectualization, and (2) counter-phobic activities such as hyperactivity, sublimation, and acceptance. Frequently, one sees unusually active elderly people who are traveling restlessly or are frenetically engaged in various hobbies and civic responsibilities. It is true that some artistic older people can remain creatively active late in their lives; Grandma Moses and Imogen Cunningham are two excellent examples, the former a well-known painter and the latter a gifted photographer.

Butler's life review, which he describes as "a universal, normal experience, intensifying in the aged, and occurring irrespective of environmental conditions," is a coping mechanism frequently used by the dying person (Butler, 1964). Findings in a study on reminiscing done by McMahon and Rhudick (1967) indicated that reminiscing is not directly related to intelligence or intellectual deterioration. Two-thirds of the total responses to the interview showed preoccupation with the past. The researchers stated that reminiscing is positively related to freedom from depression and personal survival. Ebersole developed reminiscing as a focus in group work with the aged to facilitate their adaptation to aging (Ebersole, 1972a, 1972b). Burnside, in her group work with aged patients, found that the group members did not shy away from talking about their own deaths (Burnside, 1970).

IMPLICATIONS FOR NURSING

Krant has described organized care of the dying patient at a state institution. Some of the major points of the paper have been pulled out since they have implications for nurses who are in a position to alter the attitudes of the caretakers and to improve the quality of the nursing care of the dying patient (Krant, 1972):

1. The crisis of dying demanded an intimacy from staff that they had not given previously.
2. A new unit was established to help patients "die well"; and also to help the staff become more secure with the crisis of dying and to change their attitudes about dying.
3. Doctors were asked to release their dominance over other staff members.
4. Home care in the community was part of the plan.
5. Conferences included therapeutic moves based on psychological and social needs of the patient as well as biological needs.
6. Open discussion of death and dying by everyone is encouraged.
7. A bereavement clinic is being considered to facilitate the adjustment of the family of the deceased.
8. The staff receives and gives support to one another during complex problems.
9. Communication with the patient is important. "The art of telling is the art of supporting."

The paucity of material written by nurses about the dying person, aged or otherwise, perhaps does not do justice to the amount of work and time that many in this profession spend with dying, aged people. Quint has pioneered the work in nursing the dying patient. Roberts wrote about aged patients in an intensive care unit who actually wanted to die (Roberts, 1973).

There are some areas in which nurses could concentrate efforts for improvement of the dying:

1. Provide better psychosocial care to the dying aged patient.
2. Assist patients to die in their own residences if they wish.
3. Assist dying patients to withdraw during their dying process if they so desire.
4. Find ways and means by which an aged person can die with dignity.
5. Examine the impact of institutionalization in nursing homes on the dying aged; e.g., some nursing homes conduct the funeral service within the nursing home—what effect does this have on other residents in the home?
6. Begin discussion groups and in-service programs to help nurses to handle many of the feelings they have about the aging and the dying process.
7. Encourage further research done by nurses in the area of death and dying.

Krant (1972) writes, "In recent years, as we have come to appreciate that dying is an inherent part of the life cycle rather than just a failure in medical technique, the dying person's needs as a human being have evoked more and more medical concern."

Death is a universal phenomenon about which very little is presently known. Dying can be described as a process occurring in definite stages. The process which occurs before final death may often be an extended one in the aged and may have many components. If the phenomenon of death can be viewed as a natural, normal, and inevitable event and its occurrences can be discussed with the dying patient, a long step has been taken toward the enrichment of life by the acceptance of death.

A quote attributed to Leonardo da Vinci is apropos with which to end a chapter about death and dying: "All the time I thought I was learning to live, I was learning to die."

REFERENCES

Breed, Warren (1967): "Suicide and Loss in Social Interaction," in E. S. Schneidman (ed.), *Essays in Self Destruction,* Science House, New York.

Burnside, Irene M. (1970): "Loss: A Constant Theme in Group Work with the Aged," *Hospital and Community Psychiatry,* June, pp. 173–177.

Butler, Robert N. (1964): "The Life Review: An Interpretation of Reminiscence in the Aged," in Robert Kastenbaum (ed.), *New Thoughts on Old Age,* Springer Publishing Co., Inc., New York.

Carden, Norman L., and Irene M. Burnside (1969): *The Role of a Crisis Intervention Telephone Service in a California Community,* Unpublished paper.

Duff, Raymond, and August B. Hollingshead (1968): *Sickness and Society,* Harper & Row, Publishers, Inc., New York.

Ebersole, Priscilla (1972a): *Developing the Use of Reminiscence in Group Psychotherapy with the Aged,* Unpublished paper, March.

———(1972b): *Preliminary Report on the Use of Reminiscence in Group Psychotherapy for the Aged,* Unpublished paper, June.

Erikson, Erik (1959): "Identity and the Life Cycle," *Psychological Issues* (monograph), vol. 1, no. 1, International Universities Press, New York.

Feifel, Herman (1959): "Attitudes toward Death in Some Normal and Mentally Ill Populations," in Herman Feifel (ed.), *The Meaning of Death,* McGraw-Hill Book Company, New York, p. 126.

Glaser, Barney, and Anselm Strauss (1964): "The Social Loss of Dying Patients," *American Journal of Nursing,* June, pp. 119–121.

Jaeger, Dorothea, and L. Simmons (1970): *The Aged Ill,* Appleton-Century-Crofts, Inc., New York.

Jeffers, Frances C., and Adriaan Verwoerdt (1969): "How the Old Face Death," in Edward Busse and Eric Pfeiffer (eds.), *Behavior and Adaptation in Late Life,* Little, Brown and Company, Boston, pp. 163–181.

Jourard, Sidney (1970): "Suicide: An Invitation to Die, *American Journal of Nursing,* pp. 269–275.

Jung, Carl (1959): "The Soul and Death," in Herman Feifel (ed.), *The Meaning of Death,* McGraw-Hill Book Company, New York, p. 5.

Kalish, Richard A. (1965): "The Aged and the Dying Process: The Inevitable Decisions," *Journal of Social Issues,* vol. 21, pp. 87–96.

———(1970): "The Onset of the Dying Process," *Omega,* February, pp. 57–69.

Kastenbaum, Robert (1969): "Death and Bereavement in Later Life," in Austin Kutscher (ed.), *Death and Bereavement,* Charles C Thomas, Springfield, Ill., p. 31.

Krant, Melvin J. (1972): "The Organized Care of the Dying Patient," *Hospital Practice,* January, pp. 101–108.

Kübler-Ross, Elisabeth (1970): *On Death and Dying,* The Macmillan Company, New York.

———(1971): "What Is It Like to Be Dying?" *American Journal of Nursing,* January, pp. 54–61.

McMahon, A. W., Jr., and P. J. Rhudick (1967): "Reminiscing in the Aged: An Adaptational Response," in Sidney Levin and Ralph J. Kahana (eds.), *Psychodynamic Studies on Aging: Creativity Reminiscing, and Dying,* International Universities Press, Inc., New York.

Mervyn, Frances (1971): "The Plight of Dying Patients in Hospitals," *American Journal of Nursing,* October, pp. 1988–1990.

Pattison, E. Mansell (1967): "The Experience of Dying," *American Journal of Psychotherapy,* January, pp. 32–43.

Quint, Jeanne C. (1969a): *The Nurse and the Dying Patient,* The Macmillan Company, New York.

———(1969b): "The Threat of Death: Some Consequences for Patients and Nurses," *Nursing Forum,* pp. 287–300.

Rachlis, David (1969): *Suicide and Loss Adjustment in the Aging,* Paper presented to the Second Annual Conference, American Association of Suicidology, New York, Mar. 29.

Roberts, Sharon L. (1973): "To Die or Not to Die: Plight of the Aged Patient in ICU," in Irene Mortenson Burnside (ed.), *Psychosocial Nursing Care of the Aged,* McGraw-Hill Book Company, New York.

Schneidman, Edwin (1970): "The Enemy," *Psychology Today.*

Strauss, Anselm, and Barney Glaser (1965): *Awareness of Dying,* Aldine Publishing Company, Chicago, Ill.

Swenson, Wendell M. (1965): "Attitudes toward the Dead among the Aged," in Robert Fulton (ed.), *Death and Identity,* John Wiley & Sons, Inc., New York.

Tillich, Paul (1959): "The Eternal Now," in Herman Feifel (ed.), *The Meaning of Death,* McGraw-Hill Book Company, New York.

Wahl, C. W. (1959): "The Fear of Death," in Herman Feifel (ed.), *The Meaning of Death,* McGraw-Hill Book Company, New York.

Wolff, Kurt (1967): "Helping Elderly Patients Face the Fear of Death," *Hospital and Community Psychiatry,* May, pp. 142–144.

Worcester, Alfred (1961): *The Care of the Aged, the Dying, and the Dead,"* 2d ed., Charles C Thomas, Publisher, Springfield, Ill.

PART THREE

Models of Treatment

9

MODELS OF PSYCHIATRIC TREATMENT

Marion E. Kalkman

In approaching the subject of treatment in psychiatry, the health professional is confronted by a constantly increasing number of therapeutic methods. It seemed to the writer that rather than try to discuss such a variety of treatments, it might be more helpful to devise models or analogies of a few of the current and most influential approaches to treatment. Such models could provide the mental health professional with a frame of reference or orientation to a particular way of perceiving mental illness, and characteristic methods of treatment based on the result of such perceptions and theories.

For the purposes of this discussion, four models have been chosen which represent four very different points of view and philosophy, from the standpoint of both theory and practice. Most current methods of treatment either can be included in one of these categories or may have components of one or more of them. The four models to be discussed are the medical model of psychiatric treatment, the behavioral model, the psychodynamic model, and the unitary concept model. These are presented briefly with no attempt to instruct the reader in the technique and practice of the particular type of therapy.

The goal of all methods of therapy is to change some unsatisfactory component in an individual's own personality or some unsatisfactory interaction with his environment. People who are contented with their life style do not seek therapy, no matter how unhappy, ineffectual, or strange this way of life may seem to others. In the four models selected for this discussion an attempt will be made to see if it can be determined how this change is effected by each type of therapy and what some of the theoretical assumptions are upon which the therapeutic model is based.

It is the writer's belief that a general knowledge of the basic philosophy of these four models of treatment and an understanding of the goals of therapy and methods for achieving these goals can provide the health professional therapist with several frames of reference within which he can work. As one reads the literature, one becomes aware of the fact that treatment practices are not well delineated in any of the first three models and not yet developed at all in the fourth. Regarding this paucity of information, Ford and Urban (1963, pp. 667–668), discussing the ten therapies which they critiqued wrote, "One wonders why these therapists as a group have specified so little in the way of principles and techniques for producing behavioral change." They suggest that several possible reasons for this are that the techniques may be misused by uninformed people; that many intangible variables intervene; and that further specification presents impossible problems. However, they believe that "a clear specification of principles and procedures for change is essential so that verification of their effectiveness becomes possible." Incomplete and undeveloped as these models are, nevertheless they afford the therapist with four very different frameworks for sytematically developing his own concepts of treatment.

THE MEDICAL MODEL

The medical model approach to mental illness is the oldest and still one of the most influential approaches currently operant in the treatment of mental illness. It had its beginning in the Renaissance period when men first began to question the concept that mental illness was due to possession by witches, demons, and other evil spirits. Johann Weyer (1515–1588), who is regarded by many medical historians as the first psychiatrist, carefully observed and investigated many reported cases of witchcraft and proved that the patients' behavior could be explained by naturalistic causes. Although Weyer was unable to develop a theory of the etiology of mental diseases, he crusaded for the idea that mental illnesses were not supernatural in origin, but were due to physical causes and should be treated by a physician (Alexander and Selesnick, 1966).

In the seventeenth century the clinical observations of Sydenham led him to the systematic investigation and identification of a number of disease entities, including hysteria, hypochondria, and St. Vitus' Dance. Also during this period, Harvey described the effect of psychological tensions on the circulation of the blood. In the eighteenth century, the Period of Enlightenment, the quantity of scientific and medical data became so great that systematization and classification became imperative in botany, chemistry, and physics. By 1800, mental symtoms also were categorized into disease entities, but the number of patients studied was small. Since the psychiatric classification was not necessarily related to an understanding of the psychological causes, but merely named the disease entity, psychiatric treatment was unaffected by the diagnostic designation of the disease. In 1761, Morgagni published his famous report, *On the Seats and Causes of Disease Investigated by Anatomy.* He was particularly interested in brain pathology and believed that disease could be localized in particular organs of the body. Neuroanatomists, neurologists, and physicians interested in discovering the causes of mental illness were strongly influenced by Morgagni's concepts and began making detailed investigations of the brain (Alexander and Selesnick, 1966, p. 150). This search to identify the causes of mental illness as based in an organ or organ system has continued up to the present time. One of the outstanding contributors to medical knowledge in this area is Dr. Harvey Cushing (1869–1939), who pioneered in developing modern neurosurgical procedures which made research in this field possible. Recently there has been a renewed interest in brain anatomy, physiology, and pathology in such problems as cortical organization and localization, the reticular activating and limbic systems, and problems of consciousness, sleep, and pain. Among the contributors to such research are Wilder Penfield, Horace W. Magoun, Ralph W. Gerard, and Stanley Cobb (Mora, 1959, p. 43).

The name of Emil Kraepelin (1856–1926) stands out in any discussion of the medical model of mental disorder, for it was his monumental work of systematic descriptive categorization of psychopathological conditions which is acknowledged to be the first comprehensive medical model of mental illness. Sarason and Ganzer regard this system as a true medical model or analogy in the strict sense in that the etiology was organic, that is, based in the central nervous system, and that the prognosis followed a predictable course. Kraepelin also believed that appropriate treatment should be based on accurate diagnosis (Sarason and Ganzer, 1968). Kraepelin derived his organically oriented system from painstakingly collected clinical observation of the behavior of hundreds of patients during the 19 years that he was director of a large mental hospital in Munich. Most of these patients had been hospitalized for years, with the result that their physical and mental condition had deteriorated and their symptoms had become rigidly fixed. Kraepelin's observations led him to the conclusion that mental illness followed an inevitable downward course which made the possibility of recovery highly unlikely. This was particularly the case with his observations of dementia praecox or, as it later came to be called, schizophrenia. Although his classification system of mental disorders has long since fallen out of use in favor of more modern ones, nevertheless his brilliant clinical observations and accurate description of symptoms can still be observed in mental patients today. His organic orientation to mental illness, which seems more related to the physical sciences, and hence more open to methods of experimental scientific research than the psychological approach, still holds great appeal for many clinicians and researchers in the field of psychiatry.

Assumptions of the Medical Model The medical model of mental illness used in psychiatry functions according to a number of assumptions or suppositions analogous to those in medicine. Griesinger stated, "Mental diseases are brain diseases" (quoted in Menninger, 1963, p. 26). One of these common assumptions is that the individual suffering from a mental illness, like the individual who has a physical illness, is regarded as "sick," that is, that he has an illness, or disease, or defect; and that this illness can be located in some part of the body, generally but not always in the central nervous system. Other common assumptions include that illness has characteristic mental symptoms or syndromes which can be diagnosed, classified, and labeled as a specific disease entity; that it generally runs a characteristic course and carries a prognosis for the prospect of recovery; that it is amenable to treatment by such physical means as drugs, chemicals, hormones, electricity, hydrotherapy, and diet; and that interventions are essentially those of adding something, taking something away, or counteracting or replacing something in the body.

Treatment in the Medical Model In the treatment of mental illness according to the medical model, the methodology closely follows that used in general medical practice. History taking, diagnosis, and classification play important roles and are the initial steps in the treatment process. The patient's psychiatric history is taken as soon as possible after the patient has been accepted for treatment and is generally completed in one or two interviews. These interviews follow a fairly structured pattern, including chronological events in the life history, previous medical or psychological problems, current presenting problems, onset of symptoms, and evaluation of present mental status. History taking is generally followed by a general physical examination with special attention to neurological aspects, and by referrals for such laboratory, physical, and psychological tests as seem indicated. From the data derived from these sources and from observation of the patient's behavior either directly by the psychiatrist in the interview situation and/or by other psychiatric personnel, a diagnosis is made.

Arriving at a diagnosis constitutes a critical decision. In the medical model, the psychiatrist either alone or in consultation with fellow psychiatrists assumes this responsibility. The diagnosis determined upon classifies or puts a label upon the patient as well as on the illness, and implies treatment methods in keeping with the specific diagnosis. Because diagnosis often carries with it a certain prognosis, it may have implications for the patient's future. The diagnosis made by the psychiatrist is regarded as "official" not only for legal and statistical purposes, such as insurance claims, hospital records, and government reports, but also by members of other psychiatric professionals and paraprofessionals even though privately they may not concur. A given diagnosis, however, may be revised or changed by the patient's psychiatrist during the course of his supervision of the patient's treatment. When the care of the patient is transferred to another psychiatrist, he is free to reevaluate the patient's condition and to change the diagnosis.

The interventions used in treatment consist of a variety of physical methods, of which by far the most prevalent is the administration of drugs and other substances such as vitamins and hormones. Drugs can be used for many purposes in the treatment of mental illness. Alexander had identified five different categories of use, namely (Alexander and Selesnick, 1966, pp. 353–366):

1. Drugs used not for any medicinal properties they may have but which act through suggestion to make the patient feel better, that is, the placebo effect
2. Drugs to correct a deficiency or to combat infection, as, for example, vitamin replacement in a vitamin deficiency, or penicillin in syphilis
3. Drugs used as sedatives or stimulants to modify exaggerated emotional states or mood swings
4. Drugs to facilitate verbal communication or the expression of emotion, as, for example, sodium amytal and other barbiturates
5. Drugs prescribed to ameliorate specific mental conditions, such as tranquilizers and anti-depressants in schizophrenia and lithium carbonate in manic-depressive psychoses, as well as hallucinogens such as LSD for research into psychotic states

Other forms of physical intervention once used extensively but now only infrequently are electroshock therapy and psychosurgery, principally in the procedure known as *leucotomy*. Recent advances in research in the fields of microbiology, biochemistry, and human genetics may develop new somatic methods of treatment in the future. *Medical Model: Implications for Nursing Practice* The psychiatric nurse first became involved in the treatment of mentally ill patients because, other than the psychiatrist, the nurse was the only health professional directly concerned with patient care who had a knowledge of drugs, their uses, and their desirable and undesirable effects. This attribute took precedence over any knowledge of psychology or psychiatry that a nurse might have. In the late nineteenth and early twentieth century the extent of this knowledge was very little or none. The traditional doctor-nurse relationship obtained in this period, in which the physician diagnosed and prescribed the drug and the nurse administered the drug to the patient and reported its effects to the physician. The list of drugs commonly prescribed was limited and fairly similar in all psychiatric institutions. It included sedatives such as paraldehyde, chloralhydrate, and barbital, and a few laxatives and cold remedies. In the 1930s the rise of the somatic therapies, such as deep sleep therapy induced by sodium amytal and Pentothal and insulin and metrazol therapy, increased the number and importance of nurses in psychiatric treatment programs.

The ataraxic drug revolution of the mid-twentieth century swept the country and popularized drug therapy to such a degree that psychiatrists were hard pressed not only by the constantly increasing stream of new drugs from drug manufacturers, but also by the great numbers of patients, mostly in large state hospitals, clamoring to be treated. As a result of this stress, the relationship between the physician and the nurse began to change. The nurse as a member of the treatment team became more of a colleague than an agent of the physician. When patients who were still on a drug regimen, and often still somewhat confused, were discharged into the community, the need for a nurse to follow up their adherence to their drug schedule was apparent. New drugs of all kinds for mental disorders continued to flood the market. In the sixties came the problems of the drug abusers or drug addicts and self-administered psychedelic drug users as well as the users of prescribed drugs.

The role of the nurse is becoming one of increasing independence and responsibility in psychiatric nursing practice. In rural areas and in city slums where physicians are in short supply, specially prepared nurses are carrying out many functions traditionally reserved for physicians only. Some of these duties include primary interviewing of prospective patients, history taking, examination, diagnosis, and referral to an appropriate treatment agency, discharge planning, and follow-up care. In many instances the nurse utilizes a physician as a consultant but is responsible for direct medical and nursing care. This arrangement is not uncommon with the mentally retarded, geriatric senile patients, and long-term schizophrenic patients. The psychiatric nurse may supplement the medical treatment by providing psychological nursing care for patients suffering from psychosomatic or medical conditions accompanied by severe psychological distress.

Because of manpower shortages in all the psychiatric health disciplines at the higher levels of training and competence, the psychiatric nurse specialist has assumed many responsibilities for training paraprofessional personnel. Such trained personnel can free the psychiatrist and other professionals from routine tasks. Mental health legislation and popular demands for more and better mental health services are taxing the time and energy of all mental health professionals to the utmost. The medical model of psychiatric treatment is in many ways best suited to meet these increased demands for service because it is the most economical treatment model in terms of time (length of treatment), cost, and personnel. Highly trained professionals can be used to teach less well-prepared personnel and to supervise treatment for a far greater number of patients than is possible if these professionals limited their practice to direct care. The medical model is liked by medical organizations because it maintains the prestige and authority of the medical profession, and it is popular with the public because taking a pill is less painful than many of the introspective techniques of psychotherapy. Most important of all, there is no other alternative model available that is practical for large numbers of patients (Albee, 1968, pp. 317–320).

THE BEHAVIORAL MODEL

The behavioral model of treatment is based on theories related to the learning process and has its roots in the two sciences of psychology and physiology—more particularly, neurophysiology. One of the earliest and most important contributions from physiology came from Pavlov (1849–1936), who in 1902 discovered the phenomenon which he called the "conditioned reflex." The basic principle of the conditioned reflex is that the same response in a stimulus-response reaction can be obtained if a new and different stimulus is presented just prior to the original stimulus. If, then, this double-stimuli situation is repeated frequently, eventually the new stimulus can replace the original one, as, for example, in Pavlov's classical experiment with a dog. In this experiment the sequence was as follows: (1) perception of food leads to salivary reflex; (2) sound of bell plus perception of food leads to salivary reflex; (3) sound of bell alone leads to salivary reflex. This conditioned or learned response was seen as the basic unit of all learning. From this basic unit more complex behavioral patterns could be built. Pavlov made many investigations to determine how conditioned reflexes could be reinforced or inhibited. He believed that such higher brain functions as thinking inhibited action because thought processes must take place before action can be initiated. Reinforcement occurred when a spontaneous, successful, and need-satisfying behavior pattern was discovered and repeated. Pavlov accounted for conflicts in terms of neuronal patterns that had been either overstimulated or inhibited (Matson, 1967, pp. 83–93; Alexander and Selesnick, 1966, pp. 203–204).

Pavlov's theories achieved international acclaim when they first became known and have continued to have great influence to the present time, not only in the Soviet Union, where Pavlovian psychology became the official psychology of the state, but also in the United States, where it was proclaimed as "the key to the comprehension and control of the whole range of human behavior" (Matson, 1967, p. 83). Pavlov and his associates "tried to explain conditioning on mechanistic-neurophysiological grounds avoiding psychological concepts as much as possible. Their aim was to objectify psychology and reduce it to neurophysiology, so that dealing with data on subjective awareness is made superfluous" (Alexander and Selesnick, 1966, p. 382).

The simplicity, concreteness, and objectivity of Pavlov's theories made a great appeal to a number of American experimental psychologists including J. B. Watson, the founder of behaviorism, who stated, "The time has come when psychology must discard all reference to consciousness. . . . Its sole task is the prediction and control of behavior; and introspection can form no part of its method" (quoted by Koestler, 1967, p. 5). Clark L. Hull, who held to a mechanistic view of man, said that "adaptive behavior operates ultimately according to the principles of the physical world" (Matson, 1967, p. 109). B. F. Skinner, who is presently the most notable exponent of behaviorism, is the author of a number of stimulating and provocative books on this subject (Skinner, 1938; 1953; 1971). The application of the principles of behaviorism to behavioral therapy have been made by Wolpe (1958), Gericke (1965), Lovaas (1967), Bandura (1965), Schaefer and Martin (1969), and many others.

Assumptions of the Behavioral Model of Therapy   Behavioral therapy is based on the concept that behavior is what an organism does. Behavior can be observed, described, and recorded. Not only the behavior is recorded, but also the conditions and circumstances under which a specific behavior occurred; thus it is possible to predict under what conditions the same behavior may be expected to reoccur. The aim of behavioral therapy is to change overt behavior, that is, to develop or reinstate behaviors which are necessary for effective functioning in a social context. Undesirable social behavior is regarded not as a symptom of mental illness, but as behavior which can and should be changed. The concept of mental illness as a disease is regarded as a hindrance to the patient's recovery, and psychiatric diagnostic labels are considered as possibly necessary for legal classification but as providing no assistance in prescribing treatment.

Another basic assumption of behavioral therapy is that men constantly control the behavior of other men whether they want to or not. Such control affects both the person applying the control and the person controlled. Control of itself is neither good nor evil. The goal in behavior therapy is to change unacceptable behavior to acceptable behavior, and this is brought about by the application of the principles of control. The therapist accepts the fact that he exerts control over his patient willingly or unwillingly, whether or not he is aware of this fact. The therapist also accepts responsibility for the moral and ethical implications of his interventions and for the patient's behavior while under his care. He makes no pretense that "it's up to the patients to make their own decisions to do what is 'right.'" On the other hand, the therapist is expected to relinquish his own wishes and inclinations in favor of the patient's manner of doing things (Schaefer and Martin, 1969, pp. 3–13).

Treatment in the Behavioral Model   The goal of behavioral therapy is to change those behaviors of the patient which interfere with his effective functioning in his social milieu. Such undesirable behaviors are perceived as learned disorders which develop as a consequence of acute anxiety in a given set of circumstances. Therapy, therefore, is based on the knowledge and application of principles of learning—that is, the unlearning or extinction of undesirable behavior and the substitution of new learning sequences and/or reinforcement of desirable behavior. The applicability of these principles is based on the assumption that the learning process is the same for all people. Consequently, all types of disorders are acceptable for treatment except organic conditions, which are not deemed suitable since the pathological behavior is not considered to be a learned behavior but a malfunctioning of the central nervous system.

The therapist determines what behavior should be changed and what plan of treatment should be followed. Change in behavior is effected by the therapist identifying what events in the patient's life history are crucial and arranging therapeutic situations in which the patient is confronted by these events. The therapist then may use a variety of therapeutic interventions or methods to effect the desired change. These interventions include therapeutic interviews in which the patient tries to recall the critical events and the precipitating circumstances, discussion of current life situations, simulated situations, and desensitivation techniques. In treating neurotic patients, Wolpe considered the first step in recovery not a changed way of thinking, but a changed way of acting. He also suggests that anxiety states may be prevented by avoiding environments in which anxiety-evoking stimuli or situations are present, such as elevators, fear-inspiring individuals, or attention-focusing situations. On the other hand, anxiety can often be controlled by seeking new and non-threatening environments in which the patient can become engrossed in activities which are satisfying to him and in which he can function comfortably (Ford and Urban, 1963, p. 288). For essentially nonverbal patients, operant conditioning and successive approximation, or hand-shaping, may be used to effect behavior changes. Adjunctive methods include relaxation therapy, hypnosis, and drugs such as tranquilizers, barbiturates, and alcohol (Ford and Urban, 1963, pp. 273–303; Schaefer and Martin, 1969, pp. 3–61).

The Environment as a Behavioral Change Agent   The environment plays an important role in behavioral therapy. "Environments are not passive wrappings, but are, rather, active processes which are invisible" (McLuhan, 1967, p. 68). In any description or recording of a specific behavior, the context or setting in which the behavior occurred is very carefully noted. Wolpe defines environment in behavioral therapy: "Only those events to which the individual responds or reacts are considered his environment, while the totality of events at the time are considered his surroundings" (Ford and Urban, 1963, p. 286). This difference is illustrated by the following incident. For an experiment, a group of nurses wore civilian clothes on duty. The first day, staff personnel whom they had known for years apparently did not see the nurses or respond to their nods of greeting but looked past them, as the staff customarily did with patients in their environment (Schaefer and Martin, 1969, p. 48).

Behavioral therapists often use environmental factors to effect behavior change. One such use is that of *control stimuli.* The effectiveness of this procedure is based on the fact that every behavior occurs in a real environment which contains a number of stimuli which remain more or less constant throughout the period of acquisition and which become control stimuli for the manifestation of this particular behavior. If the therapist substitutes a new stimuli complex and institutes a schedule of continuous reinforcement, the desired behavior can be established. When the patient moves to a new environment, the therapist searches this environment for stimuli which will maintain the control of the newly established behavior.

Behavioral therapists also create special environments for the treatment of groups of patients with common problems, such as the mentally retarded (Miron, 1966) and schizophrenic children (Lovaas, 1967). In many of these controlled therapeutic environments patients follow prescribed schedules for daily living. Token economy is also often used; that is, patients are rewarded for desired behavior by token reinforcers such as food, candy, money tokens, and verbal approval. Special environments and programs may also be devised for individual patients with severe, idiosyncratic behavior problems (Bandura, 1965; Gericke, 1965; Ayllon, 1963; Schaefer, 1966; Schaefer and Martin, 1969, pp. 46–49).

Behavioral Therapy: Implications for Practice To practice behavioral therapy, the therapist must have a good understanding of the learning theories upon which treatment is based, and also knowledge and skill in the specific interventions and stratagems which will produce the desired change. More emphasis is placed on the accuracy and correctness of the principles underlying a particular strategy and on its use in the appropriate situation than on the idiosyncratic personality traits of the patient. Doubtless the "robot theory of man" developed by Hull, whose theories of learning were so influential in the development of behavioral therapy, as well as B. F. Skinner's behavioral theories derived from the animal experimentation, has given an impersonal orientation to this form of therapy (Hull, 1943, p. 26; also quoted in Matson, 1967, p. 107; Skinner, 1953). These concepts have been criticized not only as presenting an oversimplified view of the complexities of the human personality, but also as having some very authoritarian implications for the therapist-patient relationship (Bertalanffy, 1967, pp. 6–14 and pp. 116–121; Bertalanffy, 1966, pp. 705–706; Koestler, 1967, pp. 5–15). The terms *molding* and *hand-shaping,* referring to techniques for modifying behavior, reflect the passive, submissive role of the patient and the active, dominating role of the therapist. One well-known paper describing the role of the nurse in behavioral therapy refers to the nurse as a "behavioral engineer" (Ayllon and Michael, 1959, pp. 323–334). It is the opinion of this writer that the behavioral therapist must be constantly aware of the ethical responsibility he assumes for the protection of the patient's personal rights and the preservation of his individuality during the practice of this method of treatment. This is not to deny the usefulness and effectiveness of behavioral therapy for some mentally ill persons, especially those who have become so alienated from society or so functionally incapacitated that they are unable to interact with or respond appropriately to others. For such severely traumatized persons behavioral therapy may serve to break through their isolation and provide the first step to a return to useful living.

The practice of behavioral therapy requires close and sometimes almost continuous observation of the patient's behavior, on-the-spot intervention and correction of undesirable behavior, and frequent recording of clinical data. If the patient is an outpatient, the therapist has to rely on his observations of the patient's behavior during the therapeutic session and also on the patient's self-observations during the interval between sessions. If the patient is receiving in-patient treatment, most of these functions are carried out by the nursing personnel. The effectiveness of behavioral treatment depends in large part on the intelligence, creativeness, tact, and persistence of the professional nurse or nurses responsible for the patient's care. Since well-prepared nurses are difficult to find in adequate numbers, another responsibility of such a nurse is the teaching and supervision of less well-prepared nursing personnel. In this manner, his knowledge and skill can be made available to a greater number of patients than would otherwise be possible.

Because behavioral therapy is based on learning theories and because the shortage of medical personnel at all levels will probably not be eliminated in the foreseeable future, several psychologists have suggested looking for other alternatives for the delivery of treatment. Bandura (1967, p. 86) writes, "The day may not be far off when psychological disorders will be treated not in hospitals or mental hygiene clinics but in comprehensive learning centers, when clients will be considered not patients suffering from hidden psychic pathologies but responsible people who participate actively in their own potentialities." Albee believes that as long as the illness model prevails, all available funds, planning, and resources will be devoted to psychiatric treatment, mental hospital beds, and the treatment team. He has suggested as an alternative utilizing the model of the educational system and developing institutional structure where the treatment and administrative policies are based on research findings in behavioral modification. These facilities would be staffed with nonprofessional people with a bachelor's degree supported by consultants in specialized areas of expertise. He visualizes these centers as places "where technicians, non-professionals, rehabilitation workers, of all kinds could be used to maximize human potential" (Albee, 1968, p. 319).

THE PSYCHODYNAMIC MODEL

The psychodynamic model of treatment was developed by Sigmund Freud in the closing years of the nineteenth century when the medical model as developed by Kraepelin was at the height of its influence and popularity. Although a number of predecessors of Freud, including Reil, Moreau, Carus, and Herbart, introduced the concept that psychological methods were necessary for the understanding and treatment of mental illness, it was Freud who developed both a theoretical model of psychology that provided a basis for understanding psychiatric symptoms, and a workable psychological method for treatment. The key concept underlying both theory and treatment is the same— Freud's outstanding discovery of the unconscious mind, its structure, and its influence on man's behavior. This was a contribution of inestimable value not only to psychology and psychiatry but to many other fields of knowledge as well.

Freud started his career with six month's apprenticeship in physiological research methodology in the laboratory of Dr. Ernst Brücke, a renowned Viennese physiologist. This experience was followed by appointments as assistant professor in neurology and later in neuropathology in a neuropsychiatric institute, by the publication of a number of articles in neuropathology and two books, one on infantile cerebral paralysis and one on aphasia. When in later years Freud was engaged in the private practice of psychiatry, he became dissatisfied with the methods of psychiatric treatment then prevalent. When he began his search for better methods of treatment, he applied the same rigorous research criteria and methodology that he had used in his physiological investigations. These were the scientific research principles of careful observation, rigorous reasoning, and testing the findings by replication of observations, which he had learned in Brücke's laboratory (Alexander and Selesnick, 1966, pp. 242–243). For concrete data, Freud utilized information derived from the intensive study of individual patients. "He created the science of psychobiography by reconstructing not only the history of the patient's symptoms but also the history of the person, which threw light on the origin of his mental symptoms. He made operational what others before him . . . postulated in vague general terms; that mental illness is the outcome of a person's life experiences" (Alexander and Selesnick, 1966, p. 236).

Freud, however, was not satisfied merely to develop a medical or psychobiographical method for understanding the patient and his symptoms, no matter how carefully and scientifically these data were obtained, but he also added another dimension—the dynamic aspect.

This was the concept that mental phenomena, normal and/or pathological, are produced by the interplay and interaction of psychological forces. Freud wrote (1966, p. 67), "We seek not merely to describe and to classify phenomena, but to understand them as signs of an interplay of forces in the mind, as a manifestation of purposeful intentions working concurrently or in mutual opposition. We are concerned with a *dynamic view* of mental phenomena." The concept of dynamic forces operative in the production of many types of psychological behavior is characteristic not only of Freudian psychoanalytical theory and practice but also of post-Freudian and other derivative so-called psychoanalytically oriented methods of psychotherapy.

Assumptions of the Psychoanalytic Model of Therapy The concept of the existence of the unconscious mind and its great influence on the life and behavior of an individual is of paramount importance in psychoanalytic theory and practice. Psychoanalytic therapy is based on the assumption that psychopathology or symptom formation arises from neurotic conflict. This occurs when the unconscious forces of the id, insistently seeking the satisfaction of innate needs, come into conflict with the conscious, reality-oriented forces of the ego, which seeks to control or inhibit the id's overt expression at the expense of the self-preservation instincts of the individual. When the forces of the id threaten to overwhelm the ego, the ego brings into action defense mechanisms which are manifested behaviorally in the individual as symptoms.

In therapy, an attempt is made to resolve the conflict by uncovering its roots in the unconscious. Little attention is placed on the symptoms per se, but rather attention is placed on the modification of the total personality. Only psychoanalysis attempts to resolve the neurotic conflicts underlying the symptoms "by making the patient aware of all the different unconscious impulses, fantasies, desires, fears, guilts, and punishments that are expressed in a condensed way in [the] symptom" (Greenson, 1967, p. 3).

Mental illness is not regarded as disease but rather as unhealthy or underdevelopment of ego functions. Relatively little emphasis is placed on diagnosis or classification of the disorder. Instead stress is placed on self-realization and maturity of the total personality. The individual develops and achieves maturity, that is, health and well-being, not so much from the biological growth of the organism, as in the medical model, nor in response to stimuli in the current, immediate environment, as in the behavioral model, but from his relationship with "significant other" persons. A crucial assumption is that the first and most important of these relationships is the mother-child relationship in the first few years of life. The success or failure of subsequent relationships is based on the degree to which the child's basic emotional needs for security, acceptance, and love were satisfied.

Treatment According to the Psychoanalytic Model In psychoanalytic therapy, one of the most important components, or in the opinion of some analysts the most important component, is considered to be the long-term therapist-patient relationship (Chessick, 1969, pp. 6–12; Alexander and Selesnick, 1966, p. 398). This relationship, which develops great depth, intensity, and strength, provides the patient with an enveloping, protective psychological climate in which he is able to reveal himself to the therapist. When the patient has achieved this degree of trust in his therapist, then together with his analyst he is able to reexamine traumatic events of his life. In this latter aspect of the relationship, the patient is said to have entered a working relationship with the therapist. In a greatly simplified presentation of a very complex process, the following is an outline of the way psychoanalytic psychotherapy works.

The work which the patient and the therapist are engaged in is to identify unsatisfactory ways of coping with life situations and to change them for more satisfying ways. In psychoanalysis, this is accomplished not only by examining all the circumstances of the present situation, but also by looking for and examining the origins of such behavior or situations in the past, especially in early childhood, for currently unavailable data buried in the unconscious. Two important techniques which the analyst uses to help the patient retrieve these data and make them available to the conscious mind are free association and dream interpretation. These additional data recalled from the past and brought into juxtaposition with a present situation often result in a shift, or change of focus, in the way the patient now views those events. A kind of enlightenment or sudden new understanding or reevaluation of the present situation in the light of the past occurs. This is one aspect of the phenomenon which in psychoanalysis is called "insight." It is not within the province of this outline to argue the question so bitterly debated, of whether or not insight is essential to behavior change, but its importance in psychoanalytic therapy lies in the fact that it very frequently precedes change of behavior. Chessick writes, "Insight may come as primarily an intellectual or primarily a sudden emotional experience in therapy. How it comes is not as important as how it is used. If it is used in a meaningful way in changing life patterns—'emotional insight'—it is of prime value" (Chessick, 1969, p. 56). "The psychological work which occurs after insight and which leads to a stable change in behavior is called *working through*" (Greenson, 1967, p. 29). Fromm-Reichmann emphasizes the importance of training patients to test out each new insight and understanding by applying it to situations in everyday living and to new ways of relating to others. It is in this way of working through in a wide variety of interactions and situations that the new changed behavior becomes assimilated and stabilized. This process effects a reorientation of the total personality toward a more satisfactory life. Alexander describes the course of treatment as a "long series of corrective emotional experiences, which follow one another as the transference situation changes its emotional content and different repressed childhood situations are revived and reexperienced in the relationship to the therapist" (Alexander, 1956, quoted in Chessick, 1969, p. 91).

Greenson states that the aim of psychoanalytic therapy is to resolve the patient's conflicts, including the infantile neurosis. This is accomplished by bringing into consciousness parts of the id, the superego, and the unconscious ego which had been excluded from the maturational processes of the healthy remainder of the total personality (Greenson, 1967, p. 26). According to Anna Freud, "Psychoanalytic technique is aimed directly at the ego since only the ego has direct access to the id, to the superego, and to the outside world. Our aim is to get the ego to renounce its pathogenic defenses or find more suitable ones" (Anna Freud, 1936, pp. 45–70; quoted in Greenson, 1967, p. 29).

Termination of treatment comes about by the dissolution of the transference relationship between patient and therapist. Patients and their therapists should agree on the time set for the termination of treatment. One of the criteria for termination is the development of sufficient insight by patients into their interpersonal processes to be able to see people and situations as they are, rather than seeing them in the light of their past experiences. They also must learn to see the therapist without distorted values. At termination, patients should be able to meet current situations without undue anxiety or return of symptoms and be free for further growth and maturation (Fromm-Reichmann, 1950, pp. 188–191).

Although validation of the psychoanalytic model is not possible by the methods of experimental psychology, Ford and Urban believe that validation of a different kind can be demonstrated by the fact that patients found Freud's explanations similar to their own observations of self, and the result of the interpretations brought about a resolution of the patients' disorder. "The theory was verified if it worked; the patient's behavior changed" (Ford and Urban, 1963, p. 176).

Psychodynamic Model: Implications for Nursing Practice Nurses have rarely practiced as qualified psychoanalysts. The most notable exception to this statement is the Swiss nurse psychoanalyst, Gertrud

Schwing, whose work with hospitalized schizophrenic patients made a major contribution to the application of the psychoanalytic principles to the treatment of psychotics at a time (1940) when other psychiatric nurses were permitted to give such patients only custodial care (Schwing, 1954). In the United States, a nurse needs a medical degree as well as psychoanalytic training to qualify as a psychoanalyst. However, a number of psychiatric nurses as well as social workers have received psychoanalytically oriented training in such institutions as the Washington School of Psychiatry, The William Alanson White Institute, and the Chicago Psychoanalytic Institute. In some states, for example, California and New Jersey, nurses may be licensed to practice independently as counselors. The role of the nurse as primary therapist is becoming increasingly common in community mental health centers and in psychiatric outpatient departments. The nurse's ability and willingness to make home visits is often much appreciated by other members of the psychiatric treatment team. Nurses have also served as adjunct therapists with psychoanalysts to give generalized support, to make interim visits between interviews with the analyst, to give additional psychological and physical care of the patient, and to assist the patient with practical problems of daily life. Analysts and other psychotherapists sometimes like to have an additional qualified therapist to provide psychotherapy for one or more members of their patient's family who need help.

It is not always easy or rewarding for a nurse to work in conjunction with a psychoanalyst; there is often a feeling on the part of the nurse of being somewhat isolated and distant. The reason for this is inherent in the nature of the psychoanalytic model. The close and deep analyst-analysand relationship tends to shut out everyone else. Analysts are very loath to share any information about their patients, even with professional colleagues. It is often difficult for an analyst to find time for a brief conference concerning the patient or his family, even if he is willing to do so, because of his tightly scheduled time. Because the emphasis in psychoanlysis is to work through the conflicts that interfere with the patient's optimum functioning, everything else is of secondary importance and the nurse may feel that the analyst is totally disinterested in external problems. This requires that a nurse be very secure and competent and be able to work with a patient in analysis without expecting approval or reassurance from the analyst.

THE UNITARY MODEL

The unitary concept of the human mind is a present-day development which arose from dissatisfaction with the narrowness and inadequacy of older theoretical models, notwithstanding the immeasurable contribution of Freudian theories to the understanding of the human mind. L. L. Whyte believed that a single method of approach which avoids the mind-matter problem and deals with the changing structure of relationships could be developed. He stated, "It will therefore be assumed that a unified theory is possible, and lies ahead, in which 'material' and 'mental,' 'conscious' and 'unconscious,' aspects will be derivable as related components of one primary system of ideas" (Whyte, 1960, p. 19). He predicted that "Freudian and Neo-Freudian psychological conceptions will only be replaced by a more reliable and comprehensive theory of the human mind after exact science has established a valid theory of biological organization" (Whyte, 1960, p. 180). Although it is impossible to determine at this point in time whether this biologically derived unitary theory will develop from physical biology, biological physics, or a more neutral science such as a general system theory, it will need some guiding principles of organic order such as are derived from the objective study of simpler organisms than man. Whyte also thought that the study of interactions will become more important than the study of isolated objects, as has already occurred in contemporary physics. The world of today is a very complex one, in which everything is not only interrelated but also intrarelated, so that it is unreasonable to ask for simplicity, clarity, or certainty. Instead, a provisional working hypothesis should be sought to find some kind of order in each complexity (Whyte, 1960, pp. 180–184). "The two great tendencies apparent in the universe: toward order and toward disorder, seem to be locked in a cosmic opposition . . . and within this universal warfare there are here and there human brain-minds impatiently reducing everything to order" (Whyte, 1960, p. 184).

Bertalanffy approaches the unitary concept from the general system point of view. He defines *general system theory* as "a discipline concerned with the general properties and laws of 'systems.' A system is defined as a complex of components in interaction" (Bertalanffy, 1967, p. 69). In another article he speaks of an organism as a system, that is, "a dynamic order of parts and processes in mutual interaction." The components of the system may be material or nonmaterial; therefore, system theory can be applied to problems in many fields, such as engineering, biophysics, biosociology, economics, mathematical description, and the prediction of social trends. In a discipline such as psychology, with multivariable components which cannot be adequately dealt with by traditional scientific concepts such as one finds in physics, system theory can prove very useful. Particularly in psychopathology these diverse components can be dealt with as categories, and by generalization can provide principles rather than detailed explanations and predictions. The system approach is eminently suited to provide new ways of conceptualizing problems in psychology and psychopathology (Bertalanffy, 1966, pp. 707–709). "Unifying concepts, such as those of general system theory, appear able to bridge fields traditionally subsumed under the title of science and humanities, and herald syntheses without obliterating or minimizing the profound differences that do exist in entities of the realm of science and the sociocultural field" (Bertalanffy, 1967, p. 114).

Whereas Whyte and Bertalanffy are primarily concerned with a unitary concept to further knowledge and understanding of the human mind, a number of psychiatric clinicians have been searching for a unified theory applicable to mental illness. Menninger credits Heinrich Neumann as the pioneer in the development of the unitary concept of mental illness. Neumann believed that there is only one kind of mental illness, and that it proceeds in stages on a continuum from health to illness. These various stages present characteristic clinical pictures of increasing severity of symptoms. Neumann wanted to abolish the classification of mental disorders because he regarded the classes as false and misleading and a barrier to the true understanding of the patient's illness. This point of view, from Neumann's time to the present, is in direct opposition to the emphasis placed on classification in the medical model. Henri Ey, a modern French psychiatrist, perceives mental illness more as "pathological reactions resulting from a multiplicity of factors" than as specific disease entities (Menninger, 1959, pp. 521–522).

Karl Menninger himself is a strong supporter of the unitary concept of mental illness (Menninger, 1958; 1959; 1963). He states that everybody has mental illness in some form or other and at some time in life. He writes (1959, p. 526), "If one sets up a scale of well-being—in other words—a scale in the successfulness of an individual-environment adaptation—at one end of the scale would be health, happiness, success, achievement, and the like, and at the other end misery, failure, crime, delirium, and so forth." The degree of an individual's well-being depends upon the amount of stress brought to bear upon him from instinctual urges, bodily needs, environmental threats, and cultural demands balanced against the strength and effectiveness of his coping mechanisms. Menninger (1959, pp. 526–527) regards mental illness as "an impairment in self-regulation whereby comfort, production, and growth are temporarily surrendered for the sake of survival at the best level possible, and at the cost of emergency coping devices." He perceives mental illness as dysfunction of both personality and environmental adjustment, and mental patients "as human beings obliged to make awkward and expensive maneuvers to maintain themselves, somewhat isolated from their fellows, harassed by faulty techniques of living, uncomfortable themselves, and often to others" (Menninger, 1963, p. 5). The practice of classifying and pejoratively labeling persons as mentally ill is deplored by Menninger. He also believes that members of the psychiatric professions should be able to describe and specify various psychological phenomena without resorting to esoteric professional jargon, on the basis that a holistic, humanistic, unitary concept of mental illness makes unnecessary many technical terms which carry extremely compressed but ambiguous information (Menninger, 1963, p. 5).

Assumptions of the Unitary Concept for Treatment At the present time it is impossible to identify any special therapeutic techniques or interventions unique to the unitary concept of treatment. According to Menninger, the unitary concept does not dispense with descriptive designations of an illness. He sees such diagnostic designations as necessary to provide a sound basis for formulating a treatment program and planned therapeutic interventions. The principal dynamic force which leads to illness is the disturbance of the total economy of the personality which causes loss of ego control. Menninger identifies two types of malfunctioning of control: (1) dyscontrol, or impaired, inefficient, and expensive control, and (2) disorganization, or lost or destroyed control. There are five levels of disorganization of the personality, ranging from (1) slight impairment of adaptive control and coping ability, usually called nervousness; (2) use of psychologically expensive compensatory mechanisms to reduce tension and anxiety characteristic of the so-called neuroses; (3) use of regressive mechanisms manifested by emotional outbursts and antisocial behavior characteristic of personality disorders; (4) more severe ego failure manifested by loss of reality sense, thought disturbances, and confused perception characteristic of psychotic behavior; and (5) total ego failure and loss of will to live (Menninger, 1963, pp. 33, 162–163).

The process of successful treatment includes progressive reintegration of the personality with the environment, reduction of inner tension and anxiety, relinquishment of symptoms, and recovery of ego control. Menninger says that this is accomplished by identifying both the positive therapeutic and negative pathogenic factors at work in the struggle for control, and by expediting and supporting the positive factors and combating the negative ones. He also recommends determining what things men cannot bear, or what they can bear only with the greatest difficulty, and how their ability to bear stress becomes impaired. This knowledge should be used to improve living conditions and thereby prevent mental illness (Menninger, 1963, pp. 271, 402–403).

Bertalanffy believes that general system theory can provide a very useful framework for a unified treatment model. He sees mental illness as "essentially a disturbance of system functions of the psychophysical organism. For this reason isolated symptoms or syndromes do not define the disease entity." Therefore, psychiatric disturbances can be defined in terms of system functions. Disintegrations of one or more systems, or parts of systems, produce mental illness. Some of the specific applications system theory has for psychiatric treatment include action-oriented therapies such as recreational and occupational therapy, as well as other adjunctive therapies necessary for a psychophysically active organism. Assiduous development of the patient's creative abilities is stressed rather than permitting a passive adjustment to illness. Emphasis in treatment is on the present and on current conflicts; on restoration of impaired system functioning and subsequent reintegration of the restored function into the psychosocial organism; and on goal orientation to the future by means of "symbolic" anticipation rather than dwelling on past events. Bertalanffy suggests that for patients suffering from meaninglessness of life or existential neurosis, Frankl's logotherapy may prove helpful (Bertalanffy, 1966, pp. 715–716; Frankl, 1965).

Unitary Model: Implications for Practice   The unified concept of mental illness applied to treatment would eliminate the dichotomy between body and mind, that is, the old Cartesian dualism which has hampered man's thinking about the nature of his mind for more than three centuries. One of the results of this dichotomy has been to place a barrier between the medical and the psychological treatment of the hapless patient who may receive either one or the other type of treatment but seldom the two combined in an integrated way. A unified method of treatment could be developed by utilizing the theoretical framework of general system theory which would enable persons to be treated as whole human beings and receive necessary treatment from health professionals who understood and were sympathetic to the concept of the interrelatedness and interaction of the biophysical, psychological, and ecosociocultural components of man. The current growing awareness of the importance of these social and environmental factors has complicated greatly the number of factors which must be evaluated in determining treatment for a given patient.

Therapists who utilize the unitary system in their psychiatric practice will need to broaden their vision and enlarge the parameters of their professional and extraprofessional knowledge to be able to cope with the many aspects of the clinical problems they will encounter. Professional schools for the preparation of mental health practitioners will be compelled to take into account these new trends and modify their curriculums accordingly. Duhl and his colleagues advocate and are developing programs in which students preparing to practice in a variety of health professions can acquire a new orientation to the problems of mental health and can learn together a broad basic body of knowledge and skills which will be essential for all mental health practitioners to have in the future whether they practice as physicians, nurses, social workers, or psychologists or in other disciplines (Duhl, 1971).

Another implication of the unitary concept of treatment is that it does not focus its attention exclusively on the individual patient. The illness of the individual is regarded as affecting the health of the community, and the healthy or unhealthy factors in a community affect each member in that community. Therefore, far greater emphasis is placed on prevention and on making life healthier for the community as a whole than is practiced at the present time. Health concerns will involve all levels of society, and all social structures—that is, family, neighborhood, community, nation, and the world. The parameters of the problem of illness and health are also enlarged to include more than the care of the sick. George Wald, discussing the problem of national health, notes that it involves the entire operation of our society. He writes, "It has to be concerned with minimal incomes, nutrition, clean air and water, sewage disposal, adequate public transportation, better schools, better housing. It demands a civilian economy that meets these needs, rather than our present military economy, wholly inflationary, and geared to killing and destruction" (Wald, 1971, p. xv).

REFERENCES

Albee, George W. (1968): "Conceptual Models and Manpower Requirements," *American Psychologist,* vol. 23, no. 5, pp. 317–320.

Alexander, Franz (1956): *Psychoanalysis and Psychotherapy,* W. W. Norton & Company, Inc., New York.

———and Sheldon T. Selesnick (1966): *The History of Psychiatry,* Harper & Row, Publishers, Inc., New York. Paperback edition, Mentor Books (1968), The New American Library, Inc., New York.

Ayllon, Teodoro (1963): "Intensive Treatment of Psychotic Behavior by Stimulus Satiation and Food Reinforcement," *Behavior Research and Therapy,* vol. 1, pp. 53–61.

———(1965): "Operant Conditioning on Trial in the Treatment of Schizophrenia," *Roche Report: Frontiers of Hospital Psychiatry,* Oct. 2, pp. 5–6.

————and Jack Michael (1959): "The Psychiatric Nurse as a Behavioral Engineer," *Journal of Experimental Analysis of Behavior,* vol. 2, pp. 323–334.

Bandura, Albert (1965): "Behavioral Modification through Modeling Procedures," in L. Krasner and L. P. Ullmann (eds.), *Research in Behavior Modification,* Holt, Rinehart, and Winston, Inc., New York.

————(1967): "Behavioral Psychotherapy," *Scientific American,* vol. 216, no. 3, pp. 78–86.

Bertalanffy, Ludwig von (1966): "General System Theory and Psychiatry," in Silvano Arieti (ed.), *American Handbook of Psychiatry,* Basic Books, Inc., Publishers, New York, vol. 3, pp. 705–721.

————(1967): *Robots, Men and Minds,* George Braziller, New York.

Chessick, Richard D. (1969): *How Psychotherapy Heals,* Science House, Inc., New York.

Duhl, Leonard J. (1973): "Education in a Diverse Society with Emphasis on the Mental Health Professions," in Esther A. Garrison et al. (eds.), *Doctoral Preparation for Nurses with Emphasis on the Psychiatric Field,* printed at the University of California, San Francisco, pp. 94–105.

Ford, Donald H., and Hugh B. Urban (1963): *Systems of Psychotherapy: A Comprehensive Study,* John Wiley & Sons, Inc., New York.

Frankl, Viktor E. (1965): *The Doctor and the Soul: From Psychotherapy to Logotherapy,* Alfred A. Knopf, Inc., New York. Paperback edition, Bantam Books, Inc. (1967), New York.

Freud, Anna (1936): *The Ego and the Mechanisms of Defense,* International Universities Press, Inc., New York.

Freud, Sigmund (1966): *The Complete Introductory Lectures on Psychoanalysis,* W. W. Norton & Company, Inc., New York.

Fromm-Reichmann, Frieda (1950): *Principles of Intensive Psychotherapy,* University of Chicago Press, Chicago.

Gericke, Otto L. (1965): "Practical Use of Operant Conditioning Procedures in a Mental Hospital," *Psychiatric Studies and Projects,* vol. 3, no. 5. Published by the Mental Hospital Service of the American Psychiatric Association.

Goldstein, Kurt (1959): "The Organismic Approach," in Silvano Arieti (ed.), *American Handbook of Psychiatry,* Basic Books, Inc., Publishers, New York, vol. 2, pp. 1333–1347.

Greenson, Ralph R. (1967): *The Technique and Practice of Psychoanalysis,* vol. 1, International Universities Press, Inc., New York.

Hull, Clark L. (1943): *Principles of Behavior: An Introduction to Behavior Theory,* D. Appleton-Century Company, Inc., New York.

Koestler, Arthur (1967): *The Ghost in the Machine,* The Macmillan Company, New York.

Lovaas, Ivar (1967): "A Behavioral Therapy Approach to the Treatment of Childhood Schizophrenia," in J. T. Hill (ed.), *Minnesota Symposia on Child Psychology,* vol. 1, University of Minnesota Press, Minneapolis.

Matson, Floyd W. (1967): *Being, Becoming, and Behavior: The Psychological Sciences,* George Braziller, New York.

McLuhan, Marshall (1967): *The Medium Is the Message: An Inventory of Effects,* Bantam Books, Inc., New York.

Menninger, Karl (1959): *A Psychiatrist's World: The Selected Papers of Karl Menninger, M.D.,* The Viking Press, Inc., New York.

————(1963): *The Vital Balance,* The Viking Press, Inc., New York.

————et al. (1958): "The Unitary Concept of Mental Illness," *Bulletin, Menninger Clinic,* vol. 22, January, pp. 4–12, reprinted in *Pastoral Psychology,* vol. 10, May, 1959, pp. 13–19.

Miron, Nathan (1966): "Behavior Shaping and Group Nursing with Severely Retarded Patients," *California Mental Health Research Monographs,* no. 8.

Mora, George (1959): "Recent American Psychiatric Developments," in Silvano Arieti (ed.), *American Handbook of Psychiatry,* Basic Books, Inc., Publishers, New York, vol. 1, pp. 18–57.

Sarason, Irwin G., and Victor J. Ganzer (1968): "Concerning the Medical Model," *American Psychologist,* vol. 23, no. 7, pp. 507–510.

Scahefer, Halmuth H. (1966): "Investigations in Operant Conditioning Procedures in a Mental Hospital," *California Mental Health Monographs,* vol. 8, pp. 25–39.

———and Patrick L. Martin (1969): *Behavioral Therapy,* McGraw-Hill Book Company, New York.

Schwing, Gertrud (1954): *A Way to the Soul of the Mentally Ill,* translated by Rudolph Ekstein and Bernard H. Hall, International Universities Press, Inc., New York.

Skinner, B. F. (1938): *The Behavior of Organisms,* Appleton-Century-Crofts, Inc., New York.

———(1971): *Beyond Freedom and Dignity,* Alfred A. Knopf, Inc., New York.

———(1953): *Science and Human Behavior,* The Macmillan Company, New York.

Wald, George (1971): Foreword, in Allan Chase, *The Biological Imperatives: Health, Politics, and Human Survival,* Holt, Rinehart and Winston, Inc., New York.

Whyte, Lancelot L. (1960): *The Unconscious before Freud,* Basic Books, Inc., Publishers, New York.

Wolpe, Joseph (1958): *Psychotherapy by Reciprocal Inhibition,* Stanford University Press, Stanford, Calif.

10

MENTAL RETARDATION

Marion E. Kalkman

"Mental retardation ranks as a major national health, social and economic problem. It strikes our most precious asset—our children." These stirring words, spoken by President John F. Kennedy in his Message to Congress on February 5, 1962, brought the problem of mental retardation to the attention of the entire nation. These words also brought hope for better understanding and more enlightened treatment to millions of mentally retarded persons in this country. For years the problem of mental retardation had been largely ignored by the health professions. Dr. Malcolm J. Farrell (in Ewalt et al., 1957) states the situation very aptly:

> Probably no other field of medicine and psychiatry has suffered from so many professional misunderstandings and misconceptions. Until recently, one of the great stumbling blocks in the way of better understanding and investigation has been the almost universal notion that mental subnormality is hereditary in origin. Because no immediate and direct cause could be found, it was easy to blame heredity and to say that nothing could be done. Many professional people thought of mentally subnormal persons as comprising a stereotyped group of individuals so limited in understanding that they could not be taught even the rudimentary care of themselves and their bodies. They were regarded as being in a hopeless condition for which little if anything could be done. Such a belief is far from the truth.

Definition

Even the term used to characterize this condition has not been agreed upon. Among the names by which it is commonly known are "mental subnormality," "feeble-mindedness," "mental deficiency," and "mental retardation." The term *mental retardation* is gaining acceptance both as a more inclusive and as a better descriptive term. Tarjan defines mental retardation as a condition characterized by a basic abnormality of the mind—an intellectual deficiency which interferes with the ability to adjust to the demands of life. It manifests itself in poor learning, inadequate social adjustment, and delayed achievement. The condition is either present at birth or starts during childhood. The term *mental retardation* also applies to those individuals who may not have an inherent mental deficiency but who, as the result of gross physical disabilities or cultural deprivation, are not able to function intellectually or socially at the level expected by their chronological age (Tarjan, 1964).

Criteria

Satisfactory criteria for the diagnosis and classification of mental retardation are not agreed upon by authorities. Since this condition is essentially the arrest or retardation of the normal processes of growth and development, various criteria for determining physical, psychological, and social growth patterns are used.

However, the single criterion which is most commonly used to determine the degree of retardation continues to be the Intelligence Quotient or IQ determination, though this test often does not give a true evaluation of the intellectual potential of many retarded individuals. It particularly discriminates against the psychologically and culturally deprived and also the individual with a severe physical or neurological handicap. Mentally retarded children who have no obvious physical signs of retardation at birth or during early childhood are often not recognized as retarded until they enroll in school, where the achievement demanded of them is primarily academic. Some retarded persons, on leaving school and entering the working world, make a satisfactory adjustment and no longer constitute a social or medical problem in the community.

The other criterion commonly used to determine mental retardation is social adaptation, that is, the individual's ability to adapt to his environment and relate to other people. Generally, social adaptability is seriously impaired in the mentally retarded. However, impairment of intelligence and of social adaptability are not necessarily of the same degree for a given individual. Some persons with a low IQ may be able to adjust fairly well socially, and some with a higher intelligence score may rate low on social adaptation. Although a number of standardized intelligence tests are available, none measures social adaptability accurately. It is estimated that about 3 percent of the general population have impaired intelligence and social maladaptation of such an extent that they can be considered mentally retarded.

CLASSIFICATION

Intelligence

The mentally retarded individual may be classified in a variety of ways: according to his intelligence quotient, his ability to participate in an educational program, his social adequacy, and his medical diagnosis. In classifying the mentally retarded person according to his intelligence, terms commonly used have been *idiot, imbecile,* and *moron.* The World Health Organization proposes replacing these terms with the following classification:

WHO	Current Use	Intelligence Quotient	Mental Age
Severe subnormality	Idiot	0–19	0– 3
Moderate subnormality	Imbecile	20–49	3– 8
Mild subnormality	Moron	50–69	8–12

Similar to this classification is that offered by the U.S. Department of Health, Education, and Welfare Committee on Mental Retardation:

Level	Intelligence Quotient
Profound	Below 20
Severe	20–35
Moderate	36–52
Mild	53–68

Another classification is based on educational potential, useful in determining the type of educational program appropriate for a mentally retarded individual:

Level	Intelligence Quotient
Custodial	Below 25
Trainable	25–50
Educable	50–75

Custodial refers to individuals who are considered too retarded to benefit from any educational program. *Trainable* refers to individuals who are able to benefit from a program which includes habit-training and the mastery of simple motor skills. *Educable* refers to those individuals who are considered to be able to benefit from some type of school program (Ewalt et al., 1957).

Social Adequacy

The British Mental Health Act of 1959 has only two categories for the mentally retarded—severe subnormality and subnormality. *Severe subnormality* is defined as a state of arrested or incomplete development of the mind so severe that the individual is incapable of leading an independent life or of guarding himself against serious exploitation (or, in the case of a child, that he will be so incapacitated when adult). *Subnormality* is defined as a state of arrested or incomplete development of the mind, the subnormality of intelligence being such that the individual requires special care of training but not to the same degree as in severe subnormality (Adams, 1960).

Medical Diagnosis

According to Tarjan, of the 3 percent of the population who are mentally retarded, 75 percent appear indistinguishable from other people. However, their intelligence and/or social adaptability is below normal, that is, below 70. The cause of mental retardation in this group is unknown. They cannot be classified according to any system of medical diagnosis; mental retardation seems related to psychological, social, and cultural factors such as poor prenatal care, inadequate diet, psychological neglect in infancy, lack of sensory, interpersonal, and cultural stimulation, and, in general, absence of those conditions necessary for healthy growth and development in infancy and childhood. The majority of these individuals remain in the community and rarely receive any form of medical treatment.

The other 25 percent of the mentally retarded are noticeably deviant from normal individuals in physical appearance. They are small at birth, often premature, and as infants may show gross abnormalities such as very small or very large heads, deformed limbs, spinal bifida, missing or extra digits, and other types of malformation. They may also have a wide variety of stigmata such as mongoloid eyes, thick tongues, dry scaly skin, webbed fingers, sunken nose, and other anomalies characteristic of a particular disease. Feeding difficulties are very common during infancy. Speech, vision, and hearing are also frequently impaired. As they grow older they often remain undersized and appear much younger than their chronological age. For the majority of this group, who comprise about 15 to 25 percent of the total number of diagnosed cases of mental retardation, causes or agents can be determined.

Classification by Specifically Identified Conditions or Diseases

In the small group of 15 to 25 percent of cases of mental retardation in which a specific causal agent can be identified, infections play a prominent role. German measles in the mother in the first trimester of pregnancy is one of the most common infectious agents, and is one cause of mental retardation which is preventable. Good prenatal care, including determination of whether the mother has been exposed to measles before pregnancy and special precautions to protect her if she has not been exposed, can do much to eliminate this cause of retardation. Nurses can play a significant role in case-finding of susceptible mothers and instituting the necessary preventive measures. Severe infections in infancy and childhood can also cause mental retardation. Many of these cases of mental retardation could be prevented by prophylaxis, early diagnosis of the infection, and adequate treatment.

Toxic agents such as Rh blood factor incompatibility at birth, carbon monoxide, and lead poisoning also account for some cases of mental retardation. A common cause of lead poisoning in children can be ascribed to lead in the paint used on toys, bed-cribs, and other objects which the child sucks or chews on. A number of metabolic disorders such as phenylketonuria and galactosemia, which produce mental retardation if untreated, can also be prevented by early diagnosis and special dietary therapy. Neurological disorders such as tuberous sclerosis, neurofibromatosis, congenital hydrocephalus, microcephalus, and macrocephaly are known to cause mental retardation. Down's disease or Mongolism is a disease of unknown prenatal origin in which mental retardation is frequently a prominent symptom. Mental retardation also commonly occurs in many cases of idiopathic epilepsy (Ewalt et al., 1957; HEW Committee on Mental Retardation, 1962).

TREATMENT

Specific Therapy

Those who suffer from one of the small group of medical conditions for which specific treatment is known can be given the appropriate treatment to arrest or, in some cases, to ameliorate the mental retardation. For example, the use of a special diet in phenylketonuria and galactosemia and the administration of thyroid in cretinism not only arrest retardation but promote definite improvement in the patient.

Supportive Drug Therapy

Tranquilizing drugs such as Serpasil and Thorazine have proved helpful in calming noisy, hyperactive, and destructive mentally retarded individuals and have thus increased their ability to utilize psychotherapy. Mildly retarded individuals with interpersonal difficulties have shown improvement in their social adjustment when given tranquilizers. Several investigators have found Thorazine beneficial for mentally retarded patients who also had epileptic seizures. These patients responded favorably to the drug and had fewer behavior disturbances and no increase in seizures (Ewalt et al., 1957).

Psychotherapy

Mentally retarded individuals not only are subject to the same mental illnesses that normal individuals suffer from but have a far higher incidence of mental illness than do the general population. Depression and paranoid trends are very common. The mentally retarded are also prone to transient emotional episodes which are usually triggered by some situational incident. During these episodes they are highly excitable. In spite of the high incidence of emotional disorders in the mentally retarded, psychotherapy has not been widely used. In the past, many therapists believed that the mentally retarded were incapable of establishing a therapeutic relationship. This belief was based on the mentally retarded individual's well-known difficulties in understanding and utilizing verbal forms of communication, his inability to view his behavior objectively, his lack of problem-solving skills, and his inability to tolerate frustration and control his emotional responses. However, in recent years, a number of studies have indicated that the mentally retarded can benefit from both individual (Thorne, 1957; Yepson, 1957) and group therapy (Cotzin, 1948; Snyder and Sechrest, 1963).

Other Methods of Treatment

A number of other forms of therapy have proved useful in the treatment of the mentally retarded. *Play therapy* has been utilized by a number of therapists with beneficial results. Play equipment should be easy to handle, simple in construction, and sturdy so the child will not be frustrated by toys that are easily broken or too difficult for him to enjoy. Play therapy groups should be small, consisting of not more than three children. *Psychodrama,* engaged in either individually or in groups, has also been used with good results. *Speech therapy* is another useful method of treatment. *Occupational* and *recreational therapy* can play a very helpful role in treatment, particularly since activity therapies are more appealing to these patients than verbal therapies. A wide range of simple projects, such as finger painting, clay modeling, playing in rhythm bands, singing, dancing, acting, and caring for pets and plants, can be developed to offer patients enjoyment as well as the experience of accomplishment and success. Finger painting and art therapy can be used as psychotherapy as well as for the patient's personal pleasure and for socialization. *Industrial* and *vocational therapy* are also beneficial, especially in the treatment of the less severely handicapped patients. Programs which help to condition patients for a work situation, including the development of work habits, are very useful. Many patients can be taught to do useful and remunerative types of work in special job training classes.

PSYCHOLOGICAL NURSING CARE OF
THE MENTALLY RETARDED

Individual Nursing Care

In the nursing care of the mentally retarded, individual nursing care, or nurse-patient relationship therapy, has been utilized very little. Professional nurses employed in institutions and agencies for the care of the mentally retarded have usually been in administrative or supervisory positions. Direct patient care has been left generally to attendants, aides, and orderlies, whose duties are largely custodial. Recently, however, a number of nurses have become interested in improving the nursing care given to the mentally retarded and have been experimenting with the use of relationship therapy with these patients. Nurse-patient relationship therapy can be of great therapeutic benefit to the mentally retarded child or adult, and it can also provide a most satisfying professional experience for nurses, not only because it gives them the opportunity to work intensively with patients, but also because it enables them to develop new and creative approaches.

In general, individual relationship therapy with the retarded follows the same principles as those employed with other types of patients. However, nonverbal communication techniques play a far more important role than with most other patients. Nurses caring for the mentally retarded patient must also utilize many general nursing skills because these patients often suffer from concomitant physical disabilities. In individual relationship therapy with the mentally retarded, it is possible to combine psychological and general nursing skills in a way that can be highly effective (Wright, 1963; Wright, 1965).

SPECIFIC PRINCIPLES OF NURSING PSYCHOTHERAPY WITH THE MENTALLY RETARDED

There are a number of principles of psychotherapy which are particularly pertinent to the nursing care and treatment of the mentally retarded patient. According to Adams (1960), the aim of therapy is to develop as far as possible the mentally retarded individual's potential capacities, and to make the most of his assets so that the handicap of his subnormal intelligence does not become a crippling disability. She sees the role of the therapist as essentially a parental one in which the special emotional needs which were missing in the actual parental relationship could be provided. These emotional needs could be supplied very appropriately by the nurse in a nurse-patient relationship, with the nurse providing not only gratifying experiences but also inhibiting and controlling ones. Adams stresses the importance of the patient's having one helping person to whom he can turn in time of trouble or stress. The development of a strong relationship with this significant figure is essential to provide security and stability for the patient.

De Martino emphasizes that the therapist should use simple, easily understood language and be able to perceive and acknowledge the patient's nonverbal cues. Believing that the therapist should have a special feeling for the mentally retarded, De Martino (1957) writes: "They [the mentally retarded] are markedly deficient in the basic need for gratification. Through counseling and psychotherapy, i.e., the imparting of praise, encouragement, support, affection, attention, respect, etc., it is therefore possible to create a highly effective situation through which basic gratification can occur."

Objectives of Nursing Psychotherapy

Frederick C. Thorne (1957) one of the pioneers in the use of psychotherapy in the treatment of the mentally retarded, has stated some basic objectives for counseling the mentally retarded. Thorne's objectives offer a most useful guide to nurses and others who are engaged in the direct care of the mentally retarded and, with some suggestions for achieving them, are outlined as follows:

1. *Accept the mentally retarded as worthy in spite of his defects.* Acceptance may be demonstrated by treating him as an individual who is liked and respected, by addressing him by name, by greeting him with a smile (since children react more to expressive gestures than to words), and by commenting favorably on some aspect of his appearance and behavior. Misconduct should be treated as an understandable mistake which, hopefully, will not be repeated. The child should be encouraged to express his individuality in dress and action, and be given the amount of freedom and responsibility that he can manage. The therapist should accept him as a person and show tolerance even in periods when he is experiencing acute behavior upsets.
2. *Permit expression and clarification of emotional reactions.* This may be accomplished by listening quietly to his initial outbursts of feeling, by reflecting and clarifying feelings nondirectively, and by discussing ways of solving difficulties.
3. *Teach stratagems for resisting frustrations and achieving emotional control.* Some of these stratagems include analyzing the situation in which the child lost his temper, encouraging him to disregard teasing by laughing or walking away, and encouraging the child to devise his own stratagems.
4. *Provide standards of acceptable behavior within the ability of the individual child.* This may be accomplished by making friendly comments on more acceptable ways of behaving and avoiding blunt suggestion, persuasion, or advice.
5. *Buid up the child's self-confidence and respect.* These attitudes may be developed by finding something to praise him for and by placing him in a situation where he can achieve success.
6. *Teach the child to seek help when he is in difficulty.* This may be done by teaching him to talk over problems before they become serious, by encouraging him to see his therapist at any reasonable time, and by informally inquiring how things are going. This is especially important with shy children.

GROUP THERAPY TECHNIQUES
USEFUL IN NURSING

Among the particular advantages that group therapy offers the mentally retarded individual are opportunities to achieve a feeling of acceptance, to develop interpersonal and social skills, and to find an outlet for his aggressive, hostile impulses. Group therapy has also proved very effective in reducing the sensitiveness common to many mentally retarded individuals. It may also help to ameliorate guilt and suppressed feelings of worthlessness and hatred, thus facilitating communication and greater trust in the therapist.

Group therapy offers considerable promise as a method of treatment that could be utilized by nurses who have had some training in the theory and practice of group therapy. However, some modification of standard group therapy techniques is required. Some group therapists who have reported good therapeutic results with mentally retarded patients stress that the inclusion of various kinds of activities, such as action games, calisthenics, volleyball, clay modeling, and story telling, can be very effective in mobilizing the children's interest and holding their attention (Cotzin, 1948; Snyder and Sechrest, 1963; Stacey and De Martino, 1957). Fisher and Wolfson encouraged the members in their groups to act out their problems; this was then followed by group discussion (Stacey and De Martino, 1957). This method, too, proved effective.

Some degree of structuring of the group is apparently helpful, for example, role-playing in situations like conducting a meeting, electing officers, enacting a courtroom scene, or making a purchase in a shop. The size of the group should be kept small, not more than five or six members. The therapist must be able to set limits without being overly rigid; destruction of property, throwing objects, or direct physical attacks on group members or the therapist should not be permitted. In general, the therapist must play a more active role than he would in most other types of group therapy. It is also the therapist's responsibility to create a warm, relaxed, and pleasant atmosphere in which group members can feel secure and be productive. It is important that nurses be encouraged to conduct types of group therapy which could be utilized by mentally retarded patients, for very little therapy is available to the majority of patients, especially to those in large institutions.

Providing a Therapeutic Milieu

To a great extent it is the nurse's responsibility to create a therapeutic environment, that is, an environment which promotes the goal of treatment. Tarjan (1956) defines this goal as helping each patient to reach the maximum of achievement and independence that his mental capacity will permit. The patient has to accomplish this goal in the context of the environment in which he finds himself. Nurses are in a strategic position to influence the patient's environment since they are active participants in it. But in order to utilize their strategic position they must be aware of the various factors in the environment which influence the behavior and mold the personality of their patients. They should evaluate these factors as therapeutic or untherapeutic, and in planning the patient's nursing care, utilize the therapeutic aspects of the environment while protecting the patient from the effects of the untherapeutic ones.

A nurse may find that such intangibles as patterns of organization, hospital traditions, cultural norms of the staff, and ideas about treatment, discipline, etc., are more influential than the physical factors in the environment. Tarjan (1956) says that a routine, protective, and pathology-oriented milieu may act as a deterrent, or even a regressive force. To make changes in a well-established milieu is not easy. If the ideas for change originate with the nurse, her first step is to discuss these ideas with the physician in charge of the ward. When they have reached an agreement on the desirable changes, or even an agreement that some changes are indicated, support should be obtained from the proper hospital administrative authorities. Then the entire ward personnel should be involved in a discussion of the proposed changes and staff cooperation secured before the changes are put into operation.

One factor in developing a therapeutic milieu is that the ward unit be furnished in as comfortable and homelike a manner as is possible within institutional limits. Meals can be served family style with a member of the nursing personnel sitting at the table with the patients. A special ward or, better yet, a cottage where patients soon to be discharged can live for a while is often very helpful in smoothing the awkward transition from institutional to community life. The patient should not be so "hospitalized" that he faces a drastic readjustment to living outside of the hospital when he is discharged. For example, words for common objects should be those generally used, rather than special institutional jargon such as "head" for *toilet,* "day room" for *living room.* Patients should wear the same type of clothing and hair styles as are current in the local community. Commonly observed social customs should be taught to patients and practiced. Patients should have facilities for keeping personal possessions. Opportunities for learning social skills, good manners, the care of clothing, the use of money, and the use of public transportation should also be made available.

Motivation

One of the primary tasks in the treatment of the mentally retarded individual is to motivate him to achieve the maximum degree of functioning of which he is capable. Most mentally retarded persons have been understimulated throughout their lives; that is, either there has been some malfunctioning of their sensory organs so that they have been unable to receive sensory stimuli with the degree of acuity of normal individuals, or they have been culturally deprived of stimulation in the form of sights, sounds, human contacts, and life experiences common to others. The culturally deprived include institutionalized children, persons living in remote, isolated areas, and children reared in severely underprivileged homes. Occasionally, a mentally retarded person suffers from overstimulation; that is, he has been so excessively stimulated that he has difficulty in organizing or integrating his input of sensory stimuli.

Sensory deprivation is one of the commonest causes of lack of motivation. Sometimes sensory deprivation is caused by impairment of hearing, sight, or one of the other sensory organs; sometimes it is the result of growing up in an environment singularly lacking in sensory stimulation. As infants and young children these retarded individuals were not caressed, rocked, smiled at, or talked to. They were not exposed to music and other interest-arousing sounds, nor to the sight of flowers, pictures, and brightly colored objects, nor were they permitted to handle and play with toys. However, once the type of sensory deprivation is identified, efforts can be made to make up the deficiency. A whole new world can open up for a child when a defect in vision or hearing is corrected or improved by appropriate medical treatment. The same exciting experience can occur when a child is awakened to the beauty of color, sound, form, and motion in his environment. The nurse can play an important role in introducing suitable toys, attractive furnishings and decorations, becoming clothes, and new experiences to the culturally deprived child. In all instances she should attempt to meet the specific needs of the particular child in a way which will be of greatest therapeutic benefit to him.

Operant Conditioning

One of the most promising new developments in the motivation of the mentally retarded is the use of operant conditioning techniques. Operant conditioning focuses on the behavior of an individual. It is a technique of the scientific control of human behavior developed by B. F. Skinner and derived from his theory of operant behavior (Skinner, 1953). According to Skinner, operant behavior is behavior of an individual which operates on the environment to generate specific consequences. For example, if A behaves in a specific way in situation B, the consequences are C. However, A's behavior can be modified by (1) operant conditioning, or (2) operant extinction, this modified behavior resulting in changed environmental response. For example, if Johnny throws his food on the floor, his mother's response is to send him from the table. If, however, Johnny's propensity to throw food can be changed, his mother's response to him will also change.

Operant conditioning is the operational method designed to reinforce desirable patterns of behavior, and operant extinction is the operational method designed to eliminate undesirable behavior. Operant conditioning is achieved by rewarding desirable behavior; operant extinction is achieved by absence of reward, i.e., ignoring the behavior. For example, Johnny enjoys desserts very much. He learns that he receives a large helping of dessert whenever he displays good table manners at dinner. If, however, his table manners are unacceptable, he receives no dessert. Note that he is rewarded for good behavior, and attention is drawn to the desired behavior rather than to the undesirable behavior. Behavior that brings no rewards quickly tends to be eliminated.

In operant conditioning there are three ways in which the reinforcement of desirable behavior can be achieved: (1) by a positive reinforcer, that is, by adding something pleasurable to the situation such as food, money, affection, or praise, as in the above illustration, and (2) by negative reinforcer, that is, removing something unpleasant from the situation, such as loud noises, extremes of heat or cold, lack of privacy, hostile or unfriendly influences (for example, Johnny's table manners might also be improved by removing him at meals from exposure to the teasing of a sibling), and (3) by adverse stimuli, that is, by applying punishment. For further explanation of these principles the reader is referred to Chapter V, "Operant Behavior," in Skinner's book, *Science and Human Behavior* (1953).

Operant conditioning has enabled many of the severely retarded, who have been almost totally dependent on others, to dress themselves, feed themselves, become toilet-trained, and otherwise achieve a degree of independence and self-care heretofore impossible for them. Hundziak, Maurer, and Watson (1965) reported a study to test the efficacy of operant conditioning for toilet training. Twenty-nine severely retarded boys participated in this study. The boys were divided into three groups, eight boys in an operant conditioning group, eight in a conventional training group, and thirteen boys in a control group. No effort was made to train the third group. The other two groups of boys were placed on a commode every 2 hours and whenever they expressed the need to eliminate. This training schedule operated on a special research unit for 7 hours a day, 5 days a week for a period of 27 days. In addition to this training schedule, the boys in the operant conditioning group received positive reinforcers in the form of candy and praise. The results of the study showed that the operant conditioning technique was superior to the conventional training method in that the boys in the former group showed a significant increase in the use of bathroom facilities and that they were able to transfer the ability to use these facilities when they returned to their home units.

A number of excellent articles on the use of operant conditioning techniques with the mentally ill suggest how this technique could be used for mentally retarded patients who are not so severely handicapped as those described here (Ayllon, 1965; Ayllon and Michael, 1959; Gericke, 1965; Hundziak et al., 1965). A number of projects in various parts of the country are in operation, whose studies have not yet been published. Dr. Nathan Miron and Mrs. M. Grey Darden set up a pilot study at Sonoma State Hospital, California, to explore the use of operant conditioning techniques in improving the social behavior of a group of severely retarded preadolescent girls (film, *The Poppe Project*). Mrs. Darden, a child psychiatric nurse specialist, was responsible for the application of operant conditioning to the nursing care given to the patients in this group. She developed nursing interventions for her own direct care of patients and also supervised the care given by the psychiatric technicians assigned to the project. The reinforcers used in this project were candy, approval, and affection. During this exploratory experimental project, some of the social skills developed by these patients included learning to dress themselves, feed themselves, use the toilet, make some efforts at improving their personal grooming (combing their hair, brushing their teeth, applying deodorants, etc.). The patients also learned to engage in some organized games and recreational activities—which they had been unable to do previously—and to make some attempts at interpersonal interactions. According to the investigators, the results of this pilot study are encouraging in that they further define the nurse's role in the utilization of operant conditioning and also in the application of these techniques to other areas of the patients' lives, such as school, vocational, and industrial training.

MANAGEMENT OR CONTROL

Discipline

No discussion of the care of the mentally retarded is complete without some mention of discipline, strange as this word may sound in the context of a treatment program. However, discipline, or training the mentally retarded individual to conform with the rules of society, presents a major problem to the mentally retarded themselves and to their families and caretakers. In the past, physicians considered discipline a necessary part of the total treatment plan but offered only some simple guidelines, leaving the responsibility for the direct implementation of these rules to the families or the caretakers in the institutions. Nurses, if any were employed by the institution, were given this responsibility, but it was most frequently the attendants and other nonprofessional personnel who were involved in imposing discipline sanctioned and delegated by the physician and the hospital administration placed the attendant in a position of great power. Gareth Thorne (1965) writes:

> Group living in institutions makes unusual demands upon the individual to conform to routines and codes of behavior essential to managing groups living closely together. It must be stated again that herein exists one of the very valid criticisms of institutional life. In order for the results of such a life to be free from tragic results, the kind of discipline administered by the attendant is of great importance.
>
> Discipline is a psychological problem, that is, it involves an attempt to modify or change behavior, or, at least, this should be the objective. Unfortunately, some people apply disciplinary measures to others, not for the purpose of modifying behavior or modes of adjustment, but rather to satisfy their own personal feelings of indignation or anger.

There is no question that in many instances discipline is imposed to satisfy personal feelings and to gratify feelings of power, but in many other instances it is also imposed by individuals of good intentions who are frustrated by some behavior of the mentally retarded and know of no other way of coping with this behavior than by applying punitive measures. Discipline then becomes inextricably bound up with punishment.

Counseling

A change occurred in the management of institutionalized retarded patients when psychologists joined the professional staffs of hospitals for the mentally retarded. At first, psychologists were concerned primarily with the psychological testing of retarded patients, but some psychologists, trained in clinical psychology, became interested in the problems of the patients' behavior on the wards. Their sphere of interest included the attendant-patient conflicts provoked by some of the unacceptable behavior of the patients and the disciplinary methods used by the attendants to correct this behavior. A number of counseling programs for mentally retarded patients were developed by clinical psychologists. Although it is difficult to draw the line between counseling and psychotherapy, psychotherapy may be thought of as focusing primarily on psychopathology or internalized emotional conflicts from which the patient suffers. On the other hand, according to Yepson (1957) " 'counseling' is a word used to describe the interpersonal relationship which takes place when one or more persons seek to influence the behavior and attitudes of another person or persons."

257

Since the psychological makeup of a retarded person is not different from that of a normal person except that the retarded person functions at a much lower intellectual level, and since many of the problems of the mentally retarded are concerned with the influencing of behavior, counseling can be very useful in their treatment.

The aim of counseling is to help an individual adjust to new situations as they occur in his daily life. Counseling differs from conventional disciplinary measures in that it seeks to understand the reasons for the specific behavior or difficulty and attempts to help the individual find a successful solution to the problem rather than to impose penalties for the infraction of rules. In some institutions, each psychologist is responsible for counseling the patients in a given area of the hospital; in others, each psychologist's case load consists of patients referred to him by the ward physician or the caretaking personnel.

In a few institutions, nurses and attendants have learned some counseling skills and utilize them in their care of patients. This is an important trend, and a growing one. It is important because there are not, and will not be in the foreseeable future, enough psychiatrists and clinical psychologists employed in hospitals for the mentally retarded to provide an adequate counseling program for the many patients who desperately need some form of counseling. Furthermore, in substituting counseling methods which stress the importance of understanding the patient for the traditional rule-oriented discipline, the whole philosophy of nursing care and treatment changes from a punitive to a therapeutic one. For a discussion of methods of counseling and specific techniques which attendants and other caretaking personnel can utilize, the reader is referred to Chapter 5, "Counseling and Guiding the Metnally Retarded," in Gareth Thorne's book, *Understanding the Mentally Retarded* (Thorne, 1965). Nursing personnel engaged in counseling should have regularly scheduled supervisory support, either individually or in group conferences, and should also have ready access to a consultant whenever needed. Nurses well prepared in interpersonal and counseling skills are qualified for this purpose, as well as psychologists, psychiatrists, and social workers.

Operant Conditioning versus Punishment

Operant conditioning, which is so useful in motivating new behavior and reinforcing present desirable behavior, is also a good technique for eliminating undesirable behavior. This method provides a far more effective way of controlling and correcting unacceptable behavior than the usual disciplinary methods. Conventional discipline depends upon two deterrent measures: the first is by the deprivation of something pleasurable, e.g., loss of freedom, income, or status; and the second, by the imposition of something disagreeable or unpleasant, e.g., corporal punishment. This method of correction emphasizes the undesirable behavior and controls it by a series of prohibitions directed against the unwanted behavior. This strategy gradually limits the range of the child's behavior and offers him nothing in its place. In some emotionally disturbed children this process reaches a stage at which the child is completely immobilized.

Operant conditioning, on the other hand, works on diametrically opposite principles. The emphasis is not on the undesirable behavior, but on the desired behavior. The desired behavior is achieved by rewarding it (positive reinforcer), or by removing something disagreeable or inhibitory (negative reinforcer). Skinner (1953) says that initially deterrents to behavior (punishments) are effective. However, in time, not only does their effectiveness decrease but, because of the constant emphasis on the undesirable behavior, they actually reinforce it. For example, one can spank a child for stealing candy. At first this punishment has some deterrent effect. Later on, as the desire for candy persists, the prospect of the spanking after theft becomes less fearful, and eventually, punishment loses all deterrent value as stealing may continue as a well-established habit, or even a game.

FACILITIES FOR CARE

Home Care

In the past, when a child was diagnosed as mentally retarded, medical authorities usually recommended institutionalization. This recommendation was based on the hopeless prognosis accompanying the diagnosis, the burden the care of such a child would impose upon the mother, and the supposedly detrimental psychological effects the presence of a retarded child would have on the other children in the family. However, the current trend is to recommend that the child be cared for at home until school age or until he is about seven years of age if this is at all possible. This reversal of attitude has been brought about by the more optimistic outlook of the medical profession regarding the treatment of mental retardation and the recognition that the mentally retarded child needs the emotional support of his family during his early developmental years as much as, if not more than, the child of normal intelligence.

Mothers can receive help in caring for the special needs of the mentally retarded child from home visits by a public health nurse or the mental retardation nursing specialist. Special community agencies which provide temporary or part-time household workers, or places where a child can stay for a few hours while the mother does her shopping, are available in some communities. Homes where the child can be boarded for a few days while the mother is ill or takes a much-needed, brief vacation are now available in many English communities and are gradually being introduced in this country (Adams, 1960).

Certain advantages in home care are superior to care in the best of institutions. In a home where the retarded child is lovingly accepted as a member of the family, where his parents talk to him, give him their attention, show concern, and patiently train him, and where the other children in the family play with him, he is stimulated to use his capacities to a degree that is not possible in institutional life (Adams, 1960). Parents are also often happier and are not haunted by feelings of guilt for having sent away their defective child. The other children in the family learn consideration and concern for their less fortunate sibling. Many mentally retarded children are deeply loved and valued members of their families, for they frequently have very winning personalities (Buck, 1950).

Foster Home Care

Some families cannot provide a suitable home environment for their mentally retarded member. Such families include those in which the parents cannot tolerate the presence of their mentally retarded child in the home and display rejection and hostility toward him. Some families are too overprotective, while others put such pressure on the child to achieve that he is immobilized. Still other families present special problems, such as an invalid in the home, or economic or cultural deprivation so severe that it is impossible for the parents to keep their retarded child at home. In these cases, foster home care may be utilized if the mentally retarded child is otherwise able to benefit from home care. Foster homes should be carefully selected and regularly supervised. The selection and supervision of foster homes are usually done by social workers.

The child chosen for foster home care should fit in easily into the family life. Generally, the placement is most successful if the foster parents and the child have somewhat similar socioeconomic backgrounds. The public health nurse and the mental retardation nurse specialist may provide the same assistance to foster home parents and child as would were the child cared for in his own home. New foster parents often need considerable assistance from these nurses in the early days of the placement. Foster home placement has also been very successful with mentally retarded adults after their discharge from a hospital for the mentally retarded. These adults can perform useful tasks in the foster home or be employed in the community while maintaining residence in the home.

Hospitals and Hospitalization

Hospitals for the mentally retarded were formerly thought of as places of permanent residence. The mentally retarded were regarded as a threat to the community, and it was therefore believed that they should be permanently segregated for the protection of society. Stanley Davies quotes from the 1915 report of the New York State Commission to Investigate Provision for the Mentally Deficient, "The mentally defective man or woman at liberty constitutes a serious menace to the State. In many cases, the mental defect is hereditary and is likely to be transmitted . . . to succeeding generations. This danger is in turn aggravated by the well-known propagating tendency of the feebleminded, and because they are in most cases potential delinquents or criminals, peculiarly susceptible to the suggestions of evil-minded associates" (Davies, 1959). Present knowledge of mental retardation has changed these ideas radically. The mentally retarded have been found to have a very low fertility rate; hereditary factors can be specifically proved to etiologically significant in only a very small number of diagnostic categories. The present trend is to provide necessary treatment for the mentally retarded person in his own community if this is at all possible.

Today, the hospital for the mentally retarded is regarded not as an asylum, but as one of a variety of treatment agencies (Roos, 1969). Tarjan (1956) perceives the role of such a hospital as providing care and treatment for those mentally retarded individuals whose condition requires psychiatric or somatic therapy, constant nursing care, or close observation. This would include individuals so severely handicapped that they could not survive without expert medical and nursing care, and also individuals only mildly retarded whose emotional or social problems are such that they would benefit from a period of hospitalization. Hospitalization should be regarded by staff, patient, and family as a phase of the patient's total treatment plan. During the patient's hospital stay every effort should be made to maintain family and community contacts to make return to the community easier for the patient. Careful planning and preparing the patient for discharge are important aspects of treatment.

Role of the Nurse in the Hospital

A hospital for the mentally retarded needs a well-trained and competent staff representing a wide variety of specialties, including a well-prepared and numerically adequate nursing staff. Unfortunately, in the past, a good professional staff was not always considered essential. In addition to their professional qualifications, staff members should be warm, friendly, and understanding of the problems of the mentally retarded. Nurses who have this knowledge and understanding have an important role in such a hospital, both in caring directly for patients, and in teaching and supervising nursing technicians, attendants, and aides.

Direct patient nursing care for which the skilled nurse is needed includes care of the most severely handicapped patients, many of whom are infants or very young children. Many have multiple disabilities; most of them are bed patients. The nurse's observational skills are valuable, too, and can be of use to the physician in both treatment and research programs. While developing her own clinical skills, the nurse can also make it easier for the patient to function, perhaps by devising aids to offset or ameliorate the effects of the patient's handicap. For example, the nurse may design individualized devices to help the child feed himself, hold tools and other objects, walk more easily, and so forth. For young children deprived of their mothers, the nurse may be able to provide some form of psychological mothering. Slightly older children who are able to be up and about the ward may be helped to achieve self-mastery skills such as feeding, dressing, and toileting themselves, developing speech, and learning to walk. The nurse may work directly with the child or help an attendant or aide to work with the child.

Day Centers and Other Facilities

The great majority of mentally retarded children and adults do not need to be hospitalized. One of the newer trends in the care and treatment of the mentally retarded centers around the development of a variety of community facilities. Some of the community facilities now available include day care centers, special nursery schools, diagnostic and evaluation clinics, training centers, and community mental health centers. Day care centers are designed primarily for very young or handicapped children who require nursing care. At the centers, children may be taken care of for the entire day and returned home in the evening, or they may spend only a part of the day at the center. Day care relieves the family of the constant care of these children, and also provides the children with greater variety of experiences, stimulation, and social contacts than are available at home. These centers are generally staffed by qualified nurses assisted by nursing aides and volunteer workers.

Nursery Schools

Special nursery schools are very helpful for less severely retarded children under the age of seven who do not require nursing care. Nursery schools are useful in encouraging the retarded child to develop his potentialities and in preparing him for possible future attendance in some type of training or educational program (Appell et al., 1966). Adams comments that a well-run nursery school is a godsend to the mentally retarded child (Adams, 1960). It offers him an opportunity to experience the society of other children, to learn games and songs, to try out various art media, and to practice simple social skills. The emphasis in nursery school is on social experience and not on academic learning. The nursery school should prepare a child for later school experience. Adams recommends that enrollment in a regular kindergarten be delayed as long as possible in order that the retarded child enter this new experience with the best possible preparation and under the most favorable conditions. A good nursery school for mentally retarded children should be staffed by a nursery school teacher specially trained to meet the needs of the mentally retarded along with an adequate number of competent assistants. A nurse with psychiatric and pediatric background is also a valuable adjunct to the staff. Supervision and consultation by a child psychiatrist are also a necessary component of a well-organized nursery school program.

Diagnostic Clinics

Diagnostic and evaluation clinics are most useful community agencies for the prevention, care, and treatment of the mentally retarded. These centers are usually staffed by a variety of specialists, including pediatricians, child psychiatrists, child neurologists, mental health and maternal-child nursing consultants, speech therapists, diet therapists, psychologists, social workers, and public health nurses. Among the many services these clinics offer are medical and psychological evaluation, family counseling, planning of care and treatment, and follow-up care. Some of the larger diagnostic clinics send out traveling teams to hold clinics in the more remote communities in their area (Koch and Gilien, 1965). The members of these teams include a pediatrician, a psychologist, a social worker, and a public health nurse. In communities where there are no diagnostic clinics, the outpatient departments of large general hospitals can often provide a number of these services (Fackler, 1966).

Special Educational Programs

For mildly retarded children educational programs are often beneficial. Special classes may be set up in existing school systems. About 2 percent of the children enrolled in elementary schools require instruction in special classes. Often, the special classes are ungraded classes in which the student is permitted to learn at his own pace. Special teaching methods are employed, emphasizing the concrete, the practical, and the functional rather than the abstract. Both public and private schools designed to meet the needs of retarded children are available in many of the larger communities. Much research is in progress regarding the development of new teaching methods for the mentally retarded, including experimentation with programmed teaching, and use of audio-visual aids and other teaching devices. Borderline retarded children can often attend regular school classes if given some additional assistance and support.

Training Centers

For children who cannot benefit from an educational program a training program is indicated. Such a program can best be developed in a training center. "Training centers give the child training and occupation to keep him happy and develop latent faculties" (Adams, 1960). The special benefits for the retarded child attending a training center, according to Adams, are that he goes to school like his siblings; he learns the social skills of leadership, mixing with others, and excelling in some activity; he produces something to take home and show off; others become interested in him as he improves; and he learns that he has a place in his family and community. Programs in training centers may cover a wide range of activities and skills which can be taught through activity teaching, or learning by doing, to the moderately retarded child. The Montessori method of teaching, or modifications of it, can often be used effectively with these children. Classroom activities may include handicrafts, physical training, dancing, singing, rhythm bands, speech and sensory training, training in simple household chores, and social behavior.

Community Mental Health Centers

Community mental health centers are being developed for the care and treatment of the mentally retarded and multiple-handicapped. These are larger and more complex agencies, designed to serve a larger segment of the population, and to care for patients with a wider range of disabilities, than the smaller agencies described above. Such centers would also be able to provide many more services, including public health nursing services, better follow-up care, facilities for teaching students from various health professions, and opportunities for research. Some authorities believe that there should not be separate community health centers for the mentally retarded but that larger health centers should provide care for all types of mental health problems.

SOME RECENT TRENDS IN THE CARE OF THE MENTALLY RETARDED

In view of recent scientific advances in genetics, endocrinology, biochemistry, nutritional therapy, and developmental, social, and educational psychology, many changes are taking place in the field of mental retardation. Several such trends will be discussed here. One such trend is the recognition of the importance of the first three years of life in the optimal development of a person as a member of society. It is known that there are critical periods for the development of specific organ functions; that developmental time limits exist; and that if the right type of stimulation does not occur, optimal development does not take place (Lourie, 1971). Methods are now available to detect many kinds of dysfunction even at this very early age. In the mentally retarded such dysfunctioning frequently is not detected until the child reaches school age. By this time patterns of dysfunctioning are well established and have also affected other organs and/or body systems. Lourie writes (1971, p. 4), "Those concerned with the problems of human behavior must be concerned with the first 3 years of life if the roots of later pathology are to be identified in the interest of prevention and early modification."

Another trend in mental retardation is the trend of mental health professionals to reject the medical model which considers mental retardation as a disease, and to turn to the behavioral model or learning theory concept, which considers mental retardation as due to a deviation of cognitive development. Patterson and Rowland (1970) believe that the medical model reinforces and augments and dehumanization of the mentally retarded person. They state (Patterson and Rowland, 1970, p. 534), "Retardation is not a sickness, and our programs are not therapy. Retardation is a complexity of human existence often physiologic in origin, but essentially a matter of decelerated and/or impaired cognitive functioning. In many instances it is remarkably responsive to certain types of educational programs." These writers also would like to see the role of the nurse for the mentally retarded redefined to include not only traditional medically oriented nursing functions but also a broadened and more relevant description of nursing functions. This more comprehensive conception would relate nursing to education and developmental psychology as well as to medicine.

Patterson and Rowland state that there are much new knowledge and skill available for the care of the mentally retarded that are not being utilized. In fact, only about 10 percent of current knowledge is made use of. "Many professionals are convinced that if we could bring a small percentage of our intellectual and financial resources to bear upon the problem of cerebral dysfunction, we could work miracles in salvaging the vast human potential currently going to waste in some of the human warehouses we call institutions" (Patterson and Rowland, 1970, p. 533).

Weiner (1971) also stresses the usefulness of the behavioral model in developing an educational program for the mentally retarded child in the school. Problems arise when the retarded child uses some form of emotional disturbed behavior to avoid realities of daily living, with the result that it becomes impossible for him to function in his environment. This is essentially a problem of interpersonal relationships and is as relevant and applicable in home settings or any other social situation. The concepts utilized to solve this problem are those of learning theory. This is accomplished, according to Weiner, by providing "an understandable environment for the educable emotionally disturbed child through stressing reasonable limits and boundaries under which the child can operate effectively, safely, and securely; and to provide an atmosphere in which educational goals can be met" (Weiner, 1971, p. 30).

The role of the nurse is expanding greatly in the home care of the mentally retarded. Jane Maxwell (1971) writes, "We are in a stage of progress and hope as increasing numbers of professional people are helping to open up the world for the retarded child. The public health nurse can be a prime catalyst in implementing this changed and changing attitude toward mental retardation." She perceives three areas of special responsibility for the nurse—prevention, case finding, and home management. Prevention and case finding are not new functions, but home management is. There has been little or no guidance or assistance for mothers in caring for and training their mentally retarded children.

Maxwell describes a program originating in a state hospital for the mentally retarded to send a team which included a public health nurse into the homes of retarded children awaiting admission to the hospital. Parents were helped to provide for the special nursing needs of their retarded child, such as walking, feeding, toilet training, and behavior problems. They were also counseled in regard to other problems which arose while waiting for admission. A number of parents learned to care for their children with such success that hospitalization became unnecessary. The nurse established a good relationship with all members of the family. Maxwell writes, "The family must have confidence in the nurse's knowledge and ability to teach their child, but this is not enough; they must also develop confidence in themselves as they actively participate in the training." In the course of working with the family, the needs of other family members become the responsibility of the nurse as well. All the children in this program made progress, some of them dramatically. Because this was a state hospital program, retarded children were often brought only as a last resort. Maxwell believes that if assistance could be provided sooner, it is certain that more parents would be able to maintain their retarded child at home. She also stresses the need for the development of community and regionally centered home care programs.

In regard to community involvement she says (Maxwell, 1971, p. 114),

> The implications for educating not only parents, but the community too, in the philosophy that the severely retarded child *can* learn are far-reaching. Acceptance of this philosophy would mean that countless retarded children would be enabled to successfully live out their lives in their own homes and communities instead of in institutions. It would also mean that parents would not be denied the guidance they need in order to maintain their retarded child within the family circle and to help him to develop to his fullest potential.

REFERENCES

Adams, Margaret (ed.) (1960): *The Mentally Subnormal,* William Heinemann, Ltd., London.

Appell, Melville J., Clarence M. Williams, and Kenneth N. Fishell (1966): "A Day Care Center Training Program for Preschool Retarded Children," *Mental Retardation,* April, pp. 17–21.

Ayllon, Teodoro (1965): "Operant Conditioning on Trial in the Treatment of Schizophrenia," *Roche Report: Frontiers of Hospital Psychiatry,* October, pp. 5–6.

————and Jack Michael (1959): "The Psychiatric Nurse as a Behavioral Engineer," *Journal of the Experimental Analysis of Behavior,* vol. 2, pp. 323–334.

Buck, Pearl (1950): *The Child Who Never Grew,* John Day Company, Inc., New York.

Chidester, Leona, and Karl A. Menninger (1936): "The Application of Psychoanalytic Methods to the Study of Mental Retardation," *American Journal of Orthopsychiatry,* vol. 6, pp. 616–625.

Cotzin, Milton (1948): "Group Therapy with Mentally Defective Problem Boys," *American Journal of Mental Deficiency,* October, pp. 268–283.

Davies, Stanley Powell (1959): *The Mentally Retarded in Society,* Columbia University Press, New York. p. 66.

De Martino, Manfred F. (1957): "Some Observations Concerning Psychotherapeutic Techniques with the Mentally Retarded," in Chalmers L. Stacey and Manfred F. De Martino (eds.), *Counseling and Psychotherapy with the Mentally Retarded,* The Free Press of Glencoe, New York, pp. 461–472.

Ewalt, Jack R., Edward A. Strecker, and Franklin G. Ebaugh (1957): *Practical Clinical Psychiatry,* 8th ed., McGraw-Hill Book Company, New York.

Fackler, Eleanor (1966): "Community Organization in Culturally Deprived Areas," *Mental Retardation,* April, pp. 12–14.

Gericke, Otto L. (1965): "Practical Use of Operant Conditioning Procedures in a Mental Hospital," *Psychiatric Studies and Projects,* vol. 3, no. 5, published by the Mental Hospital Service of the American Psychiatric Association.

HEW Committee on Mental Retardation (1962): *Mental Retardation, Activities of the U.S. Dept. of Health, Education, and Welfare,* published by U.S. Dept. of Health, Education, and Welfare, Departmental Committee on Mental Retardation, Washington, D.C., May, pp. l, 3.

Hundziak, Marcel, Ruth A. Maurer, and Luke S. Watson (1965): "Operant Conditioning in Toilet Training Severely Retarded Boys," *American Journal of Mental Deficiency,* July, pp. 120–124.

Koch, Richard, and Nancy Ragsdale Gilien (1965): "Diagnostic Experience in a Clinic for Retarded Children," *Nursing Outlook,* June, pp. 26–29.

Lourie, Reginald S. (1971): "The First Three Years of Life: An Overview of a New Frontier of Psychiatry," *Mental Health Digest,* vol. 3, no. 10, pp. 1–4.

Maxwell, Jane E. (1971): "Home Care for the Retarded Child," *Nursing Outlook,* vol. 19, no. 2, pp. 112–114.

Patterson, E. Gene, and G. Thomas Rowland (1970): "Toward a Theory of Mental Retardation Nursing: An Educational Model," *American Journal of Nursing,* vol. 70, no. 3, pp. 531–535.

The Poppe Project (film), University of California Extension Medical Center Film Distribution, 2223 Fulton Street, Berkeley, Calif. 94720.

Roos, Philip (1966): "Changing Roles of the Residential Institution," *Mental Retardation,* April, pp. 4–6.

Sarason, Seymour B (1959): *Psychological Problems in Mental Deficiency,* 3d ed., Harper & Row, Publishers, Inc., New York, p. 263.

Skinner, B. F. (1953): *Science and Human Behavior,* The Macmillan Company, New York.

Snyder, Robert, and Lee Sechrest (1963): "An Experimental Study of Directive Group Therapy with Defective Delinquents," in Max Rosenbaum and Milton M. Berger (eds.), *Group Psychotherapy and Group Function,* Basic Books, Inc., Publishers, New York, pp. 525–533.

Stacey, Chalmers L., and Manfred F. De Martino (eds.) (1957): *Counseling and Psychotherapy with the Mentally Retarded,* The Free Press of Glencoe, New York, pp. 186–201, 208–276.

Tarjan, George (1964): Unpublished lecture, Continuing Education Program, "Nursing

Care of the Mentally Retarded," University of California School of Nursing, San Francisco, Calif., Summer.

———(1956): "What Hospitals for the Mentally Retarded Can Achieve," in *Children,* May–June, Children's Bureau, Dept. of Health, Education, and Welfare, Washington, D.C., pp. 95–101.

Thorne, Frederick C. (1957): "Counseling and Psychotherapy with Mental Defectives," in Chalmers L. Stacey and Manfred F. De Martino (eds.), *Counseling and Psychotherapy with the Mentally Retarded,* The Free Press of Glencoe, New York, pp. 75–84.

Thorne, Gareth D. (1965): *Understanding the Mentally Retarded,* McGraw-Hill Book Company, New York, pp. 102–103.

Weiner, Lawrence H. (1971): "New Concepts in Educating the Emotionally Disturbed Retarded Child," *Mental Health Digest,* vol. 3, no. 7, pp. 29–30.

Wright, Margaret M. (1963): "Care for the Mentally Retarded," *American Journal of Nursing,* September, pp. 70–74.

———(1965): "Rumination: Study of a Nursing Problem in Mental Retardation," Unpublished paper read at National League for Nursing Convention, San Francisco, Calif., May 4.

Yepson, Lloyd N. (1957): "Counseling the Mentally Retarded," in Chalmers L. Stacey and Manfred F. De Martino (eds.), *Counseling and Psychotherapy with the Mentally Retarded,* The Free Press of Glencoe, New York, pp. 65–75.

11

ORGANIC BRAIN SYNDROMES

Marion E. Kalkman

The category "organic brain syndrome" includes all the psychiatric disorders which are caused by some physical agent or condition, as opposed to functional disorders, those psychiatric disorders for which no physical etiology can be found. The causes of organic brain syndromes are many and varied. They include such etiological agents as brain deterioration due to senility, cerebral arteriosclerosis, head injuries, and brain tumors; infectious diseases such as syphilis and encephalitis; alcohol and other drugs, intoxicants, and poisons; as well as endocrine, metabolic, and nutritional disorders; and many other neurological and physiological conditions. These etiological agents have one thing in common: they all affect the central nervous system and interfere with its normal functioning. Engel (1967, pp. 706–707) describes this deleterious process as follows:

> The fundamental process in organic brain syndromes is damage or destruction of neurons. It is this destruction rather than the nature of the noxious process that is responsible for the characteristic clinical picture. When the damage is diffuse and widespread, the basic disturbance in psychic function is the same, regardless of whether the underlying condition is heart failure, hypoglycemia, a head injury, bromide intoxication, or diffuse senile degenerative changes. When damage is to systems or regions of the brain concerned with particular psychic functions, this localization, rather than the nature of the organic factor, yields the characteristic syndrome.

Injury to the nervous system constitutes a severe trauma to the personality because the nervous system is the communication system of the individual. Perception of the environment, orientation to the environment, awareness of self and body functions such as breathing and heartbeat, and the mechanisms for thought, speech, memory, and judgment are all dependent on the proper functioning of the nervous system. Anything that endangers the nervous system can pose a threat to the integration of the personality. Impairment of the nervous system can also be damaging to the individual's social functioning, such as disturbed interpersonal relationships with family and friends, decreased employment capabilities, narrowed recreational interests, and more limited life style. Psychological symptoms frequently play a more prominent role in the clinical picture of organic brain syndrome than the medical and neurological symptoms.

According to Engel (1967, p. 706),

> Every patient with an organic syndrome requires prompt and thorough medical and neurological study with reference to drugs, alcohol, exposure to toxic materials or anesthesia, previous episodes of disturbed consciousness including syncope, cardiac arrest, shock, stroke, concussions, neurological symptoms and diseases, and every category of serious medical and surgical disorders in which physiological or biochemical processes can directly or indirectly affect adversely the metabolism or structure of the cerebral neurons.

ACUTE AND CHRONIC BRAIN SYNDROMES

Organic brain syndromes can be divided into two broad subgroups: (a) acute brain syndromes, and (b) chronic brain syndromes. In acute brain syndromes, damage to the nervous system may be temporary and normal function may be later restored; hence the term *reversible* is often applied to this subgroup. In chronic brain syndromes, there is generally destruction of brain tissue which is irreplaceable; hence the process is *irreversible,* resulting in permanent damage to the nervous system. In individual cases the symptomatology may vary according to the etiological agent, the location of the affected central area in the nervous system, and the ability of the body's defensive mechanisms to cope with the trauma or utilize alternate neural pathways. However, two general reaction patterns can be identified which characterize these two subgroups. In acute organic conditions, the reaction takes the form of a delirium, and in chronic conditions the reaction is that of deterioration or dementia. It should be noted that in clinical practice the lines of demarcation between these two subgroups are not always so sharply drawn. In some patients, an acute organic syndrome may develop a chronic irreversible course, and in some chronic organic syndromes the patient may recover partially or totally if the underlying etiological agent is effectively treated (as, for example, in pernicious anemia). Other chronic cases may remain at an arrested state or obtain partial remission (as, for example, in multiple sclerosis). An understanding of these two clinical reaction patterns, delirium and dementia, may be helpful to the nurse both in planning the nursing care of a patient with a rare-type organic brain syndrome and in providing a general frame of reference for the nursing care of all patients with organic disorders.

ACUTE ORGANIC SYNDROME: DELIRIUM

In acute organic brain syndromes, the essential clinical picture is that of delirium. Delirium is characterized by fluctuating states of consciousness, ranging from drowsiness, torpor, and transient states of awareness to stupor and coma; fear, ranging from apprehensiveness to panic; disorientation in all spheres; visual and auditory hallucinations and illusions; transitory delusions; and confused thinking. Engel states that suspiciousness is essential for a diagnosis of delirium. He also believes that any patient with major physiological or biochemical derangement should be considered as possibly delirious (Engel, 1967, p. 711). Engel describes several different types of delirious patients. One type is the quiet, torpid patient who does not recognize those caring for him or his visitors and is unable to feed himself, bathe, care for his excretory needs, or cooperate in his medical treatment. He tends to excuse his inabilities by complaining of being sleepy, weak, or tired. Another type is the blandly confused patient who appears normal at first and will reply appropriately to general questions but, if questioned in detail, appears puzzled, tries to avoid answering by joking or becoming irritable, and becomes angry if pressed for an answer. Still another type is the anxious, panicky patient who is aware of, and distressed by, his impaired sensorium. His physical symptoms include restlessness, tachycardia, tremors, sweating, and rapid respirations. Mental symptoms include disorientation, extreme fear, startle reaction to unexpected sounds, and brief and troubled sleep periods. Hallucinating patients are characterized primarily by illusions, hallucinations, and other psychotic symptoms. And, finally, there is the patient who is in an advanced stage of delirium, who shows signs of gross disorientation and disorganized thinking, and who often mutters and is incoherent in speech (Engel, 1967, p. 711).

Treatment in Acute Organic Brain Syndromes

Treatment should first be directed to combating the specific etiological factor if there is one, such as an infectious agent; or a toxic agent such as drugs, poisons, or alcohol; or hormonal or other metabolic deficiencies. Along with the treatment of etiological factors, any other distressing symptoms, such as acute pain or restlessness, should be treated also. General supportive measures include adequate elimination (bowel, bladder, and skin), adequate fluid intake, maintenance of body fluid and electrolyte balance, skillful nursing care, elimination of irritating stimuli in the environment, and protective measures to prevent accidents and self-injury. Psychotherapy may be helpful and needed, especially if evidence of an underlying psychosis develops (Ebaugh and Tiffany, 1959, pp. 1244–1245). According to Noyes and Kolb, sometimes incipient delirium may be aborted by the skillful reassurance of a nurse, the application of an icecap to the head, or the administration of chloropromazine or paraldehyde (Noyes and Kolb, 1968, p. 152). Measures directed to the treatment of the delirium are of major importance. Ebaugh and Tiffany (1959) in their discussion of the treatment of delirium state that sedation, properly utilized and with full appreciation of its dangers, is important. Hydrotherapy in the form of continuous tubs, though not used as much as formerly, is still a good form of sedation. However, cold packs and forms of hydrotherapy which involve restraint are contraindicated because of the lability of the autonomic nervous system and the intense fear which restraints often induce in delirious patients. Chemical sedation, provided there is no medical contraindication, can be very effective. Acutely disturbed and delirious patients can often tolerate relatively large doses of sedation, and such doses are often required to achieve effective sedation, although the cumulative effects and possible synergistic effects of the drugs prescribed must be kept in mind and guarded against.

Nursing Care

The nursing care of the patient with an acute brain syndrome is crucial to his future as well as to his current physical and psychological well-being. Frequently, in head injuries, acute poisoning, and intracranial or systemic infections, the onset is sudden and the symptoms grave. Symptoms such as high fever, shock, intracranial pressure, and acute anxiety should be watched for and given prompt attention and appropriate medical and nursing intervention. The patient with an acute brain syndrome generally appears extremely ill, and his symptoms and general condition can change rapidly. He requires constant and highly perceptive observation and skillful physical and psychological nursing care. The quality of nursing care often is an important factor in determining whether the patient makes a full or partial recovery and whether or not his condition becomes chronic.

General Nursing Measures Most patients with delirium require bed rest, and this is sometimes difficult to secure when the patient is disoriented and restless. The use of physical methods of restraint is very undesirable for delirous patients and should be avoided. The disoriented and fearful patient tends to become more frightened by the restriction of his physical movements and fights against the restraints. This struggle tends to increase his pulse, respirations, and blood pressure and can be very dangerous in his already exhausted and toxic condition. In most cases chemical sedation can be very helpful, but in those cases in which drugs are contraindicated or prove ineffective, constant attendance by a nurse is necessary. Whenever possible, the same nurse should be assigned each day to the patient so that he can relate to the nurse and be reassured by his presence. The physical presence of the nurse can in itself help to calm the patient. Some other ways that can be used to quiet the restless patient is to keep his room cool and quiet and to see that he is disturbed as little as possible. If he is febrile, an alcohol sponge bath may be helpful. If he attempts to get out of bed, he can usually be prevented from doing so by the nurse placing a restraining hand on him. The nurse's voice can also be instrumental in calming and reassuring the fearful and apprehensive patient.

The administration of adequate fluids is one of the most important points in the nursing care of delirious patients. The intake of fluids is more important than the intake of food, and the nurse should offer the patient fluids at every opportunity, taking advantage of any brief periods of lucidity when he is most able to cooperate by taking fluids orally. It is often difficult to get delirious patients to accept solid food; therefore, a high-calorie liquid diet supplemented by a soft, bland diet can give the patient the calories he needs in a form that is easy for him to take.

There is considerable danger of accidents, injuries, and suicide with delirious patients. The danger in regard to suicide is generally not due to suicidal intentions or depression, but rather the result of the patient's general state of disorientation, confusion, and apprehension and to his hallucinations and illusionary and delusional experiences. A common example of such mishaps is that of the delirious patient who walks out of an unguarded window under the impression that he is going into the bathroom. Other common accidents include drinking antiseptic solutions or medications that have been left in the vicinity of the patient, falling out of bed, removing surgical dressings, sutures, and clips, and accidentally strangling himself with bedclothes, bandages, or various electric cords and tubing which generally surround the bed patient.

Delirious patients are often very irritable. This irritability should not be responded to by impatience or reproof but by endeavoring to find out the source of irritation and removing it if possible. Sometimes it is better to allow the patient to express his irritability without comment. Irritability may be a transitory occurrence, but occasionally it may persist. If it is not dealt with in the early stages, it can build up into a state of excitement. If the early signs of it can be recognized, measures may be instituted to prevent the occurrence of a more severe and prolonged reaction.

Hallucinatory and delusional experiences which are unpleasant in nature tend to increase the patient's fearfulness and anxiety. This anxiety can sometimes be reduced by diverting his attention away from his fantasy world and making him more aware of the world of reality. Increasing the amount of lighting in the room so that the patient can see the objects in his environment more clearly, touching him in a quiet, reassuring manner, speaking to him calmly and addressing him by name, responding to his verbal and nonverbal attempts at communication, and making him aware of the constant concern and availability of those caring for him are some of the measures that may lessen his anxiety and help to keep him in touch with reality.

Fluctuating states of consciousness are characteristic of most patients with an acute organic brain disorder. There are times when the patient is so confused and disoriented that he is unable to cooperate with the medical and nursing care being given to him, and in some instances he may even actively oppose such ministrations. At other times, he may be entirely lucid and respond appropriately and cooperatively in the efforts of the treatment personnel to help him. These lucid periods should be utilized to the utmost. If medications or treatments are ordered for a time when the patient is confused or out of contact, it is often possible to postpone their administration until a lucid interval occurs. Such periods of lucidity can also be used to give psychological reassurance and information feedback to the patient.

ACUTE BRAIN SYNDROME ASSOCIATED WITH TRAUMA

One form of acute brain syndrome which is becoming increasingly frequent and which requires medical and surgical nursing treatment of a special nature is that associated with trauma, especially trauma associated with head injuries. These head injuries are primarily the consequence of high-speed automobiles and the shocking number of traffic accidents, as well as industrial accidents, especially those involving heavy construction equipment. Acute brain syndrome due to trauma generally develops immediately after head injury produced by external trauma of a gross physical nature. One of the results of such head injury is an immediate but transient loss of consciousness or concussion. Brosin defines *concussion* as caused by a head injury and resulting in an interruption of brain functions, accompanied by loss of consciousness of brief duration followed by spontaneous and complete recovery. There may be brief posttraumatic amnesia for events just prior to injury. In other cases there may be more prolonged loss of consciousness without psychiatric sequelae upon awakening. Still other patients with concussion may suffer traumatic amnesia, confusion, and disorientation or perseveration of routine activity engaged in just previous to trauma. Other symptoms in patients with head injury include headache, apathy, dizziness, dullness, inability to concentrate, defective memory, irritability, fatigue, insomnia, and decreased tolerance for noise, light, heat, and alcohol. Generally these symptoms disappear within 6 weeks after injury. If not, the patient should be reexamined for further evidence of brain damage (Brosin, 1967).

Emergency Treatment and Nursing Care

Brosin believes that the most effective emergency treatment is given in trauma centers in general hospitals specially designed and staffed with well-trained multidisciplinary teams for the diagnosis and emergency treatment of head injuries. In addition to physical and neurological examinations and electroencephalogic and laboratory tests, a psychiatric examination should be an integral part of the diagnostic work-up. Such a psychiatric evaluation when followed up with psychiatric interviews can improve the patient's chances for a good recovery (Brosin, 1967).

Following emergency treatment, of crucial importance is the supportive physical and psychological care given by the medical, nursing, and other hospital staff, particularly in the early stages of the illness. Brosin states that it is generally recognized as a fact that comprehensive and concerned care can eliminate or, at least, diminish the undesirable sequelae of head injuries. He also thinks that the attitude of the patient's family and friends is an important factor in the recovery of the patient. Injury to the head is more likely to produce anxiety in a patient than injury to any other part of his body because of the high value that our culture and society place on the head and the precious organ within it, the brain. Hence, according to Paul Schilder,

> In susceptible patients, the daily impact of the minor pain or transient disability produced by head injuries may lead to anxiety, discomfort, and fatigue, which in time may be organized into patterns of neurosis and invalidism [Brosin, 1967, p. 750].
> As we listen to patients describe their experiences during the acute period immediately after an accident, we learn that the attitudes and words of physicians, nurses, and attendants make a lasting impression on them which takes weeks or more of reassurance to correct if they gained a false impression of their injury. Relatives and friends can communicate their anxieties and hidden wishes for compensation and thereby needlessly, increase the burden on the patient [Brosin, 1959, p. 1179].

Nursing care includes rest in bed, constant and careful observation, with special attention to vital signs, blood pressure, bleeding, and increased intracranial pressure, and with reporting of critical signs or changes in the patient's condition to the surgeon or physician. Narcotics or stimulants are generally contraindicated, but paraldehyde may be given for restlessness. Brosin comments (1959, pp. 1179–1180),

> Too much emphasis cannot be placed upon excellent nursing care as the major requirement for good recovery, with minimal dependence upon mechanical restraints and sideboards. . . . Manipulation of the patient should be done skillfully to avoid sudden, unexpected movements. Brief reassurance and explanation are helpful when doing blood-pressure readings, venipuncture, spinal puncture, or injections and infusions. Tube feeding can usually be avoided by gentle persuasive spoon feeding. Rectal temperature determinations and rectal installations or enemas are poorly tolerated by some patients, especially if they are delusional.

The patient should also be watched for such psychological symptoms as acute anxiety, depression, and preoccupation with morbid or self-destructive ideas.

In any discussion of acute brain syndromes one must consider those individuals who are seen in emergency rooms or at the site of an accident without obvious signs of head injury but who nevertheless may be suffering from the effects of an accident or catastrophe. Sometimes they appear to be in a state of shock, unable to speak, disoriented, dazed, confused, and suffering from memory loss, usually for the traumatic event itself and for the incidents leading up to it. However, some often appear quite normal and will declare that they are unhurt. Nevertheless, they should be taken to an emergency center for physical and psychological examination. Some symptoms, such as amnesia, may be easily overlooked on superficial examination. This situation is well illustrated in the case of Michael Shaw, who wrote of his subjective experiences following an automobile accident in an article published in the *American Journal of Nursing* entitled "Hangman's Break." Shaw, a young college student, was admitted to the hospital with a broken neck. When he regained consciousness, he asked a doctor what had happened, and the doctor, concerned with the patient's immediate physical condition, told him only that there had been an accident on the freeway and that he was not to worry. The patient was afraid that he might have killed someone. He describes his efforts to get information from the hospital personnel about the accident. He writes (Shaw, 1970, p. 2566):

> I felt miserable. There was no place to turn. No one would tell me about the accident. What had happened? I was lost. I thought that by reconstructing the day I might remember what had happened. I reviewed the day skiing, the trip home, our stop in San Bernardino for something to eat. I remembered being on the San Bernardino Freeway, but couldn't remember driving on the Riverside Freeway where the accident had occurred.

> I went over the process time and time again. It was always the same. I thought, wondered, and tried for what must have been two hours. Each time I failed, my frustration increased. I closed my eyes.

> The sun's rays are filling my room as a nurse dries the sweat covering my body. The night has passed, but the same incessant fear still possesses me.

> My thoughts are clearer today. But no one seems to know what happened in the accident; they all say not to worry. How can I not worry? Have I killed someone?

> How can I get someone to pay attention? I'll scream. Yes, I'll yell.

> "Help! Let me out! I didn't do it. Let me go!"

This cry for help brought a nurse, who was able to get the needed information to him, but after what anxiety and suffering!

CHRONIC ORGANIC BRAIN SYNDROMES

Included in the category of chronic organic brain syndromes are many disorders, some of which are very rare and others of which constitute a large and important component of psychiatric practice. In this latter group are included the senile and presenile dementias, cerebral arteriosclerosis, epilepsy, intracranial neoplasms, chronic alcoholism, Korsakoff's psychosis, paresis, central nervous system syphilis, pernicious anemia, multiple sclerosis, and other chronic brain syndromes associated with metabolic, endocrine, and degenerative central nervous system diseases. There are, however, some commonalities that characterize this group of disorders. The onset of an illness is generally slow, and the course of the illness may become stabilized; in rare instances there may even be a remission of symptoms; but the general course is one of increasing deterioration.

Dementia

The general clinical picture which the patient with a chronic organic brain syndrome presents is that of dementia. *Dementia* refers to the condition produced by the degeneration of the nerve cells of the central nervous system which results in a permanent, irreversible loss of intellectual functions. Some of the symptoms of dementia include disorientation, severe loss of memory, calculation, and judgment. There is also a loss of capacity to learn and to maintain attention, as well as a decrease in motivation, interests, and self-concern. When a number of these symptoms are present to any degree, one may see a marked personality change in the person, with loss of inhibitions, lability of mood, irritability, and explosive behavior. As the person's ego defenses break down, underlying neurotic and/or psychotic symptoms may appear. According to Noyes and Kolb (1968, p. 91), the causes of dementia may be grouped as follows:

1. Atrophic changes of the brain resulting in senile dementia
2. Vascular disorders of the brain, including arteriosclerotic dementia and hypertensive encephalopathy
3. Inflammatory disorders of the brain, particularly syphilis and epidemic encephalitis
4. Degenerative diseases of the brain, notably Alzheimer's disease, Pick's disease, and Huntington's chorea
5. Deficiency diseases, including Korsakoff's psychosis, Wernicke's encephalopathy, pellagra, and pernicious anemia or vitamin B_{12} deficiency
6. Neoplasm
7. Trauma

The mental symptoms associated with chronic organic brain syndromes do not necessarily parallel the physical symptoms in severity in the course of the degenerative process. Some persons with serious neurological involvement maintain their intellectual and emotional faculties and are able to cope with their physical disabilities amazingly well. Other persons with only minor involvement of the central nervous system may develop overt neurotic and psychotic symptoms. Ferraro's comments in discussing the mental symptoms associated with old age are equally applicable to many persons suffering from other chronic organic brain conditions. He writes (Ferraro, 1959b, p. 1024),

In the precipitation of mental diseases in old age, all factors and influences related to the past lifetime of the individual—training, success, failure, immediate environment, economic status, acceptance or rejection by family and society play an important role. Tissue damage, per se, does not produce psychosis. It is rather the person's capacity to compensate for the damage, as well as present social and situational stresses, which impair the individual's ability to withstand the cerebral damage. Obviously, a long history of prior personality difficulties and emotional instability is more apt to lead to maladjustment in old age.

Mental symptoms which are most common in chronic organic brain syndromes are depressions of all types, including reactive, psychotic, agitated, and suicidal depressions. Depressions are especially prevalent in senile psychoses, Huntington's chorea, and pernicious anemia. Anxiety is another symptom which occurs frequently in cerebral arteriosclerosis as well as in many other organic conditions. Paranoid ideas are also common, and in the more advanced stages of organic disease hallucinations, illusions, and delusions occur.

Treatment in Chronic Organic Brain Syndromes

Medical Treatment Medical treatment in chronic organic brain syndromes is directed toward the recognition and treatment of the underlying cause if one is known, and the administration of specific medications and/or treatments, as, for example, low cholesterol diet, thyroid extract, iodides, nicotinic acid, and lipotropic compounds in arteriosclerosis (Ferraro, 1959a, p. 1102); penicillin in neurosyphilitic conditions; dilantin, phenobarbital, and other anticonvulsant drugs in epilepsy; Leva-dopa in Paralysis Agitans (Fangman and O'Malley, 1969); replacement therapy in some of the metabolic, endocrine, and nutritional disorders, such as niacin in pellagra, vitamin B_{12} in Wernicke's encephalopathy and pernicious anemia, and thyroid in hypothyroidism and myxedema. In many chronic organic syndromes, however, there are no known causal agents and/or specific medications available. Some such conditions are the senile psychoses, Alzheimer's and Pick's diseases, Huntington's chorea, and multiple sclerosis. Various tranquilizing and energizing drugs are sometimes prescribed to ameliorate the patient's symptoms and make him more comfortable.

Psychiatric Treatment Until recently psychiatric treatment has not played a prominent role in the treatment of chronic organic brain syndromes in spite of the frequent occurrence of mental symptoms in these conditions. Its importance seems to have been first recognized in the treatment of senile psychosis.

The realization that psychogenic factors play as important a role as do the organic factors in mental illnesses of later life has prompted the present-day emphasis on psychotherapeutic procedures in the handling of geriatric patients in private or state institutions, in contrast to the defeatist attitude of past years—that in the presence of organic cerebral damage, therapy was useless [Ferraro, 1959b, p. 1040].

Much psychiatric treatment is still symptomatic in nature; for example, sedatives for restlessness and insomnia, tranquilizers for agitation, hyperactivity, and acute anxiety, and electric shock for marked excitement, depression, or paranoid states. However, individual psychotherapeutic interviews are beginning to be used to reduce anxiety in some patients to help them cope with the consequences of their illness on their lives and in their relationships with others. In some hospitals and nursing homes group pyschotherapy is proving to be a valuable therapeutic adjunct. According to Ferraro, a psychological evaluation should be a part of the treatment procedure to determine the patient's psychological endowment, his life experiences, and his habitual ways of reaction to his environmental situations and stresses, particularly as they may influence his behavior, affect, and personality.

Appropriate psychological evaluation of the patient's total personality may, besides, assist in any psychotherapeutic approach, no matter how limited in scope. Attempts at stimulating the patient's interests in the life which surrounds him, at home or in the hospital, and the awakening of the desire to participate in various activities could be helped by such knowledge [Ferraro, 1959a, p. 1102].

According to Busse (1967, p. 728),

Supportive psychotherapeutic measures restricted to contact with a psychiatrist are not sufficiently remembered to be carried over into the living experience of these patients. Therefore, if one expects to alter affect and behavior, it is necessary to provide continuing supportive measures in the patient's milieu. Routine patterns of living provide a measure of security, but routinization should be limited to major events, and efforts should be made to vary constantly the intervening daily activities so that they provide both mental and physical stimulation. Objectionable behavior and the expression of exaggerations should not be ignored; they should be discussed with the patient and placed in proper perspective. Group meetings with patients with organic brain disease are valuable measures if the psychiatrist participates actively, frequently instructing as well as maintaining focus and balance. Statements made by the patients in such a meeting can often be clues to insights which result in better ward management.

Prevention of Psychiatric Reactions   Although chronic organic brain syndromes can occur at any age, the probability of their occurrence increases with age. Some psychiatrists believe that preventive psychiatry in the form of promoting general good mental health in the early and middle years of life may not only do much to prevent or mitigate psychiatric symptoms commonly present in organic illnesses such as anxiety, depression, and feelings of being unloved and unwanted, but also help the patient to cope with the increased disability occurring during the course of an illness which require changes in life style. Ferraro comments (1959, p. 1040),

> The modern trend of emphasizing the importance of psychological factors in the precipitation of senile psychoses has focused our attention on these factors, although no statistics, as yet, exist on the value of prevention along these lines. Nevertheless, a serious effort should be made to accumulate data concerning the value of mental hygiene in the prevention of senile psychoses during the course of physiological senescence.

Rehabilitation Treatment   Rehabilitation therapy plays a crucial role in the therapeutic treatment plan for patients with chronic organic brain syndromes. It is the ladder by which the disabled, discouraged, and dependent patient can climb back to some form of useful and rewarding life. The goals of physical rehabilitation are (Feldman, 1972):

1. To prevent the development of additional disabilities arising as sequelae to the original trauma, for example, muscle degeneration from disuse because of loss of nerve stimulation, or decubiti from the inability of the patient to change his position
2. To attempt to restore the traumatized part of the body to its maximum function
3. To find ways of substituting for the function which cannot be restored
4. To minimize the importance of the disability by focusing on other abilities
5. To help the patient to learn new ways of coping with his environment

Any comprehensive rehabilitation treatment plan should include physical, psychological, and social restoration.

Psychological Rehabilitation   The awareness of having a chronic organic brain syndrome often comes as a great shock to the patient. One patient recalls his initial shock as follows, "I couldn't comprehend what had happened to me. I denied the reality and extent of my injury" (Perrine, 1971). The following comments made by patients are descriptive of their reactions on learning their diagnosis: "When I heard the diagnosis, I actually had the physical feeling of being shot in the neck. . . . I was stunned." "I feel as though there is a sword hanging over my head swinging very slowly and lowering itself on me." "Even after they told me the diagnosis, it wasn't too much help for me because I didn't know what to expect and nobody could seem to tell me" (Davis, 1970).

Feldman cautions that in any rehabilitation therapy one should never forget that he is dealing with a man and not a machine. It is easy for therapists to concentrate on physical disabilities on which they can utilize their special technical knowledge and skills, either forgetting the person who is the recipient of such skill or hoping that the amelioration of the physical disability will automatically take care of any psychological discomforts with which they do not feel as knowledgeable or as competent to deal. Many patients with chronic diseases have stated that on the whole their physical needs were well met, but that their psychological needs were neglected.

Psychological Reactions to Chronic Illness One of the psychological reactions that occur as the result of severe disability is fragmentation of the self-concept. A patient who ordinarily functions well in his various vocational and social roles soon discovers that he cannot maintain these roles as successfully as previously. This failure is very threatening to his self-concept. The feeling of usefulness to others, and even of being a desirable member of society, is also threatened by chronic illness. Denial is an almost universal reaction, particularly in the early stages of chronic illness. At first, it serves to protect the patient from ego disintegration by buying him time to cope with the catastrophic knowledge and its implications. However, later the continued use of this mechanism will interfere seriously with progress in treatment.

Denial is not a coping mechanism that can be maintained indefinitely. In spite of himself, the patient eventually becomes aware of the realities of his disability. This realization is accompanied by a mood of depression, from which he emerges into either the acceptance of the sick role or a determination to avoid becoming dependent. The rejection of the sick role necessitates a restructuring of his self-concept and his life style to meet the realities of his changed situation. Feldman (1972) states that the patient who does not do this will not get well. The sick role, however, has considerable strength of appeal for a number of patients, namely, those who are without hope and believe that their disabilities are so great or that their prognosis is so poor that it is not worth the effort to try to get well. The sick role is also useful to patients for many other reasons. For many of the disabled, poor, homeless, friendless, and/or socially rejected persons, the sick role can become a way of life, and sometimes illness becomes the only way of existence possible for them. As long as they are sick, these people know that they will be cared for (Roth and Eddy, 1967). There are also the psychologically dependent persons who seem to enjoy the sick role and use their disability as a way of getting love and attention from family and friends. And, lastly, there are those patients who have learned to live with their disabilities and for whom the prospect of having to change their well-structured accommodation to their disability is so painful that they resist any efforts to rehabilitate them.

Southern Missionary College
Division of Nursing Library
711 Lake Estelle Dr.
Orlando, Florida 32803

The secondary advantages of the sick role make the problem of motivation to change one of the most difficult problems of rehabilitation therapy. Even for those patients who are eager to get well and who cooperate willingly with the rehabilitation plan the way is not easy, for it entails developing a new self-image based on an assessment of the patient's current postdisability assets and liabilities. Although the consequences of the disabilities need to be evaluated realistically and accepted by the patient, the major focus should be on recognizing and giving greater importance to the patient's assets and discovering and utilizing latent abilities. This is a difficult task for the patient, and he should have access to persons outside the team who are able to give him as much psychological assistance as he will accept.

A number of writers (Feldman, 1972; Ferraro, 1959b; Goldstein, 1959) have stressed the importance of a continuous relationship with a particular person for successful rehabilitative results. This relationship may be with a physician, a member of the rehabilitation team, a nurse or other member of the nursing personnel, a chaplain, a member of the family, a friend, or another patient. The important factor is the continuity of the relationship and the significance of that person to the patient. If the person is someone whom the patient knew and trusted before his disability occurred, and if the relationship can be continued during the patient's illness and convalescence, then it can be utilized immediately for treatment purposes. On the other hand, a relationship which begins after the disability occurs will take some time to develop to the point at which it can be utilized as a factor in rehabilitation therapy.

When a relationship develops between a patient and a therapist, a phenomenon materializes which in psychoanalytical terms is called *transference.* Kurt Goldstein calls this phenomenon *communion,* or a state of mutual trust and understanding. He believes it is the basis for all therapy. The brain-injured person, in his opinion, is unable to develop such a relationship voluntarily; therefore, it is the responsibility of the therapist to create a climate in which it can develop. The therapist himself must also participate in the communion. Goldstein writes (1959, p. 1340),

[This participation] demands a deeply sympathetic attitude toward the patient. The physician must see him as a human being like himself. . . . Only if he achieves this kind of countertransference will the physician be able to communicate with the patient and behave in such a way that the patient not only feels protected against the occurrence of catastrophes but understands the significance of the physician's procedure for using the psychic capacities still at his disposal for his existence in the future.

The complementary roles of the physician and patient in the

therapeutic relationship are described by Goldstein as follows (1959, p. 1346):

> With organic patients, the physician is the guide and careful observer during the whole treatment—and afterward, in so far as he helps the patient to organize life in the future. But the patient must not play a passive role; he must understand that he has to be active, he must learn to bear difficulties for the sake of the best form of self-realization.

The benefits to the patient of such psychotherapeutic experience can have a lasting effect on the patient's life (Goldstein, 1959, p. 1345).

> This valuable experience of the significance of mutual human relationship, which he has realized in the transference situation, he will take away with him when later on he has to live without direct contact with the therapist. He will no longer need the physician as a person; the mutual relationship between patient and physician—whether or not they later meet again—will never cease. The experience is important in that it can shorten the time of treatment, but perhaps as important is the fact that it is still effective after the treatment is ended.

Change of Life Style Some patients with disabilities resulting from an organic brain syndrome can function well with minimum changes in their customary life style; others must make major adjustments and accommodations. Considerable progress has been made in minimizing physical disabilities by means of prostheses, electrical stimulators and monitors, walking aids, electric wheelchairs, and various other devices. Loss of sensory faculty presents a more difficult problem, and generally an attempt is made to compensate for its loss by retraining one or several other sensory faculties, as, for example, hearing and touch for lost vision. Loss of motor function can be very frustrating, especially for a patient who previous to his disability was very active physically with interests such as sports, manual labor, muscular types of occupation, and other activities which involve expenditure of physical energy. Such persons generally have little interest in intellectual or sedentary types of activity or occupation. When their motor functions become incapacitated, they often become either extremely depressed or else angry and bitter. Therapists, however, must be very cautious in suggesting substitute types of activities for them. It is better to get to know the patient well and to watch and wait for clues from the patient, such as his first expression of interest in a particular activity before proposing one to him. Sometimes motor-oriented patients may discover latent intellectual, artistic, musical, or other creative abilities of which they were previously unaware or which they had no time to develop. If they pursue one or more of these new interests, they may derive great satisfaction from them. Patients whose life interests have always been in cerebral-oriented activities find it easier to adjust to their disabilities psychologically because their self-image is not so threatened as the person who is motor-oriented (Feldman, 1972). However, they often need help and encouragement in making necessary modification in technique, such as the substitution of one body-part for another, or adjustments in work habits. The lives of many artists with disabilities demonstrate the success with which they have been able to continue their lifelong interests. The well-known American musician Ferde Grofe at the age of seventy suffered a stroke that paralyzed his entire right side, including his right hand. By means of rehabilitation therapy he was able to walk again and in 6 months he was back at his piano, composing with his left hand.

Educational and Vocational Rehabilitation   Stimulation of many varieties is important in organic brain syndromes to prevent atrophy of the unaffected areas of the brain. It is also important psychologically to prevent apathy, boredom, and depression. One of the best methods of stimulating the mind and one that is not utilized as much as it could be is through educational rehabilitation. Various kinds of educational activities are helpful not only to improve the patient's morale by demonstrating to him that he is still capable of learning, but also to make it easier to facilitate the acceptance of new ideas and change. Educational activities can also make life more interesting to him. Vocational rehabilitation has many of the same effects as educational rehabilitation, and in addition it may help him to learn new skills, which, in turn, help him to feel useful and wanted. The fact that he may or may not receive monetary rewards for his efforts is not as important as the fact that he can regard himself again as a functioning member of society. Feldman says that the goal of rehabilitation may not be for economic gain but for self-worth (Feldman, 1972).

Rehabilitation treatment should be started as soon as the diagnostic evaluation has been made. Far too often rehabilitation measures are postponed until the acute phase of the illness has subsided or a plateau in medical treatment has been reached. Weeks or even months of valuable treatment time can be wasted. The earlier rehabilitation is started and the more consistently a treatment plan is carried out, the better the chances are for success. Delayed treatment permits the patient to become discouraged and depressed and also fosters some of the fixed antitreatment attitudes mentioned earlier in the chapter. The longer the delay in initiating treatment, the more difficult it is to motivate the patient to a new attitude toward rehabilitation. When the rehabilitation team is formulating the treatment plan, it is important to have the patient himself included in the planning. Participation in planning can promote cooperativeness with treatment by means of helping him to understand the rationale for the various procedures. The patient can also be taught to do those treatment procedures which are feasible for him to do by himself. If he is on a hospital ward, the nursing personnel should have sufficient knowledge of rehabilitation techniques so that they can provide necessary assistance to the patient when the rehabilitation staff is not available. The family should be involved and kept informed of the patient's progress. Before he is discharged, the family should be included in the postdischarge plans; in some instances, they may need to be taught how to carry out some parts of the rehabilitation program at home.

Nursing Care

The nursing care of patients with chronic organic syndromes can be divided into three different, but often overlapping, phases of care. Phase I is the period of diagnosis, planning for immediate, short-term treatment, and the administration of both life-supporting and disability-related nursing treatment and care. Phase II is the period of the assessment of the patient's disability and the institution of an intensive rehabilitation program to maximize his physical, psychological, and social capabilities. Phase III is the period of the patient's return to his family to face the reality of living with the residual disabilities of his illness or the reality of dying from it, as the case may be.

Phase I Included in the first phase are those chronic patients who are often very ill, whose nursing needs are both physical and psychological in nature, and who have recently learned that they are suffering from an illness from which they may not recover. These patients are generally treated in a hospital, often on the neurological or neurosurgical units. The treatment process begins with the admission of the patient to his unit. Frightened, worried, and often in pain, sometimes confused and disoriented, the patient is very sensitive to his hospital environment. Fortunately, the trend in the modern hospital is for a cheerful and homelike environment, in contrast to the colorless, impersonal hospital wards of the past. More important, however, is the warmth, kindness, and concern of the hospital staff that even the sickest patient can sense in the nurses and other personnel caring for him. "The initial atmosphere in which the patient finds himself, will have much bearing on his entire rehabilitation program. . . . The great responsibility of helping to create the introductory atmosphere is that of the nurse in the general hospital" (Martin, 1970, p. 818).

Martin stresses the fact that it is imperative for the patient to have confidence in the nurse's competence. "Unless the nurse is capable of meeting the patient's physical needs, and meeting them well, her efforts in other areas of concern (emotional, social) will be of little value" (Martin, 1970, p. 818). Knowledge and skill of a high degree in medical and surgical nursing are a prerequisite to nursing the very ill patient with a chronic organic brain syndrome. Other requirements include some experience in neurological nursing, a good working knowledge of psychological nursing, and a basic knowledge of and skill in physical therapy techniques. Perseverance, hopefulness, and the ability to work well with members of other disciplines are also very necessary. Dolores Craig, a nurse in the neurology department of a veteran's hospital, cooperating with other members of the ward staff, family, and friends, cared for a young Vietnam veteran with a traumatic head injury who lay in coma for 9 months before he responded to efforts to awaken him. He was turned in his rotating bed every 2 hours for 9 months. His lungs remained clear and he was free of bedsores. However, during all this time he made no response to the endless parade of treatments, medicines, and personal attention given to him; nevertheless, nurses and others stopped to talk to him. Craig (1972) writes, "We neurology nurses are convinced that someone in this type of deep sleep needs stimulation: talk, sound, touch. We do not know the medical reasons for our conviction, but comatose patients seem to respond best when there is constant activity around them." She gives many examples of various forms of stimulation, such as people dropping in for brief chats, radio, music, bright posters and flowers in his room, postcards, and tape recordings. Finally, after 9 months a faint smile appeared; at 10 months, his first movement—he tapped his foot against the footboard; at 11 months he spoke his first word, and by 12 months he had fully responded.

In caring for very ill patients, Read reminds nurses that these patients have very little courage or energy, and, therefore, greater sensitivity is required of nursing personnel to meet their increased psychological needs, including their needs for feedback to maintain their contact with reality. To these patients common sensory experiences can become terrifying. A tired patient generally withdraws from the environment, sleeps, accepts everything listlessly, and finds communication difficult and exhausting. Many very ill patients are annoyed by small talk and the pleasantries of nursing personnel. Read says that the best approach is often through touch. She believes that physical care given with dignity and gentleness can convey feeling to the patient and is a means of communication of an elemental and very fundamental nature. The patient can show his acceptance of this feeling by responding, not with words, but by a gesture, such as moving some part of his body to cooperate with the nurse caring for him (Read, 1970, pp. 733–734).

Psychological Problems   The very ill patient is often very anxious and afraid that he will not recover. Since his sensory faculties are generally impaired, he has no way of getting feedback by himself and must seek the help of others to give him this information in order to make the necessary adjustments to his current situation (Read, 1970). With Craig and others writers, Read also stresses the importance of stimulation to motivate the patient to regain some of his lost faculties. She writes that recovery of motion and speech will be very difficult if nurses handle the patient as little as possible and give meager care in silence. Without stimulation and continual awareness, perception is disrupted; attention gives way to distractability, interest to boredom, and behavior becomes stereotyped (Read, 1970, pp. 733).

Coping with the Patient's Reaction to His Illness   Sometime during Phase I, and usually after many tests and examinations, the patient learns the nature of his illness and the diagnosis. Generally his physician gives him this information. Depending on the diagnosis, what connotations this has for the patient, his preparation beforehand, and the manner in which he is given this information, at the moment of learning his diagnosis this knowledge elicits an emotional reaction of some kind. Typical reactions include surprise, anger, denial, depression, and deep shock; but whatever the reaction, the patient needs support in coping with his feelings. It is part of the nurse's role to give this support and to help the patient begin the long process of learning to adapt to his illness. Crate (1965), following the model developed by Engel (1964), conceptualizes this process as a grieving one and stresses the fact that it is the nurse's function to listen and try to understand the patient's feelings, and to help him to express his feelings. Denial is usually a patient's first reaction on hearing his diagnosis. Even when he seems to accept it, he may avoid recognizing his feelings by intellectualizing his situation or concentrating on factual details of his treatment. Crate comments (1965, p. 74),

> The nurse's function during this phase is to allow him to deny his illness as he needs to. . . . In this respect, the nurse functions as a noncritical listener, she accepts the patient's statement of how he feels, helps him to clarify how he says he feels, but does not point out the reality to him. She accepts his expressions of denial but does not join him in behavior to avoid treatment.

The succeeding phases in the process of emotional adjustment of the patient to his illness include: his developing awareness of what happened to him and acceptance of his illness; the reorganization of his relationships with others; the resolution of his sense of loss and the consequences of his illness; the development of an altered identity;

and adaptation to a changed life style. The role of the nurse in this process is to observe and understand the patient as he experiences the various phases of adaptation. Crate writes (1965, p. 76),

> The process of adaptation has been shown as a fluctuating but generally ordered change during which nursing is being focused on thorough understanding of how the patient is experiencing the change. The nursing is therapeutic to the extent that the nurse is able to allow the patient to experience the illness rather than to repress the experience. In this respect she also becomes a teacher. The patient has learned about being sick. . . . [The nurse's] role as a therapist over an extended period is not to force, push, or try to change the patient but to develop a relationship in which he can use her as a guide as he makes the necessary changes within himself through the normal process of adaptation.

Phase II The emphasis in Phase II is on an assessment of the disabilities which result as a consequence of the patient's illness and a therapeutic program to minimize these disabilities. This phase is one of intensive rehabilitative treatment, generally planned and carried out by a rehabilitation team. The nurse may function as an integral member of the rehabilitative team working in a special rehabilitation hospital, center, or hospital unit; or she may play a complementary role to the rehabilitation team by providing for the patient's general nursing needs on a general hospital ward.

The Role of the Nurse in a Rehabilitation Setting The nurse in a rehabilitation center functions as part of the rehabilitation team. According to Martin, King, and Suchinski (1970), the nurse, along with other members of the team, estimates the patient's capabilities and establishes treatment goals, which are then discussed in team conferences. At these conferences joint decisions are reached on treatment goals and priorities for treatment are also determined. The nurse also initiates contacts with other therapists who are involved in the treatment of a particular patient and serves as the liaison person with whom members of other disciplines communicate regarding the patient. As a member of the team the nurse evaluates patients' progress and presents these evaluations with recommendations for treatment goals at interdisciplinary conferences. He also makes observations regarding the patients' abilities to socialize and to adapt to their disabilities.

The nurse also has specific nursing responsibilities. These include nursing care and teaching in the areas of nutrition, fluid intake, skin care, personal hygiene, problems of elimination, rest and sleep difficulties, pain control, and problems in interpersonal relationships and ability to socialize. The nurse is also responsible for helping the patient to clarify his ideas about the information and instruction he has received from other members of the rehabilitation team and to assist him in carrying out his treatment instructions correctly. The nurse also gives the patient encouragement and emotional support in cooperating with his total treatment plan (Martin, King, and Suchinski, 1970). Plaisted also stresses the importance of involving the patient in treatment. She states, "Motivation for rehabilitation is within the patient himself and he must be actively involved in his own care program if his rehabilitation potential is to be reached" (Plaisted, 1969, p. 563).

One of the tasks of the patient in this phase of his treatment is to deal realistically with his disability and to maximize his residual functions and capacities. This requires a change in life style as well as a change in self-concept, and often produces great psychological stress. Norris states, "Many illnesses require reintegration of one's body image or somatic ego. Scarring, deformity, impaired functioning, or loss of a body part must be dealt with, and, if possible, made a part of the self." Many patients struggle with the problem of reintegration by themselves. Others turn to those caring for them for help. Sometimes they are successful in getting help and sometimes not. Norris (1969, p. 2119) writes,

> If, however, the persons around the patient—including nurses—can recognize and allow the expressions of real concerns, the patient will get down to work. A nurse who accepts a patient's humanness will make it easier for him to reveal his concerns and examine his life experiences. But when a patient does open up the nurse's own anxiety can be provoked.

Such anxiety may immobilize the nurse, who then avoids the patient as much as possible. Perrine (1971, p. 2130), writing of his experiences in a rehabilitation hospital, says,

> What could the professional staff who were constantly around me for those eight months have done? What would have helped me through this period more quickly and easily? I think a unified approach of honesty and emotional support would have worked wonders. If I had been confronted again and again with the truth delivered in love, if I had felt supported enough to ventilate my anger and release my tears, if I had been enabled to see the commonality of my hurt with the hurts of the patients around me, I believe that I would have moved through the period of protest months sooner.

Perrine indicates two specific ways in which a professional could have helped him, namely, as "a compassionate waiter," and as "a pattern-activator." Regarding the role of compassionate waiter, he writes, "Having done all he can do the professional person frequently must offer a loving relationship and then wait and wait until the patient is ready to receive his help." He stresses the point that the patient in need is never given up, even if a second professional has to take over from the first one. It may take a long time for the patient to develop sufficient trust to want to change. In the role of a pattern-activator, the professional "can directly aid the detached person to repattern his relationships and activities." He also believes that the patient is often ready to engage in various therapeutic activities earlier than most health professionals consider him ready. For example, group therapy, activity groups, and sensitivity groups early in the treatment plan would have been very helpful to patients in their developing trust and experiencing support from peers as well as staff. "The reevaluation of my physical patterns helped me to repattern many of them and to understand my need for exercise and for more usable activities of daily living. The detached person is looking for new patterns of life; he just doesn't know how to go about establishing them" (Perrine, 1971, p. 2132).

One special nursing problem in caring for the patient with chronic organic brain syndrome in this phase of treatment is communication with aphasic patients. These patients not only are unable to convey their needs or express their feelings, but also are often not able to understand or remember what has been said to them. This disability cuts them off from others and makes them feel isolated. They react to this isolation by withdrawal. Those caring for such patients must try to counteract this tendency to withdraw by helping them to keep in touch with others. Fox, in her very helpful paper, "Talking with Patients Who Can't Answer," gives some practical and very specific ways of providing such help. Some of the general principles that she stresses include: providing opportunities for the patient to communicate; allowing the patient sufficient time to retrieve words and formulate ideas; not talking *for* patients; not hurrying the patient when talking to him; being relaxed and leisurely and making it easier for him to find words; including him in conversation but not overwhelming him (Fox, 1971).

Phase III After the patient has completed his course of intensive rehabilitation therapy and has achieved his maximum benefits from such a program, he is discharged to the community—to either his own home, a boarding home, a nursing home, or some other extended care facility. A physician generally assumes the major responsibility for making the decision to which agency in the community the patient shall be discharged. In order to make such a decision, the physician must evaluate the patient's life outside the hospital, both before hospitalization and as it potentially might be after discharge. He needs to know the patient's relationships with various members of his family, what kinds of patients with what kinds of disabilities an agency will or will not accept, and the financial resources available to support the patient. For this information he relies heavily on the social worker. Frequently the social worker also helps to process the discharge, arranges for casework follow-up, and makes any other necessary referrals (Roth and Eddy, 1967).

Role of the Nurse in Home Care

Teaching the patient and the patient's family various nursing procedures essential to the patient's care at home constitutes an important facet of the nurse's role. Patient and family may also need some assistance in planning a daily schedule for home treatment. They occasionally may wish to talk to some member of the treatment team when questions or problems about treatment or management arise at home. Often they feel most comfortable about telephoning the nurse about such matters. A visiting nurse or community health nurse may also prove very helpful in the difficult task of reintegration into community life by preparing the patient to function outside of the protective home environment. They can be aware of the patient's reactions to returning home, observe his progress, giving him support and encouragement if the rehabilitation process is a slow and difficult one, and motivating him to work up to his potential. The patient and his family can also be helped to learn to cope with the consequences of his disability in community living (Martin, 1970, p. 819).

Although the patient in Phase I, the period of diagnosis and medical treatment, and Phase II, the period of intensive rehabilitation, was confronted with psychological and social problems, these problems were generally related to his physical disabilities either directly or indirectly. However, in Phase III, the postmedical and postrehabilitative period, the importance of the physical disabilities recedes as the patient has learned to cope with them and come to terms with them. In other words, he has learned "to live comfortably or resignedly with his illness" (Crate, 1965). In his home and community environment, the patient becomes more concerned with the psychological and social problems that face him in his daily living, as, for example, the disruptions in family relationships, friendship patterns, work, and recreational opportunities. It is not only the patient, who is faced with psychosocial problems, but also the members of his family who must make adjustments when the patient reenters the family circle.

Disturbances in Family Relationships If the patient is the father of a growing family, he may have to give up some of his prerogatives as head of the family, such as seeing his wife take over the role of breadwinner while he may have to assume some of the childrearing and household duties. This role reversal may be very difficult for him to accept. On the other hand, if the mother is the patient, especially the mother of young children, very serious disturbances may arise in the mother-child relationship. Davis found in her study of patients with multiple sclerosis (Davis, 1970, p. 72) that

> Problems in the rearing and care of children arose when there was a misalignment between the mother's diminishing capacity to perform in her role as mother and the demands which arose from the child's continual physical growth and psychological maturation. Even though she herself was a patient, responsibility for the physical care of the child continued to devolve onto the mother.

With school-age children, the problems related to the children's unfulfilled expectations of the mother. For example, they became resentful when asked to do household tasks which the mother was physically unable to do (Davis, 1970, pp. 75–76).

The person with a chronic illness who lives at home also has social and environmental problems. These include the necessity to make modifications in the home itself to accommodate the patient's disabilities, such as via special equipment, railings, handles, and sometimes architectural changes. Outside the home, problems related to transportation include high curbs and stairs, if walking, narrow doors and lack of ramps, if by wheelchair, availability of taxicabs or lack of their availability, difficulties of getting on and off buses and streetcars, locating restrooms, and the necessity of trying to anticipate difficulties and plan routes before leaving home (Davis, 1970).

Perhaps the greatest psychological and social problem which the chronically ill patient in the home has to face is social isolation, that is, the gradually diminishing contact with friends and the consequent contraction of his social world. As time goes by without amelioration of the patient's condition, friends begin to lose interest or move away or die. Opportunities are few for the chronically ill person to make new friendships to replace the lost ones. This limitation of social contacts outside the home makes the person increasingly dependent on the members of his family to meet his social needs for human companionship. It also lowers still further his concept of himself and his feelings of self-worth. Financial problems also become more serious with time. Davis (1970) writes, "It is not uncommon for persons with progressively worsening chronic illness who once had steady incomes and savings to slowly go bankrupt. These patients' incomes have stopped at some point because of the illness and their life savings are slowly drained away. Such patients are forced to seek welfare and medical care at the least possible expense to them."

The Nurse as Therapist For the patient who is unable to make a satisfactory adjustment to care at home, who has difficulty in accepting a revised self-concept, and who manifests some psychological symptoms such as anxiety or depression, individual nursing psychotherapy on a regular weekly or biweekly basis may be indicated. Such interviews may not only be helpful in overcoming some of the patient's psychosocial difficulties but can also be very supportive to him in that the psychotherapeutic relationship provides him with a concerned and trusted person with whom he feels free to discuss whatever is troubling him. Such a supportive relationship with his nurse therapist can also be instrumental not only in getting him interested in rehabilitative efforts but also in exploring plans for the future and restoring his feelings of self-worth.

For the patient whose primary problems are his interpersonal relationships with family and friends rather than strictly intrapersonal problems, family therapy which includes the patient and all significant family members may be very helpful. Davis notes that the professional nurse as a family therapist is eminently suited for the task of caring for the psychosocial needs of the chronically ill (Davis, 1970). Family therapy provides an excellent setting in which many of the problems which occur in any family with a chronically ill member can be discussed, as well as providing an opportunity for the expression of repressed feelings of various members of the family, such as fear of increasing dependency needs of the patient, fear of dwindling financial resources, and resentment of limitations put upon the family by the patient's special requirements. These family therapy sessions should be held ideally in the home with the nurse as leader. In some instances a coleader may be used to good advantage.

For instance, when individual or family therapy is not indicated or is economically not feasible, a nurse psychotherapist may provide group therapy. This form of psychotherapy could be useful in convalescent or nursing homes for the chronically ill, where patients could gather together to discuss their problems of daily living as well as their interpersonal problems with family, other patients, and staff. Group therapy can be adapted to various levels of depth and intensity, a wide range of problems, and a variety of techniques, depending on the particular needs of the group members. It has proved very helpful in a number of nursing homes where it has imparted an increased interest in living to patients and raised the morale not only of the patients but also of the staff. Group therapy has been used successfully with groups of families and/or mixed family and patient groups, especially for families that have members with a chronic illness about which little is known or that makes great demands on family members, such as severe renal disorders (Adler, 1972), brain-injured children (Hladky, 1969), or spinal bifida (Roberts and Hardgrove, 1972).

The Nurse as Mental Health Consultant   The mental health consultant is often employed by a public health agency to consult with the public health nurse who visits the chronically ill patient in his home setting. But, as Davis (1970, p. 162) discovered in her research on patients with multiple sclerosis, "It is of interest to note that these patients do not generally come to the attention of the public health nurse. . . . Once the physical aspects of the patient's care are under control, he is more or less discharged to himself. However, if there were a pressing physical care requirement, the visiting nurse would be most likely to offer this service." If this is the case with multiple sclerosis patients, how many other chronically ill patients with nonmedical problems are there in the community for whom no resource for help is available? The mental health consultant may also assist the public health nurses in an agency to gain greater knowledge and understanding of human behavior and interpersonal relationships, and to sensitize them to psychological aspects of the patients' problems (Davis, 1970). This function of the mental health consultant is particularly important in the care of the chronically ill. And to quote Davis (1970, p. 157) again, "The epitome of successful care directed to the chronically ill is that approach which considers the patient's social network as relevant to the well-being of the patient in his day-to-day living as that of a proper diet."

The Public Health Nurse as Coordinator

The public health nurse traditionally has been the nurse with the greatest knowledge of community agencies. The referral of patients to the various agencies has been one of his functions. At present, however, the public health nurse does not consider the delivery of direct patient care to the chronically ill as an area of his special concern. Davis (1970, p. 167) states, "Unless there is some change in the delivery of the services of the public health nurse to officially include this population, serious thought must be paid to developing a cadre of health persons whose main focus and work is with this population." She continues, "Based on the findings in this study, once the patient's physical care needs are brought under management, all other aspects of care are subject to a falling by the wayside when no one is directly responsible for them" (Davis, 1970, p. 168). Perhaps this situation represents one of the many lacunae in our present health care system, and the chronically ill must wait until a comprehensive national health system is developed. At such time, the responsibility for this neglected group could be assigned to specific health professions or health agencies. Davis foresees the public health nurse functioning in an expanded role as the logical person to assume this responsibility by virtue of his contacts with hospitals, clinics, homes, and communities.

The Clinical Nurse Specialist and Chronic Illness

General nursing education prepares the nurse to care for patients with illnesses most commonly encountered in general practice. But if one is so unfortunate as to contract an illness which is uncommon, where does one go for help? Among the chronic organic disorders there are many rare conditions—and some not so rare—about which little can be found in the literature that is useful in the daily nursing care of the patient. Davis in her study of patients with multiple sclerosis, one of the major disorders affecting the central nervous system, discovered that there was a dearth of information available about this disorder not only among the lay public and families of patients but also among nurses. She writes (Davis, 1970, p. 165),

> It is imperative that nurses know not only of the possibility of the patient's condition becoming progressively worse, particularly if it is a young individual, but also, as was pointed out in an earlier section, the vacillating and ambiguous nature of the symptoms should be understood by a nurse caring for a patient with multiple sclerosis to avoid her misinterpreting the patient's behavior.

The same lack of specific nursing knowledge is the case with many other chronic illnesses. As medical diagnosis becomes more precise, medical knowledge more prolific, and medical treatment more intensive, it is impossible to make any one health practitioner responsible for in-depth knowledge and skill adequate to care for patients with the variety of illnesses that man is heir to. Just as numbers of the medical profession have had to become specialists in a particular area of the field of medicine, so it will be necessary for some nurses to study in depth particular disorders and to develop effective nursing interventions. Such nurse specialists may utilize their special knowledge and skill as consultants to other nurses engaged in direct patient care. In addition to acting as consultants, the clinical nurse specialist would continue to give direct nursing care to patients needing expert care and to test out relevant nursing interventions by research. In no area of nursing is research more needed than in the care of the chronically ill with organic brain syndromes.

REFERENCES

Adler, Penny K. (1972): *The Role of the Psychiatric Nurse with Patients Suffering from End Stage Renal Failure.* Report of Asilomar Workshop, April 9–12, California Nurses' Association, San Francisco, Calif.

Brosin, Henry W. (1967): "Brain Syndromes Associated with Trauma," in Alfred M. Freedman and Harold I. Kaplan (eds.), *Comprehensive Textbook of Psychiatry,* The Williams & Wilkins Company, Baltimore, pp. 748–759.

———(1959): "Psychiatric Conditions Following Head Injury," in Silvano Arieti (ed.), *American Handbook of Psychiatry,* vol. 2, Basic Books, Inc., Publishers, New York. pp. 1175–1202.

Busse, Ewald W. (1967): "Brain Syndromes Associated with Disturbances in Metabolism, Growth, and Nutrition," in Alfred M. Freedman and Harold I. Kaplan (eds.), *Comprehensive Textbook of Psychiatry,* The Williams & Wilkins Company, Baltimore, pp. 726–739.

Craig, Dolores B. (1972): "Bringing Billy Back," *California Living Magazine,* San Francisco Sunday Examiner and Chronicle, Jan. 23, p. 17.

Crate, Marjorie A. (1965): "Nursing Functions in Adaptation to Chronic Illness," *American Journal of Nursing,* October, pp. 72–76.

Davis, Marcella Z. (1973): *Living with Multiple Sclerosis—A Social Psychological Analysis,* Charles C Thomas, Publisher, Springfield, Ill.

Ebaugh, Franklin G., and William J. Tiffany, Jr. (1959): "Infective-Exhaustive Psychoses," in Silvano Arieti (ed.), *American Handbook of Psychiatry,* vol. 2, Basic Books, Inc., Publishers, New York, pp. 1244–1245.

Engel, George L. (1964): "Grief and Grieving," *American Journal of Nursing,* September, pp. 93–98.

———(1967): "Introduction to Brain Disorders," in Alfred M. Freedman and Harold I. Kaplan (eds.), *Comprehensive Textbook of Psychiatry,* The Williams & Wilkins Company, Baltimore, pp. 706–707.

Fangman, Anne, and William E. O'Malley (1969): "L-dopa and the Patient with Parkinson's Disease," *American Journal of Nursing,* July, pp. 1455–1457.

Feldman, Daniel J. (1972): Professor, Department of Psychiatry and Human Behavior, University of California, Irvine. Personal communication.

Ferraro, Armando (1959a): "Psychoses with Arteriosclerosis," in Silvano Arieti (ed.), *American Handbook of Psychiatry,* vol. 2, Basic Books, Inc., Publishers, New York, pp. 1078–1108.

———(1959b): "Senile Psychoses," in Silvano Arieti (ed.), *American Handbook of Psychiatry,* vol. 2, Basic Books, Inc., Publishers, New York, pp. 1021–1045.

Fox, Madeline J. (1971): "Talking with Patients Who Can't Answer," *American Journal of Nursing,* June, pp. 1146–1149.

Goldstein, Kurt (1959): "The Organismic Approach," in Silvano Arieti (ed.), *American Handbook of Psychiatry,* vol. 2, Basic Books, Inc., Publishers, New York, pp. 1303–1347.

Hladky, Maryjane (1969): "Volunteer Work with a Brain-Injured Child," *American Journal of Nursing,* pp. 2130–2132.

Martin, Nancy (1970): "Nursing in Rehabilitation," in Irene L. Beland (ed.), *Clinical Nursing: Pathophysiological and Psychosocial Approaches,* 2d ed., The Macmillan Company, New York, pp. 814–839.

———, Rosemarie King, and Joyce Suchinski (1970): "The Nurse Therapist in a Rehabilitation Setting," *American Journal of Nursing,* August, pp. 1964–1967.

Norris, Catherine M. (1969): "The Work of Getting Well," *American Journal of Nursing,* October, pp. 2118–2121.

Noyes, Arthur P., and Lawrence C. Kolb (1968): *Modern Clinical Psychiatry,* 7th ed., W. B. Saunders Company, Philadelphia.

Perrine, George (1971): "Needs Met and Unmet," *American Journal of Nursing,* November, pp. 2128–2133.

Plaisted, Lena M. (1969): "The Clinical Specialist in Rehabilitation Nursing," *American Journal of Nursing,* March, pp. 562–564.

Read, Esther H. (1970): "Neural Regulation," in Irene L. Beland (ed.), *Clinical Nursing: Pathophysiological and Psychosocial Approaches,* 2d ed., The Macmillan Company, New York, pp. 703–735.

Roberts, Brenda, and Carol Hardgrove (1972): Personal communication.

Roth, Julius A., and Elizabeth M. Eddy (1967): *Rehabilitation of the Unwanted,* Atherton Press, Inc., New York.

Shaw, Michael (1970): "Hangman's Break," *American Journal of Nursing,* December, pp. 2565–2566.

12

PSYCHOSES

Marion E. Kalkman

Patients suffering from psychiatric disorders known as *psychoses* are perhaps more in need of expert nursing care than any other group of psychiatric patients. Yet until recently there was little progress in the theory and treatment of psychiatric disorders on which nurses could develop their nursing care. During the long period when descriptive psychiatry was predominant, nursing care was essentially custodial. At the turn of the century, Freud formulated the theory and principles of dynamic psychiatry and developed psychoanalysis as a method of treatment for neurotic patients. However, he was pessimistic about the value of this method in treating psychotic patients. His pessimism was based on his belief that psychotic patients were incapable of developing the strong bond of attachment with the therapist which he considered essential for psychoanalytic treatment. Although a few of Freud's followers—including Abraham, Federn, Jung, and Simmel—treated a number of psychotic patients psychoanalytically, for many years the majority of psychoanalysts preferred to use this method to treat other types of psychiatric disorders.

Somatic methods of therapy became predominant in the treatment of psychoses in the late 1930s and early 1940s. At first, these methods—which included insulin shock, metrazol, electric shock, and psychosurgery—were thought to be curative; later, it was recognized that their effect was primarily ameliorative. Electric shock is still (occasionally) used, generally in conjunction with other forms of therapy. Since the 1950s, pharmacotherapy has become the most widely used method of somatic treatment.

PIONEERS IN USE OF PSYCHOTHERAPY
IN THE PSYCHOSES

In 1931, Harry Stack Sullivan published a report of his work with a group of young schizophrenic male patients at Sheppard and Enoch Pratt Hospital in which he challenged Freud's statement regarding the inability of psychotic patients to relate to their therapists. Subsequently, a small group of psychiatrists working independently in different parts of this country and in Europe, and with different psychiatric concepts, became deeply interested in new methods of psychological treatment of psychotic patients. This small and courageous group included, in addition to Sullivan, Frieda Fromm-Reichmann, Robert Knight, John Rosen, and Marguerite Sechehaye. In recent years, the group of psychiatrists and others concerned with the treatment of psychoses has grown to include such names as Silvano Arieti, Don Jackson, Jurgen Ruesch, Gregory Bateson, Bertram Lewin, Lewis Hill, and C. A. Whitaker.

The work of these investigators in the dynamics and treatment of the psychoses has great relevance for psychiatric nurses who are entrusted with the care of psychotic patients. Many of the findings of these investigators can be very helpful to the nurse in understanding her patients better and in giving them more effective, intelligent nursing care. Moreover, some of the methods of treatment which these men developed could be adapted and incorporated into psychiatric nursing practice. To some extent the influence of these psychiatric investigators on nursing practice can be seen in the utilization of Sullivan's concepts by Peplau and others, the adaptation of Fromm-Reichmann's principles by Kalkman and Shockley, and the use of Ruesch's communication theory in teaching basic psychiatric nursing as described in Davis's paper (Davis, 1963).

IMPORTANCE OF A SPECIAL MILIEU

New studies on the treatment of psychoses also suggest the need for major changes in the environment in which therapy takes place. Psychotic patients are able to tolerate only a limited number of people around them and are far more sensitive to the pathology of other patients than are psychologically healthy individuals. It is also difficult for psychotic patients to adjust to new and strange nursing personnel. For these reasons, treatment units for psychotic patients should be kept small. Sullivan (1962) writes: "The procedure of treatment begins with removing the patient from the situation in which he is developing difficulty, to a situation in which he is encouraged to renew efforts at adjustment with others. This might well be elsewhere than to an institution dealing with a cross-section of the psychotic population; certainly it should not be to a large ward of mental patients of all sorts and ages."

Sullivan's own ward at Sheppard-Pratt was a six-bed unit consisting of three beds in two rooms connected by its own intercommunicating sitting-room and corridor. His patients were of the same sex, the same age group, and with the same diagnosis. Nursing personnel were carefully selected and trained. Rosen individualizes the treatment environment even further. He assigns one patient to a treatment unit which is a separate house with its own staff of three people. Jackson prefers to treat the patient in the patient's own home. Sechehaye at one time treated her patient, Renee, in her own home, although this arrangement proved too disruptive of the therapist's personal life to be tolerated for any length of time. Patients with manic-depressive psychoses also respond better to treatment in small nursing units. Manic patients need to be protected from overstimulation, and depressed patients tend to become confused in large, populous wards. Both manic and depressed patients require small, simply furnished surroundings with adequate nursing personnel. Other studies seem to corroborate the findings that during the acute phase of the psychosis, a small, specially planned treatment unit is of great importance (Ayd, 1961; Linn, 1962; Rosen, 1953). Sullivan (1962, p. 285) comments, "Admittedly, this is no small order, and the creation of this sort of situation is scarcely to be expected either from chance or from the efforts of a commonplace administrative agent."

IMPORTANCE OF FIRST DAYS OF HOSPITALIZATION

Sullivan also stressed the critical importance of the first 24 hours after admission of the patient to the outcome of his treatment. This statement is supported by the study of Caudill, Redlich, Gilmore, and Brody (1952), who found that patients were most amenable to treatment in the first few days of hospitalization. Ruesch, Brodsky, and Fischer (1963) have also utilized this concept in their intensive, short-term treatment of acute psychotic patients by emphasizing the need to begin intensive treatment as soon as the patient is admitted. Sullivan required his nursing personnel to devote a great deal of time to newly admitted patients. During the period immediately after admission, the nursing personnel had an opportunity to learn to know the patient, to make frequent and detailed observations, and to begin a relationship with him. This concentrated attention also gave the patient emotional support and helped to reduce his anxiety.

AVAILABILITY OF THE NURSE

Other inferences which may be drawn from these studies on the nursing care of the psychotic patient pinpoint the importance of the nurse's physical presence, her personality, and the continuity of her nursing care. The patient who is suffering from intense anxiety or loneliness, as are most psychotic patients, needs to have a nurse available in his moments of great stress. This means having a nurse who is free from other duties so that he can actually spend time with the patient when needed. An anxious patient should not be expected to postpone his requests for the nurse until such time as the nurse can get away from other duties. The mere physical presence of the nurse who remains with a patient during his periods of stress does much to relieve his feelings of fear, anxiety, loneliness, and unreality.

PERSONAL CHARACTERISTICS OF THE NURSE CARING FOR PSYCHOTIC PATIENTS

The patient's stress can be further reduced if the nurse has certain personal qualities which communicate a sense of trust and emotional support. Exactly what these personal characteristics are which prove most beneficial to psychotic patients has not been determined, but it is known that patients suffering from manic-depressive psychoses often fare better with a nurse whose personality is different from that of the nurse who is successful in caring for schizophrenic patients. Regardless of his personality type, the nurse who undertakes the care of a psychotic patient should be prepared to work with him for a far longer period of time than he would with other classifications of patients. Nursing care of the psychotic patient also demands of the nurse a great deal of patience and tolerance, the willingness to give of himself, and the ability to accept the patient's dependence on him. Sechehaye writes: "The whole problem with psychotics then, is one of finding a relationship which is often anaclitic (characterized by dependence on others) and in which the patient feels himself to be understood at the level of his regression. Only then can he receive, in a form which is specific to him, the gratification of his essential needs (Sechehaye, 1961, p. 7). Once a psychotic patient has found such a nurse, it is of the

utmost importance that he continue to work with him. Administrative-
ly, every effort should be made to facilitate this relationship, and to
give the nurse encouragement and support. A succession of different
nurses tends to increase the patient's confusion, anxiety, and sense of
unreality and to retard progress in therapy.

NURSING THE PATIENT WITH A SCHIZOPHRENIC REACTION

Schizophrenic reactions and *schizophrenic psychoses* are the terms
used to describe a group of patients who are withdrawn, lonely,
apparently indifferent to their environment, and disturbed in their
thought processes. Their behavior is often negativistic, bizarre, and
regressed. Other symptoms from which schizophrenic patients frequently suffer include faulty ideas of reference, loss of contact with
reality, hallucinations, and delusions. Schizophrenic patients may
express themselves in symbolic, condensed, and often cryptic language, which makes communication with them difficult, or, not
infrequently, they are mute.

Incidence of Schizophrenia

Patients with schizophrenic reactions, because of their strange and
often inappropriate behavior, more readily find their way into mental
hospitals than do patients with other types of psychiatric disorders.
Ewalt and Farnsworth (1963) state that about half of the mental patients
in the United States, or roughly about 350,000 patients, are diagnosed
as suffering from schizophrenia. The schizophrenic patient presents
the nurse with some challenging nursing problems, foremost of which
is his withdrawn behavior, the primary characteristic of this disorder.

The Therapeutic Task in Treatment of Schizophrenia

Ruesch (1961) says that the therapeutic task with the withdrawn patient
is to free him from living in a dream world and to bring him back to the
enjoyment of his body, of sensuous pleasure, and of other people. In
order to free him from his dream world the nurse has to be able to
reach him, to make contact with him, to communicate with him. The
schizophrenic patient has experienced many painful rejections during
the course of life. In his illness he has rejected the world of reality and
has created his own world of fantasy. He has no inclination to resume

contact with the real world. The nurse must seek the patient in his own fantasy world. The schizophrenic patient loses not only the desire but also the ability to reenter the world of reality. To accomplish his return he needs the help of a knowledgeable and concerned person. The nurse's task is to gain the patient's attention, to find some way to communicate with him, and to develop a relationship with him. By means of this relationship with him, the nurse must help him to find ways of relating to other people and to the world of reality.

Communication Problems

Communicating with a schizophrenic patient is a difficult problem. Just as the schizophrenic patient lives in his own private dream world, so he has his own private language to express his thoughts. As Ruesch has pointed out, everyone has a private language or, rather, special interpretations of certain words; but most people do not deviate from standard usage to such a degree that other people cannot understand them. Moreover, the schizophrenic patient often expresses himself in nonverbal ways that are incomprehensible to others. The nurse should recognize that the patient's communicative behavior has meaning and that the patient is well aware of the meaning. However, the nurse cannot hope to learn the meaning of the patient's behavior until he trusts the nurse enough to tell him. When the patient feels he can trust the nurse, the first step toward establishing communication has been made.

Schizophrenic patients often use abstruse or indirect methods to talk about subjects that are too painful to discuss directly. They may use symbolic expressions somewhat as a child uses riddles, in order to see if the therapist is clever enough to divine the hidden meaning. They may also try to trap the therapist into pretending to understand something he actually does not understand. Fromm-Reichmann (1950) recommends that the therapist be frank with the patient by acknowledging what is not understood or by asking the patient to clarify his meaning. Many schizophrenic patients distrust words and prefer to express themselves nonverbally. Therefore, they often pay little attention to what the nurse says. However, nonverbal means of communication by the nurse can be very effective in reaching the patient. Ruesch (1961) considers that the treatment of schizophrenic patients in the early stages is essentially nonverbal and and that the therapist should be alert to cues such as tone of voice, speech rhythm, intensity of tone, gestures, body movements, and the context in which the communication occurs rather than attempt to decipher their symbolic meanings.

Nurses have opportunities to use ways of communication that are not appropriate or permitted to other therapists. The most important of these is touch. With the catatonic patient who refuses to speak, to gesture or act, or even to see, the only avenue of communication left may be that of touch. The nurse by placing his hand on the patient may be able to communicate security, concern, and support, very much as touch may be used to "gentle" a frightened wild creature. However, touch can also be interpreted by the patient as a hostile gesture. In his role as nurse he may touch the patient in many ways, such as rubbing his back, washing his body, shaving him, putting compresses on him, and arranging and adjusting clothing and equipment. These common-place activities may be used as channels of communication to convey a variety of psychological messages to the patient (Ruesch, 1961).

The nurse may also transmit a message by gesture or body motions, or he may use objects and, for example, hand the patient a writing pad and pencil when he is unable to talk. Nonverbal communication can be a very satisfying experience for a patient who has been isolated from any other contacts. The nurse's aim should be to gradually substitute speech for nonverbal methods as the patient is able to tolerate it. Various forms of art media may be offered to the patient to encourage self-expression and interpersonal communication. Burton sees the schizophrenic patient like the artist, lonely and alienated from society in a world of his own. He writes, "Artistic movements are protests and are designed for self-healing. As such, they cure the wounds of culture. Some such expressionist process is possible—yes, necessary—for the schizophrenic" (Burton, 1961, p. 185).

Encouraging Verbal Communication

However satisfying the various forms of nonverbal communication are to the patient, the nurse's goal should be to shift the patient from nonverbal to verbal communication. Schizophrenic patients are often adept at resisting the use of speech. This can also influence the nurse. When Rose (1962) was caring for a mute catatonic patient over a period of time, she suddenly became aware that she had succumbed to the subtle but persistent nonverbal responses of her patient by gradually responding to him nonverbally. Patients can exploit the nurse's sympathy by giving the impression that they are too ill to speak. When a nurse becomes alerted to such resistance he can assist the patient in verbalizing his thoughts by a variety of methods. One method which Fromm-Reichmann (1950) used very effectively was what she called "verbalizing for the patient." She observed the patient's nonverbal behavior, then spoke aloud what she thought the patient was experiencing. This necessitated affirmation or denial from the patient, frequently in words and often accompanied by much affect. Until the schizophrenic patient is able to use speech in a way that is comprehensible to others, he has no bridge of communication to relate to others. As long as the patient expresses himself nonverbally the nurse will not know precisely what his needs are, how to help him, or how to evaluate the results of nursing care.

Nurse-Patient Relationship with
Schizophrenic Patients

Continued efforts at communication between nurse and patient, if accompanied by some degree of success, generally lead to a more stable nurse-patient relationship. With schizophrenic patients the first phase of development is the establishment of mutual trust and respect strong enough to enable the patient to move out of his isolation and toward other people. This phase is often a long and stormy one, and the nurse must be satisfied with small signs of progress. In the acute stage of his illness, the schizophrenic patient needs a satisfying relationship with one person. He generally does not profit from group experiences because group interaction is still too complex for him to cope with. If placed in a group, he may seem to be participating, but he is simply using one of his well-practiced techniques of outward compliance and inward dissociation from everything that is going on around him. He is the typical introvert who is loneliest and most isolated when he is in the midst of a crowd. After he has experienced a meaningful relationship with one or more individuals, he may slowly be introduced to group situations.

Testing-out Behavior

The schizophrenic patient often puts his nurse through a difficult testing-out period before he will really accept her help. Burton describes this situation aptly. "He [the schizophrenic] must be certain that some human will make the commitment he once expected of his mother and he has an extensive testing repertory in which to ascertain this. The schizophrenic wants an intensity of relationship which matches his estrangement; i.e., love of the most unvarnished order. This is the framework within which all therapeutic effort must be set" (Burton, 1961, p. 185). In discussing the schizophrenics' testing-out behavior Sullivan states, "These patients have learned long before they appear for treatment that there is no one in the wide world who can be trusted to value and love one. They have developed a certain timelessness in these negative convictions and often wait quite patiently for the physician to prove that he is not trustworthy, either" (Sullivan, 1962, p. 313). The nurse must recognize this testing-out phase of the relationship, appreciate the reasons for it, and patiently and intelligently wait until the patient has satisfied himself about the nurse's trustworthiness. Some of the ways in which he can demonstrate his dependability include regularity in seeing the patient and faithfulness in keeping appointments with him no matter how difficult his behavior is to tolerate or how unresponsive he is. The nurse should be clear and unambivalent in his verbal and nonverbal messages to him and, most importantly, respect him as a person and show concern for his welfare. It is also helpful for the nurse to remember that schizophrenic patients are notoriously literal-minded. For this reason care should be taken about joking or using expressions which are intended to be taken figuratively.

The Nurse as Facilitator

After the nurse has successfully passed the testing-out phase, there are many ways in which he can be helpful to the patient. The schizophrenic patient, either through insight gained by working with his psychiatrist or through his own efforts, may want to move toward a more satisfying adjustment to living but finds himself frozen, unable to take the necessary steps to accomplish this alone. He needs the help and support of a person whom he trusts and who either figuratively or literally goes along with him. This person could very well be his nurse, who by taking a participant role in the patient's daily life and by professional training is well suited for this task. Insight alone is not sufficient to make any change in the patient's behavior. He must translate this new insight into action and repeat this new behavior until it becomes integrated into his personality. The following example taken from Rose's report of her nursing care of a catatonic patient illustrates the patient's use of the nurse to enable him to translate a wish into action (Rose, 1962, pp. 22–23):

> Mr. L. and I had been sitting together for a few minutes when he said, "I'm going home Thursday morning . . . on the bus, myself." He was wringing his hands and he had an anxious look on his face. . . . I asked, "Have you ever been to the bus station in San Francisco?" "No," he replied, "I never have." He seemed to be getting more anxious yet I felt that he needed to make plans for the trip. . . . I then said, "I could go with you tomorrow morning to the bus station in San Francisco since you have never been there." He smiled and said, "Would you? The station is probably very big. Will you go with me to the bus station?" I replied, "Yes." He sat relaxed for about five minutes, then started wringing his hands again. I decided we needed to do some

further planning of the trip. I said, "How about money for the ticket?" He blurted out, obviously with great difficulty, "I—don't have any." "Have you any way to get the money?" I asked. He sat for about three minutes and then very rapidly said, "Could I borrow a dollar from the ward fund? I could pay them back when I return." "I'm sure you can if you ask the ward nurse," I said. "Will a dollar be enough?" He replied, very sure of himself, "Yes, it's 60 cents for a one-way ticket and 15 cents streetcar fare. I don't need a return ticket. My brother-in-law will bring me back, so a dollar is enough." He was able to ask the ward nurse for the money and phone his mother to tell her he was coming home and the plans he had made. I went with him to the bus station the following morning but allowed him to decide which city bus to take to the station and to purchase his ticket.

The Schizophrenic Patient's Need for Permission to Participate

Another way in which the psychiatric nurse can free the schizophrenic patient from the frozen social state in which he so frequently finds himself is to give him permission to participate in an activity. For example, in his early childhood experiences a patient may have learned to refrain from engaging in many activities because his mother became angry with him or very anxious when he did so. Action came to represent danger to him and the loss of his mother's love. However, in the nurse-patient relationship, when the patient has learned to trust the nurse, he may utilize this confidence to expand his range of activities. This may be done by indicating to him that an activity which seems dangerous or taboo, out of bounds, or forbidden to him is, in fact, safe for him to try and available to him. The patient may also be encouraged to participate in new activities. A permissive attitude provides him with an experience quite different from his mother's restrictive attitude in childhood.

Many patients are unable to derive any pleasure from their senses or from their body. They may need to have specific permission to enjoy such pleasures as dancing, good food, sports, sunbathing, use of cosmetics and perfumes, etc. When an opportunity occurs for the patient to experience something new, the nurse can stand by to give encouragement and to protect the patient from inappropriate or excessive participation. Because of his inexperience, the patient is often unable to set limits for himself. In addition to giving the patient permission to do things, the nurse can provide opportunities for him to engage in activities. Arieti (1955) believes that the patient wants tasks given to him and demands made on him, and that this is one important way in which the patient can raise his self-esteem. Care should be taken that the nurse does not make these demands or assign tasks to the patient before the nurse-patient relationship is strong enough to tolerate it. Some of his basic affectional needs must have been met by the nurse previously. Arieti noted improvement in a number of schizophrenic patients in the back wards of a state hospital and discovered that the nurses "offered the patients an image of a good mother by appearing warm, strong, and kind. The patients responded to this atmosphere of consistent warmth by becoming more active. The nurse or female attendant then would give the patient tasks, which the patient certainly was able to perform and then would praise the patient, who felt an incentive to do more. The patient felt that he deserved the praise of the nurse, and in this way his self-esteem increased" (Arieti, 1955, p. 466). The work was seen by the patient not as an exploitation on the part of the nurse but as a method of self-improvement.

Schizophrenic Patient's Inability to Cope with Tasks of Daily Life

For the schizophrenic, inhibition of activity in childhood often results in his never learning to perform many of the simple actions of everyday life which have become almost automatic for most adults. Therefore, one of the useful functions of the nurse is to teach him these skills. He also has unexpected and surprising gaps in his knowledge of the world which the nurse can supply for him. One common area of ignorance and/or misinformation is about the way his body functions. The nurse can often allay anxiety by giving the patient pertinent information. When faced with a new situation the patient often has no idea how to get the necessary information or how to proceed to solving the problem. A perceptive nurse can help him with these difficulties. It is because of the type of behavior just described that schizophrenic individuals often appear lacking in intelligence and are judged to be mentally defective.

Social situations are almost always difficult for a schizophrenic patient to tolerate. A sensitive and sympathetic nurse can provide social activities in which the patient can feel reasonably comfortable and at ease. One can gauge the moment when anxiety sets in and help him to withdraw from the group without losing face. Ruesch (1961, pp. 302–303) says:

> The patient will have to experiment with practical implementations [of his restricted social activities], perhaps rearranging his occupational life so that he will participate to a minimal degree in all those activities that are necessary in the pursuit of a career. He might learn to attend parties, to talk shop with colleagues, to drop in on the neighbors. The withdrawn person is in no way capable of keeping up a sustained social effort. Unlike the organization man, he cannot keep up year in and year out

with entertainment, occupational meetings, drinking bouts, and the like. If he drinks, he often drinks alone. But showing him good will is often enough to get him out of his isolation and to permit other people to approach him.

Low Self-Esteem of Schizophrenic Patients

It is only after one has spent a great deal of time with a schizophrenic patient that he becomes increasingly aware of the depths of the patient's self-hatred. The patient sees himself as so vile, unlovable, and strangely different from others that he often avoids his nurse, believing that no one can be sincerely interested in helping him. The nurse's protestations that he does not regard him as unlovable are of no avail, but by his actions and other nonverbal behavior it can be demonstrated to the patient that his evaluation of himself is not accepted. The nurse's response will vary with each patient, but some examples might include listening quietly without comment, continuing to see him at the customary times and places, appearing unshocked by his disclosures, and indicating that his ideas and feelings are not so very different from those of other people, in kind at least, if not in degree.

Maneuvers which will help the patient to be less introspective and to focus on people and things about him help him to modify his distorted poor opinion of himself. Listening to the conversations of other patients, observing characters in plays, television, or movies, and discussing individuals described in newspapers and books often help the patient to feel less isolated, less different from others, and not nearly so "bad" as he once thought.

Loss of Reality-Testing Ability

Loss of the ability to be certain of what is real and what is imaginary is one of the causes of greatest distress to schizophrenic patients. Loss of the reality-testing ability occurs in the schizophrenic patient when unconscious thought and feelings break through into consciousness in the course of the psychotic process, so overwhelming him that he is unable to utilize the various clues in the external environment which other people generally use to validate their experiences. When no validation occurs, distortions of sensory perceptions and though processes, such as hallucinations and delusions, may result. These symptoms are characteristic of the schizophrenic process. If the nurse has a good relationship with his patient, he may be accepted as someone whom the patient can use to test the reality or unreality of his experiences. The nurse may be able to offer him a different point of view or focus by which to examine the phenomena occurring to him.

Acceptance by another person, someone to whom he can relate his experiences, provides the patient with a new frame of reference and enables him to look at his own experiences objectively and not be subjectively overwhelmed by them.

Hallucinations and Delusions

Hallucinations and delusions are very real to the schizophrenic patient and are often more vivid than his reality-based experiences. Reasoning, arguing, or attempting to prove the patient mistaken are worse than useless; such attempts only serve to entrench the symptoms more strongly. Hallucinations and delusions may disappear in the course of treatment without the therapist's calling attention to the symptoms themselves. Many authorities advocate handling the problem this way, and it seems to work very well in nursing, too, if the patient is not made anxious by his hallucinations and delusions or if they do not interfere with his satisfying his biological needs nor disrupt his daily activities or communication with others.

Many patients with chronic schizophrenia have learned to live with their symptoms without much difficulty. However, this is not generally true of patients in the early or acute stages in which these symptoms arouse a great deal of anxiety and must be dealt with. A good relationship between nurse and patient is a prerequisite for a nurse who is trying to help a patient suffering from a hallucination. The patient must have confidence in the nurse, be able to trust him, and be aware of his concern for him before he will even admit to the symptom and, certainly, before he would be willing to talk about it. Arieti (1961, p. 84) writes, "Hospitalized patients approached with the old routine questions, 'Do you hear voices? Who is persecuting you?,' are unable to give up their hallucinations. As long as an atmosphere of unrelatedness exists, the patient cannot make an effort to see and hear things as other people do, and it is unwise to attack the problem directly.

In daily contacts with a patient, the nurse may observe cues that suggest that the patient is hallucinating. It is often a good idea to wait without comment to see whether this behavior is repeated, and, if it is, under what circumstances and in what context. Is it perhaps before visiting hours, when there is a great deal of noise, when certain topics are brought up, or when certain people are present? The nurse may then want to wait longer to see if the patient will talk about what he is experiencing, or may wish to tell the patient that he has observed his behavior by stating, for example, "I notice you are staring at the wall," or, more fully, "I notice that you began staring at the wall when the room became noisy." The nurse's comment makes the patient focus his attention on his behavior and requires some kind of reply from him. An attitude of concern makes it easier for the patient to talk about an experience which may seem very frightening. It may be a great relief to the patient to be able to tell someone he trusts that he suffers from hallucinations. Such information is also helpful to the nurse—both in understanding the patient better and in planning his care. The nurse may also wish to know if the patient has discussed these experiences with his psychiatrist, and may suggest that such a discussion could be helpful.

The Nurse's Interventions in Behalf of the Hallucinating Patient

The attitude of the nurse as he listens to the patient describe his hallucinatory or delusional experiences is of great importance. The advice given to resident psychiatrists by Fromm-Reichmann seems equally useful for nurses. She writes (Fromm-Reichmann, 1950, p. 175), "The psychiatrist should not argue about their [the experiences] hallucinatory, delusional, orillusionary character. He should state quite simply and clearly that he does not see or hear what the patient professes to see or hear or that he does not share the patient's hallucinatory, delusional, or illusional interpretation or evaluation of the facts." Arieti also believes that it is unwise to give the patient the impression that the therapist hears his [the patient's] voices and shares his unusual private experiences. The therapist should simply tell the patient that he does not hear these voices but that he will be glad to listen to the patient's experiences (Arieti, 1961, p. 84).

The therapist's permissive, nonjudgmental, neutral attitude, together with a differing set of data, allows the patient to look objectively at two points of view at the same time and to provide the possibility of a choice for the patient. The element of doubt of the veracity of his perception of the phenomena is allowed to enter into the patient's deliberations for the first time. The nurse who is able to maintain this attitude offers the patient a safe way of validating the reality or unreality of his current experiences.

The Listening Attitude

Burton and Fromm-Reichmann have observed that preceding a hallucinatory experience there is usually a set of circumstances which evoke memories or a special mood in the patient. This is then followed by a period of expectant listening which Arieti calls a "listening attitude." Fromm-Reichmann recommends that the psychiatrist try to get the patient to recall past events or experiences in the patient's past life that occurred about the same time the hallucination was first experienced to see if any elements of the early event serve as a trigger for the present hallucinatory experiences. Any nurse who has had experience caring for schizophrenic patients will recognize the "listening attitude" as a familiar one. Arieti describes this process as follows (1961, pp. 84–85):

> For example, the patient may, when he goes home, *expect* the neighbors to talk about him; then he hears the neighbors. He puts himself in what I call the "listening attitude." If the patient is related to the therapist he will be able, under his direction, to distinguish two stages: that of the listening attitude and that of the hallucinatory experience. At first he may deny the existence of the two stages, but later he may say, "I happened to think so and what I thought was confirmed. They were really talking."
>
> Later he may admit that there is a very brief interval between the expectation of the voices and the voices, but that that sequence is purely coincidental. Finally he sees the connection between putting himself into the listening attitude and his actually hearing them. Later on he also admits that he expects to hear the voices and puts himself in the listening attitude in particular situations. (Of course, this does not occur in very sick patients who hallucinate all the time.) . . .
>
> Patients learn to catch themselves in the act of putting themselves into the listening attitude at the least disturbance several times during the day. At first they recognize the phenomenon as almost an automatic mechanism which is very difficult to control and which requires an unpleasant effort, a strong determination not to succumb. Later it becomes easier to control, especially if the relatedness with the therapist and the understanding of the historical dynamic mechanisms have at the same time diminished the anxiety.

A nurse who is aware of the listening phase of the hallucinatory process could intervene in time to forestall the onset of the hallucinatory experience by helping the patient to become aware of his listening attitude and to give him support in trying to control it.

The Nurse's Interventions in Behalf of the Delusional Patient

Many of the same measures that are helpful to patients with hallucinations are also effective with their delusions. Ruesch believes that it is often helpful to try to shift the patient's area of interest from one which involves him in difficulties in his daily life to one which is less harmful to himself or others. He states (1961, pp. 303 and 320), "To accomplish such shifts, the therapist has but one tool at his disposal: the interpersonal relationship. If the relationship becomes gratifying, the patient will incorporate all significant transactions and confine himself on the outside to impersonal matters and to transactions that deal with his immediate entourage. And this is exactly what the normal person does." Fromm-Reichmann also makes the suggestion that delusional patients often benefit from information. She writes, "The psychiatrist can give enlightening explanation of facts and data about which patients were misinformed either in childhood or later, if their misconception of such facts seems to be in part responsible for the contents of the delusion" (Fromm-Reichmann, 1950, p. 181).

Regressive Behavior

Next in difficulty to the problems of communicating with a schizophrenic patient is the problem of coping with the patient's regressive behavior. Under the stress of anxiety the patient's adjustment mechanisms break down in those areas of his personality in which he is most vulnerable. He reverts to behavior patterns which were successful in earlier periods in his life. However, as Arieti (1955) expresses so well, "no matter how much a schizophrenic regresses he can never become a healthy infant." In other areas of his personality his behavior is that of an adult. The schizophrenic patient operates on several developmental levels at the same time; his nurse has to distinguish his adult behavior from his regressed behavior and to treat him accordingly. This is not always easy to do. Nurses and other therapists tend to regard the schizophrenic patient as totally regressed and to treat him in a far more infantile manner than is appropriate or beneficial. The common practice of addressing these patients by their first names in only one of the many examples of this attitude of the personnel.

Though it is often necessary to make contact with the patient at the level of his regressed behavior and on his terms, once this contact has been established, one then tries to motivate the patient to bring his regressed behavior into alignment with his more adult behavior. In addition to providing emotional support, one can also attempt to inculcate in the patient a sense of responsibility for his own progress. The feeling that he has some control over his own welfare and that he also has the help of his psychiatrist, his nurse, and the other members of the therapeutic team can be a strong incentive for his improvement. Unfortunately, the patient may not be willing or able to cooperate with his therapists.

Resistance to Therapy

One of the most effective ways of blocking therapeutic progress is to develop negativistic behavior. When the nurse or other therapists make too many demands on the patient or make them too soon, the patient may react with negativistic behavior. The therapist's only method of coping with negativism is to wait patiently and good-naturedly until the patient is ready to make the next step toward recovery. When a patient regresses further during his treatment, it is often regarded as an unfavorable sign by his therapists. Frequently this is not the case and does not warrant the discouragement and disappointment it frequently engenders. When patterns of maladjustment in behavior are firmly fixed, it may be necessary for the patient to regress to a lower but better-integrated level of adjustment in order to reach a sounder basis for improvement. Flexible patterns of behavior permit greater opportunities for better integration than do well-entrenched static ones. In other words, the therapist should not be overly concerned about the patient's short periods of increased regressive behavior. However, such flare-ups of psychotic behavior may require increased nursing time and personnel, increased attention from the psychiatrist and other therapists, and supportive measures, such as appropriate medication, treatments, activities, and a special environment.

Problems of Termination with
Schizophrenic Patients

Termination of nursing care—especially of the nurse-patient relationship with a schizophrenic patient—differs in certain important respects from termination with other kinds of patients. The schizophrenic patient needs more time and more intensive preparation for termination than other patients. The time required for termination is in direct ratio to the length of time of nursing treatment with a given nurse and the intensity of the relationship. The date of termination should be brought up by the nurse well in advance and repeated at intervals; gradually, the patient should be drawn into some discussion of his reactions to it. Schizophrenic patients often suppress any recollection of the discussion of the topic, or else they use denial to avoid talking to the nurse about it. They need time to get used to the idea, before they can discuss it. In one sense, a therapeutic relationship with a schizophrenic patient is never completely terminated even though the actual contacts between therapist and patient are terminated.

In the course of the relationship the patient has used the therapist as a model or example and has unconsciously incorporated many of the therapist's attitudes and concepts which he needs for support in maintaining his own improvement. Patients are reassured by the knowledge that the therapist will continue to be concerned about the patient's welfare. Therapist and patient should plan how the patient can apply for help if he needs it at some future time. The therapist should not set up rigid termination procedures, but should make them as gradual and painless as possible for the schizophrenic patient. The patient is often gratified by some symbolic representation of a continued relationship: an occasional postcard, the gift of a small memento, or an invitation for a return visit if needed.

NURSING THE PATIENT WITH AN AFFECTIVE REACTION

Affective states of depression and elation in a mild form are experienced by everyone in the course of a lifetime. Only when these affective states become severe enough to incapacitate the individual is he considered to be suffering from a psychiatric disorder. Individuals with severe mood disturbances are generally classified as having an affective reaction or manic-depressive psychosis. Clinically they may exhibit two very different types of behavior; namely, depression and elation, which, however, are considered to be manifestations of the same condition. The depressed state is characterized by a depressed mood, poverty of ideas, slow speech, and sometimes muteness. Generally, motor activity is also retarded, but occasionally patients may be agitated. Feelings of worthlessness, hopelessness, and guilt are almost always present, and may become so severe as to be classified as delusions. Hypochondriacal ideas are common, and suicidal ideas and suicidal trends are an omnipresent danger in depressed states. In the manic state, the patient is elated—talks volubly and in a loud voice. He is physically hyperactive, very responsive to environmental stimuli, aggressive, extroverted in his behavior, and highly distractible. Expansive ideas, delusions of grandeur, and flight of ideas characterize his thought processes.

Depressive Reactions—Treatment

Depressions are the most common psychiatric condition encountered in the general population. Yet, the literature on the treatment of depressions is very meager compared with the voluminous amount available on the treatment of schizophrenia. Also, according to Grinker, treatment in the past has not been very consistent. He writes (Grinker et al., 1961, pp. 233–234),

> Psychiatrists treated depressions with a variety of intuitive methods: some were supported and encouraged during weekly visits; others were handled in a directive, sometimes punitive manner. Some were placed in the then-popular "rest cures," while the seriously depressed were incarcerated in sanitariums away from their home

317

cities to wait out a spontaneous recovery. In general, depressions were considered to be self-limited and therapy at best only palliative alleviation of misery with reassuring words and sedation.

As time went on, the psychoanalytic theories encouraged psychiatrists to utilize psychoanalytic techniques either in the classical form or in modified psychotherapy, with many fine successes in the treatment and prevention of further attacks in neurotic or mild depressive patients. Yet with the advent of psychiatric units attached to general hospitals, the preponderance of admissions consisted of seriously depressed patients who were agitated, suicidal, withdrawn, or psychotic. For many of these psychotherapy offered little promise and electric shock therapy and recently pharmacotherapy became the treatment of choice.

Psychotherapy

Most authorities concur that psychotherapy is important in the treatment of the affective psychoses. However, there is little agreement on what kind of psychotherapy is most effective. Weigert (1961), representing the psychoanalytic point of view, says that "the hope of the psychotherapist to change the character basis of the psychosis and to prevent the recurrence of pathological cycles is dim." Linn (1962) believes that the therapist should strengthen the "fragile or depleted ego" of the patient by long-term psychotherapy in the course of which the permissive therapist would replace the harsh superego of the patient. He would also help the patient to cultivate self-esteem and better interpersonal relationships by means of correctional emotional experiences and attempt to curb his provocative behavior by stressing the realities of the therapeutic relationship. Kraines (1957) has formulated a basic triad of psychotherapy for the depressed patient: (1) that he is sympathetically understood, (2) that he must have hope that he will be cured, (3) that he will fare best with a definite plan for recovery. He utilizes ventilation to relieve tension, symptom management to deal with current physical or psychological symptoms which are troublesome, improvement of faulty life patterns, and intensive psychotherapy.

Hospitalization

The severely depressed patient often required both intensive nursing care and hospitalization. Ayd (1961) states that a depressed patient should be hospitalized on the basis of a real need for the facilities and the advantages this offers, and not just because the patient is ill. Some of the indications for hospitalization include suicidal trends in the patient, difficult interfamily relationships, and a home environment unsuitable or inimical to therapy. Linn states that hospitalization is imperative for suicidal patients. He recommends special nurses, if possible, and warns that suicidal patients should never be left in seclusion or kept in private rooms, but should be with other patients where they will feel less isolated and abandoned. On the other hand, Linn does not want a number of suicidal patients on the same unit because this has a tendency to intensify the patients' anxiety and depression. Severely depressed hospitalized patients should have around-the-clock availability of the services of a physician and a nurse. Linn also advocates the flexible use of hospital facilities so that patients can be discharged and readmitted without difficulty, as their conditions require. Ayd recommends short periods of hospitalization, which he believes may expedite recovery. In his experience, hospitalization in the general hospital is usually well accepted by the patient and his family. In the general hospital, the depressed patient, who is often in poor physical condition, can receive a thorough physical checkup and necessary medical care. If, for any reason, the patient objects to hospitalization, Ayd attempts to find other ways of treating him outside of the hospital.

Physical and Psychological Protective Measures

Until recently there was a tendency to regard the physical aspects of the protective environment, that is, the locked doors, screened windows and stairways, and the many safety devices and precautionary routines, as the principal value of hospitalization. However, the importance of providing an environment which offers the patient psychological security outweighs mere physical protection and makes many of the elaborate protective measures formerly considered essential unnecessary. In other words, the personnel may be far more important than the physical surroundings in providing the temporary protection which the patient needs. The psychological protection by the nursing personnel goes beyond mere surveillance to include concern for, and understanding of, the depressed patient and his suffering. Methods of providing psychological support and nursing care for depressed patients outside a hospital setting are also being tried in various parts of the country. Such plans include having the nurse remain in the home with the patient during an agitated or very acute depressive phase; frequent and regularly scheduled visits to the patient at home by psychiatric nurses or psychiatrically oriented public health nurses; and having the patient attend daily some type of community mental health center or day hospital.

Need for Good General Nursing Care

The severely depressed patient often needs not only physical and psychological protection but also considerable nursing care to see that his basic biological needs are met. These needs include adequate intake of fluids and food, sufficient sleep, some exercise, and attention to personal hygiene and general health. Since depressed patients are often very indifferent to these needs and neglectful of symptoms of illness, their physical condition may be very poor, particularly if they have been depressed for some time before treatment was started. In some instances, malnourishment, dehydration, lack of sleep, and neglect of infections or other symptoms may reach such a point that patients are physically ill as well as mentally ill. The nursing care of such patients is essentially the same as for any acutely ill patient, though the depressed patient may be more difficult for a nurse to care for because of his inability to cooperate in his own care. The patient's slow speech, soft voice, and, occasionally, complete muteness make communication with him difficult. He may be so slowed down in all his actions that even simple procedures such as swallowing a pill take a great deal of effort, time, and patience for both patient and nurse. Loss of appetite makes eating a particularly difficult problem. Fortunately, in recent years drug therapy and electric shock treatment have done much to shorten the acute phase of depression.

Individualization of Care, Attitudes of the Nurse

Nursing care of the depressed patient should be individualized for each patient according to the depth of his depressed mood and the degree of retardation. Depression has often been compared with mourning, and depressed patients seem to need a period of time to experience some sadness. They tend to respond badly to attempts to cheer them up or to engage them prematurely in recreational activities. On the other hand, the nurse's overly sympathetic attitude could help sustain or even increase the patient's depressed mood. A kindly, understanding, but emotionally neutral approach is often most helpful to the patient.

Communication with Depressed Patients

Simple, direct information, especially regarding the practical aspects of his illness that cause him concern—effects of drugs, electric shock treatment, prognosis, cost of treatment, sick leave, home responsibilities, possible loss of employment—when given, often helps to reduce anxiety. Ayd says that depressed patients need and expect to be told simply and repeatedly words of comfort and reassurance. Such patients get temporary relief from these reassuring words but they must be repeated as anxiety again mounts. Most depressed patients are confused to some extent and cannot remember all that is said to them. Therefore, the nurse must often give him repeated instruction in simple, concise language. Jacobson (1971) advises that in talking with depressed patients one should not allow gaps of silence to develop, for this may make the patient more anxious. Nor should one talk too rapidly or too emphatically. She also recommends that the therapist should not give too much or too little, and notes that the depressed patient demands from him flexibility of mood, warm understanding, and unwavering respect. If the patient should withdraw from the therapist, the latter must not allow him to remain withdrawn but should reestablish contact with the patient. Ayd sums up the effects of the therapist's efforts to allay the patient's anxiety and distress in the following words (Ayd, 1961, p. 118), "Regardless of how indifferent he [the depressed patient] may be and how irksome these measures may be to the doctor, the patient is grateful for sympathy and attention. When improved, many depressed people remark that their faith in the doctor's promise of recovery and his constant reassurances prevented suicide and made tolerable an otherwise intolerable existence."

Depressed Patient's Problems about Decision-Making

Ruesch (1961) recommends that the severely depressed patient be protected from coercion and the necessity of making decisions. Depressed patients because of their motor and mental retardation have great difficulty in making decisions and initiating action. No patient should be expected to make an important life decision about marriage, divorce, or a change of employment when he is in a state of emotional turmoil, but there are many minor decisions of a practical nature which must be made during the course of a day. Since the depressed patient all his life has deferred to the wishes of others, at first glance it might appear that one of the things a depressed patient needs most to learn is to become more aware of his own likes and dislikes and to be able to assert himself. This is a desirable therapeutic goal for the depressed patient at a later stage of his treatment. However, in his deeply depressed phase the ability to keep in mind the possible choices available to him, and the effort and mental anguish required to reach a decision are beyond his abilities. If the patient can find someone whom he can trust, he can temporarily delegate the authority to make decisions and be relieved of this onerous burden. This does not mean that everyone who comes in contact with the patient should decide what is best for him. Only those few people whom he trusts—his psychiatrist, his nurse, his special attendant—should be able to determine when the patient is well enough to assume responsibility for making his own decisions, and they should then encourage him to do so.

Lack of Well-Defined Self-Concept

According to Medard Boss, who represents the point of view of existential psychiatry, the depressed person is one "who has never unfolded into being himself in the sense of taking responsibly upon himself the possibilities of living which are his and with which he is entrusted. He has not been able to appropriate them to a strong, genuine, authentic, independent, and free self-being" (Boss, 1963, p. 209). Because of this the depressed patient attempts to live up to the expectations and wishes of others in order to gain their love and protection. The dilemma of the depressed patient is that the more he tries to please others, the more he strangles his own potentialities for living his own life. This leads to deep feelings of guilt, self-accusation, frustration, and anger. Boss (1963, p. 211) states that "a highly permissive attitude on the part of the therapist is indicated with these patients because . . . their illness originates essentially from their having given in ever since infancy to the demands of the people around them and from their consequent inability to discover their own genuine demands and expectations."

Communication Problems

Mabel Blake Cohen and a group of colleagues (1959) published a report of an intensive study of twelve cases of manic-depressive psychosis. The purpose of this study was to further the knowledge of this condition and to arrive at some effective therapeutic interventions. The primary problem in treatment was discovered to be a communication problem. These patients tended to say what they thought would be pleasing to others, gave stock or stereotyped replies, and avoided saying anything that would indicate their real feelings or reveal that they were in any way emotionally involved. They were adept at talking fluently without really telling anything about themselves. Words were used as a medium of social exchange without much inherent meaning. One therapist in the study found it helpful to convey her meaning to the patient primarily by her tone of voice and by gestures rather than by the specific words used. Another therapist used sudden or unexpected actions to startle the patient out of his conventional and trite responses. The use of psychiatric terms was avoided by the therapist because of the patient's tendency to use them as a screen. Instead, efforts were made to get the patient to talk about his thought and feelings, and to involve him in a more genuine emotional interaction.

Dependency

Dependency problems proved difficult for both patients and therapists. Patients made many demands but could not accept gratification or were not satisfied by the therapists' attempts to fulfill them. In this study, "demand" was used to denote unrealistic and inappropriate requests, as distinguished from those requests which were appropriate in the treatment situation. The demand type of request seemed to spring from a need that was essentially unfulfillable, either because there was no realistic action which the therapist could take or because when the request was granted the patient was still unsatisfied. This demanding attitude in time evoked anger and frustration in the therapist.

Demanding Behavior

Some of the findings of the Cohen study and concepts of treatment of other psychotherapists have important implications for nurses who are engaged in caring for patients with affective psychoses. Nurses are very familiar with the feelings of anger and frustration which the demanding behavior of the patient evokes in them. The Cohen study indicates that one way of coping with this behavior is to set limits on the patient and refuse to meet excessive or unreasonable demands. The nurse-therapist needs to be aware of her own limitations in her ability to give and not overextend herself. However, in a study of need-fulfillment, Schwartz, Schwartz, and Stanton (1951) found that when nurses did try to fulfill the patients' needs as far as possible, the number and urgency of the demands decreased.

This insatiable demanding behavior seems to have its origins in severe frustrations in the infant-mother relationship in early life. Boss states that all depressive patients in therapy show a tremendous desire to make up for what they missed during infancy, and that they need to remain in the oral-erotic, infant-mother relationship for long phases of therapy with a very permissive therapist. In this connection Ruesch says that during the severely depressed phase the patient should have

24-hour-a-day care and support. He writes (Ruesch, 1961, p. 308), "The patient becomes very demanding in these phases—so demanding that he is afraid of his own appetite and possessiveness. He has to be reassured and permitted to be demanding; and when he discovers that the other person is not afraid, he improves." It is interesting to note that the Cohen study group tried 24-hour-a-day nursing care and found it unsuccessful, but the writers speculated on the possibility of greater success with a "therapist," that is, a person with more training in psychotherapeutic skills than the traditional nurse has. Very likely, a psychiatric nurse with training in some of these skills could meet Ruesch's criterion of being able to tolerate the patient's demanding behavior without feeling threatened and would prove very helpful to the patient.

Demanding Behavior in Depressed Patients

Nurses often have difficulty coping with the many demands of both depressed and manic patients. This is partly due to the variety of ways demands are used by different patients in different phases of their illness. Many demands are reasonable, ordinary requests, but others are fraught with all kinds of covert implications. For example, many depressed patients ask for things that they do not really want in lieu of some deeper need which they themselves cannot identify. Sometimes this demand takes the form of wordless, imploring looks which by their intensity and persistence often make the nurse feel guilty and uncomfortable. One's first impulse is to avoid such a patient as much as possible. The patient generally responds to this avoidance behavior with anger, which he represses. The repressed anger is then converted into still deeper depression. If instead of avoiding the patient, one could respond to his spoken or unspoken demand by remaining with him, or could encourage him to share his thoughts and feelings, one could help to allay his anxiety.

Manic Reactions

Demanding Behavior in Manic Patients and Nursing Interventions   Manic patients, on the other hand, can be very aggressive in making their demands and in getting others to fulfill them. Depending on the therapeutic needs of the patient and the circumstances of the situation, the nurse may decide to set limits on the patient by refusing him; to postpone the decision; or to fulfill the demand in totality, in part, or by token fulfillment. Many nurses are afraid to set limits on a manic patient, who is frequently aggressive, lest they provoke a rage reaction by refusal. However, this, in fact, does not generally follow. The firm setting of definite limits often results in greater calmness in the patient. He experiences a greater sense of security, a lessening of anxiety, and a feeling that the nurse has concern for him and is competent to assume control.

Setting Limits   Setting limits, however, requires that the nurse himself be personally unafraid and sure of the validity of his decision. He may convey this sureness and self-confidence to the patient by the tone of his voice or poised manner, as he gives the patient a simple explanation of his reasons for denying his demand. The explanation should be simple and direct, to guard against providing an opening which would permit the patient to start an argument. Argumentation is a type of testing-out behavior frequently employed by manic patients and should be avoided whenever possible.

Postponement   Another form of intervention often effective in dealing with the unreasonable or inappropriate demands of manic patients is postponement. In employing postponement, the nurse listens attentively, maintaining a neutral attitude, but does not permit himself to be put on the spot for an immediate decision. Postponement can be particularly useful when the nurse surmises that he does not have sufficient information to make a decision or when he is not sure of the patient's real reasons for the demand. When one maintains a neutral and reasonable attitude, in a surprising number of instances the patient will agree to postponement. Postponement can also be used to cope with the unreasonable demands of the labile manic patient whose focus of interest changes from moment to moment. Frequently, when the patient's request is reconsidered at a later time, he is no longer interested in it. This strategem can sometimes painlessly avoid a situation which could well develop into a power struggle between nurse and patient.

Fulfillment   Sometimes it is both expedient and therapeutic in a given situation to grant a request which would not seem advisable in general practice. For example, if a nurse is working very hard to set limits for the patient in one area of his behavior, he might be more lenient in regard to lapses in behavior in other areas for the time being. It is impossible for a manic patient to accept restrictions in all areas of behavior at the same time. Therefore, the nurse must decide whether granting the request might have an over-all beneficial effect on the patient. Nurses who are experienced in nursing manic patients are aware of the importance of tempering firmness in important issues with flexibility in minor ones. Both the nurse who is a perfectionist and the overly permissive nurse often find it difficult to care for manic patients.

Partial Fulfillment Partial fulfillment is another intervention which is useful in coping with the demands of manic patients. This is often applicable when the expansiveness of the demand can be cut down to size either by reducing it in scale or by granting some part of the total demand. In this way the patient does not suffer total refusal. Sometimes requests of manic patients are impossible to grant because they are too grandiose, too unrestricted in scope, too bizarre, or too inappropriate. Modification of the demand by joint agreement of patient and nurse is sometimes feasible. Often the patient is able to recognize the inappropriate or unrealistic aspects of his demands and is willing to modify them in order to get some measure of gratification. A patient who is able to do this has taken a long step toward recovery.

Manipulative Behavior in Manic Patients In the manic patients' anxiety that his needs will not be met, he frequently attempts to use other people in a rather impersonal way as instruments to get him what he needs. This kind of behavior is often referred to as manipulative behavior, and it often presents the nurse with many difficulties in the course of caring for the patient. Contrary to the impression of self-sufficiency given by his arrogant attitude, the manic patient often has such a poor opinion of himself that he cannot believe that he can get his needs met on the basis of his own worth. Therefore he tries to make someone else get him what he wishes. This maneuver not only protects him from the danger of personal failure but gives him a sense of power over another individual. It also depersonalizes that individual to the status of agent or tool. If the first person asked refuses him or fails, the manic patient is driven by his anxiety to go to another person. Going from one person to another for gratification further increases the patient's anxiety, and consequently the intensity of his demands.

Coping with Manipulative Behavior Every psychiatric nurse recognizes this pattern of manipulative behavior. The anger and frustration one experiences on becoming aware that he is the victim of the patient's manipulative behavior make it difficult to deal rationally with the problem. On the operational level, the problem is how to interrupt the cycle of destructive behavior in which the patient is caught. This can be done only with the close cooperation of all members of the treatment team and the maintenance of good communication among themselves. Group cohesiveness makes it impossible for the patient to play one person against another. Each member of the team must also learn to recognize the pattern of manipulation characteristic of the particular patient and be on guard to deal with it.

In spite of the therapist's best efforts it is not unusual for him to be caught off guard and fall victim to the patient's manipulations. It is important that the therapist not become too angry with the patient or with himself, because then he would lose control of the situation. With experience it becomes easier to become aware of the patient's manipulative pattern. This awareness can destroy the effectiveness of the manipulation and prevent the patient from sabotaging therapy. It also serves to keep the patient's anxiety from spreading. When the patient's anxiety is controlled, he is able to discuss his behavior with his therapist, and may also gain some insight into how his anxiety is manifested in manipulative behavior toward ward personnel and other patients. The nurse can help the patient in his attempts to change this behavior if he is not caught up in his own hostile feelings. Cohen's study (1959) indicates that when the patient's anxiety is reduced he is also better able to see his therapists as individuals, to react to them with more feeling, and to be less likely to treat them as objects.

Acting-out Behavior in Manic Patients   Another pattern of behavior which is difficult for many nurses to cope with is the manic patient's propensity for acting-out. This behavior often occurs when the patient is angry and frustrated. Manic patients, characteristically, have a very low frustration tolerance. Instead of talking over his difficulties with the appropriate person, the manic patient escapes into action of some kind—usually a dramatic, and frequently a dangerous or destructive, type of behavior. Most psychiatrists frown on acting-out behavior because it is another way the manic patient can avoid facing his problems or gaining some understanding and control over them. Another aspect of acting-out behavior in manic patients is its element of hostility toward others. Acting-out behavior can be a very effective device for controlling others by frightening them, making them feel guilty, or immobilizing them with threats. This type of behavior is used by depressed patients as well. The most extreme example of this is the act of suicide.

Coping with Acting-out Behavior   When a manic-depressive patient utilizes acting-out behavior, close collaboration between the medical and the nursing staff is required to control it. However, there is a growing tendency to place increased responsibility on the patient himself to control his impulses to act out. A sudden impulsive fear (which in some patients may reach the intensity of panic) may trigger acting-out behavior. Therefore it is often helpful to warn patients of the possible occurrence of such feelings so that they can try to control them. To give added support to the patient, swift and coordinated intervention by medical and nursing personnel is essential. After the critical phase has passed, the patient should be given an opportunity to talk about what he was experiencing. The nurse should make it as easy as possible for the patient to communicate his thoughts and feelings.

Termination of Treatment in
Affective Reactions

In the later phases of treatment when the acute depression or manic reaction has subsided, the patient should be prepared for the termination of treatment and the resumption of participation in family and community living. Self-awareness and the responsibility for the direction of his own life are important goals for the patient in this phase. One way to help patients to achieve these goals is to encourage them to make their own decisions. This includes providing them with opportunities within the treatment setting to gain experience in making decisions which are realistic yet contain some degree of self-realization and gratification. Patients who are not by nature introspective can learn to develop greater awareness of their own inner thoughts and feelings and those of others. The patient's increased awareness can be very useful in improving future interpersonal relationships. It can also help the patient to recognize incipient signs of illness and to seek help in time. These patients should be aware of the good prognosis for the present attack but also of the possibility of a recurrence. They should be given information about therapists and agencies to contact if help is needed in the future.

Review and Revision of Patterns of Living

Another effective way of preparing the patient for discharge is to review pretreatment patterns of living to see in what respect they have been faulty. Many patients who develop manic-depressive reactions have patterns of living in which one interest has been pursued intensively to the detriment of all other aspects of living. Examples of this pattern would include the businessman who is so completely involved in his business affairs that he neglects his children, or the wife who has devoted herself exclusively to her home and family to the detriment of her personal fulfillment or her responsibilities to her community. During the convalescent period the patient has the opportunity to review his life pattern in its totality and to revise it so that it will be better balanced and more satisfying to him in the future. The manic-depressive patient frequently has a tendency to assume more duties and responsibilities than are beneficial for him. Such a patient may have to limit his participation in those activities in which he has overextended himself. On the other hand, he may need to enrich his life in areas which he has formerly neglected, and to make his life pattern more flexible where it has been rigid and overly conventional.

SOME RECENT TRENDS IN THE TREATMENT OF MANIC-DEPRESSIVE PSYCHOSIS

Somatic Therapy

Somatic therapies play an important role in the treatment of both severe depressions and manic attacks. Before the introduction of the ataraxic drugs, the most widely used form of somatic treatment was electroshock therapy, which is still occasionally used for severe depressions. Now drugs have become the principal agents in the treatment of the affective disorders. Since the introduction of the antidepressant drugs (the tricylic compounds and MAO inhibitors), it has been possible to treat most patients who have depressions effectively with these drugs. Although they do not work for all depressed patients, they have helped many patients who formerly would have received electroshock therapy. The phenothiazines and related neuroleptic drugs have been used successfully for manic attacks in certain patients, but if large doses are required to control the hyperactivity, a number of undesirable side effects appear, such as sluggishness and torpor (Fieve, 1970, pp. 182–183).

With the discovery of the psychoactive properties of lithium by the Australian psychiatrist, John F. J. Cade, in 1949, a new agent was introduced for the specific treatment of manic attacks. However, this discovery was largely ignored by the American medical profession until 1960, when Dr. Samuel Gershon, an Australian psychiatrist on a research fellowship at the University of Michigan, encouraged Michigan doctors to try the drug. Lithium did not come into widespread knowledge and acceptance by American psychiatrists as a specific treatment for mania until 1965. Research studies indicate that 70 to 80 percent of manic patients respond well to lithium. It has proved effective for all types of manic disorder—chronic, recurrent, and hypomanic. Lithium is often effective when other drugs fail. It has also been used as a prophylactic agent to increase the intervals between cyclical recurring attacks. The duration of the episodes was also decreased (NIMH, 1970, p. 50). Lithium is only partially effective in the treatment of depressions (Fieve, 1970, p. 186).

Psychotherapy

Primal therapy is a method of psychotherapy developed by Arthur Janov (1972) and recommended by him as particularly applicable to the treatment of manic-depressive psychosis (Janov, 1972, pp. 173–176).

Primal therapy is concerned with the release of traumatic childhood experiences (Primal pain) resulting from parental denial of a basic need, subsequently repressed. The experiences of Primal pain often occur before the development of speech. In later life, unidentifiable sensations of tension, anxiety, and pain may, in the course of therapy, be connected to their early origins and conceptualized. They then become Primal feelings. Janov believes that these Primal feelings lie at the bottom of mania and depression and must be resolved. He writes, "One of the reasons conventional psychotherapy has been so unsuccessful with the manic-depressive is that there has been an attempt to build a defense rather than to take it apart" (Janov, 1972, p. 175). Since this method of psychotherapy is so recent, there is not a sufficient number of manic-depressives treated by Primal therapy to warrant an evaluation of its effectiveness.

SOME RECENT TRENDS IN SCHIZOPHRENIA
New Concepts of Schizophrenia

The concept of schizophrenia is burgeoning out into a whole range of concepts both broader and deeper than the rigid delineation of Kraepelinian schizophrenia. According to Scheff, (1970, p. 18)

> Schizophrenia is the single most widely used diagnosis for mental illness in the United States, yet the cause, site, course, and treatment of choice are unknown, or the subject of heated and voluminous controversy. Moreover, there is some evidence that the reliability of diagnosis is quite low. Finally, there is little agreement on whether a disease entity of schizophrenia even exists, what constitutes schizophrenia's basic signs and symptoms if it does exist, and how these symptoms are to be reliably and positively identified in the diagnostic process.

Mosher (1970, p. 16) writes,

> A number of scientists have begun to view the disorder in other than a medical disease framework. To these investigators, the personality disorganization of schizophrenia may be viewed as a stage in a process of personality development with subsequent reintegration. From such a framework, schizophrenia is conceptualized as a positive growth process with potential for healthful adaptation rather than as a "disease" with its "defect" implications.

Arieti (1959, p. 501) defines *schizophrenia* as "a specific reaction to an extreme state of anxiety, originated in childhood and reactivated later in life by psychological factors. The specific reaction consists of the preponderant adoption of mental mechanisms which belong to lower levels of integration. Inasmuch as the result is a regression to, but not an integration at, lower levels, a disequilibrium is engendered which causes further regression." Thus Arieti also sees schizophrenia as an interruption and malfunctioning of the personality developmental process.

The British psychoanalyst, Ronald D. Laing, defines the term *schizophrenia* in an even broader context, stressing the social influences as well as the internal conflicts (Laing, 1967, p. 70).

> In using the term schizophrenia, I am not referring to any condition that I suppose to be mental rather than physical, or to an illness like pneumonia, but to a label that some people pin on other people under certain social circumstances. The "cause" of "schizophrenia" is to be found by the examination not of the prospective diagnosee alone, but of the whole social context in which the psychiatric ceremonial is being conducted.

Laing sees schizophrenia as a reaction to an impossible life situation such as Bateson's (1956) double-bind phenomenon, which engenders a split between the inner and outer world of man, and which in turn precipitates the psychotic process (Kalkman, 1970, pp. 39–40).

A growing number of psychiatrists, including Lidz, Bowen, Jackson, and Langsley, among others, theorize that schizophrenia is not an illness of a single individual but a manifestation of a family disorder (Massie and Beels, 1972, p. 25). Scheff, a sociologist, defines schizophrenia as a label which may be applied to those members of society who break its accepted social and cultural rules and whose deviant behavior does not lend itself easily to inclusion in the usual categories of socially deviant behavior (Scheff, 1970, p. 18).

Psychotherapy

Laing's Model Laing has developed a method of psychotherapy which is attracting considerable interest and attention in the United States. It is based on the hypothesis that schizophrenia is the result of cultural pressure on the schizophrenic to be "normal," that is, like other people in his society. As a consequence of this pressure the schizophrenic becomes alienated from his inner experience of himself and feels fragmented and lost. Laing sees psychotherapy as "an obstinate attempt of two people (therapist and client) to recover the wholeness of being human through the relationship between them" (Laing, 1967, p. 32). Schizophrenia is regarded, not as an illness, but as an experience or voyage into madness and return. Laing thinks that the schizophrenic experience can be a natural way of healing the distressing state of alienation and a potentially liberating and regenerative force (Laing, 1967, pp. 87–90; Siegler et al., 1971, p. 181).

According to Laing, the normal person is usually totally unaware of his inner world and generally really knows very little about the outer world. When the psychotic process starts, he suddenly becomes aware of the split between his inner and outer world. He confuses the two, loses the capacity to function in ordinary relations, and becomes terrified. Laing (Laing, 1967, pp. 80–81; Kalkman, 1970, p. 40) describes the behavior which can result from such an experience:

> It is hardly surprising that the person in terror may stand in curious postures in an attempt to control the irresolvably contradictory social "Forces" that are controlling him, that he projects the inner onto the outer, introjects the outer onto the inner, that he tries in short, to protect himself from destruction by every means that he has, by projection, introjection, splitting, denial, and so on.

Laing sees the process of entering the other world (inner world) from this world (reality) and returning to this world from the other world as a normal and natural process. However, the newly schizophrenic person cannot do this unassisted. For this Laing prescribes the following treatment. "We need a place—a sort of reservicing factory for human breakdowns—where people who have traveled further and, consequently, may be more lost than psychiatrists and other sane people, can find their way *further* into inner space and time, and back again." Laing also prescribes an initiation ceremony for those entering a schizophrenic breakdown, with experienced guides to enable them to move into inner space and time and to emerge to self, a new ego, and an existential rebirth (Laing, 1967, pp. 88–89).

Research in the Treatment of Schizophrenia

Methods of psychotherapy in the treatment of schizophrenia have grown in number and variety in the past 20 years, yet as a modality, psychotherapy has never enjoyed as secure a position as drug therapy in the consideration of either the medical profession or the public. Research on the effectiveness of psychotherapy, particularly with schizophrenia, has been extremely difficult because of the almost impossible task of defining either schizophrenia or the psychotherapeutic process. However, in spite of these difficulties there are currently in process a number of research studies to determine whether the human factor, as opposed to drugs or other somatic therapies, plays an important role in the prevention, treatment, and rehabilitation of schizophrenia.

Feinsilver and Gunderson (1972) report on a research study in which a number of investigators reviewed five studies which attempted to assess the effectiveness of psychotherapy by comparing psychotherapeutically treated schizophrenic patients with appropriate control groups. The psychotherapeutic methods used varied in the five studies: Program I used Rosen's direct analysis; Program II, Roger's client-centered therapy; Program III, ego-supportive therapy; Program IV, analytically oriented psychotherapy; and Program V, direct or ego-analytic psychotherapy. In three of the programs some patients in the study groups received drugs as adjuncts to psychotherapy. The control groups received routine hospital treatment, active milieu therapy, drugs, electroshock therapy, or treatment in a different setting from the study group.

Although results can be stated only in a highly qualified and restricted manner, the findings were as follows: that drugs alone are the single most powerful and economical treatment for schizophrenic patients within 1- and 2-year time limits; that certain qualities in the therapist and his relationship to the patient improve prognosis; that the failure of controlled studies to demonstrate psychotherapy's effectiveness may stem from insufficient knowledge of the critical variables of the psychotherapeutic process; that the five studies reviewed neither proved psychotherapy ineffective nor provided any strong evidence of its helpfulness (Feinsilver and Gunderson, 1972, pp. 20–21).

Implications of this review study include the recommendation that it might be advisable in future research to concentrate on correlational studies aimed at better understanding of patient variables, therapist variables, and process variables which define the therapy before launching into large-scale comparative studies. It was also noted that "research on psychotherapy with schizophrenics has for some time been in a state of semi-paralysis," and that it is incumbent on psychotherapists to demonstrate whether or not psychotherapy is indicated in the treatment of schizophrenia, of what it should consist, who should deliver it, and who should receive it (Feinsilver and Gunderson, 1972, p. 22).

Family Therapy in the Treatment of Schizophrenia

Within the past 5 years, family therapy has become an accepted method of treatment for schizophrenia, and it is predicted that in the near future it will become a major modality for treatment. This is not surprising, in view of the fact that in current psychiatric thinking schizophrenia is considered a disorder of the total family and not of an individual. In an attempt to determine the effectiveness of family therapy in the treatment of schizophrenia, Massie and Beels reviewed eight studies, widely separated geographically and in a variety of settings including hospitals, homes, and clinics, in which families were treated by family therapy. The results of therapy were then evaluated. The investigators note that these eight studies should be regarded as exploratory investigations rather than as systematic research. Nevertheless, some generalizations can be made, of which perhaps the principal one is that family techniques do give indications of effectiveness in treating schizophrenia. All eight studies reported positive results. Specifically, it was noted that in crises of family disorganization "a therapeutic team working with the whole family could restore the family members to a functional level equal to or better than before the crisis." It was recommended that a study of intensive, long-term family therapy should be made for research purposes, although for clinical practice or determining therapeutic efficiency, short-term or infrequent meetings may be desirable (Massie and Beels, 1972, pp. 24–36).

REFERENCES

Arieti, Silvano (1955): *Interpretation of Schizophrenia*, Robert Brunner, Publisher of Psychiatric Books, New York, p. 466.

————(1961): "Introductory Notes on the Psychoanalytic Theory of Schizophrenia," in Arthur Burton (ed.), *Psychotherapy of the Psychoses*, Basic Books, Inc., Publishers, New York, chap. 3, pp. 69–89.

————(1959): "Schizophrenia: Other Aspects; Psychotherapy," in S. Arieti (ed.), *American Handbook of Psychiatry*, Basic Books, Inc., Publishers, New York, vol. 1, chap. 24, pp. 485–507.

Ayd, Frank J., Jr. (1961): *Recognizing the Depressed Patient*, Grune and Stratton, Inc., New York, p. 118.

Bateson, Gregory, et al., (1956): "Toward a Theory of Schizophrenia," *Behavioral Science*, vol. 1, no. 4, pp. 251–264. Reprinted in D. D. Jackson (ed.), *Communication, Family, and Marriage*, Science and Behavior Books, Inc., Palo Alto, Calif.

Boss, Medard, (1963): *Psychoanalysis and Daseinanalysis*, Ludwig B. Lefebre (trans.), Basic Books, Inc., Publishers, New York, p. 211.

Burton, Arthur (1961): "The Quest for the Golden Mean: A Study in Schizophrenia," in Arthur Burton (ed.), *Psychotherapy of the Psychoses*, Basic Books, Inc., Publishers, New York, 1961, pp. 172–207.

Caudill, William, F. C. Redlich, H. R. Gilmore, and E. B. Brody (1952): "Social Structure and Interaction Processes on a Psychiatric Ward," *American Journal of Orthopsychiatry*, April, pp. 314–334.

Cohen, Mabel B., G. Baker, R. A. Cohen, F. Fromm-Reichmann, and E. V. Weigert (1959): "An Intensive Study of Twelve Cases of Manic-Depressive Psychosis," in Dexter M. Bullard (ed.), *Psychoanalysis and Psychotherapy*, The University of Chicago Press, Chicago, pp. 227–274.

Davis, Anne J. (1963): "The Skills of Communication," *American Journal of Nursing*, January, pp. 66–70.

Ewalt, Jack R., and Dana L. Farnsworth (1963): *Textbook of Psychiatry*, McGraw-Hill Book Company, New York.

Feinsilver, David B., and John G. Gunderson (1972): "Psychotherapy for Schizophrenia—Is It Indicated? A Review of the Literature," *Schizophrenia Bulletin,* issue no. 6, Fall, pp. 11–23.

Fieve, Donald R. (1970): "Interdisciplinary Studies of Manic-Depressive Psychosis," in *Mental Health Program Reports—4,* National Institute of Mental Health, Chevy Chase, Md., pp. 175–194.

Fromm-Reichmann, Frieda (1950): *Principles of Intensive Psychotherapy,* The University of Chicago Press, Chicago, pp. 175–176.

Grinker, Roy R., J. Miller, M. Sabshin, R. Hoonan, and J. C. Nunnally (1961): *The Phenomena of Depressions,* Harper & Row, Publishers, Inc., New York, pp. 233–234.

Jacobson, Edith (1971): *Depression,* International Universities Press, Inc., New York, pp. 284–30l.

Janov, Arthur (1972): *The Primal Revolution toward a Real World,* Simon, and Schuster, Inc., New York.

Kalkman, Marion E. (1970): "The Development of a Treatment Program in a Private, Non-Profit Psychiatric Day Treatment Center," Unpublished study.

Kraines, Samuel H. (1957): *Mental Depressions and Their Treatment,* The Macmillan Company, New York.

Laing, Ronald D. (1967): *The Politics of Experience,* Pantheon Books, Inc., New York.

Linn, Louis (1962): "Depression: Broadening Concepts in Theory and Practice," *Psychiatric Quarterly Supplement,* pt. 1, pp. 1–13.

Massie, Henry N., and C. Christian Beels (1972): "The Outcome of Family Treatment of Schizophrenia," *Schizophrenic Bulletin,* issue no. 6, Fall, pp. 24–36.

Mosher, Loren R., et al. (1970): *Special Report on Schizophrenia, April, 1970,* National Institute of Mental Health, U.S. Department of Health, Education, and Welfare, Washington, D.C.

NIHM (1970): *Lithium in the Treatment of Mood Disorders,* National Clearinghouse for Mental Health, Publication no. 5033, U.S. Department of Health, Education, and Welfare, Washington, D.C.

Rose, Williamina G. D. (1962): "Management of Dependence-Independence Factors in a Nurse-Patient Relationship with a Catatonic Patient," in *Monograph no. 7, Innovations in Nurse-Patient Relationships: Nursing the Patient with Problems of Response,* American Nurses Association, New York, pp. 5–28.

Rosen, John N. (1953): *Direct Analysis,* Grune & Stratton, Inc., New York.

Ruesch, Jurgen (1961): *Therapeutic Communication,* W. W. Norton & Company, Inc., New York, pp. 303, 320.

———, C. Brodsky, and A. Fischer (1963): "The Acute Nervous Breakdown," *Archives of General Psychiatry,* February, pp. 197–207.

Scheff, Thomas J. (1970): "Schizophrenia As Ideology," *Schizophrenia Bulletin,* Issue no. 2, Fall, pp. 15–19.

Schwartz, Charlotte G., M. S. Schwartz, and A. H. Stanton (1951): "A Study of Need-Fulfillment on a Mental Hospital Ward," *Psychiatry,* May, pp. 223–242.

Sechehaye, Marguerite A. (1961): "Introduction," in Arthur Burton (ed.), *Psychotherapy of the Psychoses,* Basic Books, Inc., Publishers, New York, pp. 1–9.

Siegler, Miriam, Humphrey Osmond, and Harriet Mann (1971): "Laing's Models of Madness," in Robert Cancro (ed.), *The Schizophrenic Syndrome: An Annual Review, 1971,* Bruner Mazel, New York, and Butterworths, London, pp. 170–188.

Sullivan, Harry Stack (1962): *Schizophrenia as a Human Process,* W. W. Norton & Company, Inc., New York, 1962, pp. 272–294, 313.

Weigert, Edith (1961): "The Psychotherapy of the Affective Psychoses," in Arthur Burton (ed.), *Psychotherapy of the Psychoses,* Basic Books, Inc., Publishers, New York, pp. 349–376.

13

PSYCHONEUROSES

Marion E. Kalkman

Stress and the anxiety which accompanies it are universal conditions of life. Individuals who try to cope with excessive anxiety by repressive measures, including the use of the common defense mechanisms, generally manifest some type of psychoneurotic behavior. To this extent, everyone is somewhat psychoneurotic. Psychoneurosis is diagnosed in those individuals who manifest quantitatively more than an average amount of psychoneurotic behavior, or qualitatively, more aberrant behavior than the average individual.

Types and Morbidity of Psychoneuroses

The psychoneurotic disorders include anxiety reactions, dissociative and conversion reactions, obsessive-compulsive reactions, and depressive reactions. The degree of severity of psychoneurotic symptomatology extends from behavior which is so mild as to be indistinguishable from so-called normal behavior to symptomatology which is so pathological as to be difficult to distinguish from psychosis. The psychoneurotic person may be able to carry on his vocational, social, and family activities with only slight limitation of his functioning, or he may be so disabled by his disorder that hospitalization is necessary. Although the psychoneuroses are generally regarded as less malignant than the psychoses, some neuroses are more disabling than some psychoses. For example, an individual with a severe obsessive-compulsive neurosis can become totally incapacitated by his symptoms.

Clinical Picture

The clinical picture in psychoneurosis is generally a mixed one; that is, any one of the psychoneurotic reactions is likely to include admixtures of symptoms characteristic of other psychoneurotic reactions. An individual suffering from an obsessive-compulsive reaction may also suffer from anxiety and depression. Psychoneurotic symptoms can also occur in psychoses, psychosomatic disturbances, and personality disorders.

Socioeconomic Factors in Treatment

Cultural, social, and economic factors play a significant role in the diagnosis and treatment of psychoneurosis. Many people who have psychoneurotic symptoms do not consider themselves to be in need of treatment and do not seek it. Others, who may be aware of their psychoneurotic difficulties, do not seek treatment for what they consider a minor ailment. The psychoneurotic patients who seek psychiatric treatment are usually from the higher economic and social classes, while those who seek medical rather than psychiatric treatment are usually from the middle-class socioeconomic group and are found in large numbers at the outpatient clinics and offices of general practitioners (Ewalt and Farnsworth, 1963). There is some evidence that cultural, social, and economic factors play a role in the type of psychoneurosis an individual develops. In military psychiatry it has been noted that in World War I, enlisted men who came from the lower socioeconomic groups had a high rate of conversion reactions (shell shock) whereas the officers suffered from anxiety reactions. In World War II, the enlisted men, who were recruited with a larger percentage from the middle class than in World War I, had many psychosomatic complaints and very few conversion symptoms.

Role of the Nurse in Treatment

The role of the nurse in the treatment of the psychoneurotic patient has not been nearly so important as it has been in the treatment of the psychotic patient. The psychotic patient generally requires hospitalization, and he needs a nurse for his physical care as well as for psychological support. In the acute phase of the psychosis, when many patients do not talk and the psychiatrist is unable to conduct psychiatric interviews, the nurse is often able to establish effective contact with the nonverbal patient. In later phases of his treatment, when the patient is responsive to psychotherapy with the psychiatrist or psychologist, the nurse continues to be a valued member of the therapeutic team.

In the Past—Minimal Role

In the past, most psychiatric nurses practiced in large, public psychiatric hospitals in which very few patients were classified as psychoneurotic. In 1950, psychoneuroses represented only 4.6 percent of first admissions to state mental hospitals in the United States. However, in 1964 this admission rate rose to 11.3 percent. The psychoneurotic patients who were hospitalized in state hospitals often suffered from long-standing, intractable symptoms such as phobias, obsessions, compulsions, hysterical paralyses, and other bizarre hysterical phenomena for which very little in the way of psychiatric treatment was available. Nursing care was largely nonspecific. The majority of private patients with psychoneuroses were treated by psychiatrists, psychoanalysts, and psychologists in out-patient clinics or mental health clinics. In the latter, they constituted more than 30 percent of the total case load. Nurses rarely saw these patients.

Present Involvement of Nurse
in Treatment

Ewalt and Farnsworth state that the most widely used method of treatment for psychoneurosis is psychotherapy based on psychoanalytical principles (Ewalt and Farnsworth, 1963). Psychoanalysis, when available, is considered by many authorities to be the treatment of choice. Occasionally tranquilizers or sedatives may be used in conjunction with psychotherapy, but many psychiatrists try to use drugs as little as possible. Although in the past, the services of a psychiatric nurse were rarely utilized, this situation is now changing. With the rapid growth of psychiatric units in general hospitals (it is now estimated that more than 50 percent of all general hospitals in the United States have psychiatric in-patient facilities), an increasing number of acutely ill psychoneurotic patients are being admitted to these units. These patients require the skilled psychiatric nursing care which can be given only by adequately prepared nurses. Directors of mental health clinics who formerly could see no role for a nurse on the treatment team, are now becoming aware that a well-prepared psychiatric public health nurse could be very useful in the treatment of the psychoneurotic patient in the community.

Dynamics of Psychoneurosis

According to Horney (1950), the psychoneurotic patient suffers from basic anxiety, which she describes as a feeling of intrinsic weakness and helplessness toward a world which he perceives as potentially hostile and dangerous. Anxiety makes it necessary for the patient to find ways to cope with life with some degree of security—which may be accomplished by his neurotic behavior. Unconscious neurotic conflicts underlying feelings of anxiety are responsible for the patient's inability to make choices. Hence decision making is one of the patient's primary areas of difficulty. He is also obliged to use his rigidly structured neurotic behavior patterns because only by following these patterns can he avoid danger. Neurotic behavior has a very limiting effect on the patient's life experiences.

Supportive Role of the Nurse in Therapy

The primary task of the therapist is to help the patient to become aware of his neurotic behavior, to recognize its crippling effect on his life, and to motivate him to change it. Because this behavior is unconsciously motivated, and the preferred method of treatment is some form of intensive psychotherapy, the role of the psychotherapist, who may be a psychoanalyst, psychiatrist, or clinical psychologist, is primary in the treatment of the psychoneuroses. The nurse of necessity must play a complementary or supportive role in therapy. Since the psychotherapist is the key figure in the treatment of the psychoneurotic patient, the nurse who is engaged in the nursing care of the patient must collaborate closely with him. The nurse is under obligation to keep him informed of nursing therapy and of the general progress of the patient. On the other hand, the nurse needs to know what the goals of the psychotherapist are. Psychotherapist and nurse may work at cross purposes unless treatment plans are carefully worked out and good lines of communication are kept open.

Establishing a Nurse-Patient Relationship
with the Psychoneurotic Patient

It is usually rather easy to establish contact with a psychoneurotic patient. Communication, too, is easier than with psychotic patients. However, the nurse may find it difficult to explain to the neurotic patient his role in the total treatment plan. The nurse must be quite specific in defining this role to the patient if he intends to utilize one-to-one nurse-patient relationship therapy or nursing group psychotherapy, both of which require an understanding or contract with the patient before beginning to work with him. It is not easy to maintain a professional role with neurotic patients. They often are skillful in their attempts to draw the nurse into a social relationship, a maneuver which may undermine subsequent therapeutic interventions by the nurse.

Observation and identification of neurotic behavior take more time and require greater acuity than the more obviously pathological behavior of some other psychiatric disorders. For this reason, in the initial stages of contact with the neurotic patient the nurse, although friendly, should maintain a degree of detachment which will permit him to observe the patient objectively. Time is needed to learn as much as possible about the patient before determining the goals of nursing therapy for a particular patient.

Anxiety, the Basic Symptom in Psychoneurosis

Psychoneurotic patients are often assailed by an upsurge of anxiety when they first begin psychiatric treatment. Anxiety, as has been mentioned, is basic to all psychoneurotic conditions (Horney, 1939). The underlying anxiety is frequently increased by fear of the therapeutic situation, that is, fear of facing the psychiatrist alone in the interview and fear of self-revelation. If the neurotic patient must be hospitalized, this adds to his initial anxiety the fear of the hospital environment itself, fear of other patients, fear of being mentally ill, and fear of the attitudes of family and friends. The patient's heightened anxiety may be the first nursing problem the nurse encounters. It can be very reassuring to a patient to have the nurse identify himself as *his* nurse and inform him that he will be available at definite periods of time.

Nonspecific Methods for Reducing Anxiety

There are many techniques which the nurse can use during contacts with the patient to decrease his anxiety. Some of the well-known, nonspecific methods include the mere physical presence of the nurse, an attitude of interest and concern for the patient, a willingness to listen attentively, and the ability to facilitate his communication. Other ways of reducing anxiety can be selected to meet the specific needs of the particular patient in a particular situation. It is well to remember, however, that anxiety is not always undesirable in therapy. Some degree of anxiety is necessary to motivate the patient to relinquish his neurotic patterns of behavior and to work toward healthier adaptations to living. It is only when anxiety reaches the stage that it inhibits therapy or even immobilizes the patient or causes him undue suffering that the nurse should try to reduce his anxiety to more comfortable limits. The need for careful and frequent collaboration between the nurse and the psychiatrist to determine the patient's level of tolerance and the methods of alleviating anxiety is obvious.

Identification of Neurotic Patterns
of Behavior

Psychoneurotic patients have characteristic ways of behaving in their relationships with other people, based on what are called *neurotic patterns.* These patterns of behavior are used repeatedly in a wide variety of situations in a rather automatic, stereotyped way; and the neurotic person depends on them more and more as time goes on. The continued use of neurotic patterns makes for the narrow range of behavior and the rigidity which characterize his interactions with others. In the initial stages of caring for a psychoneurotic patient, the nurse has the opportunity to identify a patient's particular neurotic patterns by careful and repeated observations of his behavior.

The neurotic individual himself is almost always unaware of both the sequence of events which constitute the neurotic pattern and the fact that he tends to use this same pattern repeatedly. The nurse is often in a highly advantageous position to observe this behavior directly. This fact has two important consequences for the patient's total treatment plan. One is that the nurse's observations can be reported to the patient's psychiatrist, who frequently does not have any direct or personal knowledge of the patient's interactions with other people. This information can be useful to him in his psychotherapeutic work with the patient. The nurse can also utilize these observations to help the patient become aware of his behavior at the time it is occurring by drawing attention to his behavior and giving him an opportunity to talk about it.

Verbal Interaction with
Psychoneurotic Patients

Psychoneurotic patients are repressed individuals in the sense that they suffer from conflicts which result in constricting their lives. Unlike psychotic patients, who often have difficulty in communicating verbally, most psychoneurotic patients have little difficulty in talking. However, their conversation is often vague and unrevealing as to the kind of persons they are, and their lives are not so rich or full as one might expect from their opportunities. It is often helpful in talking with such a patient to facilitate his self-expression in a variety of ways. Neurotic patients often have a very poor opinion of themselves. They perceive themselves as helpless, inferior, uninteresting to others, discontented and bored with themselves, victims of others, and, above all, unable to make decisions. When the patient is encouraged to talk about himself, he is often surprised to discover how little he really knows about himself, his likes and dislikes, his hopes and ambitions.

Fromm-Reichmann (1950) suggests that encouraging a patient to give a detailed description of his customary daily activities can be useful in giving him some awareness of the limitations his neurotic behavior is imposing upon him. The patient's conversations with his nurse can be focused on helping him to take an objective view of his present life. Discussion of events in his past can be very fruitful in his interviews with his psychiatrist, but in his talks with the nurse discussion of past events too often provides a way of escape from looking at present behavior. In contrast, discussions centered on current daily experiences can provide the nurse with leads to problems which patient and nurse can work on together, the solution of which will be of practical use to the patient in his interactions with others.

Assisting the Patient Widen His
Sphere of Interests

Severely neurotic patients frequently lead dull and joyless lives devoid of pleasure. Often they are products of a puritanical upbringing, with the result that they may be uncomfortable and unskilled in recreational and social activities. Some patients may need not only psychological support to overcome their inhibitions about enjoying such activities but they may also need varying degrees of actual instruction and assistance in order to participate. Social situations may pose problems for other patients which prevent or inhibit social interaction with others. It is part of the nurse's responsibility to be aware of these problem areas in the patient's life and to recognize their practical importance to the patient. It is not necessary, however, to take an active role in trying to meet these needs for the patient as one might do with a psychotic patient. For the neurotic patient, it is more helpful for the patient to discuss with the nurse the specific aspects of the social situation which are troublesome to him and to let him work out his own solutions to the difficulty.

The nurse can facilitate the patient's means of self-expression by stimulating his interest in social, recreational, and creative activities. Painting, sculpture, music, creative writing, and drama are all excellent media for providing outlets for the patient's self-expression, broadening his horizons, and enriching his life. Many people possess latent creative abilities they are quite unaware of or which they have had no opportunity to develop. The discovery and utilization of these hidden talents can provide a source of great personal satisfaction. A perceptive nurse may stimulate the patient's interest by accompanying him to concerts, plays, art exhibits, libraries, and book shops. If the patient shows an interest in any of these creative activities the nurse may be able to suggest ways of obtaining instruction, materials, and equipment. The nurse himself must have an authentic appreciation of the value of the creative arts in human life in order to communicate an interest in them to his patient.

Motivating the Patient Relinquish
Neurotic Behavior

The core problem in the treatment of the psychoneurotic patient, according to Horney (1939), Fromm-Reichmann (1950), and Angyal (1965) is the investigation of the actual operation of the neurotic patterns or trends and the consequences of such patterns on the patient's life. The patient must recognize the price he pays for his neurotic behavior and become so discontented with himself that he wants to change his behavior. However, at the same time that he insists he wants to change, he also would like to keep his neurotic behavior. In other words, he is afraid to give it up—afraid to be happy. This is the dilemma of the psychoneurotic patient and the reason he offers such difficulties in treatment to every member of the therapeutic team. The major burden in therapy, as has been stated, falls on the psychiatrist. The nurse can supplement the therapeutic work of the psychiatrist by helping the patient to become aware of his neurotic behavior as it occurs in the actual setting.

Helping the Patient Become Aware of
Neurotic Behavior

Patients have different ways of reacting to awareness of their neurotic behavior. For some patients anxiety is decreased by conscious awareness of it. These patients can often be taught to watch for the recurrence of the particular behavior, and when it occurs to make an effort to overcome it. Other patients tend to become more anxious. The therapist must be careful to give such patients only the degree of insight into their behavior that they can tolerate. Laughlin (1967) describes a reaction of intense hostility with which some neurotic patients respond to an interpretation of their behavior. He calls this the *King David reaction,* after the Biblical account (II Samuel 12:1–5) of King David's rage on hearing a story told to him by the prophet Nathan in which David, in a flash of insight, recognized the behavior of the leading character as similar to his own.

Helping the Patient Deal with Repressed Hostility

Some degree of repressed hostility is present in all psychoneuroses. Much of the patient's neurotic behavior revolves around his efforts to keep it repressed. The neurotic patient is very much afraid of his own hostility—afraid that if he permits any expression of it, it will get out of control. A tremendous amount of psychic energy is invested to keep hostility repressed. This impoverishes other areas of his personality and is responsible for the rigidity and constriction of the neurotic individual's life. One goal of therapy is to free the patient from his inordinate fear of hostility. If the patient has a good relationship with his nurse, he may feel comfortable and relaxed enough in his presence to make some tentative expressions of disapproval or anger without feeling threatened. He should be permitted to do this at his own pace. It is not wise to openly encourage the patient's expression of hostility, because he may interpret this as permission for uninhibited expression, or his anxiety may become so great that he is completely blocked from any expression of feeling (Fromm-Reichmann, 1950).

The nurse also needs to know how to handle his own feelings, should the patient direct his hostility toward him. In this regard, Fromm-Reichmann advises that if the patient makes accusations against the therapist, no defense should be made, nor should the therapist pretend to have no emotional reaction to the experience of anger. In the course of treatment the neurotic patient can learn gradually how to express anger in ways that are not destructive. When this occurs, he becomes more spontaneous in his behavior, and is able to expand his range of interests and activities. His nurse can be helpful in giving him support and assistance during this difficult and critical time.

Helping the Patient Make Decisions

Another major area of difficulty is that of decision making. The problems which underlie the neurotic patient's difficulties around decision making are different from those of the psychotic patient and must be treated quite differently by the nurse. In his therapy sessions with his psychiatrist, the patient investigates the obstructive forces that inhibit his psychological growth. He attempts to determine who he really is and what his feelings and beliefs are. Horney says, "Only when the patient has become interested in the question 'Who am I?' will the analyst actively try to bring to his awareness how little he does know or care about his real feelings, wishes or beliefs" (Horney, 1950). Until he is aware of his personal likes and dislikes, he is unable to commit himself to anything, and without commitment he has no real interest in the outcome of any decision.

It is of great therapeutic importance for the patient to utilize the insights gained in psychotherapy in everyday living experiences. Learning to make decisions can be one way of utilizing such insights. The nurse can encourage the patient to make his own decisions, particularly those which concern his person, his possessions, and his personal welfare. When he is hesitant or ambivalent it may be helpful to discuss with him the available choices, clarify ambiguities, supply information, or, better still, encourage him to obtain his own information and to convey to him the expectation that he will be able to make a decision. So long as he remains dependent on the decisions of others he will never achieve self-realization. The therapeutic setting— whether it is a hospital ward, day care center, clinic, or patient's home—can provide many opportunities for the patient to test his ability to make decisions and to evaluate these decisions with his psychiatrist or nurse.

Acting-out Behavior in Psychoneurotic Patients

When some neurotic patients begin to get deeply involved in psychotherapy they struggle against it by engaging in acting-out behavior. Acting-out behavior in neurotic patients is generally not as dramatic or self-destructive as the acting-out behavior of manic-depressive patients, but it can pose equal difficulties for the nurse. It should be strongly discouraged, since it undermines the acquisition of insight into neurotic conflicts. Fromm-Reichmann says that in neurotic patients, acting out is an expression of resistance against interpretative clarification, since what is acted out lends itself much less easily to interpretative investigation than what is verbalized. She recommends that when it occurs it should be curbed.

Since neurotic patients as a rule have much better self-control than psychotic patients, it is often possible to get them to see the consequences of their acting-out behavior and to assume responsibility for it. When the patient cannot develop internal controls, it will be necessary for the nurse to set limits for the patient's behavior. If this is done, other personnel should know that these limits are so that they can cooperate in maintaining these external controls for the patient.

Helping the Patient Apply Insights to Situations in Daily Life

Although the neurotic patient generally does not appear as psychologically disabled as do other psychiatric patients, progress may be slow and treatment prolonged. The neurotic patient gives up his neurotic behavior only after a stubborn battle. However, when he had made some progress, he often develops a greater incentive to change. The nurse can be supportive as she attempts to translate the insights gained in therapy into changes of behavior, applied to widely differing sets of circumstances. For example, a woman patient may learn to deal with her neurotic response to rejection from a male patient but not able to tolerate it from the head nurse. Discussion of this problem with her nurse, with amplification of details, clarification, recollection of her feelings, and similarities and differences between the two instances involving two different individuals in two different situations, may help her to become aware of the unresolved aspects of the problem which need further work.

Fromm-Reichmann (1950) believes that one should push neurotic patients who use delaying tactics to work harder in treatment toward an understanding of the central dynamics of their difficulties, particularly if they are in a protective environment. If the hospital setting the nurse can also keep this principle in mind in contacts with such patients. He can further the psychiatrist's therapeutic goal by helping the patient to become aware of the way his neurotic difficulties manifest themselves in his daily living experiences on the ward. This two-way approach, the discussions with the psychiatrist focused on the central problem and confrontation with its manifestations on the ward, makes it very difficult for the patient to avoid facing his problems. The supportive nursing care which is also available in the hospital setting enables him to tolerate a greater degree of anxiety than would be possible for him to tolerate in a less protective environment.

Helping the Patient Attain Greater Autonomy

The goal of nursing care with the neurotic patient is to help him become more self-reliant and independent. As the patient improves, the nurse should withdraw his support so that eventually his services will be unneccessary. This is the ideal way of terminating nursing care.

If the patient must leave the hospital before he is able to function independently, it would be desirable for the nurse to make some follow-up visits, gradually increasing the interval of time between visits until the are no longer necessary. Fromm-Reichmann believes that it is unnecessary for professional personnel to educate the relatives when the patient returns home. She thinks that the patient is quite capable of doing this himself.

<h2 style="text-align:center">Nursing Care of Some Specific
Psychoneurotic Reactions</h2>

Earlier in the chapter it was pointed out that the clinical picture of the psychoneurotic patient is a very fluid one; that it varies in degree from behavior that appears near-normal to near-psychotic; and that the same defense mechanisms and symptoms may occur in many types of psychoneuroses. It is, therefore, difficult to describe clear-cut sub-types of psychoneuroses. Harry Stack Sullivan (1956) believed that all dynamisms or defense mechanisms are available to patients, but that they tend to manifest one of them more frequently, and that this gives the special coloring to the particular psychoneurosis. The defense mechanisms used by psychoneurotics are used by everybody in times of stress, but certain individuals characteristically use one dynamism or defense mechanism in their interpersonal relationships with others. Sullivan thought that a psychoneurotic patient could utilize different dynamisms if need be. He wrote, "Whenever a certain type of problem is the major problem of the moment, it will call out a dynamism definitely different from the dynamism that characterizes the patient's 'basic living.'" He gave a hypothetical example of an obsessive patient who might react to a very domineering employer with a hysterical reaction. With this background in mind, some of the special problems in nursing related to the particular psychoneurotic reactions will be considered.

<h3 style="text-align:center">Anxiety Reactions</h3>

Symptomatology Anxiety reactions occur commonly in everyday life in individuals who are caught up in stressful situations as well as in patients suffering from other psychiatric and somatic disorders. Psychoneurotic patients with anxiety reactions are persons whose outstanding symptom is acute anxiety. They look anxious, feel anxious, and usually express anxious thoughts and ideas. They are often extremely tense, restless, and oppressed by a sense of impending doom. Characteristic of anxiety reaction is the fact that patients are unable to

347

identify any basis for their anxiety—the "free-floating" anxiety described by Freud. A wide variety of physiological as well as psychological symptoms may be manifested in patients with anxiety reactions. These include tremors, dyspnea, palpitation, tachycardia, excessive perspiration, frequent urination, and diarrhea, among the more common physiological symptoms, and various degrees of fear and anxiety ranging from vague feelings of uneasiness to outright panic, as well as depression, confusion, tenseness, agitation, and restlessness among the psychological symptoms.

Prognosis The prognosis in anxiety reactions is generally considered to be favorable, possibly because of the fluid character of the clinical manifestations, such as the ease with which symptoms can appear and disappear, and the absence of specific or highly organized defense mechanisms. This good prognosis, however, does not necessarily imply that patients with anxiety reaction are easy to treat. On the contrary, they often present many difficult problems in their medical and nursing care

Treatment in Acute Anxiety Reactions Most authorities agree that psychotherapy is the treatment of choice, usually psychoanalysis or psychoanalytically oriented psychotherapy. Tranquilizing and sedative drugs may be prescribed as adjunctive measures. Some patients have transient or sporadic attacks of anxiety, but other patients may suffer from a chronic state of anxiety. The treatment of these two forms of anxiety differs. The primary goal of treatment in the first instance is relief of the acute anxiety. This may be accomplished by brief, intensive treatment, which may include the use of drugs, especially if the anxiety is severe or the patient is old or has a low tolerance for anxiety.

A brief period of hospitalization may be necessary. It may be helpful to remove the patient from a stressful situation at home and also to provide the reassurance of constant nursing care and therapeutic measures such as hydrotherapy and occupational and recreational therapy. Some authorities think that hospitalization is undesirable because of the high suggestibility of these patients—that when hospitalized their anxiety is increased by the anxiety of other patients. Brief psychotherapy which offers the patient emotional catharsis and desensitization of the anxiety has been recommended.

Some Measures to Reduce Anxiety—Serenity of the Nurse In the nursing care of patients with acute anxiety reactions, it is important for the nurse not to appear anxious to the patient. Anxiety is very easily transmitted and patients are quick to detect signs of anxiety in the staff. If the patient does perceive anxiety in the personnel, it increases his own anxiety and confirms his fears of the seriousness of his condition.

Ruesch (1961) says that the anxious person expects that the therapist will be anxious. He suggests that talking to the patient in short, simple sentences in a firm, authoritative voice and appearing without anxiety can exert great therapeutic effect on the patient.

Nurse's Physical Presence, and Nonverbal Reassurance   The nurse can also lower the level of the patient's anxiety by his mere presence. An anxious patient should never be isolated from human contact to endure his attacks of anxiety by himself. The nurse's helpfulness can be increased by nonverbal communication of reassurance to the patient. Touch can often be used effectively for this purpose when other avenues prove fruitless (Ruesch, 1961).

Detecting Covert Anxiety   The observant nurse can often detect subtle indications of anxiety in a patient and intervene to prevent a full-blown attack of anxiety, or, if it is not possible to prevent an attack, at least to mitigate it. There are some patients who are very successful in covering up their anxiety. Nevertheless, something of their underlying tension is transmitted to a sensitive observer. Fromm-Reichmann says that when a therapist finds himself becoming anxious in the presence of a patient when there is nothing in the situation or in himself to account for this, he should consider the possibility that the source of anxiety is in the patient (Fromm-Reichmann, 1950).

Listening   Listening is one of the most effective methods of reducing anxiety. The nurse can often perform no more valuable aid to the patient than to take him to a quiet room and, without questions or probing, simply listen to him until the peak of his anxiety and tension has eased. If, in addition to listening, the nurse can convey understanding of his difficulties and acknowledgment of his anxiety, this further relieves his anxiety. Portnoy (1959) has summed it up very well in the following statement:

> The therapist's ability to convey to the patient, through non-verbal as well as verbal means, his sympathetic acceptance of the reality of the patient's suffering (though he is not caught up in the uses to which the patient puts his compulsive need to suffer); his refusal to view the experience as catastrophic; his ability often to protect the patient from his own self-destructiveness—these are among the psychotherapeutic approaches which may help relieve the intensity of the patient's anxiety and suffering.

Awareness of Demands as Expressions of Anxiety   Anxiety makes many patients very demanding. How the nurse reacts to this behavior may affect the course of the anxiety attack. He will have to decide whether meeting the patient's demands will allay his anxiety or whether he is asking for security rather than for the object of his request. In the latter case, it may be more reassuring to the patient to set limits on his behavior by denying his request. Anxious patients should not be asked to make decisions or to give reasons for their behavior. This should wait until such times as their anxiety subsides.

Other Measures to Reduce Anxiety Anxiety can also be relieved by activity, such as performing some routine physical task. Information giving, clarification and validation of doubtful information, and labeling or giving a name to fears and doubts can also be reassuring to anxious patients. Sometimes it is also possible for anxiety to be converted to some other affect such as anger. This, too, is effective in reducing anxiety.

Treatment of Prolonged Anxiety Reactions Patients who suffer from prolonged states of anxiety require somewhat different treatment from those suffering acute anxiety reactions. The level of anxiety is generally not so high as in the acute reactions, but in many ways patients with chronic anxiety reactions are more difficult to treat. Their anxiety is primarily one of a long-standing personality problem. The goal of treatment is a change in their basic personality. The treatment of choice is generally considered to be psychoanalysis or some other form of intensive psychotherapy.

Role of the Nurse—Supportive Measures The role of the nurse is one of giving emotional support to the patient and supplementing the insights gained in psychotherapeutic interviews with the psychiatrist by their application to everyday living experience. Abreactions may occur following the return of the patient to the unit after a psychotherapeutic interview. At these times, the patient may need special attention from the nurse—including remaining with him until he is calmer, and listening to him. Consultation with the psychiatrist regarding his suggestions for dealing with these situations is important.

In the more prolonged anxiety reactions, one of the subsidiary goals of treatment is to help the patient to identify those incidents or situations which tend to make him anxious. The nurse can help the patient with this identification by observing his signs of tension, often when he is unaware of them. It is then possible for the patient to avoid such situations until he is less vulnerable. The nurse may also be able to identify unwholesome environmental factors in the home, hospital, or community which the psychiatrist or social worker could alter for the patient's benefit.

Facilitating Desensitization During the course of psychotherapy, when the patient has gained sufficient support and insight, these critical situations lose much of their anxiety-producing effect. However, intellectual insight is not enough. Eventually the psychiatrist wants his patient to face these same situations in everyday life. It may be easier for the patient to do this at first with the emotional support of his nurse. After he has weathered one or two of these encounters successfully, he will be able to face them by himself. This process of confronting and gradually overcoming a dreaded experience is called *desensitization.* It is essentially a method of teaching the patient to endure increasing amounts of anxiety without becoming immobilized.

Planning a Daily Schedule   A daily schedule of activities can be a useful adjunct in the nursing care of the patient with anxiety reactions. This schedule should be worked out collaboratively by the nurse and psychiatrist to meet the particular needs and interests of the patient. This should not be done until the nurse has had an opportunity to become acquainted with the patient's tastes, talents, and creative abilities. Such a planned schedule seems to offer many anxious patients a feeling of security and stability. Mild recreational activities such as walking are therapeutic for the anxious patient. Games such as volley ball and ping-pong, which are fast enough to demand the patient's full attention, are also helpful. Group singing is excellent for relieving tension. Patients who respond to music find this useful. Diversional activities that will distract the patient's thoughts from his anxiety can be beneficial if not carried to excess. The patient's primary task is to work on his psychological problems. Patients also need time to think and to rest. This need is often forgotten by the staff in planning the total treatment of the patient.

Encouraging Socialization   Patients who suffer from anxiety reactions have a tendency to protect themselves from any situation that they fear may possibly reactivate their anxiety. This includes social activities, which the patient should be encouraged to attend in spite of his fears, though not until his anxiety has abated and he has established a good relationship with his nurse. When the patient first attends activities, his nurse should accompany him and reassure him that he may leave whenever he becomes uncomfortable. Another responsibility of his nurse is to protect him from overzealous personnel who may urge him to remain.

Dissociative and Conversion Reactions

Symptomatology   Dissociative and conversion reactions are character-ized by dramatic symptomatology of great variety which were formerly classified under the common term of *hysteria.* Gross disturbances of consciousness, such as fugues, fainting spells, amnesias, somnambul-isms, trances, and convulsions, are included in the dissociative reac-tions. Conversion reactions are so called because the anxiety derived from underlying intrapsychic conflicts is converted or expressed as somatic symptoms. These symptoms may resemble symptoms of known physical origin; however when examined closely they are found to be not organic but functional.

The range of symptoms is almost limitless. Among the more commonly encountered manifestations are blindness, deafness, aphonia, pain, numbness, tingling, itching, swelling, vomiting, dysphagia, globus hystericus, and paralyses of all kinds. Conversion symptoms not only are manifested in conversion reactions but can occur in conjunction with other psychiatric disorders and also with medical conditions. It is not uncommon to find an admixture of conversion symptoms with other psychoneuroses, particularly in anxiety and obsessive-compulsive reactions.

Characteristic Behavior A characteristic behavior pattern begins to emerge as the patient with a conversion reaction is observed. At the same time that he complains bitterly of pain and discomfort, he displays a peculiar calm or indifference to his symptoms (*la belle indifférence*). He tends to describe his symptoms in great detail, yet does not appear concerned. If the physician informs the patient that he can find no physical basis for his symptoms, this knowledge gives the patient no relief. He generally questions the validity of the examination and consults another physician.

Patients with this type of psychoneurosis are highly suggestible. For this reason hospitalization should be avoided if possible. If the patient with pneumonia in the next bed is breathing stertorously, the hysterical patient may develop the same symptom. If he witnesses a convulsion, he may produce one so authentic in appearance that it is difficult to differentiate from an organic seizure. Symptoms may be suggested to him during a physical examination, by reading medical texts, or even by hearing symptoms discussed that he has never seen. Conversion symptoms can sometimes be detected by the fact that they tend to follow functional rather than anatomical patterns of nerve distribution. For example, in glove and stocking anesthesia the level of anesthesia stops abruptly as though a line were drawn across the arms and legs with no regard for the actual nerve distribution.

Personality Traits Many writers are in agreement about the personality characteristics of the individual who is prone to develop a conversion reaction. Ruesch (1961) describes him as a demonstrative, exhibitionistic individual who makes every effort to obtain approval and applause. He states, "All his efforts, all decisions, and all opinions are shaped by just one desire—to make an impression. He is dependent upon his audience and willing to shape himself to the demands of the audience." Laughlin (1967) describes patients with conversion reactions as egocentric, emotionally labile or capricious, immature, attention-seeking, impulsive in their behavior with little regard for the consequences, uninhibited, dramatic, suggestible, imitative, frequently shallow in their emotional relationships, apparent dependence and helplessness combined with rebelliousness, and immature in their sexual adjustment.

Treatment Treatment recommended by most authorities for conversion reactions is psychoanalysis or psychoanalytically oriented psychotherapy. Laughlin (1967) states that this is the only approach that offers permanent relief. He writes, "In the successful case, the personality and character changes which are the consequence of the work of therapy are the basic ones." Other types of psychotherapy which have been used with varying degrees of success include suggestion, hypnosis, and reeducative and supportive psychotherapy. Occasionally, drugs such as intravenous injections of Pentothal or sodium amytal have been used, but in general the results have been disappointing.

Treatment of Disturbed Communication Patterns and Interpersonal Relationships Sullivan and Ruesch have described the interpersonal difficulties which characterize the person with conversion symptoms and have approached the problem of treatment from this point of view. Sullivan perceives the hysterical person as an immature individual who has missed out on life experiences that are commonly experienced by others. As one result of this, their communications with others are characterized by many gaps. Though their conversation sounds reasonable and logical, the careful listener is aware of these gaps. Sullivan says it is not what the hysteric says but what he omits that is important. He describes their conversation as sounding "like poor fiction— incredible or unreal." In treating such patients he recommends that the therapist give the patient correct data, tone down his extravagances while listening to him, and express skepticism of the patient's oversimplified explanations (Sullivan, 1956).

Long-term therapy which is focused on correction of distortions in communication eventually results in improvement. Sullivan warns against setting therapeutic goals too high for these patients. He sees them limited in their sensitivity to the reactions of others and in the depth of their emotional relationships. He says that one shouldn't expect the hysteric to become a great student of human personality, and advises him to choose a vocation in which relationships with others are simple and discriminating judgments are not required.

Ruesch (1957) regards the sociability of the hysterical personality an asset in therapy and the reason psychoanalysis and psychotherapy are effective with these patients. He belives that the patient's difficulty in interpersonal relationships is due to faulty patterns of communication. For example, interacting with another person, he says one thing and does another, with the real meaning in the action. On the other hand, when he is observing or perceiving another person he tends to overlook the action of the other person and focus his attention on what is being said, with special concern for possible hidden meanings. The goal in therapy is to help the patient integrate the meaning of the action and the verbal components of an event.

Acting-out Behavior In line with the observation that the hysterical person invests more meaning in what he does than in what he says, one can understand his propensity for acting-out behavior. In therapy Fromm-Reichmann and others try to prohibit acting out and encourage the patient to express himself verbally. Pearce (1963) says, "A necessary technique in therapy with these patients is the art of being pleasantly rude and incisive, with enough good nature to brush aside whole areas of the patient's verbalizations in order to focus on the genuine content of his production. One therapeutic task is to facilitate the patient's learning more about the use of words for communication, partly by clarifying that what he has done so far is not that."

The Role of the Nurse The problem of nursing these patients is not a simple one. In addition to his conversion symptoms, the patient often has personality traits that make him a difficult person to care for. In the hospital setting, he is adept at creating scenes in which he is the chief actor before a captive audience of nursing personnel and patients. He is indifferent to the needs of other patients and he is completely self-centered in demanding attention for himself. He frequently tries to embarrass the nursing personnel by maneuvering them into awkward situations. If he is frustrated he may try to gain his ends by skillful manipulation or acting-out behavior. It is often difficult to maintain composure and to treat such a patient with the kindness, understanding, tolerance, and nonjudgmental attitude that therapeutic nursing care requires.

Unless the nurse is able to cope with his own emotions he cannot nurse the patient effectively. It is often helpful to remember that the patient does not consciously produce his symptoms nor is he aware of the effects of his behavior on others. Some of the measures that can be taken to overcome negative feelings toward the patient are observing him, developing a relationship with him, reading his history, conferring with colleagues about him, and, if possible, validating impressions about him with family and friends. In the latter regard, Sullivan (1956) states that obtaining collateral information is very important. Distortions can occur very easily in evaluation of a patient with conversion reaction. This is due to his poorly developed self-concept and his tendency to give the kind of information that he thinks the other person would like to have.

Nursing the Whole Patient   In regard to the conversion symptoms *per se,* it is not helpful to focus the patient's attention on his most prominent symptom. For example, instead of trying to get a functionally paralyzed patient to walk, the nurse should try to discover the patient's psychological need for this symptom. A well-known psychiatric axiom states, "Ignore the symptom but never the patient." To concentrate on the symptom is to give greater importance to it, and hence make it more difficult for the patient to relinquish it.

Understanding the Meaning of the Patient's Symptom   The patient uses his symptoms as a plea for help, attention, and affection. His symptoms serve his deep needs for dependence which have never been fulfilled. They also satisfy his love of the dramatic and, by making him interesting to himself and others, help to raise his self-esteem. Contrary to the impression given by his assured manner, his opinion of himself is, in reality, often very low. In addition, his symptoms may absolve him from onerous duties or get him out of difficult life situations.

When the nurse who is aware of his low self-esteem gives the patient what he really wants, that is, consideration for himself as a person, his symptoms become less important to him. The attractions of illness have a strong hold on many individuals, particularly patients with conversion reactions. The importance of the role played by the secondary gains of illness in the success or failure of treatment should not be underestimated.

Evaluation of Symptoms   In apparent contradiction to what has just been said about not showing concern about particular symptoms in the patient's presence, the nurse should evaluate every symptom carefully. A patient with a conversion reaction may also develop a physical illness. By careful observation and evaluation of clinical data, the nurse should try to determine whether the patient requires immediate medical or psychiatric attention. Without arousing undue apprehension in the patient, the nurse should take the appropriate measures. Meanwhile, the general psychological treatment of the patient should not be neglected. An attempt should be made to determine what psychological incidents occurred just before the symptoms developed and, if possible, what emotional needs the symptom served.

Nurse-Patient Relationship with Patients with Conversion Reactions.- The development of sustained relationship between nurse and patient as in a nurse-patient relationship can be a very effective method of providing therapeutic nursing care to the patient with a conversion reaction. Such a relationship can provide a framework within which some of the immature aspects of the patient's personality can attain greater maturity. The nurse has many opportunities to help the patient become aware of his behavior and its reactions on other people. He may also serve as a model for more mature ways of relating to others. These patients also can benefit from group nursing psychotherapy. Like adolescents, whom they resemble in some of their behavior, patients with conversion reactions are very sensitive to group opinion. The group also serves as a stabilizer or control for some of their impulsive, acting-out behavior and emotional lability. In a sense they can experience a kind of delayed adolescence in the carefully structured setting of the therapeutic milieu or therapeutic community.

Phobic Reactions

Symptomatology A *phobic reaction* is a psychoneurosis in which the patient is harassed by uncontrollable and irrational fears which are called *phobias.* Laughlin (1967) defines a *phobia* as a "specific pathologic fear out of proportion to the apparent stimulus, which has been unconsciously attached to a specific external object or situation. A phobia is an obsessive, unrealistic fear which is inappropriate and unreasoning. It is beyond voluntary control and cannot adequately or logically be explained by the patient." A great deal of anxiety is generated in the patient with phobias. Phobias may be associated with a wide range of objects or situations from which the specific phobias derive their names. A few of the more common ones include claustrophobia (fear of closed places), agoraphobia (fear of open spaces), acrophobia (fear of high places), brontophobia (fear of thunder), mysophobia (fear of dirt), nyctophobia (fear of the dark), and photophobia (fear of light).

Morbidity A phobic reaction has a crippling effect on the life of the individual suffering from this type of psychoneurosis. The degree of limitation will depend on the number of phobias he has, their severity, the specific objects or situations involved, and the frequency with which he is likely to encounter these objects or situations in his environment. For example, a person may have a severe fear of thunder, but if he lives where thunder is a rare occurrence he will not be greatly affected. However, a person suffering from a fear of open spaces may virtually become a prisoner in his own house.

Treatment When an individual's phobias begin to interfere with the performance of his work, participation in social and recreational activities, and his interpersonal relationships, he generally seeks psychiatric treatment. Psychotherapy based on dynamic principles is the treatment of choice. Though patients with phobic reactions are generally cooperative, treatment is often long and difficult. Laughlin (1967) states that the treatment of these patients represents a major therapeutic challenge and that the completion of definitive treatment can take years of hard work. Friedman (1959) says that the phobic patient's need for dependency and protection presages a good prognosis, especially if treatment is undertaken early. He also emphasizes the importance of the therapist's skill and understanding of dynamics in enabling the patient to give up his neurotic symptoms.

Role of the Nurse—Nurse-Patient Relationship. Some of the techniques which psychiatrists have found useful in the treatment of the phobic patient would seem applicable also in his nursing care. In the early stages of treatment, it is helpful to draw the patient's attention away from his phobia and instead to focus on the patient's awareness of himself and on the occurrences of his daily life. This can be done effectively within the structure of a therapeutic nurse-patient relationship. Because anxiety often plays a prominent role in phobic reaction, the nurse should proceed slowly to develop a sound relationship.

Desensitization When the patient's anxiety has decreased and the nurse thinks that the relationship is on a secure basis he may begin to utilize the relationship for treatment purposes. After consultation with the psychiatrist, the nurse may initiate nursing interventions to supplement the insights gained in psychotherapeutic interviews with the psychiatrist in the desensitization of the patient to phobic situations, that is, to help the patient become less fearful of the specific phobic situation.

Mastering Techniques The nurse may also help the patient in relearning and retraining by helping him to meet a situation and to try to master it gradually, or to repeat an experience until it is no longer able to distress him. If the patient makes no effort to face his phobic situation or seems unready or unable to do so, the nurse should not persist but should refer the matter to the psychiatrist. He may either want to wait until the patient is less anxious or to discuss this lack of effort with the patient in an interview.

Friedman (1959), in his article on the phobias, writes, "Freud stressed the necessity of exposing the phobic patient to the dreaded situation or object, and he warned that one can hardly ever master a phobia if one waits till the patient lets the analysis influence him to give it up. He will never in that case bring to the analysis the material indispensable for a convincing solution of the phobia. Hence it is very often necessary for the analyst to intervene more actively and to insist that the patient brave the phobic situation." The emotional support which the nurse can offer the patient when he is trying to master his phobias can make things easier for him and encourage him to continue his efforts. Interested and sympathetic relatives and friends can also provide additional incentive and support.

Obsessive-Compulsive Reactions

Patients with obsessive-compulsive reactions are characterized by the manifestation of obsessions or compulsions or both. Obsessions are recurring thoughts which cannot be dismissed readily from consciousness; some obsessions may be trivial or ridiculous in nature; others are morbid or fearful, such as an obsessive thought that one might harm one's children or experience some catastrophe. Compulsions are acts which often seem meaningless or silly yet must be performed in order to relieve unbearable tension. The psychodynamics of obsessions and compulsions are closely related. Obsessions represent released unconscious instinctual impulses which have become attached to some conscious but apparently unrelated idea or ideas. Similarly, compulsions have been described as obsessions in action.

Characteristic Personality A characteristic personality type has been observed in persons who develop obsessive-compulsive reactions, known as the obsessive-compulsive personality. These individuals are neat, orderly, overly cautious, rigid in their thinking, and methodical in their ways. They have strong dependency needs, but are shy and ineffective in obtaining satisfaction for these needs. They tend to be somewhat detached and emotionally cool in their relationships with others, and because of their moralistic attitudes, stubbornly maintained opinions, and insistence on correct manners and procedures are often unpopular socially. Their considerable hostility is carefully repressed and its indirect expression appears in the form of procrastination, stubbornness, and indecision. Sullivan (1956) says that the obsessional person cries only from rage. Often, such persons are overly intellectual and tend to separate intellect from feeling. A curious air of pessimism seems to permeate their personality as though life had little purpose and offered little enjoyment.

Many of these personality traits are highly valued in our culture, and many individuals with obsessive-compulsive personalities are successful and influential members of the community. Occupations and professions in which many of these traits are very useful include banking, scientific research and scholarly investigation, curating, collecting, laboratory work, writing, editing, accounting, and library work, to name a few. Many highly skilled crafts demand some of these traits in their workers. However, when these traits are overemphasized or become too rigid, they constitute liabilities rather than assets. When the individual reaches the point that frank symptoms of obsessions and compulsions develop he may be said to suffer from a psychoneurosis. Obsessive-compulsive reactions may become so severe that the individual is unable to function personally, socially, or professionally.

Treatment   Most authorities agree that intensive, long-term investigative psychotherapy is required for effective treatment. The close cooperation between psychiatrist and patient is necessary to identify the underlying, unsatisfied needs of the patient for which the obsessive and compulsive symptoms act as defenses. These defenses, which are out of the patient's voluntary control, become so much a part of his personality that they are not easily dislodged. Laughlin writes, "They [character defenses] cannot be removed surgically as we might amputate an extremity, or by logic, or by force. They can only be modified voluntarily by the individual concerned when, through greater insight, he is ready, willing and able to forego some of the underlying psychologic needs" (Laughlin, 1967, p. 300).

Reconstructive Therapy   Rado regards the obsessive-compulsive patient as fixed at or regressed to the level of infantile dependence, and advocates *reconstructive therapy,* a type of psychoanalytic therapy in which treatment is viewed as a reconstructive process leading to greater maturity. The goals of reconstructive treatment are to remove the blocks of inhibitions to full maturation and to promote psychological development by emotional reeducation and by keeping the patient at the level of adult, self-reliant cooperation throughout the treatment. Rado (1959) sees some danger in "classic" psychoanalytic procedure in that it tends to foster dependency needs in the obsessional patient. Less intensive methods of psychotherapy and other forms of therapy such as somatic and drug therapy have not proved useful in treating these patients.

The Role of the Nurse   Since the nurse usually encounters patients with obsessive-compulsive reactions only when their condition has become incapacitating, they often present difficult problems in nursing care and make special emotional demands on the nurse as a therapeutic agent. If the psychiatrist is treating the patient with intensive psychotherapy, he should confer with the nurse, indicating how he wishes her to deal with the patient's compulsive behavior.

Coping with Compulsions   Some psychiatrists prefer to have the patient's obsessive-compulsive behavior ignored, preferring that nursing attention be directed to his total psychological needs. Other psychiatrists will allow a certain degree of permissiveness toward compulsive behavior, but place certain limits on this, modifying the degree of permissiveness with the patient's progress in therapy. For example, a patient with a hand-washing compulsion may be permitted to carry on this activity without intervention by the nursing personnel. The psychiatrist in this case relies on the work done in psychotherapy to take care of the symptom in the course of treatment. However, if the compulsion is one which could endanger the patient's life, as, for example, ritualistic behavior which prevents him from eating, some form of intervention by the nurse may be necessary. Patients with washing compulsions will frequently spend the entire day in washing activities, even refusing to take time to eat. Those who engage in elaborate rituals may keep others waiting interminably until they are ready to participate in an activity. It is usually wiser for the nurse to allow the others to go on without the patient and get him to join later.

Preventing Social Isolation Social withdrawal occurs frequently with these patients as the result of their obsessive-compulsive traits. As time goes on, their social life tends to become progressively restricted; interest in other people, in social issues, and in cultural pursuits declines. The nurse can often observe and, at the appropriate time, point out to the patient the emptiness of his life as the result of his constant preoccupation with his obsessions and compulsions. As Horney has said, he must become aware of the price he is paying for his neurotic behavior. When he is ready to change his way of life, the nurse can assist him in trying to broaden his horizons.

Coping with Negativistic Behavior One should never attempt to push or hurry an obsessive patient. He has a strong streak of negativism in his personality which may result in his becoming more firmly entrenched in his defenses. Patients with obsessive-compulsive reactions are very resistant to change. New ideas must be presented to them slowly and gradually. As with the phobic patient, whom they resemble in some respects, the nurse should develop a good relationship before she makes any demands or active interventions with these patients. An indirect approach is often more successful than a frontal attack in presenting something different or unaccustomed to these patients.

Communication Problems Communication with patients suffering from obsessive-compulsive reactions is often exceptionally frustrating. Sullivan (1956) has described a characteristic trait which he called "obsessional stickiness." This is exemplified by the obsessive behavior of the stutterer, of whom Sullivan observed, "You have to stick around to get any data from him." Of these individuals, he remarked that speech was not for communication but for defiance and domination.

Another communicative difficulty noted by Sullivan was that, according to the patient, the therapist is never able to get anything quite right. The patient constantly corrects, qualifies, or clarifies any account of the therapist's understanding of what the patient has told him. On the other hand, the patient constantly asks for more clarification, more details; yet the result of this pedantic striving for accuracy is, curiously, greater vagueness and lack of clarity, as though the patient did not want anything too clear. For these communication difficulties, Fromm-Reichmann recommends that one cut through the verbal static to them and then reformulate significant data.

Coping with the Patient's Sensitivity and Anxiety   Several authors have noted the problem of coping with the sensitivity and the quick flare-ups of anxiety which occur in patients with this type of reaction. Wolberg (1967) views them as individuals with weak egos who cannot tolerate anxiety. Interpersonal closeness often provokes such anxiety. For this reason he suggests less frequent contacts with the therapist than other patients have. The environment can sometimes be modified to minimize the opportunities for anxiety-provoking stimuli. Sullivan also refers to the fact that the patient's anxiety is often reduced when he is actually faced with an explanation of his behavior.

Building Up the Patient's Self-Esteem   The enhancement and maintenance of the patient's self-esteem is very important, for much of his extreme sensitivity is focused around this point. Care should be taken not to pressure the patient in his areas of sensitivity. Since these patients are noticeably lacking in a sense of humor, it is necessary to be particularly careful about joking or making humorous allusions in conversation with them. Teasing in any form, of course, is contraindicated. In any interaction in which one is trying to make these patients aware of their behavior, it should always be done in such a way that their self-esteem is not threatened.

Working with the Patient's Dependency-Independency Conflict   Wolberg cites another difficulty that nurses frequently encounter in working with a patient with obsessive-compulsive reaction: his dependency-independency conflict. This is expressed in a variety of ways. He longs to be dependent on his therapists, yet resists any and all suggestions. He asks for advice, then may ignore it or take the opposite path of action. He is afraid of any involvement with or possible obligation to the therapist. This kind of behavior may go on for a long time and be very difficult for anyone working with the patient to tolerate. Only time, patience, and, finally, the patient's awareness of his behavior and his willingness to relinquish it will solve the problem.

Coping with the Patient's Hostility   Management of the patient's hostility is another problem for the nurse as well as for the psychiatrist. When the patient first enters treatment, his hostility is usually well repressed. His rigid defenses take care that it is not openly expressed. However, when the patient begins to get involved in treatment, his hostility begins to be expressed more openly. Sullivan states that the therapist must accept repeated attacks of hostility because this is the way that the patient gets well. Obsessive-compulsive patients fear uncontrollable anger greatly; therefore, when the patient is able to attack the therapist, he no longer fears the utter destructiveness of this emotion. For the therapist the difficulty is not to become provoked into an expression of anger in response to the patient's hostility.

Sullivan warns, "Do not quarrel with an obsessional neurotic unless you want to have a lot of your time converted to as near nothing as the human being can convert time." Expression of anger also frees the patient from some of his rigidity and permits the emergence of spontaneity. When the patient is able to be spontaneous, a great change comes over him. He begins to look more alive and free. The nurse should be on the alert for evidences of more spontaneous behavior and encourage its expression.

Importance of a Good Experience Fromm-Reichmann believes that something good must happen before a patient can give up his obsessive behavior. He must enjoy some satisfactory experience before he can become aware of what he is missing in life by his obsessive behavior. The final phase of treatment is to translate the insights gained in therapy into action in daily life and to make it possible for the patient to function reasonably well in his interpersonal relationships. When the patient has become sufficiently self-assured that he can tolerate criticism from his peers, group therapy may be indicated.

Personal Characteristics of the Nurse The nurse who is warm and sympathetic can establish a relationship with the obsessive-compulsive patient. These qualities are very necessary for a nurse to have in order to care for these patients successfully. It is obvious that a great deal of patience and understanding are required of the nurse. It is often difficult for the nurse to overcome feelings of impatience and frustration with the patients' behavior and still retain a therapeutic attitude and feelings of genuine concern for them. A thorough understanding of the dynamics of obsessive-compulsive behavior and access to a competent supervisor or consultant should help the nurse to work with this challenging group of patients.

Depressive Reactions

Symptomatology *Depressive reaction* is the name given to a type of psychoneurosis in which the dominant symptom is depression. Other symptoms which often accompany the depression include a general slowing down of activity, a tendency to social isolation, loss of ambition, boredom, and lowered self-esteem. Patients with reactive depressions frequently have numerous physical complaints, such as fatigue, loss of appetite, sleep disturbances of both excessive sleeping and insomnia, and many other transient physical symptoms.

The psychoneurotic depressive reaction can be differentiated from psychotic depressions in that the depression usually follows some critical event in the patient's life, whereas in the psychotic depression there is usually no known precipitating event. Reactive depressions generally occur after the loss of a significant person, object, or cause (grief reaction), or following a loss of self-esteem (melancholic reaction). However, depressive reactions may also occur following what are usually considered happy events such as a promotion, the receipt of a signal honor, or the successful completion of an important work. Depressive reactions also have a number of characteristics in common with psychotic depressions, including the potentiality for suicide.

Characteristic Personality Depressive reactions may occur in individuals with differing personality types, but certain individuals are more prone to develop this particular neurotic behavior than other people are. Individuals with depressive personalities often have a pessimistic outlook on life. They tend to be chronic worriers, and they are very sensitive to slights or disappointments. Moreover, it is difficult for them to accept criticism. They are conscientious, dependable, conservative in their ideas, and conventional in their behavior. It is difficult for them to express hostility or witness it in others. Therefore they tend to placate, agree, and compromise, hiding their true feelings from others. They have inordinately strong dependency needs which they are unable to satisfy. Many of them attain positions of prominence in the community by virtue of their productiveness and sense of social responsibility. When they become depressed, they are generally not aware of their need for treatment and are often very reluctant to accept therapy.

Treatment For the treatment of patients with depressive reactions, some form of psychotherapy is recommended, but not necessarily psychoanalysis or intensive psychotherapy. In fact, Gutheil (1959) says, "Prolonged, especially orthodox, analysis is hardly ever needed to cope with this condition. Active analysis or brief psychotherapy are, as a rule, the therapies of choice." Wolberg (1967) advocates supportive therapy and group psychotherapy. Wender (1963) has found group psychotherapy helpful for hospitalized depressive patients. Laughlin and Wilson state that in the early stages of treatment ego-supportive measures are indicated. Later in the course of treatment, insight therapy may be instituted. Most psychiatrists do not use electroshock treatment, but a few still do. Drugs of the sedative and tranquilizing variety are used as adjuncts to psychotherapy but are no substitute for it. Hospitalization is generally indicated if the patient is preoccupied with suicidal ideas.

The Role of the Nurse—Development of a Relationship with the Patient Nursing care plays an important role in the treatment of the patient with a severe depressive reaction. Ruesch (1961) says that if a patient with a grief reaction is left alone, his self-destructive impulses are activated. He recommends that the psychiatrist "provide another person—for example, a nurse—to be with the patient for twenty-four hours a day. Therapy is of little help because the patient can see the doctor only for a limited period of time and what he needs is constant, benevolent, affectionate, and respectful company." In addition to being a kind and dependable companion, the nurse can go a step further and develop a therapeutic nurse-patient relationship with the patient which can be very supportive to him during the depths of his depression. Later in the course of treatment this relationship can serve to bridge the gap between the loss of the past relationship and the formation of significant future relationships.

Supportive Measures Some of the practical measures the nurse can take are to visit the patient's home, if he is not hospitalized, to see if there are morbid influences present which tend to foster his depressive mood. Fatigue can also reinforce depression; therefore, any measures that the nurse can take to help the patient get adequate rest are important. Periods of rest should alternate with periods of activity. The best form of activity for the depressed patient is work. If the patient is able to work at his usual occupation, he should be encouraged to continue. This helps him to maintain his self-esteem as well as to distract him from his morbid thoughts. If the patient is not able to engage in his customary work, the nurse may be able to find some other kind of work for him.

Encourage New Interests and New Goals for the Patient New interests should also be introduced whenever possible to counteract the boredom and staleness of life often experienced by the depressive patient. The nurse can help the patient to observe and become aware of his daily expenditure of time and to focus on the present rather than the past. He may be able to set new and more realistic goals for his life. The nurse may also be helpful to him in learning how to cope with his hostile feelings and to direct these feelings into constructive rather than destructive channels.

364

REFERENCES

Angyal, Andras (1965): *Neurosis and Treatment—A Holistic Theory*, John Wiley & Sons, Inc., New York.

Ewalt, Jack R., and Dana L. Farnsworth (1963): *Textbook of Psychiatry,* McGraw-Hill Book Company, New York.

Friedman, Paul (1959): "The Phobias," in Silvano Arieti (ed.), *American Handbook of Psychiatry,* Basic Books, Inc., Publishers, New York.

Fromm-Reichmann, Frieda (1950): *Principles of Intensive Psychotherapy,* The University of Chicago Press, Chicago.

Gutheil, Emil A. (1959): "Reactive Depressions," in Silvano Arieti (ed.), *American Handbook of Psychiatry,* Basic Books, Inc., Publishers, New York, pp. 345–352.

Horney, Karen (1950): *Neurosis and Human Growth,* W. W. Norton & Company, Inc., New York.

———(1939): *New Ways in Psychoanalysis,* W. W. Norton & Company, Inc., New York.

Laughlin, Henry P. (1967): "The Neuroses," Butterworths, Washington, D.C.

Pearce, Jane, and Saul Newton (1963): *The Conditions of Human Growth,* The Citadel Press, New York.

Portnoy, Isadore (1959): "The Anxiety States," in Silvano Arieti (ed.), *American Handbook of Psychiatry,* Basic Books, Inc., Publishers, New York, pp. 307–323.

Rado, Sandor (1959): "Obsessive Behavior—So-called Obsessive-Compulsive Neurosis," in Silvano Arieti (ed.), *American Handbook of Psychiatry,* Basic Books, Inc., Publishers, New York, pp. 324–344.

Ruesch, Jurgen (1957): *Disturbed Communication,* W. W. Norton & Company, Inc., New York.

——— (1961): *Therapeutic Communication,* W. W. Norton & Company, Inc., New York.

Sullivan, Harry Stack (1956): *Clinical Studies in Psychiatry,* W. W. Norton & Company, Inc., New York.

Wender, Louis (1963): "The Dynamics of Group Psychotherapy and Its Application," in Max Rosenbaum and Milton Berger (eds.), *Group Psychotherapy and Group Function,* Basic Books, Inc., Publishers, New York, pp. 211–217.

Wolberg, Lewis R. (1967): *The Technique of Psychotherapy,* 2 vols., Grune & Stratton, Inc., New York.

14

PERSONALITY DISORDERS

Marion E. Kalkman

The diagnostic category "personality disorders" includes a large number of conditions which differ so widely in severity and clinical manifestation that, at first glance, it is difficult to understand what they have in common. Classified in this category are (1) personality pattern disturbances manifest in persons who are abnormally shy, moody, paranoid, or eccentric; (2) personality trait disturbances seen in the emotionally unstable, the passive-aggressive, and the compulsive; (3) sociopathic disturbances, such as sexual deviations and addictions; and (4) special symptom reactions, such as enuresis and somnambulism. Diverse as the personality disorders are, they appear to have several factors in common.

Etiology and Symptomatology

The etiology of the personality disorders seems to be related to faulty or arrested emotional development in the pre-oedipal period which has interfered with the development of adequate social control or superego formation. Another commonality is that their pathology is expressed by their behavior rather than by the development of psychotic, neurotic, or somatic symptoms. In fact individuals with personality disorders appear exceptionally normal to the uninitiated person. Still another commonality is that this pathology is directed outwardly against others and does not inwardly affect the individual with feelings of guilt, anxiety, or depression, as would occur with a neurotic person.

Cleckley (1959) states that the personality disorders are regarded by many observers as chronic and deeply ingrained in what some might call the character or essence of the person.

The individual with a personality disorder of whatever type eventually comes into conflict with society. According to psychoanalytic thinking, one who in later life develops a personality disorder was in early childhood deprived of one of the basic needs for normal growth and development—the love, security, and trust of his mother, without which the child cannot tolerate the frustration of his primitive instinctual drives. Consequently, no mechanism such as the superego is developed to control and internalize the ungratified desires which are often too strong for the weak ego of the child to cope with.

In the latency period, when the child begins to interact with adults outside his family, he still reacts to them at the early level of behavior, that is, he loves them when they gratify his wishes and hates them when they frustrate him. Friedlander (1949) writes: "Since there is no functioning superego, there is no internal demand and consequently no tension between ego and superego to produce guilt feelings. The child's actions are governed by the pleasure principle, so that only direct prohibition of instinctual drives is successful, and that only temporarily. Although there may be intellectual insight into the result of actions, there is no emotional insight. The pleasure of the moment is more important than the threat of displeasures in the future." By the time the individual has reached adolescence he has transferred this same pattern of behavior to society, which brings him into conflict with the laws, customs, and conventions of the community in which he lives.

Treatment

When someone with a personality disorder comes into conflict with society, he is more likely to come to the attention of one of the law-enforcing or correctional agencies than of a health agency or the medical profession. Psychopaths especially were—and in many quarters still are—considered malefactors rather than sick people. Moreover, not only does society so regard them, but the individual himself does not consider himself ill and therefore does not seek medical treatment. Psychiatrists, on the other hand, are often loath to treat persons with personality disorders because such patients frequently prove to be difficult and unrewarding. However, in recent years, a growing number of psychiatrists, psychoanalysts, psychologists, and social workers have become deeply interested in understanding the problems of these individuals and in providing therapy for them.

Role of the Nurse

At the present time relatively few nurses have been involved in the treatment of patients with personality disorders. One reason is that such persons are generally found either in the community or in correctional institutions, where few nurses practice. The changing role of the nurse and the trend toward increased nursing care in the community makes it probably that nurses will take a far more active part in the treatment of patients with personality disorders. Also, the more civic-minded, responsible, and enlightened members of society are gradually accepting the idea that present methods of coping with these sick people are unsatisfactory and that they need treatment rather than punishment.

PERSONALITY DISORDERS AND CHARACTER DISORDERS

Under the broad classification of personality disorders is a subgroup which is also broad and vaguely defined. The clinical entities in this subgroup are variously known as character disorders, personality pattern disturbances, and personality trait disturbances. *Character disorder* is the term used in the psychoanalytic classification, whereas *personality* and *disorder* and certain other nonpsychotic mental disorders are used in the 1968 classification of psychiatric conditions prepared by the American Psychiatric Association.

In commenting on the use of the word *character* in psychoanalytic classification and the use of the word *personality* in the American Psychiatric Association classification, Michaels states that in American psychiatry the term *personality* is often used in instances where the term *character* would be used in German psychiatry. However, the terms in both classifications refer to generally mild or borderline psychiatric conditions in which the individual manifests no overt psychiatric symptoms but has personality problems which involve him in difficulties in living. The cause of these conditions seems to be the result of some interference with the process of personality growth and development. The nature of this maldevelopment may be arrested development at some stage or the overdevelopment of a personality pattern or trait.

Classification

The subtypes of character disorders take their names from the level at which psychosexual development is considered to have been fixated;

for example, oral character traits and disorders, anal character traits and disorders, and phallic character traits and disorders. Personality disorders are recognized in those whose personality is dominated by a particular personality pattern. Examples of this include the chronically unsuccessful or ineffectual members of society (inadequate personality disturbance); aloof, withdrawn, or eccentric individuals (schizoid personality disturbance); moody individuals (cyclothymic personality disturbance); and abnormally sensitive or suspicious individuals (paranoid personality disturbance). Persons with personality disturbances include the emotionally unstable, who have poor emotional control; the passive-aggressive, who propose nothing but oppose everything; the rigid, excessively orderly, overly meticulous, compulsive; and those with still other personality traits that make them difficult people for others to tolerate.

Character Disorders—A Social and Psychiatric Problem

Reiner and Kaufman, who were engaged in studying juvenile delinquency at the Judge Baker Guidance Center, found that many of the parents of these children were suffering from character disorders. They write (Reiner and Kaufman, 1959):

> It seems likely that a relatively high proportion of adults under the care of other agencies also belong in this category. The proportion is doubtless highest in agencies dealing with delinquents and "hard-to-reach" families, but a considerable number are also to be found in the case-loads of agencies providing child and family services, health care, public assistance, and so forth. Clients with character disorders present difficult and perplexing problems to all these agencies, not only because these clients are numerically frequent but because they display such an extreme degree of social pathology in all their family and community relationships. It is probably safe to say that families with members suffering from severe character disorders represent the most serious social problem in our country.
>
> In financial terms, these families account for a large part of current expenditures for public assistance, police departments, correctional systems, mental hospitals, child placement facilities, and various other institutional and welfare programs. In human terms as well, the cost of this type of psychological disorder is extremely high. The parents of these families are not only the "marginal workers" described by economists, but they are "marginal" human beings in the sense that they live on the edge of life. They are vulnerable to every wind that blows—economic, social, and physical. A child born into such a family has a negligible chance of growing into a normal, healthy, and useful adult. Although the parents may often appear to be selfish and pleasure-loving, they live their lives in the shadow of failure, defeat, and rejection. It is this paradoxical combination of pleasure-seeking and misery that often confounds the better organized persons who try to help them, as well as the public generally. Most people see only the hedonistic behavior and its results and are unaware of the misery that the behavior conceals.

Treatment

The treatment of persons with character and personality disorders is no easy matter. It is difficult to get them into treatment, and once in treatment they do not respond well to conventional psychiatric or psychoanalytic techniques. However, a number of psychoanalysts, including Reich (1945), Anna Freud (1954), Alexander (1930), Eissler (1949), Michaels (1955, 1959), Glover (1955), and others, have contributed to the greater understanding of the dynamics of character disorders and have developed variations of standard psychoanalytic technique which have proved effective in treatment. The key steps in treatment appear to be, first, to get the individual to accept treatment, and second, to help him to develop a relationship with a therapist. Treatment is usually long and complicated. Its success depends in great measure on the quality and intensity of the relationship that the patient is able to develop with the therapist.

Qualifications of the Therapist

The therapist who works with patients with severe personality and character disturbances should have special personal qualifications. Reiner and Kaufman (1959) describe these qualifications as follows:

> He must be able to tolerate the tremendous demands that these emotionally needful people make on him. He must be patient and able to curb his anxiety and resentment, and at the same time be constantly aware of his own reactions and feelings. Suppression or denial of feelings will interfere with the fluidity of communication with these clients. It is essential for the caseworker to be able to communicate both verbally and in a non-verbal symbolic way with these acting-out persons if treatment is to be successful. Such communication requires intuition, supplemented by technical knowledge about the meaning of behavior; neither one gets far without the other. The more understanding the caseworker has of his own reactions and those of the client, the better able he will be to use himself with flexibility in forming and maintaining a therapeutic relationship. He must be warm without being seductive, firm without being punitive, and accepting of the client's feelings without having to identify with his modes of behavior.

In addition, the therapist should be flexible in the choice of his therapeutic techniques, in his determination of the time, frequency, and place of the therapeutic encounter. He must be able to use authority rationally and judiciously for the patient's benefit. According to Wolberg (1954), the therapist should be able to tolerate and understand the idiom and behavior of the patient without feeling called upon to respond in kind, as, for example, by copying the patient's use of profane or crude expressions, gestures, or actions. He must be able to give unconditionally to the patient if this is therapeutically indicated.

The personal qualifications and the knowledge and skill of the therapist are of more importance in working with these patients than the particular health profession of which he is a member. The first therapists to work with patients with personality disorders were psychiatrists and psychoanalysts, and they continue to hold the foremost position in treament. However, the problems of these patients are so complex—involving almost every aspect of social living—that social workers have entered the field as therapists. In their discussion of treatment of persons with character disorders, Reiner and Kaufman (1959) write:

> We have purposely not differentiated between psychiatrists and caseworkers as therapists. . . . The dynamics of treatment are necessarily the same, regardless of the training of the therapist. In the long run, the efficacy of the treatment depends on the knowledge, skill, and patience of the person undertaking this demanding educational and therapeutic task. It is our belief that caseworkers have the necessary knowledge and skill to undertake such treatment, since the central aim is not to resolve unconscious conflicts but to further the maturation process.

Role of the Nurse—
The Public Health Nurse

The changing role of the professional nurse and the increasing trend toward the practice of nursing in the home and in community health agencies make it seem inevitable that professional nurses will be called upon to participate in the long-term treatment of individuals with personality and character disorders. In fact, certain aspects of the nursing role make the nurse especially well suited to working with such patients. Because public health nurses see the patient in his home, they have an important advantage—for one of the obstacles to treating patients with personality disorders is that they are difficult to reach, difficult to get into treatment, and difficult to keep in treatment. Public health nurses are skilled in contacting, following up, and maintaining contact with patients. Generally, these nurses are readily accepted by the patient's family and neighbors, and are not subjected to the same degree of hostility that other professional therapists are subjected.

Since these nurses work out from an agency office, going directly to the patient and his family and his neighborhood, they see the patient in his familiar environment and become cognizant of the influences of his life by direct, personal observation. They become participant-observers of the life of the patient. This direct encounter between nurse and patient makes for a more intense interaction with a higher therapeutic potentiality in a shorter period of time than generally occurs when the patient comes to the more formally structured office interview. If a nurse with background and experience in public health nursing is given the necessary psychiatric knowledge and skills and has good psychiatrically trained consultants, he can be most effective in the treatment of personality disorders.

Nurses working in the community in health agencies are rarely called upon to care for patients who are frankly diagnosed as suffering from personality or character disorders. It is far more probable that many of these patients come with physical complaints or economic or social problems. It is only when the nurse gets to know the patient and tries to understand the various factors involved in his difficulties that he becomes aware of the underlying personality problems which play such an important role in the patient's difficulties. If the nurse has not had adequate psychiatric training, he may be completely baffled when trying to understand what is going on and be frustrated in his efforts to help the patient. Even if one is aware of the underlying problem, treatment is not easy; but at least he knows the problem he is dealing with, has some knowledge of how to proceed, and can anticipate the pitfalls to avoid.

The General Hospital Nurse

Nurses working in general hospitals also encounter patients with underlying personality or character disorders. Generally, the medical diagnoses of the patients vary greatly, though one of the most frequently encountered diagnoses is a psychosomatic disorder. Nurses (among themselves) are prone to call such patients "difficult." They earn this label for the reason that, although they appear to be completely normal psychologically, they are overly sensitive, demanding, moody, querulous, uncooperative or have some other personality quirk that makes them difficult patients to care for. Nurses who are not aware of these patients' underlying difficulty are often so provoked by their behavior that they are unable to be professionally helpful to them.

The Psychiatric Nurse

On psychiatric units of general hospitals or in mental institutions the nurse may care for the patient who is specifically diagnosed as having a personality or character disorder, although hospitalized patients so diagnosed are not numerous. Most patients with a diagnosis of personality disorder are treated in private psychiatric practice or in psychiatric clinics and outpatient departments, where, generally, they do not receive nursing attention. Wherever these patients are found, in the community or in the hospital, they present the same problems in treatment and require essentially the same kind of nursing care.

Principles, Problems, and Methods of Treatment

Long-Term Treatment   The principles of treatment of the patient with a personality pattern or trait disorder do not differ greatly for the various professions, though the techniques used and their application may. One characteristic of treatment for this group of patients is that it is long-term treatment, because it is a deep-seated condition stemming from interference or distortion of the normal personality growth process. Changes in personality are made slowly and at great emotional cost and effort on the patient's part. No short-term therapy up to the present time has proved effective. Long-term treatment also demands great patience on the part of the therapist. He must be able to accept relapses in the progress of the patient and be prepared to stand by the patient during these periods.

Immature Behavior of Patients   The immaturity and infantile behavior of the patient are often another problem for the therapist. The patient is generally unaware of his immature behavior, but, because of his abnormal sensitivity to anxiety, deciding when and how to help him look at his behavior may be difficult for the therapist. In the process of becoming aware of his immature behavior the patient will need a certain amount of emotional support from the therapist in order to tolerate the accompanying anxiety. He may need also educative or reeducative measures to assist him in developing more mature patterns of behavior.

Educative Measures, Including Communication Skills   The nature of these educative measures will vary greatly from patient to patient. Some patients need realistic information, others are lacking in concepts of social responsibility, and still others may be very immature in interpersonal or social situations. Ruesch (1961) states that persons with personality disorders are unable to pick up social cues and have difficulty in self-expression. It is difficult for them to tell others how they feel or to acknowledge the feelings of others. These patients may need to be taught how to communicate with others more effectively. In addition many persons with personality disorders have difficulty in controlling their emotions. Therefore, not knowing either how to express or how to control their emotions, they make responses which are often explosive, erratic, and inappropriate. It is helpful if the therapist can be present during such crises. His physical presence during such periods has a stabilizing effect on the patient. This behavior of the therapist can provide support for the patient until he gradually learns how to cope with his feelings.

Individual Relationship Therapy   A one-to-one relationship provides a method of treatment by which many of the above-mentioned goals may be achieved. The treatment enables the patient to form a relationship with a therapist who is more mature than the patient, who is understanding of his behavior, yet who exerts certain pressures on the patient to change his behavior. The therapist may also provide a model or example of more mature behavior. In the early stages of the relationship Wolberg (1954) suggests that efforts be directed toward establishing a strong positive relationship with the patient without analyzing its sources. He also warns the therapist about the patient's excessive compliance, which is often a maneuver to gain security. By trying to please the therapist the patient can avoid examining his problems. The patient must be helped to become aware of what he is doing or no progress will be made in therapy.

Initial State Critical   Reiner and Kaufman stress that the initial stage of the relationship is the most critical one for treatment. More patients break off treatment during this stage than at any subsequent period. The treatment situation is particularly threatening to patients with personality disorders, for it mobilizes their anxiety. The reason is that the general and pervasive emotion of these people is fear, although the source of it varies. Reiner and Kaufman (1959) state:

> This fear is not like the universal fear of new situations which, in the case of the neurotic, is soon dissipated by the reality experience of a neutral or friendly response from the caseworker. In the person with a character disorder, the ghosts of old and fearful relationships are not so easily laid. He needs a long experience of testing out the worker—to find out if his worst fears will be realized—before he is free to allow himself to participate in therapeutic communication. Through his ambivalence and fears, he appears to be blocking the very relationship he so desperately seeks.
>
> His fears . . . may be due to a pathological concept of closeness, involving the threat of death or dissolution, abandonment, rejection, exploitation, control, betrayal, and so forth. The client is constantly on guard to protect himself from the danger that he sees all around him.

These writers also point out the intensive scrutiny to which patients subject the therapist and the great control the therapist must exercise over his nonverbal as well as his verbal communications with the patient.

In the initial stage of treatment it may be necessary for the therapist to give some concrete evidence of his concern and interest to the patient. Ruesch says that if the patient has many somatic complaints it may be advisable to give him medications, special food or nourishments, or physical therapy to provide the much needed sensations of physical stimulation which have been lacking in the patient's experience. When the patient's anxiety is heightened by stressful influences in his environment, the therapist may recommend environmental changes such as better working conditions, more stable living arrangements, or better planning of activities, to reduce the anxiety. It is also helpful for the patient to learn that he is not as helpless in managing his personal affairs as perhaps he had supposed. Patients tend to avoid using their own resources and try to get others to do things for them, a tendency that the therapist should counter by encouraging the patient to become more self-reliant.

Working-through Stage   As the relationship progresses, the patient is gradually able to tolerate more anxiety and can begin to look at himself and his problems. A nice balance has to be maintained in the rate of development of the relationship. If it develops too fast, the patient becomes frightened at the emotional closeness to another person and either breaks away or becomes hostile to the therapist. If the relationship develops too slowly or does not progress, the patient does not have the necessary incentive to face his problems. During this stage of the therapeutic relationship, patients are also encouraged to inhibit their acting-out behavior and to utilize verbal communication more. They are often able to use the therapist as a source of strength and support for gaining greater self-control and as a model for identification. During the course of treatment the low self-esteem which is so characteristic of patients with personality disorders gradually begins to lessen. The regard and concern for the patient as a person which the therapist has consistently demonstrated over a long period of time begins to influence the patient, who in turn begins to regard himself in a better light, and his self-hatred diminishes.

Developing Greater Maturity   With the development of a more positive and realistic self-concept, it becomes possible for the patient to continue the process of personality growth which was interfered with in his preadolescent and adolescent years. The potentiality for a healthier growth may vary greatly from one patient to another, depending on a wide variety of factors, including severity of emotional deprivation, rigidity of personality structure, ego strength and superego development, motivation to change, the vicissitudes of therapy, and many other factors. However, among the important avenues of development are the patient's growing awareness of his self-identity, his separateness from other individuals, and his desire to fulfill his unique potentialities as a person. The patient's maturation process requires considerable self-examination and self-understanding, including a realistic evaluation of his assets and liabilities as well as a decision to focus on certain of his potentialities and to develop them.

Depression in Therapy A certain amount of depression, as well as the ever-present anxiety, is not uncommon during the latter phase of treatment, and the therapist copes with it much as he would with anxiety in a psychoneurotic patient. The depression is due in part to the patient's growing realization and acceptance of his responsibility for his own behavior and his social responsibility to others. In other words, depression is the patient's emotional reaction to the price he must pay for attaining greater maturity. Depression may also arise from knowing that termination of therapy is not far off. Greater maturity implies relinquishing dependence on the therapist and ending the relationship. Some therapists find it helpful at this time to review the long course of the relationship so that the patient can see the gains he has made. Such a review also helps him to deepen his self-understanding. Planning some follow-up is also desirable for both patient and therapist.

Special Problems The different personality patterns and traits particular patients suffer from will each present their special problems in therapy and will modify the management of the treatment. Ruesch has written on the problems in the treatment of the infantile personality; Wolberg, on the inadequate, schizoid, paranoid, power-seeking, and narcissistic individuals. Michaels (1955, 1959) discusses the hysterical, compulsive, narcissistic, impulsive, and other character disorders in his writings. The reader is referred to these authors and to others for additional information.

Group Therapy Group therapy for patients with personality disorders has been recommended by a number of psychotherapists, including Schilder (1938), Wolf (1963), and Wolberg (1954). On the other hand, other therapists exclude these patients from group therapy because of their frequently disruptive influence on the group. The rationale for the utilization of group therapy with patients with personality disorders is that it offers each patient an opportunity to observe the behavior of other group members with the same problems and helps each patient gain some insight into the way his behavior probably affects others. Gaining insight in the company of other members of the group is often easier to tolerate than it is in the individual interview. The group situation also makes it more difficult for the patient to reject the observations, interpretations, evaluations, and opinions of his behavior as expressed by the various members of the group than it would be for him to reject the interpretations of his therapist.

Reiner and Kaufman (1959) believe that group therapy has special significance for patients with character disorders in that it helps them overcome their great loneliness and fear of close relationships. It is often helpful to organize the group around an activity such as sewing, craftwork, or some other congenial activity, thus giving the members a tangible incentive for joining. Reiner and Kaufman think that it is important for the success of the group that the members be approximately the same age, level of intelligence, and social status in order to avoid feelings of inferiority. Reiner and Kaufman also believe that in therapy sessions the therapist may give information when it is requested, but should not elicit discussions about the feelings until the group has met for some time. The therapist should discourage individual members from using the group to act out separation and desertion anxieties. Members are expected to attend regularly, and absent members are contacted by the therapist to determine why they have been absent.

THE PYSCHOPATH AND THE DELINQUENT

The term *psychopathic personality* is used to describe individuals with a wide variety of personality defects whose behavior involves them in a violent clash with their social and cultural environment. In general, the personality disturbance in an individual with a psychopathic personality is more serious, more deeply ingrained, and less amenable to treatment than it is in individuals with personality pattern, personality trait, or character disorders. Those with a psychopathic personality express their hostility toward others in a more direct, undisguised form. Among the many other terms which are used, or were formerly used, to characterize psychopathic individuals are *sociopaths, delinquents, constitutional psychopaths,* and *moral imbeciles.*

Cleckley (1959) has given an excellent description of the psychopath in his article, "Psychopathic States." He writes:

> The typical psychopath is a person who appears to have at least average, and often unusual, ability and who seems to be clearly aware of the amenities and to affirm the moral code. Frequently he demonstrates superior intelligence and other assets and succeeds brilliantly for a while in work, in studies, and in all his human relations. But inevitably and repeatedly, he fails, losing his job, alienating his friends, perhaps losing his wife and his children. It is difficult to account for these failures. Seldom can one find adequate motivation to explain why such a person has, in the midst of success, grossly shirked his immediate responsibilities, perhaps abandoned his work at the behest of impulses that seem to the observer no more than a trivial whim. His failures deprive him of what he tells us are his chief objectives, and also bring

hardship, shame, or disaster to his wife, his children, his parents, and to all those closely concerned with him.

In addition to such relatively passive types of failure, most fully developed psychopaths also commit aggressive antisocial acts. They forge checks, steal repeatedly, lightly indulge in bigamy, swindle, and show little or no compunction about their sexual behavior, no matter what the consequences may be. Some who have attracted wide public attention have committed murder or other shocking felonies, usually with little or no provocation, often without comprehensible motivation. The majority, despite many conflicts with the law, appear to avoid crimes sufficiently grave to result in their being removed from society for long prison terms.

Etiology

Noyes (1953) regards the etiology of psychopathic behavior as the result of frustration of the basic human needs of love, security, recognition, and respect. He states that the child who was rejected may suppress all desire for love and become resentful, rebellious, and antisocial. He writes, "In early years he is the difficult child, in adolescence he may be delinquent and in later life the criminal." Noyes sees the psychopath's behavior as an expression of an arrested or deviant development of personality which permitted primitive psychopathological drives to persist. These persisting drives account for the compulsive quality of the psychopath's behavior patterns. He thinks that possibly the pathological personality is produced by unconscious forces which are never satisfied adequately by the psychopath's acts. These acts then become stereotyped and repetitive, and are organized into behavior patterns which are integrated into the character.

According to Noyes, "Many pathological personalities are persons whose emotional conflicts of childhood and youth were left unsolved. Later, therefore, they continue to seek an emotional expression or outlet for them. The psychopath accordingly goes through life unconsciously creating situations whereby he can act out his earlier unexpressed feelings. Since, too, the emotional factors that have led to his behavior remain unchanged his behavior is not modified. He accordingly appears to others as not learning by experience. He is impelled by unconscious compulsive drives demanding a gratification that is insatiable." Psychopathic individuals are found in all walks of life and in every socioeconomic group. Wherever they are, they are usually storm centers of unrest and discord in interpersonal relationships. It is characteristic of them that they seem to thrive on the turmoil they have stirred up and are totally unconcerned by the distress occasioned in others by their behavior.

Delinquency

Delinquency is a rather loosely used term which describes a group of psychopathic individuals who, usually, first come to the attention of social workers and other community welfare workers because of the social difficulties they get into. Delinquency seems to be predominant in a certain age range, generally becoming evident in the adolescent years, flourishing in early adult life, then declining during the middle adult years. After the age of forty, the number of individuals classified as delinquent drops off markedly. The line between delinquent behavior and behavior still regarded within the range of normal adolescent behavior is often difficult to determine. In fact, it often depends on the social values of the community in which the individual lives which label is applied to a given sample of behavior. Delinquency also seems to flourish in those neighborhoods which have few channels for the expression of adolescent rebellious tendencies. Those individuals who do not outgrow their delinquent tendencies by middle age either continue their delinquent career as full-blown psychopaths or, according to their special type of social psychopathy, as, for example, alcoholics, drug addicts, sexual psychopaths, or criminal personalities.

Treatment

The treatment of delinquents and psychopathic personalities is in general quite similar. The difference primarily is that the delinquent is usually a younger individual, his psychopathic behavior is less deeply entrenched, and his prognosis for social adjustment as a result of the passage of time, changing interests, the vicissitudes of living, or of therapy is more promising than is that of the psychopath. However, the delinquent individual as well as the psychopath presents many difficult problems in treatment. For both, the first problem is that they do not see any need for treatment and, in fact, often go to great lengths to avoid it. It is their suffering relatives or outraged society in the guise of a school principal, a social worker, or a judge of the court who seeks to bring them into psychiatric treatment.

Psychopath's Resistance to Therapy

Psychotic and neurotic patients are driven by their suffering into treatment. This is not true of psychopathic individuals. Eissler (1949) writes, "The true delinquent certainly does not suffer unless he is caught and fears punishment; he denies that his behavior may be an illness; on the contrary he will claim that others who do not behave as he does are stupid and ignorant of the pleasures of life. He laughs at the idea of possibly needing that sort of help which the psychiatrist customarily gives. Last, but certainly not least, the delinquent is markedly lacking in the ability to observe himself, and he is disinclined to communicate to any other person even the little which he may know about his subjective experiences. There are some indications that delinquents and psychopaths not only enjoy their periodic outbursts of aggressive, antisocial behavior, but actually need to behave that way to achieve or restore a feeling of well-being. These individuals often report that they only feel real, alive, and vital when they have committed some antisocial act.

The initial problem, therefore, with the delinquent or the psychopath is to get him into treatment. Although generally resistant to treatment, he may agree to accept it in a moment of depression or self-recrimination or at a time when his behavior has involved him so deeply in difficulties with others that he accepts it as a possible avenue of escape from the consequences of that behavior. He may also enter therapy under covert or overt pressure from relatives or by court order. The therapeutic relationship thus starts off under the handicap of a tenuous commitment and generally with hostile feelings on the part of the patient.

Problems in Therapy

Greenacre (1947) in discussing the difficulties of treating the psychopathic patient, identifies three areas of defect in his personality with which the therapist must cope. These are his strong primitive drives, his defective sense of self, and his lack of conscience or moral values. She sees the long-range goals of treatment as "the development in the patient of a better sense of reality, a more useful conscience including realistic self-criticism and durable ideals." Most authorities agree that to achieve any effective results, therapy for psychopaths must be planned as a long-term project.

Lack of Sense of Reality and Dependence on Magical Thinking

Greenacre believes that the disturbed sense of reality of the psychopath is due to his lack of reality-testing techniques and his dependence on magical thinking. In therapy he must develop and learn to utilize reality-testing techniques. He must also give up his expectations of magical results and acquire a rational understanding of the role of cause and effect in the manifestations of behavior. Greenacre warns that magical thinking may also color the patient-therapist relationship, for the patient frequently endows the therapist with magic qualities and then by flattery attempts to subvert him.

Magical Thinking and the
Role of the Therapist

The magical thinking in which the psychopath characteristically indulges includes such expectations as the belief that the therapist will be able to get him out of his impasses, no matter how serious or complex, without any effort on his own part. He believes that the consequences of his behavior can be in some way negated or condoned without his paying the price for it, and that the effects of therapy will be instantaneous, complete, and painless. The psychopath does his best to put the therapist in this omnipotent role, and does it in such a winning manner that it is often difficult for the therapist to resist. If the therapist is unaware of what is going on or takes no active measures to reject this omnipotent role, he is heading for trouble.

When the patient begins to demand that the therapist act as a powerful agent for him and the therapist refuses or tries to point out the realistic limitations of the therapist's role, the patient, enraged and feeling betrayed and cheated, often denounces the therapist and derogates the value of therapy. It is important, therefore, that the therapist be alert to the first indications of magical thinking, identify them as such, and discuss their unrealistic nature with the patient. Greenacre also emphasizes the importance of fairness and consistency in treating the psychopath, and the need for pointing out repeatedly to him the natural consequences of his psychopathic behavior.

Importance of a Strong Relationship
with the Therapist

Eissler (1949) recommends establishing "a tight, fool-proof attachment between the psychoanalyst and the delinquent in the shortest possible time" so that the therapist can exert some control over the patient's antisocial behavior which could result in some type of incarceration and remove him from the possibility of continuing therapy. He also believes that the element of surprise is important in the treatment of delinquents and psychopaths. He states, "It is a general rule in the therapy of the delinquent never to act in the way he expects, but unceasingly to introduce new and unforeseen elements in order to keep alive his interest in the therapeutic situation."

Therapist—Available and Strong

The therapist must always be ready to stand by to help the delinquent out of the difficulties in which he inevitably becomes embroiled. The therapist can expect to be called any hour of the day or night. On the other hand, he must be careful not to be duped by the patient or to bow to the patient's whims. The therapist must maintain control of the therapeutic situation. Relapses are common in the therapy of the delinquent and it is difficult for the therapist not to be angry or disappointed or both. Often the therapist can see a sequence of events which precedes a relapse, but if he can predict it he may be able to forewarn and forearm the patient and thus prevent its happening. By repeatedly working through a number of such incidences the patient may learn to gain conscious control over his behavior. As the delinquent becomes better able to control his behavior, his psychopathology begins to resemble that of the neurotic patient, and then many of the more conventional therapeutic techniques can be utilized in his therapy. In fact, several well-known psychiatrists, among them Franz Alexander and Kurt Eissler, have stated that the goal in therapy for a psychopath is to make him neurotic and then treat him accordingly.

Active Therapy and Reeducation

The best plan for those who do intensive therapy with psychopaths, according to Diethelm (1947), is active psychotherapy combined with reeducation. He writes, "Psychotherapy without active help from the physician is contraindicated because the personality is too loosely integrated to achieve spontaneous synthesis. Environmental difficulties lead to repetitious emotional involvement which interferes with treatment." Diethelm believes that every psychopath has inherent potentialities which would permit him to function adequately if the right situations in life could be found for him. He also stresses the importance of reeducation in treatment. The psychopath has to be taught that his antisocial behavior will produce reactions from the environment which can affect him painfully and that his attempts to gain sympathy and pity will not mollify the attitudes of others. He has to learn to become self-dependent and recognize the necessity of modifying his behavior to conform with the rules of society. And finally he must come to see that his pathology is not an excuse but a handicap. During treatment the patient should work (be self-supporting) and be engaged in a variety of activities.

Outpatient Treatment

Some psychopathic and delinquent individuals can be treated as outpatients. This is possible when some degree of control over the patient's impulsive behavior can be maintained by a strong therapist-patient relationship and when the patient has sufficient ego strength to exert at least some self-control. It is desirable to have the patient remain in the community, engaged in useful pursuits such as work or school. Therapy can be focused on helping him to tolerate the social pressures inherent in community living and helping him to develop the self-discipline demanded by school and work situations.

Inpatient Treatment

Some individuals with psychopathic personalities, however, are so lacking in ability to control their impulses that they cannot adjust to community living. For them, a more structured environment, such as a psychiatric hospital unit, a special school, or a correctional agency, may be necessary. Unfortunately, inpatient psychiatric facilities that meet the special treatment needs of these patients are still very difficult to find. Many of the patients are adolescents and their admission to either adult or children's psychiatric units can create havoc. Adolescents require facilities designed especially for them, where their special treatment needs can be met.

As psychiatric facilities for adolescents and for psychopathic and delinquent individuals are developed, increasing numbers of nurses will be needed to help create the special environment needed for these patients and to participate in the total plan for their treatment. Much of what has been said in the preceding paragraphs regarding therapy is equally applicable to the nurse with some adaptation to the special functions of the nursing role. Of the greatest importance in the success or failure of a treatment program for these patients in an inpatient service are close collaboration and effective communication among all members of the treatment team.

Psychoanalytically Oriented Group Therapy

Psychopathic individuals do not, as a rule, respond well to psychoanalytically oriented group therapy. Many therapists believe them to be totally unsuitable for this type of treatment. Johnson (1963) observes that psychopaths seek therapy only if coerced or after they are involved in difficulties, and then they tend to manipulate the therapy for their own ends. Wolf (1963) excludes them in his selection of patients for group therapy on the basis that they "are always dangerous and potentially group-disrupting," and also that they have a tendency to betray group confidences. Rosenbaum (1963) has found that these patients are usually rejected by other patients as group members.

Other Types of Group Therapy

However, Wolberg (1954) states that psychopaths can benefit from some forms of group therapy. He writes:

> Experience demonstrates that it is possible to modify to some extent the immature, explosive reactions of the psychopath by an extensive training program, particularly in cooperative group work where the individual participates as a member toward a common objective. Adequate group identifications are lacking in the psychopath, and the realization that ego satisfactions can accrue from group experience, may create a chink in the defensive armor. In cases where the psychopath comes into conflict with the law, and where incarceration is necessary, a program organized around building up whatever assets the individual possesses, particularly in a group setting, may, in some instances, bring success. In young psychopaths, vocational schools that teach the individual a trade may contribute to his self-esteem and provide him with a means of diverting his energies into a profitable channel.

The Therapeutic Community

One of the more promising approaches to the treatment of the psychopath in recent years is derived from the concepts of social psychiatry. Maxwell Jones developed his method of treatment, known as the *therapeutic community,* from his efforts to rehabilitate a group of socially maladjusted individuals in Britain whom he referred to as "the psychological casualties in the struggle of everyday life." At the Industrial Neurosis Unit of Belmont Hospital, Dr. Jones created a special therapeutic environment in which these patients could have their problems investigated, receive psychiatric treatment, and be rehabilitated so that they could resume a meaningful role in the community. The treatment program was designed so that the patient was forced to examine his interactions with a small, specially structured society of the hospital unit (Jones, 1953, 1962).

A wide variety of techniques were used, including group therapy, patient government, sociodrama, work groups, recreational activities, vocational and educational training—with special emphasis on interpatient and interstaff interactions. The psychopath's insensitivity to the effects of his behavior on others and his characteristic lack of responsibility for the welfare of others could not go unchallenged in an environment where the behavior of all members was observed, examined, and discussed by the entire group. Jones writes:

> The daily examination of behavior and current problems means that the patients become aware of the factors which lie behind behavior and learn a great deal about each others' problems. In any type of hospital, they are forced to relate to other patients and staff at ward level whether they like it or not, and it seems reasonable to try to help them have a positive role to play and a much better insight into what is going on in themselves and in those around them. In my experience, it is possible to get patients and staff at all levels to appreciate some of the phenomena that occur on the unit and in the daily community meetings.

The Nurse in the Therapeutic Community

Jones regards the nurse's role as a very important one in the therapeutic community; in fact he dedicated his book, *The Therapeutic Community, a New Treatment Method in Psychiatry,* to his nursing staff. He views the nurse's role as a tripartite one—authoritarian, social, and therapeutic. The authoritarian role is called into play by the fact that, as the staff members most involved in the patients' daily life, nurses are often the first people to be confronted with problems posed by the patients' behavior. Therefore they may have to set limits on some behaviors which violate basic rules of health or safety. In emergency situations, it may be necessary for nurses to intervene actively, as, for example, when two patients are fighting; and in general they try to maintain a sense of order and discipline on the unit in order to discourage antisocial behavior and protect the unit from the disintegrative effects of such behavior. Their social role is to interact with their patients in social situations without forfeiting their professional identity; that is, they may teach a patient to play bridge because his bridge-playing ability may facilitate his social acceptance by others. They spend time each day with patients, provide them with human contacts, and help them to interact with others in socially acceptable ways.

In their therapeutic role nurses do not participate in a one-to-one relationship with a particular patient but help to transmit the unit culture and philosophy of treatment to the patient. They encourage and support him in his various therapeutic activities, including his therapeutic relationship with his psychiatrist. Occasionally they may be asked to collaborate with the psychiatrist in some phase of the patient's psychotherapy. Dr. Jones acknowledges that this concept of the therapeutic role of the nurse is a fairly simple one. One reason for this is that most of his nurses remain less than a year with him. He believes that if they were to remain longer, this role would undoubtedly become more complex. Holmes and Werner (1966) have also delineated the role of the psychiatric nurse in a therapeutic community.

Treatment Results

The results of treatment of psychopathic individuals by this method are more promising than those of any of the previously mentioned types of therapy. Jones (1953) states that the findings of his group of investigators "appear to justify the conclusion that it is possible to change social attitudes in relatively desocialized patients with severe character disorders, provided they are treated together in a therapeutic community." Six months after discharge, two-thirds of his patients made fair to good adjustments, one-third made poor adjustments, and more than one-half worked full-time after leaving the hospital. Jones comments, "We believe (but cannot prove) that the results described could not have been achieved by individual psychotherapy and hospitalization alone."

In a follow-up study, home visits were made by one of Dr. Jones's colleagues, Miss Joy Tuxford, a social worker, who came to the conclusion that the absence of any real family life was the cause of much of the desocialization which was observed in the hospital. This observation, together with the fact that the patient's families were unable to participate in the treatment situation because they lived too far from the hospital, led Dr. Jones to believe that treatment of the patient and his family in the local community would probably yield even better results.

THE ALCOHOLIC AND THE DRUG ADDICT

The alcoholic and drug addicts present two of the most serious and baffling problems with which the health professions have to cope. In the United States there are reported to be 80 million consumers of alcohol, and of this number 10 percent or 8 million are problem drinkers, that is, alcoholics. Figures are more difficult to obtain on drug addicts, but Nyswander (1956) estimates their number to be between 60,000 and 180,000. Only in recent years have alcoholism and drug addiction been regarded as illnesses rather than as moral delinquency or criminal behavior. In 1956, when the report of the Committee on Alcoholism of the Council on Mental Health of the American Medical Association was published, the medical profession first officially recognized alcoholism as an illness. Both alcohol and drug addiction are very complex and poorly understood conditions which have physiological, psychological, and social components in their etiology, symptomatology, and treatment. In both conditions, disturbances of personality play a major role.

Alcohol Addiction—Definition

Among the millions of persons who utilize alcohol for a wide variety of reasons, the term *alcoholic* is reserved for those whose continued or excessive use of alcohol results in the impairment of his health, his family and social relationships, and his economic security. Alcohol addiction develops when there is a physiological dependence upon alcohol, which is demonstrated by the appearance of true withdrawal symptoms when the ingestion of alcohol is terminated abruptly. Withdrawal symptoms may include tremors, excessive perspiration, nausea, vomiting, anorexia, restlessness, hallucinations, convulsions, and delirium tremens.

Personality Traits

The person who drinks to excess, either chronically or periodically, does so because he is mentally ill, according to Thompson. The emotional illness may be transient, due to sudden severe situational stress, or it may be basically a neurosis, psychosis, or organic brain syndrome which is accompanied by excessive drinking. For example, bouts of heavy drinking often presage a manic attack. This is often the case also with acute schizophrenic episodes, and very commonly it manifests itself either as a primary or secondary symptom in personality disorders. In all of these conditions excessive drinking seems to be used as a way of coping with acute anxiety. Zwerling and Rosenberg (1959), on the basis of a review of the psychiatric literature, point out that many authorities state that there is no specific personality type basic to alcoholism, yet there is agreement that some personality disorder is present in every instance of chronic alcoholism. Thompson (1959), however, makes some generalizations about the personality structure of alcoholics. He notes their difficulties in interpersonal relationships, their general uneasiness and dissatisfaction with life, their tendencies to excess in all areas of activity such as work, sex, and recreation, their low frustration tolerance, their extreme dependence coupled with resentment of authority, their flagrant selfishness and insistent demands for immediate satisfaction of their needs, their domineering and destructive traits, including self-destructive or suicidal tendencies. These personality traits are characteristic of many types of personality disorders and not peculiar to the alcoholic.

Etiology

The causes that underlie the development of the personality traits and symptomatology of the alcoholic are not easy to trace. There is reason to believe that genetic factors related to a specific physiologic reaction to alcohol and susceptibility to alcohol addiction are probably involved. Certainly, as has been mentioned, there are psychological components both in the early developmental experiences, especially those centering around a disrupted or distorted mother-child relationship, and the later interpersonal family interactions characteristic of the adult alcoholic and his family. The characteristic pattern of the family interactions around an alcoholic member have been well described by Eric Berne (1961) in the game of Alcoholic.

Social and cultural factors in alcoholism are also important strands in this complex problem. These factors include local customs about drinking, social attitudes toward excessive drinking, and the amount of stress and tension in the community. However, until there is more knowledge and a clearer understanding of the various factors involved in the etiology of alcoholism, prevention and effective treatment will not be possible. Nevertheless, there is no need to underrate the growing body of available knowledge which can be and is being utilized for the treatment of those individuals suffering from this condition.

Treatment

The alcoholic generally comes to the attention of the nurse when he is acutely ill from the toxic effects of the drug and in need of hospitalization. He may be hospitalized in a general hospital, a sanitarium for alcoholics, or a psychiatric hospital. If he is emotionally disturbed, he would probably be hospitalized in a psychiatric facility. Many general hospitals are reluctant to admit alcoholics and do so only when they are quiet and cooperative. There has been a growing trend to educate administrators and the medical and nursing staffs of general hospitals toward greater acceptance of the admission and treatment of those suffering from alcoholism (Connor et al., 1963). This movement seems to be achieving some measure of success.

Treatment of the Acute Phase

The alcohol addict generally comes to the hospital as an acutely ill individual in every sense of the term. His presenting symptoms are due to the toxic effects of alcohol and include nausea and often vomiting; perspiration and weakness; severe tremors, especially of the hands and face; myoclonic jerking of the arms, legs, head, and neck, which may increase to the severity of generalized convulsions, with pupils dilated. Insomnia, loss of appetite or even inability to tolerate food, and dehydration are also common. Speech is slurred and often rambling and incoherent. Motor activity may range from wild restlessness and excitability to a state of stupor. Emotional symptoms may include anxiety, depression, irritability, hypersensitivity to light and sound, impaired memory, disorientation, silly or inappropriate behavior, visual and auditory hallucinations, and greatly impaired insight and judgment.

In addition to symptoms due to alcoholic intoxication, the alcoholic patient often suffers from intercurrent respiratory infections which may rapidly develop into pneumonia. The alcoholic generally neglects his health so that the results of poor diet and poor hygiene are apparent. Nutritional and vitamin deficiencies, including polyneuritis, as well as cirrhosis of the liver, chronic brain damage, and mental deterioration, are common sequelae of prolonged addiction to alcohol.

Medical Treatment

The medical treatment of the acute phase of alcoholism includes such general supportive measures as some type of sedation or tranquilizer, adequate diet, replacement of fluids, and vitamin therapy. Insulin and hydrotherapy are also sometimes prescribed, as are antibiotics if respiratory or other infections are present. The use of the new tranquilizing drugs has drastically improved the treatment of the acute alcoholic patient. By controlling the alcoholic's uncooperative behavior with these drugs, it has been possible to care for him at home or in a general hospital rather than in a psychiatric or other special facility. These drugs also relieve the symptoms of nausea and insomnia and promote a general feeling of well-being. The patient is again able to eat a well-balanced diet, and this in turn corrects the dietary deficiencies. Mann mentions that Antabuse is often prescribed during this phase of treatment to reinforce the patient's efforts to stop drinking (Mann, 1958).

Nursing Care

Good nursing care is essential in the initial steps in treating the alcoholic patient. Because patients in the acute state are often uncooperative and difficult to care for, and also because many nurses have prejudices against alcoholic patients, there are many nurses who find it difficult to give as good care to alcoholics as they do to other patients (Wilson, 1960). Other nurses regard this phase of treatment only as a "drying out" process. Their goal is to give the patient good routine nursing care with the hope that he will be discharged as soon as possible. They consider their responsibility ended at this point. However, the experience of those who have treated many alcoholic patients and who have followed their careers as alcoholics is that the acute phase is only the initial phase of treatment. Thompson (1959) writes, "When the patient has recovered from his acute disorder, further treatment must be directed to the underlying illness or problem that caused the alcoholism."

Total nursing care of the acute alcoholic patient includes adequate psychological nursing care as well as good physical nursing care. Such psychological nursing care would provide psychotherapeutic supportive measures to mitigate the patient's emotional discomfort and help him to realize his need for further psychiatric treatment. The nurse can be helpful in preparing him to accept treatment and in easing the steps to the next phase of treatment.

Importance of Follow-up Treatment

The alcoholic, like most other individuals with personality disorders, does not consider himself in need of prolonged psychological treatment. He is prone to tell others, and often believes himself, that the present drinking episode will never be repeated. Anyone who has had experience with alcoholics knows that this is not the case. The physician or nurse who makes no provision for further treatment helps to confirm a lifelong pattern of alternate drinking episodes and remissions. One important reason psychotherapy should be started during the acute phase of treatment is that it is then easier for the patient to tolerate psychotherapy than at a later stage of treatment.

Follow-up Treatment

The second phase of treatment is primarily psychological and social. The first hurdle the alcoholic must face is realizing that he must give up alcohol for the rest of his life. Mann (1958) states that no treatment exists which can restore the alcoholic's control so that he may drink normally. Some authorities believe that to reach this conclusion the alcoholic has to hit rock bottom.

Before the second phase of treatment is begun, the patient should have regained his physical health and been treated for any intercurrent illnesses or physical complaints. Generally the alcoholic needs some help in restructuring or reinforcing his patterns of everyday living. An assessment of his psychological and social abilities is often a useful preliminary step in helping the patient to do this. Emphasis on assets of his personal and social situation is important in increasing his self-confidence and feelings of self-worth, and in encouraging his attempts to become more independent. All these efforts are geared to redirecting the patient's life and helping him to develop a satisfying life without alcohol.

Hospitalization

Some alcoholics can be treated during this phase without being hospitalized, but for a number of patients a period of hospitalization is necessary. Prout (1955) writes, "The routine and discipline of a well-ordered psychiatric hospital has much to offer, not only in terms of a regulated life or companionship, but as a model upon which the patient's life can be patterned. . . . Good hospital management will not allow the substitution of hospital dependency for addiction." Many alcoholics can also benefit from milieu therapy which can be provided in a hospital setting. Some of the components of a well-organized milieu program include patient government, group therapy, patient-planned and patient-directed social activities, and carefully selected vocational opportunities. By helping the alcoholic patient to develop self-confidence, improve his social skills, and remotivate him to engage in some satisfying type of work, milieu therapy can play an important role in his social recovery. Mann (1958) defines social recovery for the alcoholic patient as the ability to live with others in the everyday world as an accepted member of society, with every human function restored except the ability to drink.

Conflicting views are held whether alcoholics should be treated in the same units with other types of psychiatric patients or whether they should be treated separately. The rationale for the former view is that alcoholism is an emotional illness, similar in many ways to a number of other types of psychological disorders. Since alcoholics can benefit from the same kinds of treatment as other patients, there is no reason to segregate them. However, many alcoholic patients prefer not to mix with other patients. They believe that their problems are of a different nature and require different treatment methods and a different kind of treatment environment from those provided for psychiatric patients. Physicians and nurses who have had much experience in treating alcoholic patients generally agree that ward management problems are decreased and therapeutic programs proceed more smoothly when alcoholic patients are treated separately.

Individual Psychotherapy

Alcoholics generally do not respond favorably to intensive psychotherapy on a one-to-one basis. Their anxiety is often increased by the threat of closeness to the therapist. They tend to find talking about their difficulties, which involves self-examination and introspection, intolerably painful. And they become impatient with the slowness of progress observable in psychotherapy and the length of time required. Another difficulty is that many therapists are reluctant to treat alcoholic patients because of their excessive demands on the therapist, their deviousness, and their tendency toward acting-out behavior. These same difficulties arise also with the nurse who engages them in nurse-patient relationship therapy.

Group Therapy

Group therapy, on the other hand, has proved to be more successful than individual therapy in the treatment of alcoholics, according to Wolf (1963) and Standish and Semrad (1963). These writers think that alcoholic patients can be treated more effectively in homogeneous groups than in mixed groups. Gliedman (1958) states that the group offers support but also helps to keep in check the hostile impulses of the alcoholic patient, and that it is able to motivate him to look at his problems in a way that is not possible in individual therapy. Many writers note that alcoholics seem to be able to communicate with each other better than they can with other people. They have their own special language, and in groups they interact and influence each other strongly. This characteristic has been utilized by Alcoholics Anonymous, an organization of former alcoholics whose personal experience with alcohol enables them to understand the alcoholic patient's problem as no one else can.

Family Therapy

As it becomes more and more apparent that alcoholism is not an illness which involves only one individual, family therapy is increasingly being used as a form of psychotherapy for the alcoholic. The psychodynamics of alcoholism has its roots in the family constellation in the family of origin; that is, the family into which the individual who later becomes an alcoholic was born. The same patterns of interaction are repeated in the family which he establishes in his adult life. The interaction of the alcoholic and his spouse are of particular importance. Therefore, many therapists include therapy of the spouse as an essential part of the treatment of the patient.

CONCURRENT TREATMENT OF ALCOHOLIC PATIENTS AND THEIR WIVES

Gliedman, Rosenthal, Frank, and Nash (1963) report on a study in which they treated nine alcoholic patients and their wives in concurrent group therapy consisting of two sessions per week with the patients and one session per week with the wives. Evaluation of this group treatment showed the greatest changes occurred in the areas of better marital relationships and increased self-esteem of the patients. There was also a decrease in depression, irritability, and drinking behavior. Least changed was the patients' social effectiveness. Group therapy provided the alcoholic patients with a nonthreatening milieu in which they could discuss their problems. Patients were permitted to take the treatment at their own pace and to the degree of participation of which they were capable at the moment. Since it was an all-alcoholic group, mutual support was given and readily accepted. The concurrent therapy of the wives emphasized the role the wives played in the husbands' alcoholic problem.

REVERSAL OF PARENTAL ROLES IN FAMILIES OF ALCOHOLICS

Burton (1964) has described the shifting of family roles which occurs in the family of the alcoholic. She writes, "If the father is an alcoholic, the mother becomes the head of the family. The husband is eliminated as a participant in planning and decision making. If he is there, it is all right. If he is not, that is all right, too. It simply makes no difference." The reversal of parental roles is confusing and disturbing to the children, also. They see their father at home idle and their mother going out to work, and they may be fearful about bringing friends to the house. The children may have to take on added responsibilities before they are ready for them, and they may become fearful and emotionally insecure as a result of the family disorganization.

Role of the Public Health Nurse
in Family Therapy

Burton views the public health nurse as one who plays an important role in helping the alcoholic patient and his family. She may be the first person to encounter the problem of alcoholism—not yet acknowledged by the patient or his family—as she visits the family for some quite different reason. The public health nurse's primary responsibility is to make community resources available to the family; she herself can be helpful to the patient and his family by listening to their difficulties, providing them with useful informational and educational data, and by giving them emotional support.

Burton also considers the public health nurses' participation important in the total community effort to cope with the problem of alcoholism. She sees them working closely with the nurses and physicians in alcoholic clinics, with Alcoholics Anonymous members, with the nurses caring for alcoholic patients in the general hospitals, with family service agencies, the police and judicial departments, psychiatric hospitals, mental health clinics, and visiting nurse agencies.

Blane and Hill (1964) observe that the public health nurse is in a unique position to identify the problems involved in alcoholism, to provide further information and assistance to the patient and his family, and to serve as a valuable adjunct to treatment resources. However, they found that the nurses were often unsure of their role in treating the alcoholic, feeling handicapped by the lack of any psychotherapeutic skills. One nurse was quoted as saying, "Sometimes it's very difficult to appeal to a person to help him to seek help. And we're not equipped for this. All we can do is try to find out if he really wants help, and give him a little push." A supervisor who was interviewed stated, "If we're really going to help people, public health nurses need a lot more help in how to approach families."

Need for Better Preparation of Nurses
Caring for Alcoholic Patients

Few nurses at the present time have special preparation in the care of the alcoholic patient and his family. There is great need for nurse specialists with a thorough preparation in psychiatric nursing, some advanced preparation in public health nursing, and an understanding of the problems of alcoholism who could develop effective nursing care programs for alcoholic patients. Such a nurse could follow the patient throughout the course of his illness and provide some continuity and consistency in his care. The earlier this specially prepared nurse would be able to make contact with the alcoholic patient and his family, the more effective he could be. His primary function would be to plan and coordinate the nursing care program. At times, he would give direct patient care, and at times he would be a consultant to nurses less skilled or less familiar with the problems of alcoholism. That is, he would not necessarily assume the responsibility for providing all the direct nursing care needed by the alcoholic patient and his family, but would work with nurses in hospitals and public health nursing services to coordinate their efforts with the total nursing plan. Such a nurse specialist would also participate in multidisciplinary conferences, contributing the nursing point of view to the total plan of therapy. In times of crises or when intensive psychiatric nursing care was required, he would give direct nursing care.

Failures in Treatment—
Poor Follow-up Plans

Some of the causes of failure in the treatment of the alcoholic have been that the alcoholic patient characteristically gets lost between referrals or evades treatment in the intervals between his drinking episodes. When he is acutely ill and hospitalized, he receives intensive treatment. Then, in most instances, he is discharged quickly with no follow-up. Generally, the patient is not motivated to seek treatment on his own during this period. However, since his illness is a deep-seated, chronic condition, treatment must be continuous and consistent in terms of treatment plan, regularity of professional contacts, and maintenance of relationships with treatment personnel.

Unavailability of Therapists at
Critical Times

The alcoholic patient cannot tolerate delays in referrals, lack of time or availability of professional help, nor an impersonal or disinterested attitude in his therapists (Chafetz et al., 1962). When he wants help, he wants it immediately. This means that therapists who treat alcoholics must be prepared to maintain very flexible working hours. It seems logical, too, that a nurse with special training in the care of alcoholic patients would be ideally suited to follow the alcoholic patient through the vicissitudes of his episodes of drinking and periods of remission. At the present time very little is known about the patient during his periods of remission or what the circumstances are that contribute to or initiate the onset of a drinking episode.

395

Alcoholics Anonymous

Any discussion of the treatment of alcoholism would be incomplete without noting that the efforts of all the health professions to date have had only limited success. Alcoholics Anonymous, a voluntary organization of exalcoholics, has helped many alcoholics, whether as an adjunct to professional medical treatment or independently. To receive assistance from Alcoholics Anonymous, the alcoholic must have an honest desire to stop drinking and must ask for help (Mann, 1958). His family cannot ask for help for him if he is unwilling. However, when he sincerely asks for help, members of Alcoholics Anonymous will go to great lengths to assist him. They will come to him at any hour of the day or night to give help, sitting with him, nursing him through hangovers, helping him with personal or family problems, and even taking him into their own homes. There is no fee for this service.

One of the factors contributing to the success of Alcoholics Anonymous seems to be that the alcoholic individual feels that the AA member understands him and his problems in a way that a non-alcoholic, no matter what his professional qualifications are, could not possibly do. The alcoholic is also encouraged by the example of former alcoholics who have successfully overcome their drinking habit. Knowing that he is constantly supported by a group of AA members who are ready and willing to come to his assistance day or night is also a great source of strength.

Prevention of Alcoholism

Newer concepts concerning the prevention and control of alcoholism stress the importance of community responsibility and environmental factors and advocate public health approaches rather than treatment of individual cases of alcoholism (Cummings, 1963; Eissler, 1949; Plaut, 1963). McGavran (1963) writes:

> We must face alcoholism as a community problem, not as an individual problem, a community disease that can be diagnosed and treated as such in each community, every community being different from its neighbor as each individual is different from his neighbor. Diagnosis here means community research into the factors that make this disease more prevalent in one community than in another—determining environmental factors that are conducive to the disease. This has physical, social, economic, political, religious, psychological, and educational components. It is immediately obvious that no one individual, agency, profession or group can have all the skills, knowledge and competence necessary—a team of professional equals from all these disciplines is necessary—the whole team being the doctor of the body politic.

Plaut (1963) sees the major objective of a community public health program for the prevention and control of alcoholism as influencing the rate of alcoholism in the community and strengthening communitywide resistance to this disease. He also stresses the importance of community diagnosis before a realistic and effective program can be initiated. He defines community diagnosis as "the general assessment of the manner in which the community operates, makes decisions, handles conflicts and tensions, divides its membership into various categories or classes." For an alcoholism control program it would also include an analysis of the community's attitudes and concerns and involvement with the problem of alcoholism. In planning a program, decisions regarding the optimum use of funds and personnel are dependent on such a diagnosis. Because the problem of alcoholism is deeply imbedded in the socioeconomic structure of the community, any alcoholism program must be coordinated with other health and welfare agencies in the community.

Preventive Measures

Some of the nonspecific primary preventive measures which Plaut suggests include efforts to improve the general mental health of the community (adequate mental health facilities); training people to tolerate greater psychological stress and to learn improved methods of coping with stressful situations, by gradual exposure to stressful situations, as in Peace Corps training; preparing in advance for anticipated difficult or painful events (surgery, separation from a loved one); reducing environmental stress (irritating or frustrating regulations); and reducing social isolation. Specific primary preventive measures include attempts to alter alcoholic beverages chemically to lessen their addictive qualities, measures to influence their sale and distribution, educational programs in the schools on the use and abuse of alcohol, methods to provide a more objective appraisal of the psychological and social values associated with drinking by teen-agers, and attempts to change harmful attitudes in the community in regard to alcoholic consumption, for example, community attitudes toward drunkenness. Still another important specific measure is to find a satisfactory substitute for alcohol as a tension-reducing agent (Plaut, 1963).

Role of the Community in Prevention

The successful operation of any alcoholism preventive program, no matter how carefully planned, will depend to a great extent on the cooperation of the key figures in the community—those who influence public opinion or who are the decision makers. Plaut is convinced that the alcoholism specialist must enlist the cooperation of these persons, believing that both treatment and prevention programs can succeed only if expanding groups of professional workers and community groups work together. He sees an increasingly important role for the nonprofessional in alcoholism programs and states that more and more of the treatment and educational work needs to be done by people who are not alcoholism specialists. At present it is necessary to develop and strengthen alcoholism programs, but in the future, with more knowledge and understanding of the problem, these programs could be integrated with other community health and educational agencies.

DRUG ADDICTION

Drug addiction has been defined by the World Health Organization as a state of periodic or chronic intoxication detrimental to the individual and to society, produced by the repeated consumption of a drug (natural or synthetic). Its characteristics include: (1) an overpowering desire or need (compulsion) to continue taking the drug and to obtain it by any means; (2) a tendency to increase the dose; (3) a psychic (psychological) and sometimes a physical dependence on the effects of the drug (Nyswander, 1956). The addictive narcotic drugs include morphine, heroin, Dilaudid, Metopan, Demerol, methadone, codeine, and cocaine. Within recent years it has been shown that some sedative, tranquilizing, and stimulating drugs also have addictive qualities. Of these the most commonly used are the barbiturates and the amphetamines.

Differences between Alcoholism and Drug Addiction

The sale and distribution of narcotic drugs are rigidly controlled under the provisions of the Harrison Narcotic Act in the United States. Most addicts obtain narcotic drugs from illegal sources, thus complicating the problem of drug addiction by making the treatment of the addict not only a medical and social problem but also a legal and criminal one. The alcohol addict, on the other hand, can obtain alcohol without difficulty. This is only one of the differences between the alcohol and the drug addict. Another difference is that alcohol tends to release aggression whereas narcotics inhibit it. Gerard (1959) states that the drug addict is comfortable and functions well as long as he receives large enough quantities of drugs to stave off his abstinence syndrome, but the chronically intoxicated alcoholic cannot function normally as long as he maintains his intoxicating intake of alcohol.

The Drug Addict—Personality Traits

Drug addicts come from all walks of life. According to Nyswander (1956) there are no special social factors which characterize the drug addict, that is, no special social class, occupation, religion, or race. However, men outnumber women by a ratio of three to one. Social data are still very meager. Most authorities agree that drug addicts are emotionally unstable, one of their most outstanding psychological characteristics being extreme emotional immaturity; they often function psychologically at the level of a three-year-old child. Their dependence and passiveness have been commented on by many observers. Drug addicts have been described as "people without a purpose" and "rootless," who drift through life without becoming involved. Characteristically, they have a very low opinion of themselves, which is often accompanied by a strong self-destructive trend, a desire to play the role of martyr.

Nyswander notes the narcissism, inability to tolerate anxiety or pain, and need for self-gratification of drug addicts. Their interpersonal relationships become very limited; the drug takes the place of wife, doctor, priest, and friend. The addict turns to no one for help, but by administering the drug to himself he becomes his own savior—the drug does all the work. According to Yahraes (1963), "It takes three things to make an addict—a psychologically maladjusted individual, an available drug, and a mechanism for bringing them together. Contrary to general belief, the bringing-together is largely accidental. The susceptible person does not, as a rule, start out looking for a shot and he is not, as a rule, coaxed into taking one by a 'pusher' for the illegal drug trade. Ordinarily, he is introduced to drugs by his associates."

Treatment—Withdrawal Phase

The drug addict generally seeks treatment for one of the following reasons: (1) he sincerely wants to "break the habit" and return to society, (2) he finds himself physically ill or too old to keep up the struggle to obtain drugs, or (3) it has become impossible for him to satisfy his drug requirements. His treatment goal, therefore, may be either to learn to live without drugs or to cut down the dosage required and maintain his addiction. To accomplish the latter goal he may even seek arrest and a brief period in jail. Treatment for drug addiction is also provided on commitment or on a voluntary basis at two federal hospitals, the U.S. Public Health Service hospitals at Lexington, Kentucky, and Fort Worth, Texas. Lexington has 1,000 beds for both men and women; Fort Worth, which can accommodate 800 patients, accepts only men patients from west of the Mississippi.

Other treatment programs for drug addicts include state- and city-supported programs such as special narcotic units in the New York Department of Mental Hygiene system; the California Rehabilitation Center; a pilot project at Spring Grove State Hospital, Catonsville, Maryland; New York City's master plan for narcotics control; the New York Demonstration Center program; the Metropolitan Hospital After-care Program; and the special narcotic project of the New York State Division of Parole. Nongovernmental programs include private sanitariums, psychiatric hospitals and clinics, and various church-supported agencies such as the East Harlem Protestant Parish Narcotics Committee mission in New York City. Synanon and Narcotics Anonymous are two lay organizations providing help to addicts by former addicts.

Withdrawal Phase

The treatment plan for drug addiction can be divided roughly into two phases—the withdrawal phase and the rehabilitation phase. The withdrawal phase, during which the addict is weaned from his dependence on the addicting drugs, may be accomplished by one of three methods: abrupt withdrawal, abrupt withdrawal with supportive treatment, and gradual withdrawal.

Abrupt Withdrawal

In abrupt withdrawal, known as "cold turkey," the addict is taken off all drugs immediately on entering treatment. No narcotics or other drugs are administered. The patient generally experiences violent withdrawal symptoms which are not unlike those of severe influenza. These symptoms include chills, profuse perspiration, lacrimation, rhinorrhea, restlessness, tremors, gooseflesh, loss of appetite, sleeplessness, diarrhea, nausea, vomiting, a slight elevation of temperature, and increased pulse rate. Psychological symptoms include anxiety, depression, and sometimes conversion symptoms.

These symptoms are typical of withdrawal sickness in all methods of withdrawal. In abrupt withdrawal, although the patient appears sicker, the period of discomfort is much shorter than in the other methods. Regan (1958) states that the physical symptoms begin 12 hours after the last dose, reach their peak in 24 to 36 hours, subside in 72 hours, and are minimal or absent in 5 to 6 days. The individual is not socially or psychologically incapacitated during the withdrawal period and may be available for psychotherapeutic interviewing and engage in nonstrenuous social activities.

Abrupt Withdrawal with Supportive
Treatment and Gradual Withdrawal

The abrupt method of withdrawal may be modified by using supportive therapeutic measures or by substituting another drug to mitigate the severity of the withdrawal symptoms. These measures include the use of insulin, hyosine, calcium gluconate, prolonged narcosis, and electroshock therapy. Some of the tranquilizing drugs such as chlorpromazine have also proved helpful (Nyswander, 1956). The gradual withdrawal method consists of administering gradually decreasing doses of the drug or a substitute drug until the patient is free from addiction. At Lexington Hospital, methadone, a synthetic drug which can be given orally and has longer-lasting effects than morphine, has been substituted for morphine in the treatment program (Yahraes, 1963). With either method the withdrawal period may last 10 to 12 days with an additional period for convalescence. During the convalescent period, psychotherapy, occupational and vocational therapy, and social planning are initiated. Contraindications for withdrawal of addicting drugs include cardiac disease, acute infections and surgical procedures, some types of chronic disease, and terminal illness. However, even in these conditions patients fare better, according to Nyswander, if the drug dosage is kept at a minimum level for the control of pain.

Hospital Treatment

The major problem during the withdrawal phase, whatever the method used, is making sure that the addict is not receiving drugs surreptitiously. The ability of addicts to secrete drugs or to prevail on others, even medical and hospital personnel, to obtain drugs for them is well known. Therefore, many authorities state that drugs can be successfully withdrawn only in a controlled environment such as a hospital (Nyswander, 1956; Yahraes, 1963). Hospitalization also affords much-needed medical and nursing care when withdrawal symptoms are most acute. For example, some addicts react to withdrawal with severe symptoms such as high fever, rapid drop in blood pressure, persistent vomiting and diarrhea, and rapid loss of weight. Although fatalities are extremely rare, they can occur.

Role of the Nurse

Nyswander (1956) regards the nurse as playing an important role in observing and reporting to the physician such serious symptoms as rapid pulse and shallow or irregular breathing. She writes:

> An experienced nurse is of inestimable help to the physician. If inexperienced, the nurse in charge must be given specific instruction and told what to expect in terms of the patient's behavior. The nurse must watch the collection of all specimens and supervise the temperature taking. Drug addicts know how to raise a thermometer reading, prick a finger to put blood in their urine, or cause themselves to vomit. They will often swallow blood in sufficient amounts to produce a positive test in their stools in order to simulate a bleeding ulcer. The nurse's report, of decisive importance in evaluating the severity of withdrawal symptoms, should include a three-times-a-day temperature, check on weight, blood pressure, respiration and pulse rate, food and fluid intake, and consistency of the stools.

Rapid loss of weight resulting from inability to eat and from excessive vomiting and diarrhea occurs frequently during the withdrawal phase. Danger signals which the nurse should watch for and report to the physician immediately are a sudden or marked rise in temperature or blood pressure. Supportive measures during the withdrawal phase include adequate fluid intake, hot baths or continuous tubs for muscular tremors and discomfort, and nighttime sedation and other sleep-promoting measures for insomnia. Some patients require medication for constipation; others, antidiarrhetic drugs. Fluid intake and output should be noted, for it is important that the patient maintain his fluid balance.

Psychotherapy and Social Therapy

Although most physicians are primarily concerned with treating the patient's physical symptoms in the withdrawal phase, Regan emphasizes the importance of initiating psychotherapy and social therapy during this period. Psychotherapy and social therapy are aspects of treatment which have been largely ignored in the past. Common psychological symptoms which require psychotherapy are anxiety and depression. Often they are so severe that the discomfort they cause the patient overshadows the distress caused by the physical symptoms of withdrawal.

Regan (1958) believes that during the acute phase it is essential for the drug addict to become aware that he uses narcotics to cope with anxiety and depression and to realize the self-destructiveness of this method. The patient must be willing to try other ways of coping with his psychological problems if treatment is to be effective. In his treatment of drug addicts, Regan initiated psychotherapy with frequent, brief, informal, and unscheduled interviews. He often found that several interviews a day were necessary at first, but that by the end of 5 or 6 days the patient was able to engage in regularly scheduled interviews. Patients are also encouraged to attend occupational therapy, recreational therapy, and physical therapy programs, and to participate in the ongoing social activities with other patients.

Synanon

Synanon is both an agency and an organization of former addicts dedicated to the treatment of drug addiction. The management of the withdrawal phase at Synanon, as described by Yablonsky, presents an interesting approach with implications that could also be useful to nurses, especially in the psychological and social management of the addict. In fact, this is the only method used at Synanon, since the addict withdraws from his habit without the support of any drugs and without the supervision of a physician. Yablonsky (1965) writes:

In contrast with the difficulty of withdrawal symptoms under other conditions, Synanon provides a unique social setting for withdrawal. The withdrawing addict at Synanon has already taken the first step by making a voluntary decision to attempt to eliminate his habit. He is placed on a couch in the main living room, where he is in full view of all members. Also, he is in a position to visit with residents, observe the activities in the House, and become better acquainted with Synanon. Although he can leave, the newcomer voluntarily remains because of a commitment he has made to himself and partially to the people of Synanon. Moreover, he is in a reasonably pleasant environment, entirely different from a jail or prison situation.

The hi-fi is usually playing, children may be around in the room, he receives warm drinks (eggnog, hot tea), and he is physically soothed with occasional shoulder rubs. People will come over, shake his hand, welcome him, and chat. Most important, he can literally see live evidence of success at Synanon. He may see "clean" ex-addicts with whom he personally used drugs. He is encouraged to achieve the healthy physical and emotional condition of the people he sees before him. He begins to learn about Synanon from people who have experienced his current emotions. He sees role models of achievable success around him. He is interacting with people who understand how he feels, since they themselves were at one time in his shoes. In addition to understanding his feelings, they sketch for him a positive future which they themselves are literally experiencing. In his confused state, these solid reference points provided by other Synanon members help to minimize his psychic and physical withdrawal pains and speed his involvement in the group.

Rehabilitation Phase or
Aftercare Treatment

The withdrawal phase, when the addicted individual is being freed of drugs or "kicking the habit," is not nearly so difficult as the problem of keeping him free from his dependence on drugs, i.e., preventing readdiction, and rehabilitating him for a useful role in society. The length of time required for rehabilitation has not been determined, varying in different treatment programs from 3 months to 5 years. A number of state hospitals have a 90-day program for addicts somewhat comparable to the 90-day program for alcoholics.

At Lexington, the rehabilitation phase is the 4-month period following the termination of drugs, but many patients do not remain for the full period. More than one-third of the voluntary patients leave within 2 weeks, or as soon as they have gone through the withdrawal period, and by the end of 4 weeks more than half have left. Only one-third complete the 4-month stay (Yahraes, 1963). In California, voluntary or committed patients at the California Rehabilitation Center must stay for at least 6 months, and even a voluntary patient may be required to stay as long as 5 years. After discharge from the Center the patient is released on parole and must remain free of drugs for 3 consecutive years before receiving complete discharge. Dr. Nyswander estimates that complete rehabilitation takes between 1 and 3 years. Synanon has determined that a period of $2^{1}/_{2}$ years is the length of time required for successful rehabilitation.

Types of Rehabilitation Programs

The various patterns of rehabilitation programs can be divided roughly into two groups. In the first, the patient is treated in a controlled environment, such as Lexington and Fort Worth, Riverside Hospital, N.Y., Metropolitan Hospital, N.Y., California Rehabilitation Center, special narcotic units in state hospitals, private sanitariums, and Synanon. In the second group, the patient is treated in a noncontrolled environment such as general hospitals, the New York Demonstration Center, East Harlem Protestant Narcotics Committee Mission, and Narcotics Anonymous.

Controlled versus Uncontrolled
Environments

Those authorities who advocate the controlled environment believe that it protects the patient at a time when he is particularly vulnerable to the temptation to revert to drugs. It also provides the patient an escape from family contacts and other stresses in the home, help from individuals with special knowledge and understanding of his problem, and an opportunity for objective examination of his difficulties and the establishment of new patterns of behavior. Those who advocate the noncontrolled environment include Dr. Nyswander, who states, "Any treatment center which brings active drug addicts together in large numbers is bound to fail in its purpose." Other authorities think that the interaction of the addict with other general hospital patients helps to provide a more wholesome climate. Still other authorities think that taking the patient out of his accustomed environment for treatment does not prepare him to cope with problems in that environment when he returns to it following treatment. However, the increasing use of day and night hospitals, halfway houses, and carefully planned home visits before discharge help to overcome this latter objection.

Preparation for Rehabilitation Treatment

Transition from the withdrawal phase to the rehabilitation phase is made smoother and proceeds more rapidly when preliminary psycho-therapeutic and sociotherapeutic measures are initiated in the withdrawal phase. Psychotherapy with drug addicts differs in some respects from psychotherapy with other types of patients. In the New York Demonstration Project it was found that the first year of treatment was essentially an introductory or preparatory phase. During this year a supportive, counseling type of psychotherapy was used because the patient could not tolerate the traditional interview techniques. He also could not maintain a scheduled pattern of interviews, nor could he face up to an examination of his problems during the interview. What the patient needed was to develop a supportive, dependent relationship with the therapist without exploration of his feelings. The patient also wanted the therapist to be available when needed, and to be able to give assistance of a practical nature—such as provision for food, shelter, or medical attention.

Improving the Patient's Ability
to Communicate

Another important purpose which the preliminary year of psychother-apy accomplished was to improve the drug addict's ability to com-municate. Generally speaking, addicts are very inarticulate. Among themselves they tend to use a special addict's jargon which reduces communication to a few stereotyped terms. Those who have been addicts for many years use even this type of communication sparingly. Conversation becomes restricted to topics related to their addictive habit. In Synanon, new patients are discouraged from using the addict's language; and in some cases, to break them of this habit, they are banned from speaking for a period of time. Yablonsky (1965) quotes a new Synanon member as follows:

> We were just not permitted to discuss drugs and all that gutter talk that was so common in Lexington. In Lexington, for one thing, most of the addicts were officially getting drugs. So, there you were, living in a place with many loaded addicts. Naturally, when you get addicts together like that, they'll talk about their connections, different scores they've made, and using drugs. I found that Synanon was refreshing change. I always had an inner desire to talk about art and intellectual matters. Because of my past life, it was seldom appropriate, except in a phony way. In the dope-fiend world, in Lexington, and in jail, it was always the same monotonous garbage. Who you fixed with, how much time you got, the quality of the junk, and all that nonsense.

Therefore, one of the therapeutic tasks of this initial stage is to help the patient become accustomed to talking and to expand his range of interests.

Helping the Patient Overcome
Boredom and Loneliness

Workers in the New York Demonstration Center speak of the chronic boredom and stimulus-hunger which characterizes so many drug addicts (Brill, 1963). Many addicts try to overcome their boredom by developing a dull apathy; others, by aimless and incessant activity. Boredom is often relieved when they are admitted to an institution where a structured environment and planned routine are provided. Other addicts are driven back to the use of drugs by boredom. One former addict describes her feelings as follows (Yablonsky, 1965), "I remember one time, when I got out of jail, I went for three days without using. Then I began to get lonely. I suddenly realized the only people I knew to call and talk to were dope fiends. I didn't have any non-addict friends, and I surely didn't know any addict who would admit trying to quit using. Finally, I broke down and called some weed-head (marijuana smoker) I knew, out of sheer boredom and loneliness. Naturally I was back on heroin in a few days."

Drug addicts have very few inner resources. They are very immature, limited individuals. Contrary to popular opinion, they are not creative. The social workers at the Demonstration Center found that as a general rule the typical addict had been "constricted and unimaginative all his life, unable to use himself effectively in any way, so that even his illegal activities become stereotyped (Brill, 1963). To overcome boredom, loneliness, and lack of imagination, it would seem that some forms of educational therapy could be very beneficial in a treatment program for drug addicts. Activities might include discussion groups on current events, lectures on topics of special interest, opportunities to appreciate and participate in dramatics, music, and art, and classes of academic, avocational, and vocational interest.

The therapist working with addicts must be skillful in creating an interest in these activities and must also support the patient's interest once it is evoked. Like other individuals with behavior disorders, these patients have a very short attention span and are easily frustrated and discouraged. Therefore assistance should be available whenever the patient needs it. Patients should also be cautioned not to attempt too much at one time nor to set unrealistic goals for accomplishment.

Psychotherapy

Most addicts do not respond favorably to the conventional methods of psychotherapy, either individual or group therapy. However, some patients do benefit from individual psychotherapy if the therapist is nonmoralistic yet firm, authoritative, understanding of the problems of addiction, and sincerely interested in his patient, and when the patient, on the other hand, really wants to be helped. Nyswander (1956) also stresses the fact that the therapist must be prepared for relapses to the use of drugs and that he must be able to cope with these crises without becoming unduly alarmed, even if a few days of hospitalization is indicated.

Another element in successful psychotherapy is the ability of the therapist to achieve an important role in the patient's life as a stabilizing, supportive, authoritative figure. Like the alcoholic patient, the drug addict cannot tolerate changes of therapists. It is difficult for the patient to establish a working relationship with a therapist, but once established, the relationship can be used as a kind of safety line to support him during the vicissitudes of treatment. The drug addict requires frequent and regular contacts with his therapists. Some authorities recommend daily communication of some kind. Telephone calls are often a useful way of maintaining contact between patient and therapist between interviews. Such contact makes it possible for a patient to receive individual psychotherapy on an outpatient basis.

Group Therapy

Although drug addicts do not seem to benefit from the permissive types of group therapy that have proved helpful with other patients, they can benefit from certain special types of therapy such as those developed by Synanon and Narcotics Anonymous. The type of group meeting utilized in Narcotics Anonymous is patterned after the group meetings in Alcoholics Anonymous. The meeting is attended exclusively by addicts or ex-addicts and is held in the local community. Charles Dederich, the founder of Synanon, has devised several types of group therapy suitable for the treatment of addicts in the various Synanon establishments. These establishments are located in Santa Monica, San Francisco, and San Diego, California; Westport, Connecticut; and Reno, Nevada.

The Synanon treatment program could best be described as a type of milieu therapy. That is, in a given setting, such as a large house, former factory, etc., which is staffed by exaddicts, everything possible is done to create a climate in which addicts can live and be treated. The goal of treatment is to free them from their dependence on drugs and to return them to the community as useful members of society. The word *synanon* is a neologism coined by an early member of the group when he tried to pronounce simultaneously the words "symposium" and "seminar." The term has been kept and is used to mean both the Synanon establishment and also, spelled with a small *s,* a particular type of group therapy.

The Synanon

The basic form of synanon consists of twelve to fifteen people. Synanons are generally held three times a week. One radical difference between a synanon and other types of group therapy is that the membership of a synanon is different at each session. That is, each member faces a totally different group at each synanon. The rationale behind this is that a member cannot, by tacit mutual agreement, protect another member from revealing painful material as could be possible in a long-term therapy group. Yablonsky (1965) describes a typical session as follows:

> Everyone in the group settles down, as comfortably as possible, in a circle, facing one another. There is usually a brief silence, a scanning appraisal as to who is present, a kind of sizing one another up, and then the group launches into an intensive emotional discussion of personal and group problems. A key point of the sessions is an emphasis on extreme, uncompromising candor about one another. "No holds or

statements are barred from the group effort at truth-seeking about problem situations, feelings, and emotions of each and all members of the group," I have been
told.

The synanon is, in some respects, an emotional battlefield. Here an individual's
delusions, distorted self-images, and negative behavior are attacked again and
again.—Attack therapy in synanon has the effect of "toughening up" the person. It
helps him to see himself as relevant others do. He gains information and insights into
his problems.—A participant in a synanon is forced to examine positive and negative
aspects about himself, as well as some dimensions he would never have considered
on his own. This often leaves him with a clearer view and a greater knowledge of his
inner and outer world.

The process of a synanon also involves learning something about the norms of the
overall Synanon society. The synanon helps to socialize the person and fosters a
learning of interpersonal competence. This set of experiences seems to be useful for
interaction situations both in Synanon and in the larger society.

A synanon is led by a synanist, who is one of the older and more
experienced members of the Synanon. A house synanon is a group
session of all the members living in a particular establishment and may
be called when a crisis occurs or a problem arises involving the total
membership. Another type of group therapy used only in special
situations is the "haircut." This is an attack form of therapy used to
counteract particularly undesirable behavior. The "haircut" is planned
and admininstered by several expert synanists to the erring members.
Ridicule, exaggeration, and direct attack are used to puncture the
self-image of the culprits and to cut them down to size. Even the most
hardened tough guy generally succumbs to this treatment. However,
the "haircut" also offers support to the positive behavior of the
recipients and, according to Yablonsky, "goes beyond the bad behavior of the moment and into a more serious problem which is also
revealed in the session."

In addition to synanons, there are weekly seminars at which outside
speakers are invited to address the membership on a wide variety of
topics followed by general discussion. There are also seminars at
which the philosophy synanon treatment is discussed by one of the
members of the top echelon of Synanon, and Open House, a weekly
discussion group for members, family, and visitors.

Employment as Therapy

An important aspect of rehabilitation is employment. Many drug
addicts are quite unable to get and hold a job. While on drugs, most of
their time and energy have been spent meeting the demands of the
habit—getting money to pay for drugs, obtaining the drug, preparing
and administering it, and then repeating this routine ceaselessly. By

the time they come for treatment and rehabilitation they are literally unemployable. Their health is impaired, they have lost their work habits, their self-confidence, and their ability to persevere at a job. A period of work training to get them ready to work may be necessary; some will also need vocational counseling and possibly retraining for different types of jobs. Some authorities stress the importance of starting the addict on some simple type of work even before he has completely recovered from the withdrawal phase, so important do they regard the therapeutic value of work for these patients.

Role of the Family in the Treatment of Drug Addiction

Members of the patient's family, expecially parents and spouse, are almost always involved deeply in the emotional problems of the patient. Some authorities believe in isolating the patient from his family during the critical stages of treatment or until the patient is strong enough to cope with the neurotic patterns of interaction with significant family members. Other authorities have been successful in working with members of the patient's family, either individually or in groups, as, for example, groups of wives of addicts, or parents of young addicts. Family therapy, involving all the members of the addict's family, might also have something to offer in the treatment of some cases of drug addiction.

RECENT TRENDS IN THE TREATMENT OF ADDICTION

Training of Professionals

Earlier in this chapter it was noted that most nurses involved in the treatment of alcoholic patients had received no previous preparation for this work. Einstein and Wolfson (1970) sent out questionnaires to 601 accredited professional schools, which included medicine, pharmacy, social work, psychology, nursing, and law, to determine whether the study of alcoholism was taught in their curriculums. Of the 55 percent who responded, 307 schools, or 95 percent, included some teaching on alcoholism. All medical schools taught something—primarily in graduate programs, but very few at the undergraduate level. This was the case also in schools of social work and law. Schools of pharmacy and psychology included more at the undergraduate level, but the major teaching was at the graduate level. Only in nursing was alcoholism taught early in the professional training at the under-graduate level. All schools gave some didactic teaching, but only medical, nursing, and psychology students were given any clinical experience with patients. Field trips to agencies treating alcoholics was part of the training of medical and nursing students.

According to this study, nursing was considered to provide the most comprehensive preparation for subsequent practice. In 90 percent of the nursing schools sociological, psychological, psychiatric, and medical aspects of alcoholism were taught. In general, nursing students were taught more about the medical aspects of alcoholism than medical students were. Possibly the reason for this was that nurses were seen as the professional persons most concerned with the direct care of the alcoholic patient in the inpatient service and as often playing a decisive role in determination of the agency to which the alcoholic would be admitted for treatment.

This study also showed that there were great differences among the professions and among the various schools of a given profession regarding the importance given to the teaching of alcoholism in the curriculum, as well as great differences in the methods of teaching it. Schools of nursing and social work gave high priority to the inclusion of alcoholism in the curriculum, but generally schools of law and pharmacy regarded it as not important. The researchers concluded that the many inconsistencies in the teaching of alcoholism were probably due to the ambivalence of lay and professional groups regarding what to do with and for the alcoholic, and they suggest, in view of the seriousness of the problem to the health of the community, studying the best method for integrating the teaching of alcoholism with their professional training programs (Einstein and Wolfson, 1970).

Attitudes toward Addiction

The greatest drawback in the successful treatment of the alcoholic is the antipathy and lack of understanding of the therapists (Chafetz, 1970). Morgan and Moreno (1973) discuss the particular problems that beset the nurse in this regard and make some suggestions for overcoming these difficulties. Chafetz stresses the importance of the therapist being prepared to step outside the traditional role of the therapist-patient relationship in which the therapist waits passively for the patient to seek his help and then accept it gratefully. In Chafetz's opinion, the therapist must accept the responsibility for establishing the relationship. "From the very first meeting the therapist must be openly and warmly interested in the patient's well-being. He must reach out to the patient. Moreover, he must make his concern explicit by taking an active hand in helping the patient solve urgent problems of daily living" (Chafetz, 1970, p. 109). The therapist must also be able to withstand the incessant, insatiable demands and hostility of the alcoholic patient. Therefore, Chafetz suggests that the team approach in treatment permits this hostility to be shared by the members of the team rather than having it focused on the therapist alone.

In his clinical research studies in alcoholism, Chafetz found nurses accepting of alcoholics when they were sober, but ambivalent when the alcoholics were intoxicated. Some nurses found their work with alcoholics challenging and rewarding, but others were discouraged and thought attempts at treatment were futile. Still other nurses appeared disinterested and made no attempts to extend their knowledge or skills in the treatment of alcoholism. Nurses were often uncertain of their role when confronted with an alcoholic patient and felt limited to referral of the patient to someone else for information and/or help. Research colleagues noted that if the nurse is to work comfortably as well as effectively, she may need a chance to examine her own feelings and reactions to alcoholic patients. They saw additional training for nurses as desirable to help them become preventive agents for identifying and referring for treatment persons in the community with alcoholic problems (Chafetz, 1970, p. 118).

Drug Treatment of Addiction

Since 1964 when Doctors Marie Nyswander and Vincent P. Dole treated their first heroin addict with methadone (Nyswander, 1967; Dole and Nyswander, 1965), the treatment of addicts by the substitution of methadone has grown enormously. Methadone clinics and community mental health centers with methadone programs can be found in most of the large cities of the United States. Methadone is an addictive narcotic like heroin but, unlike heroin, it has no secondary effects. It relieves withdrawal symptoms, permits the addicted person to function normally in social and work situations, and it needs to be taken only once a day. It is also inexpensive and can be administered orally. Psychotherapy and rehabilitation therapy should be given concomitantly with methadone therapy. Methadone has proved to be a boon to many addicted persons, restoring them as useful members of society. Critics, however, point out that the person is still as addicted and dependent on methadone as he formerly was on heroin. Also, methadone users in time come to miss the euphoric experiences of heroin and often return to its use. To obtain heroin, they often sell or trade their methadone. A growing black market is also developing for methadone. There is also a tendency for patients on methadone to take other drugs along with the methadone (Morgan and Moreno, 1973, p. 501; Fink et al., 1971).

Since 1966, a number of drugs known as *narcotic antagonists* have been introduced in the treatment of opiate addiction. The rationale for the use of opiate antagonists is to free the drug user eventually from dependence on an addicting drug. This is accomplished by blocking or reversing the effects of the addicting opiate, and this in time should lead to the extinction of the drug-seeking behavior. Two of the present most satisfactory antagonists for addiction therapy are cyclazone (1966) and naloxone (1968) (Fink et al., 1971).

According to Fink and his associates, cyclazone has a long duration of action but a number of undesirable side effects. Naloxone is effective for 24 hours and has no secondary effects. However, in its present state of development it requires a relatively large dosage (3.0 gm). Fink and his associates are presently investigating the possibility of finding a way to provide for a gradual, continuous release of the drug, as, for example, by implanting it under the skin. Although present formulations of antagonists are unsatisfactory, Fink believes that "recent data indicate that the treatment is safe and rational and provides a logical and achievable endpoint. Narcotic antagonists are not easily abused nor are they salable. It is logical and feasible that the development of a long-acting, parenteral antagonist, which could be implanted under the skin to block the effects of opiates, could serve as the model for the prevention and treatment of opiate dependence in a few years" (Fink et al., 1971, p. 1363).

Social Approaches to Alcoholism

Adlestein (1970) states that the medical model of alcoholism as a disease is not adequate to encompass all aspects of the problem. Social medicine offers some new approaches. "Social medicine and social psychiatry are not only concerned with the impact of society or culture upon the development of illness in man but with the impact of the illness and its management upon society" (Adlestein, 1970, p. 27). There are indications from a social medicine point of view that possibly society could be changed to protect individual members from community influences conducive to alcoholism. He cites the Social Security Act and the civil rights movement as examples of social reforms which had great impact on the mental health of certain segments of the population although mental health was not the primary objective of either. Adlestein raises the question whether it would be more fruitful for mental health professionals to focus their efforts on changing social customs than to try to prevent alcoholism in individuals in that society. However, victims of alcohol need treatment, and he indicates some specific factors to keep in mind in developing a treatment program, such as commonalities encountered in alcoholics, multiple causation of alcoholism, the course of an alcoholic career, the need for continuity of care, and barriers to treatment. He also challenges the reader to further consideration of the complex problem of alcoholism by asking what would happen to society if excessive drinking could be eliminated; whether our society needs alcoholism; and whether the elimination of alcoholism will cause more serious problems in our society (Adlestein, 1970, p. 28).

REFERENCES

Adlestein, Joseph (1970): "Implications for Alcoholism Programming from Social Psychiatry and Social Medicine," *Mental Health Digest*, vol. 2, no. 11, pp. 23–28.

Alexander, Franz (1930): "The Neurotic Character," *International Journal of Psychoanalysis*, July, pp. 292–311.

Berne, Eric (1961): *Transactional Analysis in Psychotherapy*, Grove Press, Inc., New York.

Blane, Howard T., and Marjorie J. Hill (1964): "Public Health Nurses Speak Up about Alcoholism," *Nursing Outlook*, May, pp. 34–37.

Brill, Leon (1963): *Rehabilitation in Drug Addiction: A Report on a Five-Year Community Experiment of the New York Demonstration Center*, Mental Health Monograph #3, U.S. Dept. of Health, Education, and Welfare, Bethesda 14, Md., May, P.H.S. Pub. #1013, p. 18.

Burton, Genevieve (1964): "An Alcoholic in the Family," *Nursing Outlook*, May, pp. 30–33.

Chafetz, Morris E. (1970): "Clinical Studies in Alcohol," in *Mental Health Program Reports—4*, January, U.S. Department of Health, Education, and Welfare, National Institute of Mental Health, Chevy Chase, Md.

————et al. (1962): "Establishing Treatment Relations with Alcoholics," *Journal of Nervous and Mental Diseases*, May, pp. 395–409.

Cleckley, Hervey M. (1959): "Psychopathic States," in Silvano Arieti (ed.), *American Handbook of Psychiatry*, Basic Books, Inc., Publishers, New York, vol. I, pp. 567–588.

Conner, Ralph G., Richard Flowers, Joan K. Jackson, and H. Wallace Lane (1963): *Hospital Management of Alcoholics*, Washington State Department of Health.

Cummings, Elaine (1963): "Pathways to Prevention," in *Key Issues in the Prevention of Alcoholism*, Report of the Northeast States Conferences, Pittsburgh, published by Division of Behavioral Problems and Drug Control, Dept. of Health, Box 90, Harrisburg, Penna., March, pp. 11–25.

Diethelm, Oskar (1947): "Basic Considerations of the Concept of Psychopathic Personality," in R. M. Lindner and R. V. Seliger (eds.), *Handbook of Correctional Psychology*, Philosophical Library, Inc., New York, pp. 384–394.

Dole, Vincent P., and Marie Nyswander (1965): "A Medical Treatment for Diacetylmorphine (Heroin) Addiction," *Journal of the American Medical Association*, Aug. 23, vol. 193, pp. 646–650.

Einstein, Stanley, and Edward Wolfson (1970): "Alcoholism Curricula: How Professionals Are Trained," *Mental Health Digest*, vol. 2, no. 11, pp. 29–32.

Eissler, Kurt R. (1949): "Some Problems of Delinquency," in K. R. Eissler (ed.), *Searchlights on Delinquency*, International Universities Press, Inc., New York, pp. 3–25.

Fink, Max, Alfred M. Freedman, Arthur M. Zaks, and Richard B. Resnick (1971): "Narcotic Antagonists: Another Approach to Addiction Therapy," *American Journal of Nursing,* vol. 71, no. 7, pp. 1359–1363.

Foreman, Nancy J., and Joyce V. Zerwekh (1971): "Drug Crisis Intervention," *American Journal of Nursing,* vol. 71, no. 9, pp. 1736–1741.

Freud, Anna (1954): "The Widening Scope of Indications for Psychoanalysis," *Journal of the American Psychoanalytic Association,* October, pp. 607–720.

Friedlander, Kate (1949): "Latent Delinquency and Ego Development," in K. R. Eissler (ed.), *Searchlights on Delinquency,* International Universities Press, Inc., New York, pp. 205–215.

Gerard, Donald L. (1959): "Intoxication and Addiction," in Raymond G. McCarthy (ed.), *Drinking and Intoxication,* The Free Press, New York, pp. 33–39.

Gliedman, Lester H. (1958): "Some Contributions of Group Therapy in the Treatment of Chronic Alcoholism," in Paul H. Hoch and Joseph Zubin (eds.), *Problems of Addiction and Habituation,* Grune & Stratton, Inc., New York pp. 214–227.

———, David Rosenthal, Jerome D. Frank, and Helen T. Nash (1963): "Group Therapy of Alcoholics with Concurrent Group Meetings of Their Wives," in Max Rosenbaum and Milton M. Berger (eds.), *Group Psychotherapy and Group Function,* Basic Books, Inc., Publishers, New York, pp. 510–524.

Glover, Edward (1955): *The Technique of Psycho-Analysis,* International Universities Press, Inc., New York.

Greenacre, Phyllis (1947): "Problems of the Patient-Therapist Relationship in the Treatment of Psychopaths," in Robert M. Lindner and Robert V. Seliger, *Handbook of Correctional Psychology,* Philosophical Library, Inc., New York, pp. 278–383.

Holmes, Marguerite J., and Jean A. Werner (1966): *Psychiatric Nursing in a Therapeutic Community,* The Macmillan Company, New York.

Johnson, James A. (1963): *Group Therapy, A Practical Approach,* McGraw-Hill Book Company, New York.

Jones, Maxwell (1962): *Social Psychiatry,* Charles C Thomas, Publisher, Springfield, Ill., p. 68.

———(1953): *The Therapeutic Community, a New Treatment Method in Psychiatry,* Basic Books, Inc., Publishers, New York.

Mann, Marty (1958): *New Primer on Alcoholism,* Rinehart and Company, Inc., New York.

McGavran, Edward G. (1963): "Facing Reality in Public Health," in *Key Issues in the Prevention of Alcoholism,* Report of the Northeast States Conference, Pittsburgh, 1962, published by Division of Behavioral Problems and Drug Control, Dept. of Health, Box 90, Harrisburg, Penna., March, pp. 55–61.

Michaels, Joseph J. (1959): "Character Structure and Character Disorders," in Silvano Arieti (ed.), *American Handbook of Psychiatry,* Basic Books, Inc., Publishers, New York, vol. 1, pp. 351–377.

———(1955): *Disorders of Character,* Charles C Thomas, Publisher, Springfield, Ill.

Morgan, Arthur J., and Judith W. Moreno (1973): "Attitudes toward Addiction," *American Journal of Nursing,* vol. 73, no. 3, pp. 497–505.

Noyes, Arthur P. (1953): *Modern Clinical Psychiatry,* 4th ed., W. B. Saunders Company, Philadelphia, p. 501.

Nyswander, Marie (1956): *The Drug Addict as a Patient,* Grune & Stratton, Inc., New York, pp. 116–122.

———(1967): "Methadone Treatment of Heroin Addicts," *The Bulletin,* New York State Branches, American Psychiatric Association, vol. 9, no. 5, p. 1.

Plaut, Thomas F. A. (1963): "Translating Concept into Action," in *Key Issues in the Prevention of Alcoholism,* Report of Northeast States Conference, Pittsburgh, 1962, published by Division of Behavioral Problems and Drug Control, Dept. of Health, Box 90, Harrisburg, Penna., March, pp. 62–72.

Prout, Curtis, M. A. White, and J. Charry (1958): "Current Issues in Addiction Research," in Paul H. Hoch and Joseph Zubin (eds.), *Problems of Addiction and Habituation,* Grune & Stratton, Inc., –ew York, pp. 202–213.

Regan, Peter, III (1958): "The Psychotherapeutic Management of Abrupt Drug Withdrawal," in Paul H. Hoch and Joseph Zubin (eds.), *Problems of Addiction and Habituation,* Grune & Stratton, Inc., New York, 186–201.

Reich, Wilhelm (1945): *Character Analysis,* 2d ed., Orgone Institute Press, New York.

Reiner, Beatrice Simcox, and Irving Kaufman (1959): *Character Disorders in Parents of Delinquents,* Family Service Association of America, New York, pp. 3–4, 14, 67.

Rosenbaum, Max (1963): "The Challenge of Group Psychoanalysis," in Max Rosenbaum and Milton M. Berger (eds.), *Group Psychotherapy and Group Function,* Basic Books, Inc., Publishers, New York.

Ruesch, Jurgen (1948): "The Infantile Personality: The Core Problem of Psychosomatic Medicine," *Psychosomatic Medicine,* May–June, pp. 133–144.

———(1961): *Therapeutic Communication,* W. W. Norton & Company, Inc., New York.

Schilder, Paul (1938): *Psychotherapy,* W. W. Norton & Company, Inc., New York.

Standish, Christopher T., and Elvin V. Semrad (1963): "Group Psychotherapy with Psychotics," in Max Rosenbaum and Milton M. Berger (eds.), *Group Psychotherapy and Group Function,* Basic Books, Inc., Publishers, New York.

Thompson, George N. (1959): "Acute and Chronic Alcoholic Conditions," in Silvano Arieti (ed.), *American Handbook of Psychiatry,* Basic Books, Inc., Publishers, New York, vol. 2, pp. 1203–1221.

Wilson, Robert N. (1960): "The Nurse and the Alcoholic Patient, Attitudes and Feelings," in *The Role of the Nurse in the Care of the Alcoholic Patient in a General Hospital,* Proceedings of a Conference, Chatham, Mass., Sept. 19–21, published by the Massachusetts Dept. of Public Health, Division of Alcoholism, Boston, Mass., pp. 19–24.

Wolberg, Lewis R. (1954): *The Technique of Psychotherapy,* Grune & Stratton, Inc., New York, pp. 614–615.

Wolf, Alexander (1963): "The Psychoanalysis of Groups," in Max Rosenbaum and Milton M. Berger (eds.), *Group Psychotherapy and Group Function,* Basic Books, Inc., Publishers, New York, pp. 273–327.

Yablonsky, Lewis (1965): *The Tunnel Back, Synanon,* The Macmillan Company, New York, pp. 137–138, 198–199.

Yahraes, Herbert (1963): *Narcotic Drug Addiction,* Mental Health Monograph #2, U.S. Dept. of Health, Education, and Welfare, Bethesda, 14, Md., P.H.S. Pub. #1021, pp. 11, 15.

Zwerling, Israel, and Milton Rosenberg (1959): "Alcoholic Addiction and Personality," in Silvano Arieti (ed.), *American Handbook of Psychiatry,* Basic Books, Inc., Publishers, New York, vol. I, pp. 623–644.

15

PSYCHOSOMATIC DISORDERS

Judith M. Sitzman

Psychosomatic care represents a humanistic approach to health care delivery in that it focuses treatment on the total care of the person. It raises questions concerning the complexity of man, his nature, and their interrelationship. Underlying psychosomatic care is the basic assumption that any function or malfunctioning of either mind or body effects changes in the other. The term *psychosomatic* itself expresses the fusion of the mind-body dichotomy into a unity. Other terms commonly used in psychosomatic treatment, such as *comprehensive patient care, holistic medicine,* and *continuity of care,* also reflect movements toward bringing humanism to the bedside. Trends toward a more humanistic approach are reflected in the media and literature by a growing interest of health professionals in the knowledge and use of body language, communication theory, and individual, family, and group psychotherapy in psychosomatic treatment.

PSYCHOSOMATIC MEDICINE

Psychosomatic medicine is not a specialty field. The methods used for the study and treatment of disorders in the body organ systems have been developed by the medical specialties; the methods used for the study, interpretation, and treatment of psychological malfunctioning are the methods of psychiatry. Therefore, *psychosomatic medicine* refers to a method of approach in research and therapy which coordinates and integrates the use of medical and psychiatric methods simultaneously (Alexander, 1950, p. 50).

Psychosomatic medicine evolved gradually from the mind-body problem which has provoked philosophical inquiry for centuries. Historically, primitive psychology was fostered by demonology; and primitive medicine, rooted in religion and magic, emphasized the mind's influence on bodily functioning. Yet, minimal interest in psychological phenomena was evident during the Greek and Roman civilizations and at the time of the Renaissance, when scientific inquiry dominated. Although two famous physicians, Thomas Sydenham and William Harvey, in the seventeenth century recognized that bodily changes were associated with psychological phenomena, progress in psychosomatic medicine did not occur until the nineteenth century. Early contributions to psychosomatic medicine were provided by many, including Féré, Freud, Ferenczi, and Deutsch. For example, Freud recognized that particular physical symptoms were symbolic of emotional conflicts. Paralyses, anesthesias, pains, vomiting, and visual disturbances were described by him as manifestations of hysteria. Symptoms were viewed by him as unconscious attempts to resolve sexual conflicts. Unconscious conflict occurred when a situation presented both a wish to act and a fear of expressing the wish. The symptoms which resulted may be either a substitutive satisfaction of some wish or sexual impulse or they may reflect measures to prevent the satisfaction. Such physical symptoms were called "substitutes" or "conversions" (Schwartz and Schwartz, 1972, p. 244).

In the 1920s, Cannon noted through his laboratory experiments that particular emotional states, such as fear and anger, activated major physiological responses. His work provided information concerning the interrelationship between the autonomic nervous and neuroendocrine systems and emotions (Cannon, 1929, 1932).

In the 1940s, Franz Alexander offered a major contribution to psychosomatic medicine through using psychoanalytic concepts as a method for studying the less obvious and symbolic meaning of stressful situations for the individual. He and his associates examined particular diseases, such as peptic ulcer, ulcerative colitis, and rheumatoid arthritis, in which emotional conflicts appeared to play a significant role (Alexander, 1950). Yet he stressed that physiologic expressions of emotion are not necessarily symbolic expressions of repressed instinctual drives (Lidz, 1959, p. 651). Alexander and French wrote: "It is well known from everyday experience that emotions such as fear, anger, resentment, guilt or embarrassment have definite physiological effects. The best known examples are weeping, laughing, blushing, and losing bowel and bladder control under the influence of fear" (Alexander and French, 1948, p. 26).

Studies which examined the relationship between life situations, emotions, and particular diseases progressed in the fifties. Hinkle and others reviewed major investigations made on the correlations between life situations and diabetes (Hinkle et al., 1951). Duncan and others studied people with paroxysmal arrhythmias of whom 50 percent had structural heart disease. It was found that such irregularities occurred when the patients were under stress, and that they had common personality traits consisting of inadequately expressed hostility, compulsion, unusual ambition, and long-standing anxiety (Duncan et al., 1950). Wolff emphasized that life stresses may cause bodily organs to react in stereotyped ways, and that persistent stress results in chronic bodily changes (Wolff, 1950). A compilation of analytic and nonanalytic studies on the mind-body relationship was provided by Dunbar (Dunbar, 1954). Also, she identified particular illness states in which she thought psychosomatic relationships might exist.

CURRENT PSYCHOSOMATIC CONCEPTS

A more recent humanistic approach to health and disease is well described by Engel (1962). In viewing life as a series of adjustments within the environment, he describes a healthy individual as one who is "functioning effectively, fulfilling needs, successfully responding to the requirements or demands of the environment, whether internal or external, and pursuing its biological destiny, including growth and reproduction" (Engel, 1962, p. 240). Correspondingly, a disease state involves "failures or disturbances in the growth, development, functions and adjustments of the organism as a whole or any of its systems" (Engel, 1962, p. 240). Generally, the term *psychosomatic* does not account for the social, cultural, and economic factors which influence the cause and severity of a given illness or the patient's perception of it; however, psychosomatic care when influenced by Engel's approach may take into consideration such factors. His broad definitions of health and disease allow for the concept of multiple causation in illness rather than restricting a given disease to a single etiological factor. If one views disease as caused by a single agent, defect, or lesion, then one separates the disease entity from the patient. The single etiological factor is treated, but how a given disease affects one individual versus another and how the patient perceives his illness may be ignored. Interrelationships between psychological, interpersonal, social, biochemical, and organic factors become irrelevant.

Engel also emphasizes that diagnostic labels provide categories of information about a patient but rarely define the illness fully. Clinical diagnoses are established by experience and convention. They are broad generalizations applicable to all patients, which have statistical and predictive value; however, one cannot assume that all patients with a particular disease have all the signs and symptoms of the diagnostic category. Diagnostic categories ignore the unique differences between patients. Travelbee in writing about interpersonal aspects of nursing stresses that the term *patient* is also a stereotype and a category. She emphasizes that there are no patients but only individual human beings in need of care and particular services. When nurses perceive individuals as "patients," little emotional involvement is required, as "'the patient' is an abstraction, a set of expectations personified by tasks to be performed, treatments to carry out, an illness, or a room number" (Travelbee, 1961, p. 34). When a member of a health profession perceives a person as a room number or an illness to be treated, he may easily relate to the person in a mechanistic manner whereby he treats the disease or complication but ignores the person's perceptions, concerns, and emotional reactions. Dehumanization results.

Engel further sees health as a dynamic process, since there is a continuous need for adjustment and adaptation to the changing internal and external environment. Clinical symptoms and/or signs provide information about disturbances in adjustment or adaptation; however, the absence of symptoms may not mean the absence of a disease. In some stages of a given disease the patient may not experience symptoms, but physical signs and/or laboratory tests may reveal the presence of a defect. Also, people may not communicate their symptoms to others because of personal, social, or cultural factors. For example, a productive cough may be viewed by some people as a sign of uncleanliness; therefore, they may not mention it to health professionals. Vague and general system symptoms, such as fatigue, lack of energy, and decreased physical activity, which accompany some diseases, or psychological states such as depression may be explained away as part of the aging process, or as a result of long working hours, or they may be simply unrecognized. Other disturbances in physical and psychological processes may be kept out of consciousness so that even gross, visible changes in functioning may be denied by some individuals.

CONCEPTS OF PSYCHOSOMATIC NURSING

Adaptation

Psychosomatic nursing specialists must not only integrate knowledge related to psychopathology and pathophysiology but they must also apply knowledge of particular concepts closely related to the adjustment and the growth and development of an individual as a whole. Major concepts which must be incorporated into nursing care include: adaptation, stress, anxiety, and body image. Concerning adaptation, man's survival, growth, and development depend not only on effective physiological functioning but also on satisfactory relationships with his total environment. Man needs to live in harmony with himself and others. He needs to have physical as well as emotional nourishment. He needs to love, be loved, and create. Living exposes man to constant change. Change requires an adaptive response. Our cultural evolution is exploding, as is evident in the rapid technological changes, urbanization, and population pressures, and with this explosion come enormous problems of adaptation.

Just as there are diverse meanings for *health* and *illness,* the term *adaptation* may have various meanings. Often it is used interchangeably with *adjustment.* Lazarus defines *adjustment* as consisting of "the psychological processes by means of which the individual manages or copes with various demands or pressures" (Lazarus, 1969, p. 18). Similarly, adaptation may be viewed as a biological concept whereby physiological processes are altered, or changed, to cope with various physical demands and pressures.

Adaptation is intertwined closely with one's personality. The way one adapts within a given situation depends on a variety of factors—in particular, the characteristics of the individual. Therefore, many people may be labeled as having a given disease, but how this disease affects the individual and how it is preceived are variable. Individual and group adaptation assume high importance to health professionals, since they are involved in evaluating the adequacy of adjustment. Broadly speaking, such evaluation may be considered the diagnostic process through which therapeutic plans evolve. The process of evaluating adjustment is complex. What is healthy adaptation? When one speaks of good or bad adjustment, one is implying the choice of values. Within the medical model, symptoms and signs are viewed frequently as bad adjustment; yet the controversial question centers on whether or not healthy adjustment is judged on more than the absence of symptoms or signs. Besides being linked to the concept of change, personality, and values, adaptation is related closely to the concepts of stress and anxiety.

Stress

Man, constantly exposed to changes within himself and between himself and the environment, is taxed by a multitude of physical and interpersonal demands requiring adaptive behavior. The nature of stress can be examined from a social, psychological, or physiological perspective. Hans Selye was one of the most influential theoreticians who investigated physiological stress (Selye, 1956). *Physiological stress* refers to disturbances in the structure or function of tissues as a result of noxious stimuli. Selye emphasized that the body reacts in the same way when exposed to specific noxious stimuli. The defense against the stimuli is called the "general adaptive syndrome." As the result of stress, three stages involving major bodily changes can occur. The first stage is called the *alarm stage,* which can be followed by the *resistance stage* and later by the *stage of exhaustion.* The severity of the stimuli, the stressor, and the individual involved influence the severity of the effects on the tissues. Bodily diseases, irreversible damage, and death can result from a prolonged adaptive struggle.

From a psychological perspective, *psychological stress* may be defined as a psychological or social event perceived as harmful, threatening, or frustrating to the individual. Various theories exist in relation to psychological stress. For example, Lazarus refers to stress as any demands which tax the system and produce reactions or responses within the system. He distinguishes psychological stress from physiological stress, as he writes that in the former "the reaction depends on how the the person interprets or appraises (consciously or unconsciously), the significance of a harmful, threatening or challenging event, while in the latter it is the condition of the tissues which directly determines noxiousness" (Lazarus, 1961, p. 54). He also emphasizes the fact that adaptation is influenced strongly by the way a person copes with stressful conditions. Stress management must encourage the ways in which "successful" people cope (Lazarus, 1961, p. 55). Engel writes (1962, p. 264), "Psychological stress refers to all processes, whether originating in the external environment or within the person, which impose a demand or requirement upon the organism, the resolution or handling of which requires work or activity of the mental apparatus before any other system is involved or activated."

Major sources of psychological stress may be real or imagined loss, or threat of loss, of objects, actual or threatened injury, and frustration of drives. For example, death or loss of a loved one may engender severe stress accompanied by many unpleasant emotions. Loss or alteration in bodily functions through an acute or chronic illness may also create severe stress. Furthermore, an accumulation of stressors may result from a long-term illness. Also dysfunction or alteration of body parts may alter one's image of self. Grief and the mourning process are the major responses to object loss, whether the loss be loss of persons or loss of body functions, loss of a job, or loss of valued possessions (Engel, 1962, p. 274). A loss can also precipitate other reactions, such as depression or an increase in physical symptoms. Stress may also result from disruption in one's life style. Major changes in one's life style can be expected to occur as a result of particular illnesses, disasters, and industrial changes such as automation.

Menninger stresses the importance of the ego in regulating homeostatic processes. Furthermore, he postulates that man not only has a tendency to seek or maintain a "steady state," but he also has a tendency to search for new and unsettled states. This latter tendency is labeled the *principle of heterostasis* (Menninger, 1954, 1963).

People react to stress in various ways. According to Menninger, normal, minor emergency responses to stress include fantasy, swearing, weeping, laughing, sleeping, "talking it out," and "walking it off." However, under major stress the functions of the ego are taxed increasingly and the person may have to resort to costly expedients, such as extended use of repression, depression, excessive fantasy, somatic reactions, and detachment from reality (Menninger, 1954). Physiologic reactions to stress are related closely to the autonomic nervous system. The autonomic nervous system supplies innervation to the heart, vessels, lungs, viscera, glands, and smooth muscle. It is divided into the sympathetic and parasympathetic systems. Both of these systems carry impulses to and from the central nervous system. Both systems are involved in maintaining homeostasis. Generally, if one system inhibits a given bodily function, the other system augments it. Stress itself usually excites the sympathetic system. Sympathetic stimulation produces increased activity of many bodily functions. More recently researchers have found that the sympathetic system is activated by two types of receptors located at effector organ sites. These receptors are called *alpha* and *beta receptors*. They are stimulated by the catecholamines—norepinephrine, epinephrine, and isoproterenol, and they can be blocked or stimulated by specific drugs. Catecholamines induce various physiological effects in different bodily organs. The specific effect depends on such factors as the organ system involved and which receptor effects predominate. Norepinephrine mediates greater alpha activity while epinephrine mediates greater beta activity, and isoproterenol only mediates beta activity. The effects of alpha and beta adrenergic (sympathetic) stimulation are stated in the literature (White, 1971, pp. 12–15). For example, stimulation of beta receptor sites in the heart increases heart rate, contraction strength, and conduction velocity, while stimulation of the beta receptors in the bronchial muscle produces relaxation of the muscle.

In addition the adrenal glands play an important role in maintaining homeostasis. The adrenal medulla secretes increased amounts of norepinephrine and epinephrine in response to sympathetic stimulation, while corticosteriods are secreted by the adrenal cortex. For example, one category of corticosteriods is the glucocorticoids. Cortisol is responsible for 95 percent of glucocorticoid activity, and stimulation of cortisol secretion is activated by stress and ACTH (Guyton, 1966, p. 1059). Types of stress that stimulate cortisol secretion include trauma, increased heat or cold, surgery, physical restraint, and any debilitating disease (French and Alexander, 1941). Theoretically, it appears that any stressor could increase cortisol secretion. The effects of cortisol involve anti-inflammatory functions and the mobilization of amino acids and fats for increased energy, and increased secretion increases the blood glucose level of the body.

Stress not only increases cortisol secretion but it activates the sympathetic nervous system. Therefore, the physiological effects of stress are those which result from increased cortisol secretion and sympathetic stimulation.

Anxiety

The concept of anxiety has received wide exploration in diverse fields, such as literature, politics, religion, philosophy, and education. Prior to Freud, the problem of anxiety was a problem of religious and philosophical men, such as Pascal, Spinoza, and Kierkegaard (May, 1950, p. 17). Anxiety can be interpreted biologically, culturally, and psychologically. Subjectively it is experienced as an emotion without a specific object. When there appears to be an objective basis for the feeling state, the term *fear* is used.

The psychological meaning of anxiety has been discussed by many psychiatrists, including Freud, Rank, Jung, Adler, Sullivan, and May. For example, Freud was one of the first writers to note that anxiety is a central problem of neurosis. He spoke of the difference between objective and neurotic anxiety. *Objective anxiety* is a natural and useful emotional reaction to an external danger perceived by the ego. Although the danger is not identified by the person, the unpleasant affect alerts one to danger, thereby serving to protect the person.

Concerning *neurotic anxiety,* Freud noted that the ego perceives unconsciously the danger of inner instinctual impulses which arouse anxiety. The ego represses these impulses to avoid anxiety, and symptoms and inhibitions may be created (May, 1950, p. 118). Sullivan believed that anxiety resulted from interpersonal relations which produced threats to the self-system. He perceived anxiety as restricting awareness, growth, and effective emotional health (May, 1950, pp. 149–150).

Peplau, in writing of anxiety, summarizes the major effects of various levels of anxiety upon behavior. She states that mild anxiety is evidenced by alertness, restlessness, and an ability to probem-solve. For example, under mild anxiety the person can observe, describe, analyze, test, and integrate. As the emotion increases to a moderate level, the person's perception and ability to communicate decrease. His attention is directed toward gaining immediate relief. Relationships between details may not be seen and minimal problem solving can be accomplished. Severe anxiety is equated with a feeling of panic. Perception is scattered, and a detail preceived may be blown up. Learning cannot be expected to take place (Peplau, 1963, pp. 323–327).

Body Image

Changes or disturbances in body image may result from a variety of conditions, such as: neurologic disorders, progressive deformities, loss of body parts or functions, and personality disorders. Historically, the concept of "body image" evolved from the early observations of the phantom limb phenomenon following amputations and the work of Schilder and Head. Further information on body image disturbances was provided by psychiatrists and psychoanalysts (Kolb, 1959, pp. 750–751). The term *body image* includes the perceptions, attitudes, feelings, and personality reactions relative to one's own body. Our psychological investment in our body appears to derive from interpersonal, environmental, and cultural factors. For example, families may emphasize or value particular bodily parts and deemphasize others. The attitude of society may also affect one's body image. Persons with particular defects, such as physical disfigurement, deafness, or blindness, may be rejected or stereotyped as having particular negative attributes.

One's perceptions and attitudes toward his body and its parts can be conveyed both verbally and nonverbally. Data can be obtained through psychiatric interviews, rating scales, and projective and perceptual tests, as well as by figure drawings. Reactions to changes in one's body image may be healthy or pathological. Sudden changes produce anxiety, while loss of parts or functions results in grief and mourning. If patients willingly discuss the change which has occurred, and if they cooperate by accepting physical aids and other rehabilitative measures, healthy adaptation may be expected. Pathological responses are manifested in various ways. Some patients may use denial over an extended period of time, as may be evidenced in their refusal to accept rehabilitation recommendations. Depressive, paranoid, and psychotic reactions may occur (Kolb, 1959, pp. 763–764).

Frequently changes in body parts or functions occur with any illness; therefore, nurses need to ascertain the meaning this has for the patient so that he can be assisted to cope with the changes effectively. When body image changes are expected, patients and their families should be advised about them to alleviate panic, reduce anxiety, and promote health adaptation.

GOALS OF PSYCHOSOMATIC NURSING

A unified concept of health and disease lends itself to the study of interrelationships between psychological, social, cultural, and physiological processes. Also, this perspective views man as an open system whereby continuous transactions occur between systems and between man and the outside environment; therefore, any change within one bodily system affects another system even if the change is unmeasurable. Also, man as a dynamic being is influenced by changes within the environment as well as creating changes within it. Within this framework the broad goals of psychosomatic nursing include: (1) reduction of stress and anxiety; (2) maintanance of psychophysiological functioning; (3) restoration of equilibrium; and (4) maximization of individual potential. Particular clinical situations exemplify interventions related to such goals.

Reduction of Stress and Anxiety

The acute care setting presents a major source of stress for many patients. Generally, the patient arrives in the unit unprepared for the foreign environment and unprepared for the sudden disruption in his familiar outside world. Within the unit, stress can result from a variety of sources, such as the noisy, frightening machines, monitoring equipment attached to self and others, tubes entering and leaving body orifices, continuous bright lights, and the multitude of strange faces. Most frequently these patients are in acute physiological crisis, and, therefore, totally dependent on other people, machines, and drugs for control of their welfare. Privacy is nonexistent. A recent study of patients exposed to an intensive care unit reports, "Any patient in this environment . . . suffers from some degree of sleep deprivation, sensory overstimulation, and a frightening isolation" (Dlin and others, 1971, p. 157). The researchers emphasize that patients respond to sleep deprivation in two possible ways: emotional withdrawal and hyper-alertness (Dlin and others, 1971, p. 155). With this awareness, nurses must recognize clues indicating such responses in order to decrease the stress factors present. Emotional withdrawal is evidenced by the patient who appears to doze and lies quietly with minimal facial expression. His appearance will indicate a passive acceptance of the environment with little response to procedures and the questions of the staff. As people interrupt his environment, he may become restless and agitated. The hyperalert patient will respond with behavior opposite from withdrawal. He appears engrossed totally in his environment through close and careful observation of others. He makes frequent inquiries, and he favors any opportunity to engage people in discussion. By keeping constant vigil in monitoring his surroundings, he notes in detail any disruption or change. Through involving self, the patient hopes to control his situation.

Nursing goals involve the reduction of sleep deprivation, isolation, and overstimulation. These goals can be accomplished through the control of the environment by (1) decreasing lighting and noise when possible; (2) controlling the traffic which enters the unit; (3) providing conference space for the staff to eliminate bedside discussion; and (4) providing resources for staff—whether of time, space, or a psychiatric specialist to assist them in the ventilation of their feelings. Too frequently a support system for staff is overlooked, even though the staff is exposed constantly to a highly stressful environment. Other interventions must involve personalization of care. Since patients are unprepared frequently for the acute disruption in their life style, the nurse can smooth the transition from the past by investigating the patient's immediate concerns. Death may be an imminent concern, and most patients, especially the dyspneic, know they are dangerously ill. Empty reassurance insults patients, as the staff's concern will be conveyed nonverbally, and statements denying this concern produce a conflicting message. Honest reassurance involves verbal communication which recognizes the patient's major concern yet conveys the support being given to help him overcome the crisis. Besides honest reassurance, the nurse can reduce stress through orienting patients to the staff, the time of day, the place, and the present activity. Unorganized, hurried activity and communication should be avoided. Urgency can be communicated without arousing panic. Additionally, an attitude of competency is essential. When possible, busy, urgent routines should be planned to minimize excessive patient fatigue. Pain, a common problem of the acutely ill, must be controlled, as it leads not only to exhaustion but also to alveolar hypoventilation, which produces an acid-base imbalance.

Although acute care nurses may have minimal time to spend with patients' families, family management is vital. Patients perceive what their family feels, and family attitudes can alter recovery. For example, often the family feels considerable guilt in contributing to the patient's myocardial infarction. Repressed guilt feelings may be evidenced by relative criticism of care and questions about the events surrounding the patient's onset of symptoms. Also, relatives may have unconscious anger toward the patient for disrupting their lives in some way. In turn, the patient may feel guilt and react by denying the severity of his illness (Twerski, 1972, 67–68). Frequently outside resources, such as other clinicians and social workers, can be used to provide family support.

Surgery presents another major source of stress for many adults. Through conducting systematic studies of hospitalized adults who were required to have surgical operations, Janis examined the relationship between preoperative fear and postoperative emotional disturbance (Janis, 1958). He emphasized that surgery presents three major threats to the individual: (1) the possibility of suffering acute pain; (2) the fear of undergoing body damage; and (3) the danger of dying. If another physical situation entails the same threats as surgery, it is assumed one can generalize that similar effects will result. Also, Janis proposes that when a person is exposed to an objectively dangerous situation, he experiences three phases of psychological stress: (1) the threat phase; (2) the danger impact phase; and (3) the postimpact victimization phase. During the threat phase, the person perceives signs of oncoming danger which arouse anticipatory fear. The second phase, danger impact, occurs when the person perceives that the physical danger is near. Survival is recognized as depending on the use of one's protective actions or those of others. The postimpact phase is related to loss. Losses sustained are perceived and the experience of severe deprivations continues over a variable period of time. Janis does not describe how people cope successfully with loss over time.

According to Janis, the level of a patient's preoperative anticipatory fear appeared to have a definite influence on his postoperative emotional state. Patients with a high level of anticipatory fear manifested a high level of fear, especially of body damage, and other forms of emotional disturbance postoperatively. Those who displayed a low level of anticipatory fear also had various forms of emotional disturbance, especially rage reactions and resentment toward staff postoperatively. Generally, these patients were uninformed about the oncoming unpleasant experiences. A major finding was that a relative absence of postoperative emotional disturbance existed in those people who had experienced a moderate level of anticipatory fear. Those categorized as "moderate" appeared to be part-time worriers and experienced insomnia and restlessness occasionally.

Janis suggests that the arousal of some degree of anticipatory fear may be a necessary condition for developing effective protective defenses to cope with the physical danger once it occurs. Based on Janis's findings, preoperative teaching should involve diagnosing the patient's level of fear early in the impact phase. If the patient's level of fear is low, Janis suggests the health professionals assist him to do "worry work," thereby achieving a moderate level of anticipatory fear. Preoperative teaching which involves giving patients technical information not essential to conveying a realistic picture of what the patient will perceive postoperatively is considered useless. Such patients should be given superficial descriptive material which conveys a personalized picture of the outstanding danger events which are likely to occur postoperatively. Danger events often include unpleasant pain and treatments such as suctioning procedures and positive pressure ventilation. He assumes that this information helps the patient to worry realistically about the physical dangers, which prepares him to cope with the event and postoperative course more effectively. During such preoperative teaching, Janis suggests that a balance be achieved between fear-arousing statements and fear-reducing statements. The latter refers to communication which informs the patient about the realistic favorable aspects of the danger situation and how the health professional will be of assistance to him.

Meares (1963) presents a detailed description of how to recognize and manage the anxious patient. Common signs of anxiety can be noted by observing the patient's appearance. For example, he is alert and on guard; his posture may be stiff and his fingers may twitch; there is continuous restlessness; actions may be carried out quickly without forethought. His dress may be disorderly and he usually talks too much, tolerating silence poorly. Symptomatology involves apprehension and difficulty in describing the feeling. He may experience muscular tension, fatigue, and heart palpitations. The management of anxiety involves communication with the patient through use of the psychotherapeutic process and techniques such as environmental alteration.

Maintenance of Psychophysiological Functioning

To maintain psychophysiological functioning the nurse must have baseline information about patients under his care. The baseline is provided by the medical-nursing history, the physical examination, and the initial laboratory findings. Since nurses are responsible for 24-hour care of hospitalized patients, they need to collect and understand the meaning of baseline information if they are to evaluate changes in a patient's behavior and the effect of therapy. Baseline information also assists nurses to select and carry out particular therapeutic measures which support equilibrium. One questions whether psychiatric nurses attend to the patient's medical problems sufficiently and whether or not medical nurses recognize early clues of emotional problems. As the complexity of any specialty increases, the focus of care may narrow and the psychosomatic approach can be lost. This is the reason why a psychosomatic nurse specialist is so needed to integrate the physical and psychological components of nursing care.

Major nursing interventions which maintain psychophysiological functioning include:

1. Health teaching of patients and families
2. Preparing patients for hospital entry and discharge
3. Monitoring mental and physiological functions through the use of one's senses, equipment, and laboratory procedures
4. Supporting organ system defenses against illness and the patient's successful coping abilities
5. Maintaining homeostasis through use of various therapies

Restoration of Equilibrium

When imbalance or disturbances in functioning occur, nurses must direct their activities toward restoration of equilibrium. For example, with an acutely ill population, timing is crucial, as medical treatment must be instituted immediately. Time-limited assessments should be accomplished within minutes. Neither a complete history nor an examination should be performed, as more comprehensive data can be collected once the crisis is controlled. Using one's physical senses, interviewing techniques, and physical diagnostic skills, the nurse can collect data about the precipitating event, severity of the patient's condition, his major concerns, and the major bodily systems involved.

Particular questions which should be answered immediately are: Is the patient dead or alive? Is he conscious or unconscious? Is he in acute distress? Questions related to orientation and mobility provide initial clues about responsiveness. Restlessness, difficulty concentrating, confusion, or lack of responsiveness can indicate mental or physical pathology.

Data about the precipitating event can be obtained by such questions as, "What led you to come to the hospital?" or, "What problem brought you here?" Major immediate concerns may be elicited by such questions as, "Tell me about the difficulty you are experiencing?" If his immediate concern seems obvious, e.g., difficulty in breathing, then you want to ask, "Besides your breathing, what else concerns you?" Assessment of the major bodily systems is essential. The brain, heart, lung, and kidney regulate major functions, such as acid-base balance, which are vital to life. Vital signs and a gross physical examination can be done systematically within minutes. Particular attention should be paid to pupillary reaction to light, distension of the neck veins, chest movement, injury, absence of breath sounds, presence of wheezes and/or râles, possible abdominal distension, liver tenderness, cyanosis of mucous membranes, possible sacral or ankle edema, and calf tenderness. Kidney function can be estimated by questioning the patient's ability to micturate and eliciting the time and amount of his last voiding. Depending on the situation, the nurse may initiate treatment while continuing to obtain further information. Restorative nurse actions include: (1) assessment of the severity of disturbances in functioning; (2) support of systems through use of self and other resources; (3) monitoring changes in behavior; and (4) use of crisis therapy to reestablish equilibrium.

Maximization of Individual Potential

Another major goal of psychosomatic nursing is to assist patients in utilizing their human potentials. Too frequently people are unaware of their talents, strengths, and abilities. How often do we as health professionals discover and explore patients' abilities? How often do we commend their ability to cope with stressful situations, their effective communication, and their use of self during and following an illness?

The discovery of human potential occurs through dialogues. Only through communication with the patient, his family, and other health professionals can one ascertain the uniqueness of the individual—his likes and dislikes, his expectations, concerns, strengths, and weaknesses. Dialogue begins and ends relationships with people. As Howe (1967, p. 148) states, "Dialogue is to love, what blood is to the body.

431

When the flow of blood stops, the body dies. When dialogue stops, love dies and resentment and hate are born." Likewise, it is through relationships with patients, their families, and health professionals that nurses can reinforce effective communication and teach others more effective communication; assist people in their use of internal and external resources; provide pathways whereby another's talents can be used; facilitate a person's problem-solving abilities; explore definitions or redefinitions of one's goals; support realistic expectations of self and others; and increase a person's awareness and acceptance of self. Dialogue is not only indispensable, for as Howe states (1967, p. 151), "It is the worker of miracles."

ROLE OF THE PSYCHOSOMATIC NURSE SPECIALIST

The psychosomatic specialist centers on the relationship between himself and the patient. The relationship, being psychotherapeutic in nature, serves as the foundation for future encounters with the patient. *Psychotherapeutic* implies expertise in interpersonal relations. It involves goal-directed, purposeful behavior aimed at the development of a relationship which may be supportive and/or reeducative in nature. Within a supportive relationship, a major goal may be to strengthen a patient's adaptive qualities. Patients are encouraged to discuss more conscious, current problems. The health professional sensitive to the patient's thoughts and feelings remains with him during stressful situations and allows him to test his abilities within safe limits. Within a reeducative framework, the goals involve facilitating insight into more conscious conflicts, deliberately working toward teaching patients more mature ways of thinking and acting, and assisting them to utilize their potentials more fully in their relationships with others.

The process of a relationship begins immediately when the nurse first meets the patient. Likewise, it is at this point in time that the assessment process is initiated. The initial hour with a patient is crucial. How the nurse responds to the patient and the atmosphere he creates will influence the patient's behavior and reaction to him. If the nurse appears hurried or gives the impression that he is unprepared to listen to highly charged emotional communication, the patient may omit or distort information or shy away from painful subjects. If the patient is not approached in a spirit of getting to know him, being interested in him as a person, then the patient may be put on guard—may feel he is being quizzed and simply treated as a number among numbers. Once the patient begins to feel at ease, factual information may be more easily supplied. The nurse must constantly keep the focus of the interview in mind.

PSYCHOSOMATIC ASSESSMENT

In a psychosomatic assessment both factual information about the illness and the process of the developing relationship are significant. It is insufficient only to collect data related to the patient's physical symptomatology, as his life situation, his attitude toward living, his ego strength, and the nature of his stress and anxiety must also be considered. Quiet listening and observing become essential. How the patient communicates, his appearance, posture, glances, and gestures, convey beginning ideas about him as a person. Whether the nurse at a given moment should pursue factual information or focus on the patient's feelings or his nonverbal behavior, is dependent on the individual situation. For example, the acutely ill patient cannot tolerate long interviews, as they can be too exhausting for him. Also, in an initial acute situation, timing is crucial. Information should be collected quickly, as medical treatment will need to be instituted immediately. Data collected should involve the nature and severity of the patient's condition, his major concerns, and the major bodily systems involved. An estimate must be made about how well the patient is compensating both physically and mentally for his illness. Another situation concerns the patient for whom no positive organic disease can be diagnosed. Generally such patients respond poorly to long silences and more easily when the initial portion of the first interview follows the medical format for history taking (MacKinnon and Michels, 1971). When any patient begins to express his feelings, the nurse must decide whether or not to pursue them or to continue obtaining factual information. Several alternatives exist. If the patient pursues the expression of his feelings, the nurse must continue to pursue them until he feels relatively comfortable, for interrupting his expression can lead to anxiety. The nurse's other alternative is to recognize the patient's feelings and inform him that they will be discussed later after information vital to his welfare is obtained.

Since the psychosomatic approach examines the multiple causes of a given illness, including precipitating factors and the interrelationships which may exist between the patient's life situation and his illness, it is essential that the patient's history, with both physical and psychological data, and the physical examination be incorporated into

433

the initial assessment of the patient. Depending on the health care setting, available resources, and the expertise of nurses, these procedures may or may not be done by the nurse.

Concerning history taking, the psychiatric model must merge with the medical model. Generally, nurses have been prepared more adequately to use the psychiatric approach when interviewing patients; however, the medical history framework must blend with it if one is to collect data about physiological functioning. The medical history outline as described in textbooks of physical diagnosis consists of five divisions: personal data, present illness, past and family health, personal and social history, and a systems review. For example, the "present illness" category describes all the distant and present psychophysiological symptoms reported by the patient which led him to seek medical attention. To determine the somatic and psychic processes underlying the patient's symptoms, the physician or nurse elicits the following data about each symptom reported (Morgan and Engel, 1970, pp. 35–50):

Bodily location: Where is the symptom located?
Quality: What is it like?
Quantity: How intense is it?
Chronology: When did the symptom begin, and what course has it followed?
Setting: Under what circumstances does it take place?
Aggravating and alleviating factors: What makes it better or worse?
Associated manifestations: What other symptoms or phenomena are associated with it?

The psychosomatic perspective recognizes that particular symptoms seldom manifest themselves for the first time in adulthood but may recur when new conflict situations arise. Therefore, it is essential to ascertain the relationship of time between the first manifestation and the development, worsening, or remission of symptoms. The critical time periods of growth and development could be used as a guideline in helping to indicate this relationship. Erik Erikson's schema of personality development in which the developmental stages of childhood and adulthood are examined might serve as one useful guideline (Erikson, 1963).

Once factual information is collected about the patient's symptomatology, the nurse may focus on the patient's emotional responses which may have accompanied his symptoms. The patient, who may have no organic cause for his symptoms, may not be aware of a relationship between anxiety, fear, or anger and his physical symptoms, but he may readily admit that insomnia, fatigue, anorexia, nightmares, or sexual disturbances were present concurrently with the physical symptoms (MacKinnon and Michels, 1971, p. 367). If the patient denies any psychological factors in his illness or claims that no emotional responses accompany his symptoms, then the nurse has several alternatives. One, he can wait until anxiety is manifested and then direct the patient's attention to his behavior. Second, the nurse can focus on the way the illness or symptoms may have prevented the patient from doing particular tasks. In other situations it may be easier for the patient to develop insight by focusing on his reactions to a given symptom, rather than having him recognize that the symptom may be a manifestation of anxiety, fear, or depression (MacKinnon and Michels, 1971, p. 368).

Other information which becomes significant regarding the illness is the relationship between the onset of illness and current events in the patient's life which occurred at or around the same time. Such information seeks to explain "why" a patient became ill at a given time in history. Engel examines the central question: Why do people fall ill or die at the time they do? He emphasizes that a particular psychological state called the "giving up-given up complex" may precede the onset of illness and play a major role in modifying the capacity of the organism to cope with concurrent pathogenic factors. A characteristic feature of this psychological state seems to be a feeling of psychological impotence, a feeling of being unable to cope with changes in the environment. Coping mechanisms seem to longer effective or available. Clinically, the "giving up-given up" state appears to have five characteristics (Engel, 1968, pp. 293–300): (1) the experience of feeling helpless and hopeless; (2) a depreciated image of oneself; (3) a loss or decrease in gratification from relationships or roles; (4) a sense of discontinuity between the past, present, and future; and (5) reactivation of memories of earlier periods of giving up. The state may be transient or intermittent, but during its presence the physiologic balance may be altered and the person's ability to cope with potential pathogenic processes may be decreased. Disease can result if the predisposition to organic disease is present concurrently. It seems that this theoretical position supports the need for health professionals to engage in careful evaluations of events preceding the onset of illness, complications, or additional symptoms. Knowledge of the antecedents may direct treatment plans. Illness in the future could be prevented. Also, routine examinations which include an investigation of clues related to the presence of this psychological state in supposedly healthy populations could detect potential problems earlier, and perhaps aid in the prevention of illness through early initiation of treatment.

Besides collecting information about the patient's current symptomatology, his past health and his family's health, and other data related to major system symptoms, the nurse can focus gradually on the patient's emotional life during the initial assessment. Depending on the social context, this initial assessment may take place in one, several, or many encounters with the patient; however, particular attention must be given to the following areas if a comprehensive assessment is to be accomplished:

1. Patient's perception of self. What does he value? What does he see as his strengths and weaknesses? What are his ideals and aspirations? Has he completed successfully the stages of development? Has he experienced a sense of intimacy, generativity, and a feeling of integrity?
2. Patient's perception and attitude toward his illness and/or hospitalization. Does he feel angry, frustrated, resentful, sad, or fearful? What does he know about his illness? What does he expect from the staff and significant others?
3. Patient's perception of changes in his life style. What disruptions in his life style have resulted because of his illness? For example, how has his illness affected his daily routine, work and family role, and leisure activity?
4. Patient's perception of previous and current changing relationships. What losses has he experienced? How did he react to these events?

Within the interview, special attention should be given to the patient's nonverbal behavior, which may provide clues concerning his emotional state. Attention should also be given to his memory span, orientation, intellectual functioning, judgment, and insight. This information can be categorized under the *review of systems* in a general history or it may be included within a *mental status* examination.

In addition to history taking, a psychosomatic assessment involves performing a physical examination of the patient. The use of physical diagnostic skills—inspection, palpation, percussion, and auscultation—as well as the use of laboratory tests assists the nurse to identify alterations in physiological functioning and to monitor changes over time, thereby leading to a broader base for planning, executing, and evaluating patient care. Furthermore, a broader, more systemized method of data collection helps the nurse and physician to expand, alter, or discontinue treatment plans more rapidly.

Patient Population Requiring Psychosomatic Nursing

The psychosomatic approach can be utilized in the nursing care of any medical-surgical patient. This approach transcends the boundaries of given patient populations, and there are no disease categories considered strictly psychosomatic (Alexander, 1950, pp. 50–52). At one time such diseases as hay fever, asthma, peptic ulcer, ulcerative colitis, fluctuating hypertension, and vasospastic conditions were labeled psychosomatic diseases based on the assumption that their etiology was primarily psychological. Such labeling or categorization lends itself to stereotyping the patient and narrows the perspective of psychosomatic treatment. If one believes that the soma and psyche are interrelated, then theoretically every disease could be considered psychosomatic. Therefore, it seems more appropriate to examine the interrelationship between psychological and physiological factors present in each patient situation. The way organic diseases affect changes in the psychological state and how emotional states influence somatic processes will be discussed more fully in the following paragraphs.

Psychosomatic Nursing Care of Medical-Surgical Patients: Cardiovascular Disorders The psychological impact of any organic disease, including cardiovascular disturbances, is highly individual. It depends on various factors, such as the symbolic significance of organ function, how the person copes with fantasies about organ function, the nature and severity of the disturbance, and the adaptive ability of the person in relation to stress. Although the psychological impact is variable, two major potential psychological problems can result from any cardiac disturbance: fear of death and anxiety. As Hammerschlag (1952, p. 34) states, "The heart literally serves as the center for fears of 'suddenly dropping dead.'" Many people equate the beating of the heart with the source of life; therefore, any medical or surgical procedure on the heart may be perceived as an assault on the very essence of his life. Words pertaining to the heart are often used by people when describing their perceptions or reactions to other individuals; for example, people may be described as being warm- or stonyhearted. Cardiac rhythm occurs automatically, and usually it can be controlled only with outside assistance such as drugs or pacemakers. Changes in rhythm bring into one's awareness alteration in cardiac activity which can produce fear and/or anxiety.

Often cardiac patients have had to restrict their physical activities, and in some cases restriction may be for months or a lifetime. Activity restriction may create mandatory changes in one's life style, particularly in relation to occupation and leisure activity. Role reversal may occur whereby the woman, instead of the male, may have to be the breadwinner of the family. The patient may experience stress, anxiety, and fear from having to assume a more passive role, permitting others, such as spouses, friends, or health professionals, to take care of him. Consequently, the sense of powerlessness and helplessness may be overwhelming. If the patient was very active and ambitious to compensate for inferiority feelings, restricted activity will create additional stress.

Patients undergoing cardiac surgery may perceive it as life-threatening. Abram (1965, p. 659) cites one author's corroborating opinion, "Operating on the heart 'partakes of the touching, manipulating and cutting of an organ that even by the most ignorant or the most sophisticated subject, is viewed as the be-all and the end-all of life itself.'" One young patient having open-heart surgery for mitral valve disease described his fear of death in postoperative interviews as follows (Carrieri, 1966): After an episode of atrial fibrillation he stated, "My heart went all to pieces . . . fluttered all over the place." Later he commented, "Guess I am coming all unglued . . . guess I'm dying . . . no, not now, but in a couple of weeks." During another interview he said, "Froze all night. All I could think of was let me die warm, if I'm going to die." Helplessness and fear of dying may deprive patients of adequate sleep. Resultant fatigue depletes one's energy reserve which could be used to maintain physiological functioning. Postoperative cardiac surgical patients may have a fear of the fragility of their heart which could lead to cardiac invalidism. One cardiac surgical patient experiencing hospitalization and surgery for the first time complained of a severe backache postoperatively. A muscle relaxant was ordered; however, during an interview the patient was observed lying on her back in a rigid, fixed manner. When the nurse commented on the patient's posture, the patient expressed the fact that she was afraid of incisional hemorrhage, which she thought could occur if she changed her position (Sitzman, 1966). Another cardiac sugical patient expressed a similar fear of body fragility when he described a health professional removing his incisional dressing as being as clumsy as "a bull in a china shop" (Carrieri, 1966).

Chest pain may also be associated with a fear of death. Patients may feel a sense of panic when experiencing such pain. Often chest pain of cardiac origin is described as being knifelike, stabbing in nature, or it may be referred to as a severe pressure sensation closing down and around the heart, almost as if the source of life was being squeezed out of the individual. Perhaps pain, more than any other symptom, alerts the individual to seek medical attention. Yet, it has been observed that patients experiencing chest pain may delay seeking medical help for days or weeks (Sitzman, 1972).

Besides chest pain, there are other cardiac symptoms or signs which can produce anxiety and fear of death. Dyspnea, orthopnea, and paroxysmal, nocturnal dyspnea involve difficulty in breathing and consequent anxiety. Paroxysmal nocturnal dyspnea, which usually occurs suddenly and often several hours after a patient retires, can produce a panic state when he is awakened by a feeling of suffocation. Also changes in cardiac rhythm, including the experience of extrasystoles, can produce anxiety. Peripheral edema, which often accompanies severe congestive heart failure, can distort one's body image; and cerebral edema can impair judgment and cause irritable behavior.

Hypertension In the literature the etiology of hypertension has been a controversial subject. Some writers stress the causal relationship between chronic repressed anger and chronic vascular constriction. However, other writers note that a variety of complex factors, such as the personality structure, the state of the autonomic nervous system, organic vascular changes, and environmental circumstances, appear to play a decisive role in this problem. Furthermore, emotionally charged life situations increase peripheral vascular resistance via the autonomic nervous and endocrine systems. Therefore, such situations may contribute to the onset of the illness, symptom occurrence, and the acceleration of the disease (Reiser and Bakst, 1959, p. 671).

Nursing treatment may involve individual or group psychotherapy. As Hammerschlag (1952, p. 37) states, "One can safely state that existing hypertension with its threat of sudden death and its requirement of continuous inactivity and diet—whatever its origin may be—creates increased psychological tension and irritability . . . psychotherapy—regardless of the nature of the hypertension—can be useful." Psychotherapy must be carried out in close teamwork with the medical specialist, since these patients are on long-term medical treatment programs, and their response to them must be evaluated frequently. Within a psychotherapeutic relationship, careful consideration must be given to identifying current sources of conflict and their potential relationship to the clinical manifestations of the disease. The nurse must also explore the possibility of environmental stressors, as well as determine the patient's ego strengths, so that specific therapeutic goals can be determined. In some instances, short-term therapy may be useful, especially during crisis situations such as hospitalization and surgery.

Psychosomatic nursing care of any patient, including the cardiovascular patient, must evolve from the assessment process; however, if the nurse has a knowledge of potential causal factors and psychophysiological problems related to a given condition, he may recognize more readily early symptoms and signs of them. When fear of death or anxiety is evident in the patient, the nurse must use particular interviewing skills which allow the patient an opportunity to discuss his concerns, thereby reducing the fear and/or anxiety. He must explore with the patient the possible causes of his anxiety so that they can be examined, reduced, or eliminated. Since activity restriction can produce stress, the nurse must obtain the patient's perceptions and his reactions related to them. He must also appraise how the restriction will affect the patient's life style. For example, is the physical home environment conducive to the patient's health? Will he be forced to retire? Will the limitations create or increase social isolation? Such knowledge guides the nurse to help these patients adapt to their limitations. The patient's strengths and weaknesses must be considered as the nurse plans realistic short- and long-term goals with the patient.

Reduction of stress may occur through a variety of other treatment measures. For example, the person experiencing a myocardial infarction for the first time may know little about the nature of his illness and the death-producing complications such as congestive failure and the arrhythmias. A major nursing goal would then involve teaching him about the nature of his illness, the medical treatment regimen and the importance of following it, and how to recognize and prevent complications. Nursing actions related to reducing stress may also involve helping the family and/or significant others to understand their reactions to his illness and examining means whereby they can cope with the situation most effectively.

To maintain functioning, not only cardiovascular patients must be taught about treatment regimens and complications, but nurses must help them budget their daily routines to conserve energy, thereby decreasing the tissue demands for oxygen. Health maintenance also depends on how effectively the patient is able to communicate his needs to others. When, and under what circumstances, did the patient seek medical help?

Other psychosomatic treatment measures may involve a one-to-one psychotherapeutic relationship with the patient over an extended period of time or during a crisis situation. The cardiovascular patient may need to explore more healthy ways of adapting to his illness; how to prevent social isolation; how to maximize his strengths; and how to reduce his weaknesses through increased awareness of self and others.

Respiratory Disorders Like the cardiovascular system, the respiratory system is essential to life. The major purpose of breathing is to oxygenate the venous return of the blood, which then nourishes the cells of the body by way of the pulmonary, coronary, and systemic circulations. Man can survive for days without water, while he cannot survive more than a few minutes without oxygen. Breathing serves many other functions. It is necessary for physical activity, such as running, lifting, pulling, and pushing. It assists in regulating the acid-base balance of the body. It provides a major pathway for communication, since without the respiratory system vocalization would be impossible. Babies would be unable to cry when hungry, wet, or cold; cooing and gurgling would be impossible. People would be unable to talk, sing, whistle, or laugh. The organs of the respiratory system are also affected by psychological factors. Although sore throats and colds are caused by viruses or pathogenic organisms, it appears that they may occur at the time of a stressful situation which may lower bodily resistance.

Emphysema Dyspnea without orthopnea is a major symptom of emphysema, an airway-obstructive disease. It is one of the largest categories of chronic respiratory disease. The cause is unknown and the disease process is irreversible, two potential sources of psychological stress. Dyspnea can lead to anxiety, fear of suffocation, and death. People who experience dyspnea may appear as if they are struggling between life and death. This seems evident in their facial expressions, the use of accessory muscles, and their slow gait, forward-leaning posture, and decreased or slower verbal communication. Frequently dyspnea leads to a decrease in exercise tolerance, which may create disturbances in their life style requiring new adaptive responses. Change may be evidenced in their work role, living conditions, and social activities. The change may be characterized by withdrawal from physical activity, which may also engender social isolation and depression. Concerns about masculinity and femininity may surface. Respiratory symptoms resulting in fatigue, immobility, and dependence on mechanical ventilatory aids may alter one's body image, and this aspect of the self-concept can be conveyed both verbally and nonverbally. Any alteration in body image results in a process of adjustment which may or may not be healthy. As Hargreaves shows, in our culture the chest has a special meaning related to masculinity and femininity. Changes in the shape and size of the thorax can produce psychological reactions. Also, sputum production accompanying respiratory infections and chronic obstructive lung disease may cause feelings of shame, uncleanness, and guilt (Hargreaves, 1968).

Airway obstruction and hyperinflation are major signs of chronic obstructive pulmonary emphysema. The major complications of this condition are: infection, hypoxemia, hypercapnea, and right ventricular failure. Each complication may be life-threatening. For example, hypoxemia—decreased oxgen in the arterial blood—and hypercapnea—increased carbon dioxide in the arterial blood—produce variable manifestations, including central nervous system changes ranging from restlessness and irritability to difficulty in concentrating and coma. Systemic hypotension may occur, while tachycardia and an increased respiratory rate (tachypnea) are early clues to the presence of both problems. Since oxygen is required for myocardial contractility and conduction, lack of it leads to arrhythmias. Four major mechanisms can produce hypoxemia: alveolar hypoventilation, impaired diffusion, venous to arterial shunts, and uneven distribution of ventilation and/or perfusion. Generally, the latter is the single most frequent cause, whereas alveolar hypoventilation is the major cause of hypercapnea. A more immediate cause of hypercapnea is fatigue and pain. Although the literature focuses on the physiological causes of these conditions, one wonders about the social and/or psychological events and stressors which may influence their occurrence. Since the manifestations of these problems are similar, it is often difficult to determine whether one or both exist without the use of arterial blood gas analysis.

Infection is a frequent precipitating factor producing a respiratory crisis in the patient with chronic obstructive lung disease. It can be easily explained on the basis of airtrapping and stagnant secretions which produce a media for bacterial growth; but what other factors influence the occurrence of infection at a given point in time? Minimal research exists which examines the interrelationship between psychological and physiological factors in patients with irreversible lung disease. However, a current study was done to bring some objectivity into the area of dying behavior and its antecedents in relation to patients having severe, debilitating, irreversible, diffuse, obstructive pulmonary disease (Dudley et al., 1969). The patients studied over a 4-year period were found to "use denial, repression, and isolation to protect their failing respiratory systems from environmental inputs" (Dudley et al., 1969, p. 310). Physiologic and psychologic deterioration occurred when their defenses failed. Patients having psychosocial assets complied realistically and appropriately with treatment programs, and they were more effective in protecting themselves from dangerous symptoms. The probability of dying increased in patients having both low psychosocial and low physiologic assets. Dying was seen as goal-directed, adaptive, and comfortable behavior reflecting the best solution to an intolerable situation.

Medical treatment of pulmonary emphysema must be reinforced by nurses caring for this population. It consists of bronchial hygiene accomplished via bronchodilator drugs, increased hydration, and physical therapy procedures; early recognition and treatment of upper respiratory infection; annual influenza immunization; elimination of inhaled irritants; and use of mucolytic agents. Particular psychological problems which may occur involve: body image disturbances, social isolation, depression, stress, and anxiety, as well as a loss or decrease in respiratory functions. Early comprehensive assessments can provide clues concerning clinical manifestations of such problems so that nursing treatment can be instituted as soon as possible. These patients may need counseling, not only in understanding the nature of their illness but also in adapting to the many changes resulting from it. Crisis intervention therapy and individual supportive and reeducative psychotherapy may be useful. Nurses must consider the patient's fatigue level prior to instituting any treatment program, particularly group therapy, since some patients tire easily from verbal communication. Although the condition is irreversible, it seems that their lives could possibly be prolonged through rehabilitative measures which support both physiological and psychological functioning.

Besides dyspnea, other major chest symptoms which may produce fear, anxiety, or stress are cough, wheezing, sputum, hemoptysis, and chest pain. Although any cough is normal, people may ignore seeking medical attention for it. Bronchogenic carcinoma should be suspected in any person over fifty years old who develops a productive cough of increasing severity. Cough and spitting may also be used to attract the attention of others. Hemoptysis indicates the presence of serious disease. From a psychological perspective, loss of blood can be equated with loss of life. Oozing from an incision could be perceived as fear of rupture and death. Hemoptysis may also be associated with fantasies of violence. Chest pain, often associated with a cardiac condition, may also be neurologic, muscular, respiratory, or psychogenic in origin. Frequently pain produces anxiety and fear, and chest pain also causes splinting of the chest, which decreases aeration, resulting in infection or atelectasis.

Asthma The chief symptoms of bronchial asthma are recurring paroxysms of diffuse wheezing, dyspnea, and cough. Increased airway resistance results, and hypertrophy of bronchial smooth muscle, along with thickening of membranes in the respiratory tract, occurs. However, it is a highly reversible condition. The emotional component of asthma has received wide recognition in the literature; however, it is not understood clearly. It appears that a combination of emotional factors and allergic factors may produce an asthmatic attack. Many allergists believe that the heightened sensitivity is congenital or hereditary. The psychological approach seems to stress that these patients experience a conflict focusing on an excessive, unresolved dependence on the mother (French and Alexander, 1941). Thus, it is assumed they want a protective mother or mother substitute. Separation from this protective person produces anxiety, resulting in an asthmatic attack. Behavioral characteristics vary in these patients. Some patients may be aggressive and argumentive. This behavior may be a means of overcompensating for their dependency conflict. Others may be passive, clinging, and demanding. Several other characteristics, such as a need for confession and an inability to cry during intense anxiety, have been observed. Based on the theory of an unresolved dependence conflict, it appears that individual and family psychotherapy could be beneficial. In health care settings, patients might also benefit from a consistent relationship with a physician, but physicians must recognize that the patient's intense dependency could make them angry. Since separation from a consistent therapeutic relationship might precipitate a severe asthmatic attack, the physician should prepare the patient for this event at least several weeks in advance.

Gastrointestinal Diseases The mind-body problem is also reflected in other illness states. For example, the gastrointestinal tract is involved in early contact with others. In addition to physical nourishment, food intake can symbolize psychological nourishment and satisfaction. An examination of the gastrointestinal tract in relation to psychosomatic theory is presented in Cantor (1951). He states that particular problems which have psychological impact include: obesity, peptic ulcer, diarrhea, constipation, and ano-rectal illness. The majority of gastrointestinal problems necessitate dietary changes which may arouse unconscious anger due to the restriction. A health professional requiring dietary restrictions of the patient should consider the possible emotional impact of the diet on the patient. Although some patients may react angrily and not follow their diets, others may respond happily to special diets, which may symbolize special love or provide an opportunity for making special demands on significant others (Hammerschlag, 1952, p. 30). Other psychological implications in gastrointestinal conditions include obesity, which involves changes in body image, whereas stomach lesions may produce fears of bleeding to death or of something festering and dirty. People experiencing diarrhea may also feel dirty and embarrassed. Besides concerns about cleanliness, patients with ano-rectal illnesses are often exposed to medication, intensive procedures with instruments, or a symptom such as itching. These may fulfill pleasurable infantile needs or arouse great anger and hostility. In working with such patients the nurse must recognize that comprehensive treatment involves an exploration of the patient's emotional and social situation.

Infectious Disease Frequently, infectious problems require isolation measures; therefore, patients may feel like social outcasts. "Distancing" behavior may be reflected by relatives and staff, which increases the patient's feeling of aloneness and unacceptability. In some instances patients may view isolation techniques positively. For instance, the reverse isolation technique when explained adequately to patients may be viewed by them as a protective defense against the environment; however, this could possibly enhance fear, especially if the staff failed to follow the procedure adequately. Generally a fever accompanies an infectious illness, and this can produce feelings of unreality, strangeness, and fear of losing mental control (Hammerschlag, 1952, p. 41). Although the death rate from pulmonary tuberculosis has declined greatly in the United States, the relationship of psychological factors to the onset of this illness has received considerable attention in the literature. Fatigue and undernourishment, along with the presence of the tubercle bacilli, seem to be important factors in the etiology of tuberculosis. Misuse of energy is reflected in overwork, irregular hours, inadequate meals, loss of sleep, and overindulgence (Hendricks, 1949, p. 240). Long-term hospitalization and isolation could increase the patient's feelings of loneliness and of social rejection. Current drug treatment has decreased the need for long-term isolation within sanitariums, and emphasis is being placed on treating such patients within general hospital and outpatient settings. Hopefully, this change will decrease the stigma and social isolation which have accompanied this illness in the past.

Psychomatic Reactions to Chronic Illness Chronic illnesses must be examined from the perspective of the individual and his family. The kind of adjustment required depends on the characteristics of the illness as well as the individual's and/or family's ability to adapt in light of the many changes produced by the illness. Concerning personal tragedy and illness, Engel emphasizes that one cannot tell how the person will respond to the onset of illness from the nature of the external event (Engel, 1968). Additionally, how the person reacts to long-term illness seems to depend more on his adaptive ability than on the changing events themselves.

What does terminal illness mean to the patient? Any terminal illness, such as a malignancy or lymphoma, shortens the life-span and is often characterized by exacerbations and remissions. Besides medical-surgical problems, these illnesses present multiple emotional problems. Expected and actual loss of a loved one are also accompanied by changes in living patterns. Perceived loss of a significant other reactivates psychological and behavioral reactions associated with previous losses and may result in depression (Engel, 1962, p. 331). Patients experiencing terminal illness and their families respond to expected death by mourning and grieving.

Emotional implications of cancer are obtained through the patient's perception and attitude toward it and the meaning of the organ(s) invaded. Similar to surgery, malignancy is characterized by a: "(1) greater chance of death; (2) greater chance of destruction or removal or organs (loss); (3) greater chance of pain, suffering and fearful anticipation" (Meerloo and Zeckel, 1952, p. 46). Since the meaning of illness to the patient affects his emotional reaction, cancer may be perceived as an enemy invading the body, leaving the patient feeling passive and helpless. Patients may become preoccupied with their symptoms, and different organ invasion presents different fears. For example, pulmonary cancer may arouse a vague fear of breathing suffocation, while cancer of the larynx can disturb communication. Loss of voice could produce fear of social isolation.

Quint writes of the impact of mastectomy (1963). In her study, women undergoing a mastectomy perceived three basic changes initiated by the operation. The first change experienced by them was a period of shock and unexpected events, which was often prolonged by delayed wound healing, another complication, or radiation therapy. Second, bodily appearance changed, and this was a real concern for some women. Third, the operation initiated concerns about the future and the fear of death.

Cancer also evokes feelings in the health professional caring for a terminally ill patient. Since the professional's activities involve preventing illness and restoring health, he may feel frustrated and annoyed in his wish to help when cure activities cannot be accomplished. Frustration and annoyance may result in carrying out desperate measures to overcome his helplessness. Also, he may experience fears about death. Helping patients cope with anticipated loss and death requires reexamination of one's own philosophy and feelings about dying. This is an essential ingredient in providing support and comfort to patients and their families.

Depression Depression is a common clinical situation in medical settings which requires maintenance and restorative nurse actions. It may refer to a symptom or a group of illnesses which have common features. Depressive diseases include involutional depression and manic-depressive psychosis. Reactive depressions are perceived as a response to a traumatic experience in the patient's life. It seems that these are observed most frequently in medical-surgical patients. Often the precipitating experience involves a specific stress, such as an acute or terminal illness, prolonged recovery, the loss of a loved one, a change in life style such as forced retirement, or a direct threat to one's adaptive capacity. The clinical features are reflected in the patient's affect, thought processes, behavior, and relationships (MacKinnon and Michels, 1971). Affectively, the patient's mood is lowered. He may describe this as a feeling of sadness, gloom, fear, guilt, or emptiness. Anger may be expressed directly or indirectly. Both anxiety and agitation may be experienced. In severe or chronic depression, apathy and withdrawal occur. He may not perceive his emotional reactions and bodily functions as part of his self (MacKinnon and Michels, 1971,

p. 176). Constriction of thought processes is evidenced through preoccupation with his self and his past experiences. Happy, joyful thoughts seem nonexistent. Spontaneity and initiative are lacking. Slowness characterizes his thoughts, speech, and movements. Weight loss results from a lack of appetite. Insomnia may occur and the patient's metabolic rate is lowered. Other general physical symptoms include fatigue, loss of libido, headache, aches and pains, and dryness of the mouth (MacKinnon and Michels, 1971, p. 179). The organ systems affected often have symbolic meaning to the patient. In mild depressions the patient may seek aid from others, while in more severe depressions he may be withdrawn from others. Self-esteem and self-confidence are diminished in all depressed patients. Suicide is a major complicaton of depression. The psychodynamic mechanisms involved in depression are well described by MacKinnon and Michels (1971). Treatment involves supportive therapy directed toward "the alleviation of suffering and guilt, the stimulation of hope, and the protection from self-injury" (MacKinnon and Michels, 1971, p. 209). Also, treatment involves understanding the meaning and causes of the depression so that the problem can be resolved and future recurrences can be eliminated.

Depression must also be distinguished from sadness, which is a normal feeling experienced by many people exposed to changes in their life. Sadness reflects the absence of gratification but not yet a giving up. Emptiness and unhappiness may be felt along with pleasant thoughts. The person retains a feeling of worthiness although tears and physical distress may be experienced. Sometimes sadness is denied, as evidenced through forced cheerfulness; excessive drinking, sleeping, and eating; impulsive behavior; and physical symptoms which may be functional in origin. People sometimes fail to express emotions because they may view the expression as a sign of weakness. Health professionals may also avoid patients who express loneliness and sadness, as they may feel uncomfortable, helpless, or fearful of handling the patient's feelings. Unsuccessful dealing with sadness can lead to depression. Nurse actions should involve recognizing the patient's feeling and allowing him to discuss the feeling and its significance (Lazare, 1970).

Other Conditions Requiring Psychosomatic Nursing Care

Although specific conditions have been cited which require psychosomatic care, any medical-surgical patient can benefit from it. For example, rheumatoid conditions, skin disorders, and reconstructive surgical procedures particularly involve body image changes which may provoke various responses in the patient. In addition, the clinical manifestations of these conditions are often quite visible to others. Visible, gross deformities may cause the patient to fear rejection by others; therefore, he may refuse the use of outside resources and professional help, and he may gradually demonstrate increasing withdrawal behavior. Nurses must also recognize that gross deformities of others can evoke various feelings in themselves. Once the feelings become conscious, the nurse can examine them and hopefully prevent their interference with treatment programs.

REFERENCES

Abram, Harry S. (1965): "Adaptation to Open Heart Surgery: A Psychiatric Study of Response to the Threat of Death," *American Journal of Psychiatry*, vol. 122, p. 659.

Alexander, Franz (1950): *Psychosomatic Medicine: Its Principles and Applications,* W. W. Norton & Company, Inc., New York, pp. 50–52.

————, and Thomas M. French (1948): *Studies in Psychosomatic Medicine*, The Ronald Press Company, New York, p. 26.

Cannon, Walter B. (1929): *Bodily Changes in Pain, Hunger, Fear and Rage,* Appleton-Century-Crofts, Inc., New York.

————(1932): *The Wisdom of the Body,* W. W. Norton & Company, Inc., New York.

Cantor, Al J. (1951): *A Handbook of Psychosomatic Medicine (with Particular Reference to Intestinal Disorders),* Julian Press, New York.

Carrieri, Virginia (1966): Personal interviews of a patient undergoing open-heart surgery.

Dlin, Barney M., et al. (1971): "The Problems of Sleep and Rest in the Intensive Care Unit," *Psychosomatics,* May–June, pp. 155–163.

Dudley, D. L., et al. (1969): "Long-Term Adjustment, Prognosis, and Death in Irreversible Diffuse Obstructive Pulmonary Syndromes," *Psychosomatic Medicine,* vol. 31, no. 4, pp. 310–325.

Dunbar, Helen F. (1954): *Emotions and Bodily Changes,* 4th ed., Columbia University Press, New York.

Duncan, C. H., et al. (1950): "Life Situations, Emotions and Paroxysmal Auricular Arrhythmias," *Psychosomatic Medicine,* vol. 12, no. 23.

Engel, George L. (1968): "A Life Setting Conducive to Illness: The Giving-Up-Given-Up Complex," *Annals of Internal Medicine,* vol. 69, August, pp. 293–300.

————(1962): *Psychological Development in Health and Disease,* W. B. Saunders Company, Philadelphia, pp. 240, 264, 274, 331.

Erikson, Erik H. (1963): *Childhood and Society,* W. W. Norton & Company, Inc., New York.

French, Thomas M., and Franz Alexander (1941): "Psychogenic Factors in Bronchial Asthma," *Psychosomatic Medicine Monographs 4,* Arthur C. Guyton, quoted in *Textbook of Medical Physiology,* 3d ed., W. B. Saunders Company, Philadelphia, 1966, p. 1059.

Hammerschlag, Ernst (1952): "Psychiatry Applied to Internal Medicine," in Leopold Bellak (ed.), *Psychology of Physical Illness: Psychiatry Applied to Medicine, Surgery and the Specialities,* Grune & Stratton, Inc., New York. pp. 30, 34, 37, 41.

Hargreaves, A. G. (1968): "Emotional Problems of Patients with Respiratory Disease," *Nursing Clinics of North America,* W. B. Saunders Company, Philadelphia.

Hendricks, C. M. (1949): "Psychosomatic Aspects of Tuberculosis and Its Complications," in E. W. Hayes (ed.), *Fundamentals of Pulmonary Tuberculosis and Its Complications,* Charles C Thomas, Springfield, Ill., p. 240.

Hinkle, L. E., et al. (1951): "Studies in Diabetes Mellitus: III. Life History of Three Persons with Labile Diabetes, and Relation of Significant Experiences in Their Lives to the Onset and Course of the Disease," *Psychosomatic Medicine,* vol. 13, no. 160.

Howe, Revel L. (1967): "The Miracle of Dialogue," in Floyd W. Matson and Ashley Montagu (eds.), *The Human Dialogue: Perspectives on Communication,* The Free Press, New York, pp. 148, 151.

Janis, Irving L. (1958): *Psychological Stress: Psychoanalytic and Behavioral Studies of Surgical Patients,* John Wiley & Sons, Inc., New York.

Kolb, Lawrence C. (1959): "Disturbances of the Body-Image," in Silvano Arieti (ed.), *American Handbook of Psychiatry,* vol. I, Basic Books, Inc., Publishers, New York, pp. 749–769, 763–764.

Lazare, Aaron (1970): "The Difference between Sadness and Depression," *Medical Insight,* February, pp. 22–32.

Lazarus, Richard S. (1961): *Adjustment and Personality,* McGraw-Hill Book Company, New York, pp. 54–55.

———(1969): *Patterns of Adjustment and Human Effectiveness,* McGraw-Hill Book Company, New York, p. 18.

Lidz, Theodore (1959): "General Concepts of Psychosomatic Medicine," in Silvano Arieti (ed.), *American Handbook of Psychiatry,* vol. I, Basic Books, Inc., Publishers, New York, p. 651.

MacKinnon, Roger A., and Robert Michels (1971): *The Psychiatric Interview in Clinical Practice,* W. B. Saunders Company, Philadelphia, pp. 176, 179, 209, 367–368.

May, Rollo (1950): *The Meaning of Anxiety,* The Ronald Press Company, New York, pp. 17, 118, 149–150.

Meares, Ainslie (1963): *The Management of the Anxious Patient,* W. B. Saunders Company, Philadelphia.

Meerloo, Joost M., and Adolf Zeckel (1952): "Psychiatric Problems of Malignancy," in Leopold Bellak (ed.), *Psychology of Physical Illness: Psychiatry Applied to Medicine, Surgery and the Specialties,* Grune & Stratton, Inc., New York, p. 46.

Menninger, Karl (1954): "Psychological Aspects of the Organism under Stress," *Journal of the American Psychoanalytic Association,* vol. 2, January, April, pp. 67–106, 280–310.

———(1963): *The Vital Balance,* The Viking Press, New York. pp. 84–85.

Morgan, William L., and George L. Engel (1970): *The Clinical Approach to the Patient,* W. B. Saunders Company, Philadelphia, pp. 35–50.

Peplau, Hildegard E. (1963): "A Working Definition of Anxiety," in Shirley F. Burd and Margaret A. Marshal (eds.), *Some Clinical Approaches to Psychiatric Nursing,* The Macmillan Company, New York, pp. 323–327.

Quint, Jeanne C. (1963): "The Impact of Mastectomy," *American Journal of Nursing,* November, pp. 88–92,

Reiser, Morton F., and Hyman Bakst (1959): "Psychology of Cardiovascular Disorders," in Silvano Arieti (ed.), *American Handbook of Psychiatry,* vol. 1, Basic Books, Inc., Publishers, New York, p. 671.

Schwartz, Lawrence H., and Jane Linker Schwartz (1972): *The Psychodynamics of Patient Care,* Prentice-Hall, Inc., Englewood Cliffs, N.J., p. 244.

Selye, Hans (1956): *The Stress of Life,* McGraw-Hill Book Company, New York.

Sitzman, Judith (1972): "Interviews with Patients Experiencing Respiratory Problems." (Unpublished.)

————(1966): "Postoperative Interview of a Patient Undergoing Open-Heart Surgery." (Unpublished.)

Travelbee, Joyce (1961): *Interpersonal Aspects of Nursing,* F. A. Davis Company, Philadelphia, p. 34.

Twerski, Abraham (1972): "Psychological Considerations on the Coronary Care Unit," *Cardiovascular Nursing,* March–April, pp. 67–68.

White, Barry B. (1971): *Therapy in Acute Coronary Care,* Year Book Medical Publishers, Inc., Chicago, pp. 12–15.

Wolff, Harold (1950): "Life Stress and Bodily Disease—A Formulation," *Nervous Mental Disorders,* Proc. Ass. Res., vol. 29.

16

SOCIAL AND PSYCHOLOGICAL CRISES

Janice E. Hitchcock

In recent years "crisis" has become a common word in our vocabulary. Its usage has greatly increased not only in professional literature, but in all forms of mass media. Although *crisis* may refer to a physiological state, the use of the word relative to social and psychological phenomena has popularized the concept. Life crises are not strangers to us. Not only are we continually confronted with them in our professional work with patients, but we are not immune ourselves from personal crises. One has only to read the newspaper, watch a play, turn on the TV, or browse through a book store to hear or see a reference to some aspect of crisis.

The fact of crisis, then, is not new; what is being studied in greater detail is the crisis process as it pertains to many different life events. Theories have developed from these studies which help to conceptualize and delineate crises more fully. This chapter is about crisis theory from a psychological and sociological perspective. It describes the pertinent studies on which crisis theory is based and discusses crisis theory as it relates to the individual, family, and society. The final section will include implications for nursing and the relationship of crisis theory to the future of the individual and society.

HISTORICAL DEVELOPMENT OF CRISIS THEORY

Crisis theory has its base in the work of a number of people who have contributed theories of human behavior. Freud should be mentioned first because of his beliefs related to psychic determinism. He felt that all behavior has a cause or source, whether or not consciously operative, in the history and experience of the individual, and that the foundation for present and future behavior is laid down in infancy and childhood. The ego-analytic theorists have added a dimension to Freud's pathologically oriented view by including the study of normal and healthy behavior (Aguilera et al., 1970, p. 3).

Heinz Hartmann extended Freudian theory to include considerations of man's ability to maintain adaptation to environment in later life as well as in early childhood. Sandor Rado viewed behavior in terms of its effect upon the welfare of the individual, not just in terms of cause and effect. He attached importance to the reality of the present, emphasizing the immediate present but without neglecting the influences of the developmental past. His primary concern was with patients who failed to adapt to current problems in today's world, what caused the failures, and what patients must do to learn to overcome them. According to Rado, this is accomplished by the patient automatizing new patterns of healthy behavior through practice. This is the ultimately curative process, not insight. The automatization takes place actively in the reality of daily living, not passively in the doctor's office (Aguilera et al., 1970).

Erik Erikson (1968) adds another dimension to crisis theory. He considers the totality of the life cycle, and has identified eight major stages through which every individual passes, each of which presents a crisis. He believes in the epigenesis of the ego, that is, that the ego develops in an orderly, sequential way and that each stage that is reached is dependent upon the previous one for successful completion. He is particularly interested in identity and identity crisis, and has developed a theoretical formulation of these concepts. If growth proceeds well, it will be made up of inner and outer conflicts which the personality weathers, reemerging from each crisis "with an increased sense of inner unity, with an increase of judgment, and an increase in the capacity 'to do well' according to his own standards and to the standards of those who are significant to him" (Erikson, 1968, p. 92). Each stage is a potential crisis because it is a turning point in one's life. At the beginning of a stage, one is vulnerable because the approaches used to maintain equilibrium in the previous stage are no longer effective for use in the one that is newly developing. Until new methods of coping are fully developed near the end of a stage, the personality is in an upheaval where old methods no longer work but new approaches to the world have yet to be developed. It is during this unsettling time that the individual rapidly changes his perspective and is most open to all kinds of influences both from without and from within. How the personality develops from the initial stage of infancy—of basic trust versus mistrust—to the final stage in adulthood—of integrity versus despair—depends on the way with which each of the intervening stages are dealt. If one must move from the first stage of development with a fundamental distrust of his interpersonal relationships, he will have considerable difficulty developing autonomy in the second stage and be more vulnerable to shame and doubt. He will have difficulty integrating his life experiences because of shaky progress through the developmental stages and will be led to despair rather than fulfillment.

Another contribution central to crisis theory is that of Erich Lindemann (1944), who made a special study of one type of crisis, that of grief. His conceptualization of the grieving process is the basis for the development of crisis theory. He identified five characteristics of grief: (1) somatic distress, (2) preoccupation with the image of the deceased, (3) guilt, (4) hostile reactions, and (5) loss of habitual patterns of conduct which were usual activities tied in with the relationship to the deceased. He also indicated a sixth characteristic that borders on the pathological. That characteristic is the appearance of traits of the deceased in the behavior of the bereaved. He said that the duration of a grief reaction seems to depend upon the success with which a person does the grief work, achieves emancipation from the bondage of the deceased, readjusts to the environment in which the deceased is missing, and forms new relationships. Lindemann noted that one of the biggest obstacles to completing grief work is the attempt made by many people to avoid both the intense distress connected with the grief experience and the necessary expression of emotion. The resolution of the crisis of death can be accomplished only if grief work is completed.

If loss is defined as a state of being deprived of or being without something one has had (Schoenberg et al., 1970), most crises can be discussed in terms of loss of a loved one through death, institutionalization, or divorce; loss of a part of oneself by amputation, miscarriage, organ surgery, or plastic surgery; loss or change in role by retirement, moving in with children, military draft, unemployment, or employment or status change; loss of self-esteem that may be real, threatened, or anticipated, such as occurs in delinquency, alcoholism, imprisonment, marital failure, and academic failure. In response to these losses, the individual experiences grief and must work through this grief feeling until he is able to adapt himself to his new environment. This process may take many months or years.

Built upon the work of these theorists and studies conducted around specific crisis events, Gerald Caplan evolved his own theory of crisis and is, perhaps, its best-known proponent. Caplan's theory emphasizes the growth potential for the individual as an outcome of a crisis, in contrast to the view frequently taken that equates crisis with catastrophe and sees all related behavior as pathological. He stresses the importance of crisis periods in individual and group development and views crisis in terms of the homeostatic process analogous to the well-known concept of homeostasis in physiological functioning. Similarly, one's normal psychological pattern is maintained by homeostatic, reequilibrating mechanisms. When a pattern deviation occurs, the organism attempts to reequilibrate. This upset in equilibrium caused by some force or situation which alters its functioning is called a "problem" and, initially, will call forth a number of habitual problem-solving mechanisms which are normally used by the individual. In a crisis, since the problem is larger than usual, normal coping mechanisms are not as effective as usual within a given time range. When equilibrium is finally achieved, the new pattern may be quite different from the old. However, it will function in a similar way; that is, it will be stable and constitute an equilibrium maintained by homeostatic reequilibrating forces. A significant factor in a crisis is the fact that major pattern alterations may occur over a short period yet remain stable for a very long time (Caplan, 1964).

Caplan describes four characteristics of crisis based on the fact that tension is produced when a crisis situation occurs. The individual is faced with "stimuli which signal danger to a fundamental need satisfaction or evoke major need appetite" (Caplan, 1964, p. 37), but his habitual problem-solving techniques prove unsuccessful. The tension evoked will vary according to the degree of frustration involved. The characteristics produced by this tension are as follows (Caplan, 1964, pp. 40–41):

1. There is a rise in tension in response to the impact of a stimulus. Habitual problem-solving mechanisms are called forth.
2. If these fail, tension increases, creating an increased feeling of upset and ineffectiveness.
3. *Emergency* problem-solving mechanisms are called forth. The problem may be redefining or altering his original goals. All resources are utilized and totally new responses may be tried. As a result, one of three possibilities is likely to happen:
   a. The problem is solved to the satisfaction of the individual.
   b. The problem is solved as a result of redefinition of the problem.
   c. The problem is avoided by giving up one's goals completely.
4. If no resolution takes place, the result is a state of major disorganization.

Caplan explains this process of crisis as occurring "when a person faces an obstacle to important life goals that is for a time unsurmountable through the utilization of customary methods of problem solving.

A period of disorganization ensues; a period of upset, during which many abortive attempts at solution are made" (Caplan, 1961, p. 18).

Characteristics of Crisis

As the result of his experience and research, Caplan has found certain specific characteristics of crisis. It is self-limiting, lasting from 1 to 6 weeks, and during that time a solution is found to restore the equilibrium. The individual will return to a state that is better, worse, or the same as that before the crisis. The triggering factor is usually a fairly clear-cut event. The person in crisis feels himself involved totally in his problem to the point where it takes precedence over everything else in his life, and he emotionally hurts all over; the experience is totally subjective. At this time he is most open to intervention. This openness accounts for the fact that major changes in perception can take place and make the crisis a turning point for the individual.

Different Responses to Crisis

Crisis occurs as the result of an event that is linked symbolically with either earlier threats that resulted in vulnerability or conflict, an external disaster, or an event for which known coping mechanisms are inadequate. Defensive mechanisms may not be effective either because the event is too overwhelming or because the individual has too few responses available at that time. For instance, a fire which destroys a man's home and kills his wife and children is likely to overwhelm the coping ability of even the most mature individual. On the other hand, someone who is very tired, or old, or who has never learned to deal with his problems except by avoidance may be totally unable to deal with even a minor fire which destroys a few pieces of his furniture.

There are many factors that account for these differences, primarily sociocultural, community, and family influences. Whether or not an event becomes critical for an individual will depend on his interpretation of the event. For instance, family illness is more likely to be perceived as a crisis in a culture that rejects infirmity. Another culture that considers illness to be inevitable and offers much family support when someone is sick is less likely to experience the event as critical. Aside from culture, if one member is in crisis, all members are affected. This fact is true whether one speaks of the traditional nuclear or extended family or refers to an alternative life style such as group marriage or communal living. In crisis, the family and the community may be at the same time both a resource and a precipitating factor. Parents, spouses, siblings, work situations, school, and church may all be potentially supportive to a person in crisis, but they may also create interacting forces in the relationship which bring about the crisis.

Another variable on which crisis depends is the "supplies" described by Caplan that ensure good mental health (Caplan, 1964, p. 56). These include physical supplies, such as food, shelter, sensory stimulation, and health; psychosocial supplies, such as personal interaction, family integrity, personality development, and cognitive and affective development; and sociocultural supplies, such as community contact and involvement, education, appropriate work, and values and customs of the culture. A lack of any of these supplies constitutes a threat to the integrity of the individual.

With these factors in mind, it is clearly possible to identify certain hazards that universally are a potential threat to all individuals. Such a hazard as death, divorce, retirement, loss of job, upward or downward status mobility, and premature birth exemplify situations of challenge, loss of basic supplies, or threat of life. They represent significant life events, and for some they will precipitate a developmental or situational (or accidental) crisis. Knowledge of these hazards is necessary if preventive actions are to be employed.

Elements of Crisis

A concept that is a part of, and frequently equated with, crisis is *stress.* Lazarus (1969), in his definition of the nature of stress in relation to both stimulus and response, also describes behavior and physiological responses seen in crisis. When a stress occurs because of a circumstance external to a person which makes unusual or extraordinary demands on him or threatens him, it is called a *stress stimulus.* Examples are natural disasters, incapacitating illness, and military combat. Since different people respond differently to external stresses, another aspect of stress focuses on the responses of reaction of the person rather than the situation producing the stress; it is important to consider both aspects. People in stress exhibit both physiological and psychological reactions. In addition to stress, frustration, threat, conflict, and anxiety are also associated with crisis. Lazarus defined *frustration* as a condition in which "a course of action cannot be carried out or brought to its conclusion for some reason or other" (Lazarus, 1969, p. 173). *Threat* is defined as "anticipation of harm of some kind" (Lazarus, 1969, p. 174). The difference between these two concepts is that threat is anticipated harm and therefore future-oriented; frustration has already occurred and so is present- or past-oriented.

456

Conflict is "the presence, simultaneously of two incompatible action tendencies or goals" (Lazarus, 1969, p. 178). There may be conflict between two internal needs, between two external demands, or between an internal need and an external demand. Such a situation makes threat or frustration inevitable because to satisfy one goal necessarily threatens or frustrates the others. It is conflict that leads to crisis.

Anxiety is regarded as a response to certain stress stimuli. It is an intensely unpleasant affective state that can be only subjectively experienced. It is characterized by physical manifestations such as rapid heart beat, sweaty palms, frequency, urgency, diarrhea, restlessness, and psychological manifestations such as shortened attention span and fear of impending doom, and has no object as a causative agent. This last element differentiates anxiety from fear in that fear has a clearly defined object causing it (Lazarus, 1969).

Other Theories

Although Caplan's concept of crisis theory is the best-known and most used, another theorist not so well known in the United States has developed ideas that in many ways parallel the approach of Caplan and Lindemann. Dabrowski (1940) believes that "personality growth occurs through the disintegration of the existing personality structure, and then reconstruction at a higher level, which derives impetus from the developmental instinct" (Harrison, 1965). He differentiates between "primitive integration," which he describes as similar to psychopathology and which he views as a negative force, and the "capacity" for disintegration, which he sees as a basis for upward development. Often, he says, behaviors and feelings are interpreted as psychological illness when in fact they are a manifestation of "positive disintegration," which is a healthy, creative expression.

Dabrowski, Caplan, and Lindemann all give a very positive interpretation to many behaviors often labeled "illness" by health professionals and viewed with fear and avoidance by much of society. According to their thesis, feelings and behaviors expressed as a manifestation of a response to crisis should be encouraged and supported, not rejected, repressed, and denied, if the outcome is to be a full realization of one's personality potential.

Family Crisis Theory

In many instances, an individual in crisis needs assistance for himself alone, but frequently it is the family as a unit to which attention must be directed. Hill (1965) has developed a formula that describes a family's perception of a crisis:

A (event) interacts with B (family's crisis meeting resource) interacts with C (family definition of the event) = X (crisis).

Stated another way, it takes the interaction of several factors (A, B, and C) to constitute a family crisis. The event (A) will precipitate a crisis only if the family has few or no resources to cope with the event and/or if the event is defined by the family as a crisis. For example, a family that operates within a value system that gives health a high priority is more likely to view chronic illness in a member as catastrophic than a family that accepts illness in a fatalistic way. However, the degree of illness and the presence or absence of adequate health facilities may make the difference as to whether the event will be within or beyond the coping capacity of the family.

Hill (1965) has classified family crises in several ways: first by source—whether they are extrafamily (earthquakes or floods, fires, etc.) or intrafamily (infidelity, nonsupport, alcoholism, etc.). He also developed a form of classification by family configuration—that is, change in composition of the family, such as the loss of a family member, as happens in hospitalization, divorce, or death, or an addition to the family, such as occurs in birth, return of an absent family member, or adoption. Family crisis can also be the result of loss of morale and family unity. This demoralizing component may be seen in cases of drug addiction, delinquency, infidelity, and nonsupport. A combination of demoralization with one of the other two configurations could also develop, as frequently occurs in illegitimacy, alcoholism, divorce, runaway, imprisonment, suicide, and institutionalization. And finally, classification of family crisis may be in terms of type of an event which results in a status shift, such as sudden impoverishment, prolonged unemployment, sudden wealth or fame, disasters, migrations, promotions, and retirement.

STUDIES

Many studies related to crisis have been based upon mentally ill populations (Shellow, 1967; Langsley and Kaplan, 1968; Pearlman, 1970; Leff, 1970). None prove that life stresses lead to mental illness for the majority of people, but they do support the thesis that certain hazardous events usually precipitate either an individual or a family crisis. This is not to say that these events constitute overwhelming situations which involve personality disintegration, but they clearly put this population at risk.

Paykel (1969) studied depressed patients and developed a list of the most significant life events preceding the depression. These were (1) increase in arguments with spouse, (2) marital separation, (3) new type of employment, (4) death of an immediate family member, (5) serious illness of a family member, (6) departure of a family member from the home, (7) serious personal physical illness, and (8) change in work conditions. "On the average, depressed patients reported nearly three times as many important life events in the six-months prior to the onset of the depressive episode as were reported by controls in a comparable six-month period" (Paykel, 1969, p. 767). Wyler (1971) reported a similar finding in his study of the relationship of disease to life changes.

From these and other less significant events, Paykel developed three categories. The first group included events which involved changes in the immediate social field of the subject. Two classes of such events were defined: (1) entrances, or the introduction of a new person into the social field; (2) exits, or departures from the social field. The latter were much more frequent among depressed subjects than among normal subjects.

The second group of events was classified by social desirability or undesirability. The undesirable events, such as being fired, demotion, separation, and major financial problems, were more common in the depressive subjects than in the control group. For desired events, such as promotion, engagement, and marriage, the pattern was reversed.

The third category of events was in the area of social activity. Five categories, related to employment, legal, family, marital, and health, were derived. Again events were more likely to be found among the depressed subjects.

Not only do there seem to be hazardous life events which precipitate emotional difficulties, but they also appear to precipitate physical illness. In both instances, family conflict is involved.

Such occurrences as dissatisfaction with living arrangements, violent arguments, and threat of separation from family antedated congestive heart failure in 49 percent of one study of 105 cases (Pearlman, 1970). Another indicated that the greater the life change, the greater the disruption of bodily functions (Wyler, 1971). The most positive correlation was the relationship of hazardous events with chronic illnesses. Because of increased vulnerability, the disease which develops is of a greater magnitude because the body resists it less than it would otherwise.

Other studies show that physical loss or service injury creates crises which are resolved through the process of grief work. Hamburg et al. (1967) indicate that denial gives way to depression and then to comprehensive understanding of the situation for patients with severe burns or poliomyelitis. The manner with which key figures in their environment responded to such patients was critical.

Fitzgerald (1970) studied people who became blind and found that the loss model is in operation as a result of this crisis. There was a difference between those who faced sudden sight loss and those who knew of their impending blindness. In the former group, people had to work through the stages of initial disbelief, distress (protest), depression, and resolution or continued the process as a pathological syndrome. The latter group tended to begin working through the loss and preparing for substitute resources before the event, thus averting a crisis.

The preceding studies strongly suggest that life events have a significant effect on one's total state of being. In all the events described, human personal and family relationships are directly involved. Some events are more likely than others to precipitate depression or a somatic illness, but the actual meaning of the event to that individual is the deciding factor. One other important point to remember is that we are speaking of experiences common to us all, many of which are everyday events, not necessarily or per se catastrophic occurrences.

Smith (1971) questions whether life events or "risk-markers" can be utilized as clues to pending mental illness. He found that these events, although similar to those cited above, occurred after the beginning of psychosocial disintegration, not antecedent to it. However, early intervention can prevent further deterioration. He also pointed out that several critical events actually occurred more frequently among the general population, such as death of a family member, loss of a close friend, and onset of menopause. These findings suggest that the resolution of most crises does not result in mental illness for such individuals, but rather in some adaptation, or adjustment, to their environment. Thus, populations at risk with regard to crisis events must be recognized within the general population who utilize and seek help for life crises in agencies such as hospitals, schools, welfare, divorce courts, clergy, and police, rather than in agencies such as mental hospitals or counseling centers which focus on people who are emotionally disturbed.

It seems clear that change and loss do create stress, which may or may not lead to a state of crisis. If a crisis does occur, and resources are available, such as supportive crisis counseling, it is probable that maladaptive responses can be avoided. If resources are not utilized or are unavailable, the likelihood is that a maladaptive response, such as suicide, mental or physical illness, or violence, may be the result.

Community and Society

Crisis theory can be utilized as a frame of reference, not only in relation to individual and family events, but also events occurring to a community and in the larger society. A number of writers have expressed the idea that our technological society is moving at a faster rate than man can respond to (Slater, 1971; Milgram, 1970; Gilula et al., 1970; Toffler, 1970; McLuhan and Quentin, 1967). Toffler sees the world in a superindustrial revolution in which people are faced with ever-increasing choices in life, most of which are novel and thus require a novel reaction. In the face of these increasing choices, people are also being asked to make rapid decisions about issues which require more time for thought because of their novelty. This situation overloads the human nervous system to the point where people can see no alternatives and wish only for a way out. The tension and anxiety thus created are often manifest in violence, as in riots, or in apathy, both of which are very common in today's society (Toffler, 1970).

Polak's studies of life events preceding psychiatric illness led him to state that psychiatric symptoms must be interpreted within a framework of that individual's relationships in work, school, home, or community (Polak, 1971).

This accelerated change in life manifests itself in many events that have been shown to have crisis potential. The increase in mobility means that people change jobs and homes very frequently and do not make or maintain close personal ties with significant others. Nuclear families are changing and alternative life styles such as communes and trial marriages are developing (Toffler, 1970).

McLuhan and Quentin (1967, pp. 74–75) describe the present dilemma: "When faced with a totally new situation, we tend always to attach ourselves to the objects, to the flavor of the most recent past. We look at the present through a rear-view mirror. We march backward into the future." They further point out that we confront our world with an "enormous backlog of outdated mental and psychological responses." Our words and thoughts refer us only to the past, not to the present (McLuhan and Quentin, 1967, p. 63).

Toffler (1970) stresses that society must educate for the future and not rely on the experiences of the past to offer solutions. This means that almost every event requires a novel solution; previous coping mechanisms are no longer effective. Thus, life crises are intensified and those who cannot adapt to the accelerated demands experience "future shock."

The future-shocked society manifests itself in many ways. The pressures of mobility, increased life expectancy, and shorter relationships result in many divorces, leaving the respective spouses alone and often without the resource of family and friends that were available in the past. The extended family of grandparents, aunts, and uncles no longer exists and often the people who live in a community are strangers. Family agencies are still unable for many reasons to meet the needs of broken families, and few other resources are available. One of the major problems is the psychological impact of divorce on the children. Sugar (1970) describes its similarity to the death of a parent in its effects on the emotional growth and development of the child.

Another crisis made more difficult by our society is widowhood. Customs and economy in America make readjustment harder than in many other cultures. Expressions of grief are often not accepted by others and feelings are repressed. Many widows have no skills and find it difficult to support themselves. Most of their friends have been couples, and they no longer feel a part of their former groups, yet making new friends can be very difficult.

Silverman (1969) has reported on one attempt to deal with this problem. Widows have been trained in one Boston program in an understanding of grief and bereavement. They are able to help other widows work through their acute pain with support from someone who can understand what they are experiencing. The aides help the new widows by assisting them to find jobs, sort out finances, and gradually reestablish community relationships. These are functions formerly done by one's family, but in today's world the family members may be many miles away. Without a formalized program, making contacts with other widows in our more complex communities would be virtually impossible.

Employment is another problem made more difficult by our super-industrial society. Levenstein (1968) questions how man will adjust his attitudes toward working in an automated society. Employment can only be maintained through such strategies as early retirement and shorter workweeks. Most workers value the work ethic and are threatened with an identity crisis as work becomes less necessary and they become lost in large industrial complexes.

Cancro (1969) suggests that we may have found ways to technically deal with the work load, but have not at all addressed ourselves to the psychological impact of these transitions. Only if man can adjust his self-image to the changing environment and come to view himself as a part of a cooperative society, rather than an individual competitor, will he be able to adapt to the needs of the future.

Another outcome of the shift from industrial to superindustrial society has been the impact on the white-collar worker. Rockey (1971) reports that the rate of joblessness for professional and technical workers in 1971 was up 27 percent from 1969. For most of these workers, unemployment is a first-time crisis with no past experience from which to draw. The experience for some has been to increase their skills and abilities as they work to weather the storm, but for others unemployment has set off a series of other crises, such as marital problems, change of residence, and downward mobility. In Seattle in 1971, the crisis clinic received increasing calls, particularly from men, as the economic situation became worse (Rockey, 1971).

Other studies have demonstrated the effect of one's work situation on physical and emotional health. Kasl and Cobb (1970) studied blue-collar workers whose plant was about to be shut down. Their blood pressure was higher during the anticipation of the shutdown and tended to remain high in those men who had more severe experiences or who reported lasting subjective stress. Another study done between 1910 and 1960 showed a marked increase in mental hospital admissions during short-term changes in the aggregate level of industrial activities (Brenner, 1969). The economically insecure groups showed the greatest risk.

As a result of our increased health technology, we have, on the other hand, helped to increase the life span of individuals and created a sizable geriatric segment of society; on the other hand, we have not made old people a valid part of our society, but relegate them to an institution. Many of the stresses of middle-aged or older people can be attributed to current social and economic factors and the trend toward institutionalization (Busse, 1971). Aged people who are anticipating being institutionalized have been shown to be worse off psychologically than those who live at home or are already institutionalized (Prock, 1969). Their general anxiety and tension are greater, they have high emotional reactivity, express a sense of helplessness and powerlessness, and manifest a tone of depression accompanied by low self-esteem. Their interpersonal relationship patterns, which suggest active withdrawal from those around them, signs of ego disorganization, and a quality of "my life is over," are similar to that of social death with concomitant mourning (Prock, 1969).

In middle and late life, behavioral, psychological, and emotional changes are frequently determined by an interaction of biological and socioeconomic factors. Continuous activity throughout one's life span is beneficial and achieves greater satisfaction than early retirement. However, the elderly are not needed in our society, and pressures of unemployment have led to earlier and earlier retirement. Economic deprivation is common and devastating. This problem becomes greater as more and more people must move from a dying agrarian way of life to the urban life of a city (Busse, 1971). Increased levels of social complexity, with its demand for social conformity and group-oriented actions, lead to increased intergroup tensions.

An Australian study points up the need for better management of the patient's social environment, particularly family and employment, in order to lessen morbidity. As myocardial malfunctions in men under fifty were being studied, it became evident that invalidism was often perpetuated by the patient's attitude and the attitude of family members. With increased communication between patient, family, health personnel, and social environment, the patient is able to make a more realistic adjustment to his illness (Brown, 1969).

Environmental stress also affects lower-status groups. One must evaluate symptomatology to decide to what extent they represent personality defects and to what extent they consist of normal reactions to unusually harsh and numerous stressors in the contemporary situation (Dohrenwend, 1967). Much more research is needed before it will be possible to make this evaluation. Man's physical, social, and cultural environments are so closely interwoven that stresses which accompany them must be viewed as interdependent (Chance, 1968). Resolution in one area may promote additional stress in another. Stress associated with high rates of social interaction or crowding is felt more by previously isolated people, such as movement from rural to urban living.

Culture conflicts also create stresses. Conflicting expectations about how to behave in a given social context, lack of effective communication due to culturally dissonant values, and cultural restraints on the expression of human needs frequently lead to continuous and intense stresses. One's identity is questioned, resulting in feelings of inferiority. Discrimination often reinforces these identity conflicts. One study with Mexican-American adolescents describes the crisis of being caught between Mexican and American value systems (Ramirez, 1969). Rejecting one's system results in guilt and self-derogation. Adjustment problems are related to reactions to this value conflict. The family conflicts which frequently result often lead to health problems.

The rapid and extensive changes in our social and physical environments require major modifications which are both adaptive and maladaptive. Milgram (1970) describes some of the adaptations to city life that have resulted from urban overload. In New York City, one can meet 220,000 persons within a 10-minute radius of his office by foot or car, as compared with 20,000 persons he could meet in a similar area in Newark. This magnitude of communication possibilities has both positive and negative aspects. Overload to this extent results in adaptations which take the form of deformities in daily life: i.e., impinging on role performance, evolution of social norms, cognitive functioning, and the use of facilities. Responses to overload include allocation of less time to each input (you don't apologize when you brush past people in a crowd) and disregard of low-priority inputs (you ignore drunks in alleys); boundaries are redrawn in certain social transactions so that the overload system can shift the burden to the other party in the exchange (bus drivers no longer give change); reception is blocked off prior to entrance into the system (unlisted telephones); social screening devices are interposed between the individual and environmental inputs (helping agencies). Intensity of inputs is diminished by filtering devices, so that only weak and relatively superficial forms of involvement with others are allowed and specialized institutions are created to absorb inputs that would other-wise swamp the individual.

The consequence of these responses to overload make for the differences in the tone of city and town. The disregard for people who are not personally significant, and for their needs is increased. The extreme is seen in situations of crisis in which the bystander will not intervene. The frequency of demands gives rise to noninvolvement. There is less willingness to trust and assist strangers, often increased by the increased dangers of the city. Civilities become less. Men no longer defer to women on buses and in opening doors. Anonymity varies according to the size of the city. This offers privacy in some respects, but can also result in anomie. In cities, roles are segmented. We relate to others according to the piece of us that is relevant, not with our whole selves. These observations are similar to Toffler's (1970) comments about the "throw-away society" concept of transience, the modular man, and a diversity of life styles. His concept of the future is reflected in Milgram's ideas (Milgram, 1970).

MALADAPTIVE RESPONSES

While the previously stated adaptations may be necessary in order for people to function in today's world, there are other responses that are definitely maladaptive.

Violence is a currently prevalent maladaptive response to crisis. Gilula et al. (1970) describe violence in the context of adaptation, as a struggle to resolve stressful and threatening events. They believe that the survival value of violence is diminishing rapidly in our society, and that alternatives to violence must be found if we are to survive. These conclusions sound very similar to those of Hoagland (1969), who feels that if we do not learn to control our overpopulation of the earth and our aggressive instincts, hates, and fears, we are likely to commit nuclear suicides and become extinct. Gilula et al. differentiate between aggression and violence by defining *violence* as destructive aggression. It is not aggression in the broad sense which must be eliminated, but only its destructive component, because it is no longer an adaptive response to threatening events.

Another important differentiation is made between adaptation and adjustment. Adaptive behaviors enhance species' survival, and, in most instances, individual survival tends to be an active process resulting in an enduring alteration of behavior structure and pattern. Adjustment, on the other hand, temporarily enhances the way we fit with the immediate situation; it tends to be passive and does not result in enduring behavior and pattern changes. Because adjustment is a temporary response to an immediate need, it tends to be maladaptive in our rapidly changing society. What was adaptive yesterday may be maladaptive today and can "work against survival in 'new' or unusual environments" (Gilula and Daniels, 1969, p. 397). McLuhan's "rear-view mirror" world is clearly different from *coping,* which is defined as "the continuing, usually successful struggle, to accomplish tasks and goals with adaptive consequences," not adjustive consequences (Gilula and Daniels, 1969). Violence is viewed as a maladaptive mechanism in that it is used in situations where stress has become overwhelming to the individual or group and leads to aggression which is indiscriminate and protective. We have the equipment necessary for adapting to and modeling diverse environments, but in doing so, man changes the conditions necessary for survival. Can we adapt or will we adjust? At present, violence continues to be a greater and greater part of our world, suggesting that adaptive forms of aggression are yet to be effectively utilized. War, mass media, violence, presidential assassinations, gun control controversies, crime, and riots, all illustrate the maladaptive response to crisis we seem to take. It is not aggression in general, but our continued violent response to threat, that is society's crisis.

Suicide

Suicide must be considered briefly here as another one of the maladaptive responses to crisis. *Suicide* is a "conscious, deliberate attempt to take one's life quickly" (Farber, 1968). The frequency with which suicide is considered as an alternative to an insoluble crisis is in part related to the culture in which it occurs and the positive or negative value placed upon it in that culture. Other factors to be considered are the degree of lethality of the intention, not merely the outcome; the degree of vulnerability of the personality; and the deprivation of the situation. All of these must be examined to assess the probability of suicide as a response to crisis.

The concept of "hope" is closely related to suicide. It "entails confident expectation that a desired outcome will occur" (Farber, 1968, p. 12). Kübler-Ross (1969) considers this a vital factor in facing the crisis of dying. When hope is lost, death occurs very shortly thereafter. Hope is determined by the degree of threat leveled against the individual's sense of being able to master his environment. Vulnerability, and therefore lessening of hope, will increase as the threat overtakes the individual's sense of competence. It becomes obvious that all these factors are variable and must be assessed in a given individual at a given time to determine the degree of lethality at that moment. Suicide will be the chosen alternative only when there appears to be no available path that will lead to a tolerable existence (Farber, 1968, p. 17).

A fairly typical list of precipitating causes for suicide includes the same kinds of events previously described in other studies. The top four are (1) poor health, (2) economic distress, (3) death of a loved one, and (4) domestic difficulties. Basic to them all is that for a "given low sense of competence the conditions of life have been rendered intolerable and unmanageable" (Farber, 1968, p. 39). The part played by society in determining suicide as an alternative can be defined in terms of resources available to the individual. Lack of succorant persons and institutions, strong demands in society for the exercising of competence, demands for interpersonal giving, such as nursing and medicine, lack of a hopeful future time perspective or a constricted psychological space of free movement, and degree of toleration or prohibition of suicide in the society make up the aspects of the social surroundings which must be taken into account. Still, statistically, there seems to be no direct correlation between advancing civilization and suicide, since the rate is about the same now as it was in 1900 (Farber, 1968, p. 71). Positive expressions of aggression are probably an important factor in preventing suicide.

Extreme Stress

A final aspect of crisis has to do with those situations of extreme environmental stress faced by many people in society but which do not fall within the category of everyone's experience. Examples are concentration camp experiences, front-line war activities, earthquakes in populated areas, tornados, floods, and experiences of victims of atomic bombing. Studies have shown that certain syndromes can be associated with behavior following such events (Chodoff, 1970; Hocking, 1970; Lifton, 1964).

One study of 300 people subjected to severe stress in World War II found that all who were in a ghetto or concentration camp were characterized by a distinctive apathetic appearance (Hocking, 1970). Those who were in hiding for a period of time or escaped showed marked tension and anxiety that overlay depressive symptoms.

Chodoff (1970) studied the concentration camp experience in detail. He found that the initial sequential reactions were shock and terror, apathy, and regressive behavior. In some there developed identification with the aggressor and denial and isolation of effect. Years later, after the experience, a syndrome seemed to develop that had apparently lain dormant for many years. This consisted of depression and guilt, feelings of emptiness, despair, hopelessness, and depression at holidays or anniversaries associated with their experiences. He found parallels between concentration camp experiences and the A-bomb disease or neurosis described by Lifton (1964), as well as much of the behavior seen in people living in poverty ghettos.

According to Hocking (1970), any extreme sensory deprivation, through either deprivation or continuous stimulation for more than a few hours results in marked anxiety, irritability, agitation, depersonalization, disorientation, impairment of concentration, difficulty in problem solving, and abnormal visual sensations such as hallucinations. After isolation, the individual complains of fatigue, drowsiness, confusion, and loss of orientation to time and has difficulty readjusting to a normal environment. Hocking (1970) believes that if stress is sufficiently intense, virtually everyone will develop neurotic symptoms regardless of individual personality patterns.

In order to consider extreme stresses to the community and society, systems theory can be utilized. Miller (1964) points out that large social bodies have normal adjustment processes to control energy and information flow. Under normal conditions, neither excess nor lack is experienced. Warehouses are filled and reservoirs maintained for later use. Changes are made in the economy to keep money flowing. At times, the society can sustain stresses which upset the equilibrium, such as revolutions, wars, natural disasters such as famine, fire, and flood, and such economic disasters as in the Depression. At other times, society can be vulnerable to the same stresses, which may go to the extent of irreversibly destroying the existing structure.

Natural and man-made disasters result in a disaster syndrome in many that is characterized by anxiety, insomnia, and digestive upsets. Preexisting personality factors are important in determining the intensity of the syndrome (Hocking, 1970).

Disaster studies can be described in terms of two frameworks: time stages and spatial zones (Miller, 1964). Time stages in disaster can be identified as: warning, threat, impact, inventory, rescue, remedy, and recovery. Spatial zones are produced in society when disaster strikes: total impact (not destruction), fringe impact, filter area, organized community aid, and organized regional aid.

External disasters can be described in terms of certain attributes: (1) anticipated or unanticipated, (2) precedented or unprecedented, and (3) discriminating or undiscriminating. For instance, an earthquake is usually unanticipated and undiscriminating, but not unprecedented in places like California and Japan. On the other hand, a bombing might be anticipated, but not precedented, in America, whereas in Vietnam it has much precedent; and in both cases it is undiscriminating. The degree of disorganization that is likely to occur will be based on the novelty and intensity of the event to the victims. A crisis develops as a sudden or unexpected increase in threat brings a group to a breaking point. The breaking point can also be approached as a result of cumulative exposure to a threat. Reactions will differ accordingly. Planning cannot occur in a crisis situation as it can in a cumulative threat. On the other hand, cumulative threat requires accommodation to the threat, as well as countering demoralization related to the crisis. This prolonged anxiety that develops from waiting for a crisis can be more demoralizing than dealing with the crisis itself. Reality of danger may be denied, or behavior may displace attention from the real threat. Danger that seems manageable produces less demoralization than that which seems overwhelming or is unknown.

In many external disasters such as floods or storms, there is a great deal of advance warning about the pending event. Success of the warning depends on several factors. First of all, do the people receive it? If they do, how does the information interact with their background experiences and current social and physical situation? Whether people receive the warning also depends on the behavior of other people involved in the detection, interpretation, and relating of danger information to them (Williams, 1964). If all radio stations send out special bulletins about a hurricane and urge everyone to move to higher ground, people are more likely to respond to it if they know the danger from past experience. If hurricanes are not usually severe, or if the alert is given in a routine news announcement, there is less likelihood that it will be heeded. Warning, which includes information about a danger and what can be done to prevent, minimize, or avoid it, is not in itself enough. How an individual defines his situation seems to determine his response to the warning. This definition is made up of several interrelated factors: strength of threat, time element, cost of taking protective action, and presumed effectiveness of available countermeasures.

Lang and Lang (1964) present an analysis of the dynamics underlying many of our current societal and community crises. They point out that disaster threatened over a long period of time subjects the cohesive forces of a group to a severe strain. Mass hysteria, rioting, delinquency, and extreme social movements can be attributed to such stresses. The degree to which constructive or destructive responses are given to the situation depends on the degree of morale or demoralization. *Morale* is defined as "continued performance and coordination of roles in situations of stress" (Lang and Lang, 1964, p. 66). *Demoralization* involves the "progressive weakening of affective ties and commitment to group goals and values" (Lang and Lang, 1964, p. 67). If personal and socially structured defenses such as organizational rules are maintained, then constructive and coordinated, preventive, or remedial action will take place. However, collective responses based on an emotional reaction are likely to disrupt the group and have negative consequences. Such responses can be divided into three types of effort: (1) coping with threat on symbolic level only (shared psychopathology and mass hysteria), (2) recrystallizing group norms around hostile impulses and displacing on targets considered outside the framework of values (riots and scapegoating), (3) developing schismatic tendencies toward mutual withdrawal and increased subgroup solidarity (distrust of authority and charges of favoritism).

Nuclear attack is perhaps the most extreme of external threats with which we might be faced. Such an event is a threat to life; it may cause separation and loss, produce a feeling of helplessness like that of an abandoned infant, and imply an indefinite duration of danger, such as: radiation and unknown dangers, threat of having to defend oneself and one's family, threat of sickness and death, and speculation of what the outside world will be like afterward. Few of us react to all of these possibilities as an ever-present threat because we utilize many defenses to prevent ourselves from acknowledging such unacceptable facts (Grenspoon, 1964). If this were not so, we would become totally demoralized and unable to function effectively in the world.

THE NURSE'S ROLE IN CRISIS SITUATIONS

Incorporating crisis theory and intervention into one's nursing activity has far-reaching implications for both patient care and program and policy development. Defining the crisis, enhancing communication, exploring and implementing constructive interventions, and evaluating the results are the key elements necessary for effective nursing action. On an individual or family basis, the nurse must be able to assess the social, cultural, physical, and emotional components of the people involved (Aguilera et al., 1970). This alone involves broad background in the behavioral and social sciences as well as the biological sciences in order to have the tools with which to work.

The nurse has the responsibility for developing the strengths apparent in a crisis situation and for capitalizing on them rather than dwelling on existent weaknesses or pathology. The ability to listen is essential. Often, this is all that is necessary to help the one in crisis to become aware of available alternatives. Sometimes more intensive crisis intervention or family therapy may be necessary, and in other cases practical intervention, such as helping to find housing or employment, may provide the most effective assistance.

Since immediate intervention is so important in crisis (King, 1971; Jacobson et al., 1965), it is often a nurse who will be involved in providing the interventions. For instance, liaison nurses working between hospital, home, and other agencies that help to plan for a patient's discharge frequently become the primary interveners in any crisis which does occur. Both admission and discharge from the hospital are often seen as crisis situations to the patient and his family. The liaison nurse can prepare the patient for these events and provide resources which can avert a potential crisis.

Crisis theory can provide the nurse with a means of evaluating not only the patient, but also the entire family situation. For example, when a child who has been blind from birth is able to see following an operation, it is as necessary to be available to that family as when blindness was first diagnosed. The family must learn all over again how to relate to a child who sees and no longer needs certain supports, just as they had to learn to adapt to a blind child.

Crisis theory may have implications for changes in the hospital environment which can be initiated by nurses. Waiting rooms in clinics could be arranged to provide privacy for conferences between the nurse and patient and/or family. Other areas could be arranged to encourage group discussion which might be initiated by a nurse. The crisis of separation of a child from its parents can be averted by open visiting hours and planned parent involvement. Community health and mental health nurses can work together in providing needed ongoing support for families living with catastrophic illnesses such as terminal cancer, mutilating and emotionally charged kinds of surgery, such as mastectomies, hysterectomies, orchidectomies, and hemimandiblectomies. Nurses can also case-find other potential crises by concerning themselves with the event as defined by the individual or family, not necessarily as they might define it themselves.

In order to encourage expression of feelings as an important part of crisis resolution, rooms should be available for nurse and family to talk alone, particularly in cardiac care and intensive care units and in areas where there are terminally ill patients. When there is a death on the unit, it is the nurse who is in a position to talk with the other patients about whatever aspects of the death they need to discuss. This approach will help patients ventilate their own feelings and thereby allay their anxiety about what otherwise may be a frightening event to them.

In our changing society, the nurse's role in crisis intervention can be further developed. First aid nurses in airports and at bus terminals can deal with clients who have emotional as well as physical needs. These are contact points for people who may experience many of the crises previously discussed. Immediate intervention, so important to a successful outcome in many instances, could be available in the person of a crisis-oriented nurse. Such a nurse could also provide consultation to other health professionals who are in contact with people in crisis (Donner, 1972, p. 87). Ministers, schoolteachers, waitresses, bartenders, and hairdressers, as well as many community agencies in daily contact with distressed people, may also benefit from consultation. A consultative relationship of this kind is usually beneficial not only for the client but for both professionals involved (Deloughery et al., 1971).

Involvement in crisis on a community or societal level may affect the nurse in a more abstract way, such as becoming a member of a program planning committee, actively participating as a member of a nursing organization, becoming part of an interdisciplinary team to help to plan the nursing component of a health program, or, as a private citizen, participating privately as a member of a parent-teacher's association. In order to be aware of and participate in the solution of community crises, a knowledge of one's community and the larger society is necessary if one is to be effective in the planning for creative change. In today's world, sound nursing care is possible only when viewed within a conceptual framework that recognizes the interrelationships in individual-family-community society. Otherwise, one is working in a vacuum.

Agencies also face crisis. Nurses are often so much a part of an agency that the clues are often not seen. However, if one examines one's experiences within a theoretical framework of crisis, the symptoms emerge. Examples of resistance to change in agency members include reacting to a new policy or program as if nothing had been changed, denial of anxiety in a new situation, and not recalling decisions that had been previously made; and these frequently occur. Conflict within a committee or team often is a result of unresolved group crisis. The nurse who can assess these events and objectively evaluate what is happening can accept change more easily and learn to work effectively in changed situations.

In disaster nursing, dealing with the immediate crisis is the priority. Recognizing the behavior of people as being a response to crisis helps give perspective to the situation and suggests intervention. It is important to listen to a victim as he pours out his dilemma and decides on his next move. Furthermore, it may be necessary to help him take the next move—for example, help him find shelter, food, or clothing—before he can begin to function on his own accord. Many victims of a disaster suffer severe losses. Therefore an understanding of the grief process is vital (Lindemann, 1944). Much disbelief, denial, and anger are likely to be encountered in grief as well as sadness. When these are viewed as normal responses, it is healthy to encourage the expression of the victim's negative feeling and to provide necessary support at this time rather than have it remain as a hidden source of unresolved conflict.

When involved in crisis intervention, it is most important for the nurse to develop and utilize a personal support system. Crises are emotionally draining for therapists as well as for those in crisis. Nurses need an opportunity to talk over their problems as therapists with someone else. A colleague from the nursing or other health professions might be sufficient. However, it is often helpful to seek out consultation on a regular basis if one is consistently confronted with crisis situations in one's daily working situation. One's own resources need recharging as much as do those of people in crisis; learning to be in touch with one's own feelings and to utilize them effectively with others requires continuing effort. Nurses can be effective crisis interveners only if these factors are taken into account and a resource is provided (Deloughery, 1971).

Nursing must concentrate on developing ways of thinking that can be adapted to a future world that will be quite different in many ways from the present. Changes in nursing must take place along with the changes in society. If nursing is to fulfill its role in crisis intervention, it must be ready to cope with the society of the future or itself become a victim of "future shock."

One of the major shortcomings of crisis theory is the paucity of research which evaluates the theory itself and which studies normal subjects as well as those who already show personality disorganization. Until more data are collected in these areas, the theory must be open to challenge and modification as new input becomes known. In the meantime, such theory as exists provides an effective conceptual base from which to interpret the impact on individuals and families of many aspects of our stress-filled environment and future-oriented society.

BIBLIOGRAPHY

Aguilera, Donna, Janice Messick, and Marlene Tarrell (1970): *Crisis Intervention: Theory and Methodology,* C. V. Mosby Company, St. Louis, p. 3.

Brenner, M. Harvey (1969): "Patterns of Psychiatric Hospitalization among Different Socioeconomic Groups in Response to Economic Stress," *Journal of Nervous and Mental Diseases,* January, pp. 31-38.

Brown, L. B., et al. (1969): "Social Effects of Myocardial Infarct in Men under Fifty," *The Medical Journal of Australia,* July 19, pp. 125–128.

Busse, Ewald W. (1971): "Biologic and Sociologic Changes Affecting Adaptation in Mid and Later Life," *Annals of Internal Medicine, pp. 115–120.*

Cancro, Robert (1969): "Automation: The Second Emancipation Proclamation," *American Journal of Psychotherapy,* October, pp. 657–666.

Caplan, Gerald (1961): *An Approach to Community Mental Health,* Grune & Stratton, Inc., New York, p. 18.

———(1964): *Principles of Preventive Psychiatry,* Basic Books, Inc., Publishers, New York, p. 56.

Chance, Norman A. (1968): "Implications of Environmental Stress—Strategies of Developmental Change in the North," *Archives of Environmental Health,* October, pp. 571–577.

Chodoff, Paul (1970): "The German Concentration Camp as a Psychological Stress," *Archives of General Psychiatry,* January, pp. 78–87.

Dabrowski, K. (1940): *Positive Disintegration,* Little, Brown and Company, Boston.

Deloughery, Grace, et al. (1971): *Consultation and Community Organization in Community Mental Health Nursing,* The Williams and Wilkins Company, Baltimore.

Dohrenwend, B. P. (1967): "Social Status, Stress and Psychiatric Symptoms," *American Journal of Public Health,* April, pp. 625–632.

Donner, Gail (1972): "Parenthood as a Crisis: A Role for the Psychiatric Nurse," *Perspectives of Psychiatric Care,* April–June, pp. 84–87.

Erikson, Erik H. (1968): *Identity, Youth and Crisis,* W. W. Norton & Company, Inc., New York, chap. 2.

Farber, Maurice L. (1968): *Theory of Suicide,* Funk and Wagnalls, New York.

Fitzgerald, Roy G. (1970): "Reactions to Blindness, An Exploratory Study of Adults with Recent Loss of Sight," *Archives of General Psychiatry,* April, pp. 370–379.

Gilula, Marshall F., and David N. Daniels (1969): "Violence and Man's Struggle to Adapt," *Science,* April 25, pp. 396–405.

———, ———, and F. M. Ochberg (eds.) (1970): *Violence and the Struggle for Existence,* Little, Brown and Company, Boston.

Grenspoon, Lester (1964): "Fall-out Shelters and the Unacceptability of Disquieting Facts," in George H. Grosser et al. (eds.), *The Threat of Impending Disaster*, The M.I.T. Press, Cambridge, Mass., pp. 117–130.

Hamburg, David, and John E. Adams (1967): "A Perspective on Coping Behavior," *Archives of General Psychiatry*, September.

Harrison, Mary (1965): "Lindemann's Crisis Theory and Dabrowski's Positive Disintegration Theory—A Comparative Analysis," *Perspectives in Psychiatric Care*, pp. 8–13.

Hill, Reuben (1965): "Generic Features of Families under Stress," in Howard Parad (ed.), *Crisis Intervention: Selected Readings*, Family Service Association of America, New York.

Hoagland, Hudson (1969): "Technology, Adaptation and Evolution," *Biological Psychiatry*, January, pp. 73–80.

Hocking, F. (1970): "Psychiatric Aspects of Extreme Environmental Stress," *Diseases of the Nervous System*, August, pp. 542–545.

Jacobson, Gerald F., et al. (1965): "The Scope and Practice of an Early Access Brief Treatment, Psychiatric Center," *American Journal of Psychiatry*, June.

Kasl, S. V., and S. Cobb (1970): "Blood Pressure Changes in Men Undergoing Job Loss: A Preliminary Report," *Psychosomatic Medicine*, January–February, pp. 19–38.

King, Joan (1971): "The Initial Interview: Basis for Assessment in Crisis Intervention," *Perspectives in Psychiatric Care*, November–December, pp. 1176–1182.

Kübler-Ross, Elisabeth (1969): *On Death and Dying*, The Macmillan Company, New York.

Lang, Kurt, and Gladys Lang (1964): "Collective Responses to the Threat of Disaster," in George H. Grosser et al. (eds.), *The Threat of Impending Disaster*, The M.I.T. Press, Cambridge, Mass., pp. 58–75.

Langsley, Donald, and David Kaplan (1968): *The Treatment of Families in Crisis*, Grune & Stratton, Inc., New York.

Lazarus, Richard (1969): *Patterns of Adjustment and Human Effectiveness*, McGraw-Hill Book Company, New York.

Leff, M. J., et al. (1970): "Environmental Factors Preceding the Onset of Severe Depression," *Psychiatry*, August, pp. 293–311.

Levenstein, Aaron (1968): "Work Incentives in the Age of Automation," *American Journal of Orthopsychiatry*, October, pp. 893–899.

Lifton, Robert Jay (1964): "Psychological Effects of the Atomic Bomb in Hiroshima: The Theme of Death," in George H. Grosser et al. (eds.), *The Threat of Impending Disaster*, The M.I.T. Press, Cambridge, Mass., pp. 152–193.

Lindemann, Erich (1944): "Symptomatology and Management of Acute Grief," *American Journal of Psychiatry*, September.

McLuhan, Marshall, and Fiore Quentin (1967): *The Medium Is the Message*, Bantam Books, Inc., New York.

Milgram, Stanley (1970): "The Experience of Living in Cities," *Science*, Mar. 13, pp. 1461–1468.

Miller, James G. (1964): "A Theoretical Review of Individual and Group Psychological Reactions to Stress," in George H. Grosser et al. (eds.), *The Threat of Impending Disaster*, The M.I.T. Press, Cambridge, Mass., pp. 11–33.

Paykel, Eugene, et al. (1969): "Life Events and Depression," *Archives of General Psychiatry*, December, pp. 753–760.

Pearlman, Chester A. (1970): "Separation Reactions of Married Women," *American Journal of Psychiatry*, January, pp. 946–950.

Pearlman, Laurence V., et al. (1970): "Precipitation of Congestive Heart Failure: Social and Emotional Factors," *Annals of Internal Medicine*, July, pp. 1–7.

Polak, P. (1971): "Social Systems Intervention," *Archives of General Psychiatry,* August, pp. 110–117.

Prock, Valencia N. (1969): "Effects of Institutionalization," *American Journal of Public Health,* October, pp. 1837–1844.

Ramirez, M. (1969): "Identification with Mexican-American Values and Psychological Adjustment in Mexican-American Adolescents," *International Journal of Social Psychiatry,* Spring, pp. 151–156.

Rockey, Linda (1971): "Dark Days for the White Collar," *Today's Health,* August, pp. 16–19.

Schoenberg, F., et al. (eds.) (1970): *Loss and Grief: Psychological Management in Medical Practice,* Columbia University Press, New York, p. 4.

Shellow, Robert, et al. (1967): "Suburban Runaways of the 1960's," *Monograph of the Society for Research in Child Development,* pp. 1–51.

Silverman, P. R. (1969): "The Widow-to-Widow Program—An Experiment in Preventive Intervention," *Mental Hygiene,* July, pp. 333–337.

Slater, Philip (1971): *The Pursuit of Loneliness: American Culture at the Breaking Point,* Beacon Press, Boston, Mass.

Smith, William G. (1971): "Critical Life Events and Prevention Strategies in Mental Health," *Archives of General Psychiatry,* August, pp. 103–109.

Sugar, Max (1970): "Children of Divorce," *Pediatrics,* October, pp. 588–595.

Toffler, Alvin (1970): *Future Shock,* Random House, Inc., New York.

Williams, Harry B. (1964): "Human Factors in Warning and Response Systems," in George H. Grosser et al. (eds.), *The Threat of Impending Disaster,* The M.I.T. Press, Cambridge, Mass., pp. 79–104.

Wyler, A. R., et al. (1971): "Magnitude of Life Events and Seriousness of Illness," *Psychosomatic Medicine,* March–April, pp. 115–122.

PART FOUR

Environmental Influences on Mental Health and Mental Illness

17

ENVIRONMENTAL FACTORS

Anne J. Davis

Only by abstraction can a person be viewed apart from the environmental factors which surround him. Knowledge of any person and an understanding of his psychology must rest upon knowledge of the larger social and cultural environment in which he develops and then lives his life as an adult. Since it is within this environment that he develops and gains and maintains a sense of himself, it is only against this background that he can be fully understood.

DIFFICULTIES IN DEFINING MENTAL ILLNESS

All attempts to define mental illness in precise terms do so by designating it as a deviation from a standard referred to as "the normal." However, those making these definitions then must grapple with the difficult task of making clear what the concept "normality" means. Evolving such a definition can range from taking into account a limited number of variables, such as individual behavior, without inclusion of the social context within which that behavior occurs, to taking into account multiple variables which include such factors as economic, cultural, political, and social factors which are not specifically behavior variables per se but which influence behavior in various ways. Such definitions, simple or complex, are no small matter, since they not only have vast philosophical, cultural, social, and personal ramifications but also have pragmatic implications as well. The parameters placed on any definition of mental illness will serve operationally to include certain types of individual and social problems for consideration while simultaneously excluding others from consideration by mental health professionals and mental health funding agencies at the federal, state, and local levels.

The basis for viewing some behaviors or situations as adaptive or maladaptive may in the long run depend on who makes the judgment and from what perspective he views the behavior being judged. Mental health professionals hold a variety of views regarding mental illness. For example, some mental health professionals view mental illness primarily as a disease in which constitutional, genetic, and biological factors play the predominant role in explaining the causes of mental illness. They base their perspective on the recognition of not only maladaptive behavior as an overall category, but also more specific symptoms, such as delusions and hallucinations. From this perspective, the psychological criteria function in similar fashion to the pathological criteria utilized in diagnosing physical illness, since they provide the medical category by which the etiology and prognosis can be discussed and treatment methods can be determined.

Other mental health professionals, in contrast, view mental illness as a disturbance in personality functioning where deeply rooted, early-established patterns of feelings and behaviors, resulting from the person's social development as a child, persist into adult life, where they are deemed as inappropriate, since they lessen effective social functioning. Adhering to this point of view, these health professionals proceed on the theory that all behavior can be placed on a continuum with the optimal state of mental health on one end, mental illness on the other end, and the daily ups and downs in living fluctuating between these two extremes. Using the developmental approach, the therapist is initially confronted by the task of ascertaining what aspects of the individual patient's past experiences have led him to develop his present personality patterns which are said to underlie his psychological difficulty. The core of this view can be found in the theory that the source of disturbance lies within the individual himself and his personality development, and that, furthermore, alleviation of the problem relies on changing some aspect of his personality.

GROWING IMPORTANCE OF ENVIRONMENTAL FACTORS IN MENTAL ILLNESS

In the past, there has been a tendency to overlook environmental factors in mental illness in favor of developmental or disease-oriented factors. However, modification of these views has occurred as more mental health professionals have become more or less cognizant of environmental factors and now tend to view mental disorders as the end product of a complex interaction among constitutional factors, personality development, and environmental factors.

Although most mental health professionals now recognize that environmental influences have notable impact on the development and course of some mental illness, they differ greatly in their views of the way these influences interact with biological and psychological factors of the human personality. Some take the position that a physiological malfunction is a basic condition for mental illness and that adverse environmental influences only act to precipitate the episode of illness. At the other extreme, some view psychiatric problems as resulting from adverse environmental forces compounded by stresses which accumulate over a period of time.

Regardless of the definitions and established theories that individual mental health professionals hold regarding the etiology, diagnosis, and treatment of mental illness, the fact remains that much can be gained from bringing social science perspectives to bear on the problem of mental illness. The importance of these perspectives rests on the very basic fact that man, sick or well, can be comprehended fully only by studying his intricate relationship to himself and to other men within a social and cultural context (Plog and Edgerton, 1969).

NEW DIMENSIONS

Examining these factors can provide other ways of thinking about mental health and illness. Since our present state of knowledge of the etiology of mental illness still remains rudimentary, an examination of these environmental factors can serve not only to provide another perspective of mental health and illness, but also to require a closer look at such questions as: What role do environmental factors play in maintaining mental health or facilitating mental illness? What is the nature of the interaction between man and his environment? Can environmental factors be utilized in therapy of the mentally ill?

This approach, focusing on influences from arenas external to the individual which impinge on him in very profound ways, brings additional dimensions to other perspectives of mental health and illness. Lack of sufficient evidence, for the most part, prevents establishing a cause-and-effect relationship between these environmental factors and mental illness. However, the point of view taken here emphasizes the need for a deeper awareness and understanding of the complicated network of forces surrounding each individual. This approach then can serve to remind us that man lives his daily life in this network of external forces which influence such fundamental matters as his world view, his life style, his potential impact on societal institutions, and his accessibility to consumer goods, including health care. In no way should the discussion which follows be taken as one which implies that these environmental factors stand alone in their impact on the cause and course of mental illness or that positive change in any one or more of these factors would eliminate mental illness.

Each chapter which follows in this section takes one environmental factor and examines it, based on the evidence available, in order to assist the reader in developing an understanding of these factors and their importance in the lives of people.

REFERENCE

Plog, Stanley C., and Robert B. Edgerton (eds.) (1969): *Changing Perspectives in Mental Illness,* Holt, Rinehart and Winston, Inc., New York.

18

ECONOMIC FACTORS

Anne J. Davis

The Concept of Socioeconomic Status

Confusion surrounds the concept of socioeconomic status for two major reasons. First, as an idea which hierarchically arranges people in differentiated statuses, this concept violates the American dream of the classless society which provides all with equal opportunity to realize their potentialities. Second, and more important for research purposes, the lack of consensus among social scientists concerning this concept has resulted in controversies related to the theory and measurement of social class as a construct. Numerous examples of this confusion can be found in the literature on the topic (Svalastoga, 1964; Jackson, 1968). Some studies divide the population into three classes —upper, middle, and lower—while others use a six- or nine-class index to subdivide the three classes above into smaller units. Other researchers use such terms as *white-collar* (Mills, 1956) and *blue-collar* (Shostak, 1969) classes to describe social class position. Some studies have used a single variable, e.g., occupation, as the criterion for determining social class, while others have utilized multiple criteria, such as occupation, education, income, and neighborhood of resi dence.

Although no universal agreement exists among social scientists as to the conditions necessary to a definition of social class, most would agree that the concept of socioeconomic status refers to a mul-tifactored phenomenon, and that the one variable central to its definition is the economic conditions of those being studied. Major variables most often used to define social class standing fall into two categories: (1) economic security and insecurity, based upon the amount and stability of income, and (2) family stability, based upon family behavior and structure (Miller, 1964).

Lower Socioeconomic Status and Health

Statistics point to the interrelationship of being poor and a person's state of health; however, until recently the association of these two factors received little attention. In part, one can account for this neglect by the fact that historically we accepted the assumption that poverty and disease were inevitably linked and, furthermore, that being poor itself was thought of as an inevitable state for some people. Another, and more recent, factor has to do with what Michael Harrington (1962) refers to as the *invisible poor.* He maintains that in a highly urbanized society, the rural poor and those who live in slums of large cities remain invisible to the more affluent, few of whom live on farms and most of whom live, work, and play away from those areas of the city where being poor becomes a way of life.

The term *lower socioeconomic status* ranges over a number of categories, including that of poverty (Davis, 1971). No objective definition of *poverty* exists. Rather, society establishes the standards, which vary from time to time for a given place, and from place to place at the same time. The size of the group labeled "poor" then varies, depending on these standards and the criteria used to establish them. Because what constitutes poverty is historically relative, knowledge of the past can lead to the attitude that all people today in a given society, such as the United States, are much better off than those of previous generations. This attitude, however, misses the point. New standards of what human life should be arise as societies change, and those who suffer levels of life well below what is possible, even though they live better than people in the past, fall into the category labeled "poor." Poverty operationally for the United States, therefore, must be defined in terms of those who are denied the minimal levels of health care, housing, food, and education that the present stage of scientific knowledge specifies as necessary for life as most of our citizens live it today (Harrington, 1962).

In the larger sense, two types of poverty can be described. The first type, that of *acute poverty,* refers to reduced means due to given circumstances, such as the loss of a job or retirement without adequate funds. For example, according to a 1971 report from the U.S. Senate Special Committee on Aging, one out of every four Americans sixty-five years of age and over now is forced to live on a poverty-level income. Since the late 1960s both the number and the proportion of aged poor in our society have increased. A factor which compounds this situation is the rapidly rising health costs. The average health bill in 1969 for a person sixty-five years of age and over totaled $692, two and a half times that for those in the nineteen to sixty-four age bracket (*San Francisco Chronicle*, 1971, p. 9).

The other type of poverty implies a long-term life style in which acquisitive abilities have been chronically restricted. *Chronic poverty* breeds poverty, since low income means higher risks of illness; limited access to education, information, and training; and limited social, geographical, and occupational mobility. This type of poverty, in which lack of motivation, hope, and incentive becomes as powerful a barrier as lack of financial means, has the potential for becoming a life style transmitted from generation to generation.

Although these two types of poverty can be identified and differentiated, the practical results for the people involved differ very little. Both live in enforced dependency with little scope for action to affect events which are central to their needs and values (Haggstrom, 1964). These practical consequences take on dramatic dimensions when we realize that an estimated 25.5 million people in the United States live in poverty (U.S. Bureau of Census, 1970). Half of these reside in rural areas, while the other half can be located in metropolitan areas, most often in those sections of town populated by nonwhite groups. Poverty, already an urban phenomenon, will most likely become increasingly so and will become increasingly concentrated among the groups in which the incidence of poverty is already highest. Using flexible standards of measurement to account for regional differences, the incidence of poverty is heaviest among nonwhites, families with a very young head of household, the aged, broken families, very large families, families without breadwinners, the unemployed, families headed by farmers or unskilled workers, and unrelated persons living alone regardless of age, sex, or color.

To measure with accuracy the level of a population's health presents a complex problem, since health is a multidimensional phenomenon for which no standard definition appears to be completely satisfactory. To measure the level of physical health, such data as mortality rates, morbidity, impairments, and disability, which have been collected on the national level and correlated with family income, often serve as measurements of physical health. One systematic study (Lerner, 1969) surveyed the existing empirical data which compare the physical health of the poor in the United States with that of the rest of the population and concluded that the poverty population is today considerably less healthy than the population at large in this country. Specifically, the survey found that the poverty population still experiences higher rates of overall mortality, infant mortality, and severe illness. Infant mortality rates for the poor rise to twice that of the national average; life expectancies fall years shorter; infectious diseases, such as tuberculosis, all but eliminated for the majority of the population, still are found at epidemic levels in slum and rural poverty areas. Recent evidence overwhelmingly supports the fact that just as the poor are deprived politically, educationally, and economically, so are they also deprived medically.

Increasingly health professionals recognize that the conditions of life, including physical health, interact with the individual's mental well-being. We now turn from these physical health factors to a discussion of socioeconomic status and mental health.

Socioeconomic Status and Mental Health Research

The study of socioeconomic class-related behavior has received extensive attention, particularly in mental health research. Major research in this area includes the Yale Study (Hollingshead and Redlich, 1958), which examined the relationship of social class to the incidence and prevalence of mental disorders, types of mental disorders, attitudes toward mental illness and treatment, and types of treatment received; the Cornell Study (Srole et al., 1962), which examined the relationship of social class and the incidence and prevalence of mental disorders, history of mental disorders, attitudes regarding mental health professionals, and the outcome of psychiatric treatment in midtown Manhattan; the Freeman-Simmons Study (1963), which focused on the relation of posthospital adjustment to social class position; and finally, the Myers and Roberts Study (1959) of family and class dynamics in mental illness. These major studies, responsible for much of the increased awareness regarding the relationship between socioeconomic variables and mental illness, in concert with numerous other studies (Dohrenwend, 1966; Dunham, 1965; Goldberg and Morrison, 1963; Jaco, 1960; Langner, 1961; Lee, 1963; Mintz and Schwartz, 1964; Pasamanick, 1962; Thomas and Locke, 1963), provide extensive documentation on this topic. A recent follow-up research project of the Yale Study mentioned above focused on social class as a determinant of the patients' experience in the 10 years following the original study (Myers and Bean, 1968). Specifically, the researchers examined three hypotheses to determine the relationships between social class and treatment outcome: (1) Social class is related to treatment status in 1960 at follow-up; (2) social class is related to the patient's 1950 to 1960 treatment and readmission experience; (3) social class is related to the former patient's adjustment in the community.

The systematic tests made on the three hypotheses support the general proposition that social class relates both to the outcome of psychiatric treatment and to the former patient's adjustment in the community no matter how they are defined or measured. The details of the findings reveal the following. For both hospital and clinic patients, the higher the socioeconomic class, the less likely the patients were to be hospitalized 10 years later. In addition, the reverse relationship was found between class and treatment in that the higher the class, the greater the number in outpatient treatment. Chances of hospital discharge proved to be greater for higher-status individuals both for first discharge and for each subsequent discharge following readmission. With regard to type of treatment received, the higher the class, the more likely the patient was to receive therapies such as psychotherapy or somatotherapy associated with higher discharge rates. Upper- and middle-class patients remained in outpatient care for longer time periods than lower-class patients, more frequently received individual psychotherapy, and at the time of the follow-up study were more likely to be receiving outpatient treatment. Examining the patient's adjustment in the community, the researchers found that regardless of treatment agency or level of psychological performance, the lower-class individual who had been treated for mental illness remained isolated from formal and informal groups in the community. In summary, this study concluded that mental illness is apparently catastrophic for the lower-class person and his family in that economic and social problems characteristic of this group become magnified for the former mental patient. If hospitalized, his chances of returning to the community are less than those of patients at higher social levels. If he does return to the community or receives treatment in outpatient facilities, the impact of his illness is maximal in that it results in serious financial and employment problems and a high degree of social isolation. In general the most widespread adjustment problems are economic in nature.

These studies and similar ones concerned with social class distribution of mental disorders can best be characterized as extraordinarily consistent in their findings. With one exception (Clausen and Kohn, 1959), every research study conducted in the last 45 years has concluded that the highest concentration of mental disorders occurs in the lowest social class. Support for this finding emerges from studies conducted in eight different countries, with a variety of social class indices, including individual and ecological categories, utilizing hospital admissions as well as total community populations as the sample, concerned with incidence as well as prevalence, and focusing on specific diagnostic categories in addition to all major mental disorders collectively. These findings hold true across all ethnic groups studied and for both sexes, although the mental disorder rates for females are higher across all social classes than those for men.

Although this impressive amount of research with the consistent finding that the highest concentration of mental disorders occurs in the lowest class has been conducted, these studies have not yielded much knowledge as to the determinants of mental disorders. Each study has replicated a previous one, but no study has utilized the findings to generate hypotheses for testing which could provide a regular progression of ideas and possibly lead to major advances in knowledge as to the determinants of mental disorders. No unified theory of mental disorder causation has evolved from this research. However, a number of possible but untested hypotheses have been advanced to explain the findings.

These untested hypotheses include such concepts as the following to explain the consistent correlation between lower social class and mental illness. Social isolation, which functions to lock people out of the mainstream of society and to lessen their access to information, services, and goods, coupled with social disorganization reflected in unemployment or lack of stable employment, problems in family planning, and broken homes, has been advanced as one hypothesis. Another hypothesis put forward concerns what has been called a "value conflict." The values of a culture include the ideals, the aims and ends, the aesthetic and ethical standards, and the criteria of knowledge and wisdom embodied within it, taught to and modified by each generation (Valentine, 1968). The concept of value conflict states that lower-class individuals hold values which conflict with the values of the dominant culture. For example, there is some evidence that those in the lower class do not value health care to the same extent as those in the middle and upper classes. This, of course, may be viewed as a conflict in values between classes but also can be viewed as an understandable position for those in the lower class whose time, energy, and money are taken up with the pressures of meeting immediate, basic needs such as food and clothing.

Additional hypotheses include such concepts as that of blocked aspirations and deprecatory self-conceptions which illustrate the possibility of a circular system in which low self-esteem and the limited possibilities to achieve due to economic, social, political, and cultural factors interact with one another to maintain the individual at the same socioeconomic level. Yet another hypothesis, familial influences, points to the research evidence that the childrearing and family life patterns more characteristic of the lower socioeconomic class tend to be highly deficient in reference to the development of the child's intellectual and attitudinal preparation for school.

Economic Factors and Mental Health Treatment

Based on the reasonably reliable research evidence, certain generalizations can be drawn with regard to mental health treatment and individuals of lower socioeconomic levels. Not only are people from this group less frequently accepted for mental health treatment, but also they tend to stay in treatment for a shorter period of time and this treatment is more likely to consist of somatic as opposed to psychotherapeutic approaches. More likely to be committed to a mental hospital, they also usually stay longer, but this does not necessarily imply that they automatically receive treatment for the entire duration of their hospitalization. Since private psychiatric treatment is expensive, the argument could be made that economic factors constitute the major deterrent to persons of lower socioeconomic levels receiving mental health care other than in a government-supported mental hospital. However, much of the research on this topic has been conducted in agencies or clinics with little or no fee involved, so the cost of treatment per se does not seem to be a critical factor. However, the tenuousness of employment, the lack of child care facilities, the possibly inadequate public transportation system, etc., may be very real factors in the daily lives of the individuals of a lower socioeconomic level and may combine to inhibit their entering or continuing treatment.

Seven factors have been suggested by Miller and Riessman (1968) as contributing to the comparatively low utilization rates of mental health services by the lower socioeconomic class. These suggested factors point to the interrelatedness of economic factors with other social and psychological factors and can be listed as (Miller and Riessman, 1968):

1. Cost of services
2. Availability of services
3. Failure of the general practitioner to refer cases for psychiatric treatment
4. Failure to define distress in psychologically relevant terms
5. Attitudes toward mental illness
6. Fear of institutionalization
7. The middle-class character of the mental health movement and the associated inappropriate nature of the services offered to low-income people

Furthermore, data indicate that people who have more psychiatric facilities available to them are more likely to have received help, given the definition of the problem as a mental health one, than have people with fewer available resources. Less than half (46 percent) of the group with the least facilities available to them have gone for assistance, as compared with 60 percent or more of the groups with some mental health facilities available to them (Gurin, Veroff, and Feld, 1960). The seven factors listed above give direction for strategies in the modification of treatment approaches.

Socioeconomic Status and Mental Illness in Children

The socioeconomic status of a family has pyschosocial consequences in the development of a child's ability to function successfully in the urban, technological, and verbal society which characterizes the United States. The basic assumptions in research on sociological correlates of child behavior are that the position his parents occupy in the socioeconomic hierarchy influences the training the child receives, since that position provides a distinctive context and life experience for him, and that these experiences have an enduring if not irreversible effect in his later life. These assumptions have produced a massive but often contradictory literature on the relationships of social class to childrearing and child behavior. The greater part of the class-linked literature has focused on specific infant and child care practices; however, some earlier evidence indicates that this aspect of child rearing is least stable (Klatskin, 1952) and the least relevant to personality outcome (Orlansky, 1949; Sewell, 1952). Previous studies examining these variables have, by and large, omitted any reference to the context in which these practices and routines occur and have therefore been inconsistent and contradictory in their findings.

A clearer picture of sociological correlates involved in child behavior unfolds when studies shift their focus from these specifics to an assessment of such class-linked dimensions as patterns of affection and authority, expectations for the child, quality of family relationships, and conceptions of parenthood held by the adults. By examining such variables, these studies translate the behavioral requirements and dominant value orientation of a specific social class into what impinges on the child (Clausen and Williams, 1963).

The disadvantaged child begins to experience the impact of lower socioeconomic status even before birth. He often experiences inadequate prenatal care and then continues to be exposed to material deprivation, including the lack of ongoing and preventive health care. In addition, and compounding this situation, he may experience emotional deprivations which generate a feeling of powerlessness.

Later, the poor child is more likely to leave school early because of the financial straits of the family or the belief that school will not provide him with the tools he needs in adult life. So even though lower socioeconomic-class parents often have high aspirations for their children, until recently they also believed that their children had little chance of success (Purcell, 1964; Miller, 1964). With these data as background material, social scientists have raised questions as to whether the individual's place on the socioeconomic scale affects his state of mental health.

In an attempt to explore the possibility that a relationship between social class and mental illness among children does exist, McDermott and his colleagues (1968) examined available data from their clinical experiences at a children's psychiatric hospital. A pilot study of these data (Harrison et al., 1964) found a distinct correlation between the father's occupation and the particular kind of psychiatric diagnosis and dispositional recommendations which they made. They found the most striking contrasts between children of professional persons and those of unskilled laborers. However, this pilot study revealed one unanticipated finding regarding children of the blue-collar group. In this early part of the research, the authors had divided the blue-collar group into two subgroups, namely, children of skilled workers and those of unskilled workers. They had expected similarities in psychiatric diagnosis, since these two groups stand in juxtaposition to one another on the socioeconomic scale and share overlapping cultural factors. However, such was not the finding, and this led them to investigate the basis for differential diagnosis within the blue-collar group. They found that personality disorders, including borderline psychoses, were diagnosed significantly more often in the children from the unskilled workers' group. The most characteristic clinical description of these children included such terms as *overt hostility, impulsivity, paranoid reaction, affective disturbance,* and *withdrawal.* By contrast, the psychiatrists characterized children of skilled workers as *anxious, obsessive-compulsive,* and *with somatic complaints.* Also, children from the unskilled workers' group were far more often thought to come from conflict-ridden, unstable homes when contrasted with the skilled workers' group.

When these researchers compared the histories of the two groups, several important findings emerged. Families of both groups rated their children alike in adjustment to the home situation; however, they indicated marked differences in adjustment to school. The skilled group rated their children as doing well at school while the unskilled group said that their children were doing very poorly at school and in some cases received failing grades. Another finding indicated that the unskilled group delayed significantly longer in referral to the clinic from the time that the children's problems became obvious.

This study supports the earlier finding of Hollingshead and Redlich (1958) that blue-collar workers cannot be considered a homogeneous group, since they span at least two positions on the social scale and since particular difficulties in defining them arise from the fact that this overall classification has become blurred. The study also raises a number of questions with reference to the unskilled group.

The usual assumption that the lower the socioeconomic position, the greater the likelihood of family disruption by desertion, separation, or divorce was not supported by these data, since the majority of the children from both groups lived with both parents in an intact family unit. However, as noted above, the clinical staff rated the unskilled workers' homes as unstable and conflict-ridden twice as frequently as they did the skilled workers' home. The questions of the subjective nature of the evaluation and possible rater bias must be taken into account as a possible and potent variable which affects definitions of the situation and the recommendations for health care. The authors concluded that the professionals of that community did view these two groups of children differently both in the school and in the psychiatric setting. These professional evaluations may indeed reflect some degree of psychological differences that these children have acquired through life experiences and which become more pronounced as they enter into the larger social structure through the school. However, the possibility of the professionals' value and perspectives stemming from their own class-linked socialization skewing their view of the blue-collar group remains a fertile area for further research.

Socioeconomic Status and Mental Retardation

Current popular attitudes toward mental retardation still reflect an adherence to long-standing prejudices coupled with a degree of ignorance. The idea that an unsatisfactory environment may produce the most important cause of retardation has not, in most cases, replaced the persistent myths surrounding the subject. According to one source (Bradley, 1964) with data from 100 interviews, only one in ten persons indicated specialized information about retardation. One-fifth of this sample (twenty) confused retardation with other mental and physical disorders, and the most usual description of the retarded emphasized their mental ineffectiveness and irresponsible nature. More than half had neither read nor heard about mental retardation in the few months preceding the interview. Another study (Murray, 1964) revealed that such confusion and lack of information regarding mental retardation can also be found among college students.

The long-term and widespread prejudice and ignorance surrounding mental retardation often obscure the fact that poverty stands as one of its most significant predisposing factors. Over 10 years ago, the President's Panel on Mental Retardation (1962) said that the majority of the retarded children come from the more disadvantaged socioeconomic classes in our society, and they pointed to the fact that this heavy prevalence in these classes suggests a major causative role, not fully delineated, for adverse economic, social, and cultural factors. The Connecticut Mental Retardation Project (1966) group emphasized the important factor repeatedly found in many studies that the high percentage of people in this group are retarded in function rather than lacking in endowment. Mental retardation must be viewed, then, not only as a health problem in the narrow sense of that phrase, but also as a social pathology which thrives in the lower socioeconomic classes.

Many of those in positions to assist most with this problem have failed in the past to do so for several reasons. One of the most fundamental reasons lies in their tendency to equate poverty with genetic inferiority. This assumed correlation in the literature dates back to 1914 with the publication of *The Kallikak Family: i.e., p. 500 A Study in the Heredity of Feeblemindedness* (Goddard, 1914), which has had a pernicious and widespread influence both in later research and in clinical practice. Recently another approach to the question of genetics and mental retardation has appeared which says that an hereditary determinant of mental capacity cannot be assumed to exist until scientifically proved (Sarason, Gladwin, and Masland, 1958). They do not deny heredity as a possible factor, particularly in mental deficiency, where organic dysfunction enters the picture. However, they emphasize the need for scientific proof based on present and future knowledge of human genetics.

Much previous research in mental retardation has relied on administering routine intelligent tests to a sample of identified racial and other groups, but the potential cultural and social bias of these tests constructed by educated, middle-class, and often white, professionals has raised questions as to the reliability of these studies. The findings of most such studies reveal that blacks and people with lower socioeconomic status constitute an overrepresented percentage of the mentally retarded (Wakefield, 1964; Erdman and Olson, 1966; Knott, 1967).

Unless one adheres to the theory—which strikes many as not only scientifically without support but also potentially racist—that these groups are inherently inferior, then other avenues must be explored.

After reviewing the literature, Perry (1965) concluded that the vast majority of retardates present problems related to the socioeconomic background of the lower-class population. Other studies also raise the possibility that general environmental deprivation needs to be examined as a central factor. For example, studies (Shortwell, 1945; Gibson and Butler, 1954; Dunn, 1963; Edgerton, 1963) indicate that great numbers of individuals, most often from the lower socioeconomic class or from an ethnic or racial minority group, are confined in institutions for the mentally retarded without sufficient justification.

Summary of Research Findings

Research findings demonstrate that an individual's socioeconomic status and his state of health are interrelated. In addition, these findings show that the highest concentration of mental disorders, including mental retardation, occurs in the lowest class, or those who live below the poverty line. However, the evidence indicates that this group is less likely to receive health care in adequate amount or of adequate quality.

Implications for Health Care

Since poverty and ill health reinforce each other, several implications for health care emerge which fall into two categories: (1) structural and (2) clinical. *Structural problems* refer to the fact that many, if not most, of the major societal institutions are not geared to deal effectively with lower socioeconomic groups. In the opinion of English (1969), the health care available to the poor is inaccessible, inadequate, impersonal, and fragmented. Some critics (Bullough and Bullough, 1972) of this situation say that the United States needs to replace the nonsystem for financing health care with a comprehensive, federally run system of national health insurance which would provide all citizens with better health care. Analyzing this situation, another writer (Silver, 1971) thinks that national health insurance will fall short of solving the health care problem.

The report by the Health Task Force of the Urban Coalition (Rusk, 1969) indicated that despite the fact that this country spends a larger portion of its gross national product on health than any other country does, our medical care is not the best in the world for the majority of our people. The belief held by some people, including health professionals, that the extremes of the socioeconomic continuum receive better medical care does not gain support from the report's findings. It cites the following:

Over 45 percent of the nation's population suffer from one or more chronic diseases.

Those with an annual income of $4,345 for a family of four have from four to eight times the incidence of major chronic conditions.

We have a shorter life expectancy and a greater infant mortality rate than the people of fifteen other countries.

The ratio of doctors to residents in poverty areas is from one-eighth to one-half that of the city as a whole.

The very structure of the present health care system impedes the poor from receiving the care they need. Strauss (1967) contends that those from the lower socioeconomic group will never have anything approaching adequate health care until the present delivery system providing that care undergoes radical reforms. He argues that the reason this system has not reached the poor is simply that it was never designed to do so, since it does not take into account the way the poor think and respond to their life style—which differs from that of other socioeconomic classes. What may appear as unimportant or insignificant to others can present difficulties of monumental proportions for the poor. Such things as getting to a health facility and then attempting to deal with the complex labyrinth of that facility do not always enter into the thinking of health professionals, who may take the health bureaucracy for granted.

In a beginning attempt to change these structural arrangements which impede the lower socioeconomic from receiving adequate care, a number of experiments have been devised. For example, in New York, the Henry Street Settlement Mental Hygiene Clinic (Levine, 1964) experimented with ways to bring mental health services to low-income, multiproblem families. The major feature of this experiment lay in shifting treatment from the clinic to the home and using demonstration and intervention techniques tailored to what the families could both understand and accept. Another example (Fantal, 1964) involved a small unit of social workers who left the downtown centralized school child guidance office to live in a lower-class neighborhood. Their concern soon shifted from the traditional one-to-one relationship therapy to a broad awareness of the daily life situations of those in the neighborhood. They identified the major areas of weakness and strength of the neighborhood by comparing it with other neighborhoods; determined the social institutions, the composition of ethnic groups, and the ways in which people communicated and related with each other; and evolved a new conception of their services which seemed more realistically related to the needs of the total community. They increasingly spent more time in collaboration and consultation with some of the caretaking agents who had profound influence on the lives of the people in this neighborhood. They developed an awareness of the social distance between clients and caretakers, their bias about each other, and the communication breakdowns which defied efforts and good intentions of both parties toward positive interaction.

Other experiments can be found in the ever-increasing so-called unorthodox facilities springing up around the country. One such facility, Salud Woodville, in rural California, is a clinic for the Mexican-American farm workers and their families in that area. Many recent reports in the nursing literature describe the work nurses are doing to learn about and work with lower socioeconomic-level patients (Barker, 1972; Bellaire, 1971; Corbey, 1971; Cooper, 1971; Freeman, 1971; Henry, 1971; Joyce, 1971; Levinger and Billings, 1971; Maxwell, 1971; Pasquali, 1972; Underwood, 1971; Wilson and Fabric, 1971; Schutt, 1972).

Some who would like to see the institutions of society become more responsive to the disadvantaged put much stock in voluntary associations. As important as they can be toward influencing change, a review of the historical correlates of membership in these associations shows that the more affluent and better educated people in our society are, the more often they affiliate with these organizations. Furthermore, class-based patterns can be identified for the types of associations which people join. The upper-class person most often joins service- and change-oriented organizations, in contrast to lower socioeconomic-level persons, who prefer more intimate and particularistic relational settings (Curtis and Zurcher, 1971).

In addition to the larger structural problems, specific *clinical problems,* which also impede the poor from obtaining health care, can be identified. Health professionals may be biased against working with the lower socioeconomic-level patient (Walsh, 1969). Like all people in the United States, health professionals have attitudes which are class-linked and which have deep roots in the fabric of the country's history. Historically, the middle and upper classes have tended to dwell on the undesirable character or moral traits of the poor (Newman, 1969); however, this attitude overlooks the fact that the system of institutions in which the poor are enmeshed tends to perpetuate their poverty. For example, in the major 1969 tax reform, the poor received some relief, but the middle and upper classes got even more. The oil magnate with political clout, who might condemn the man on welfare, was a much bigger recipient of state largess in the form of huge tax benefits than were any of the poor (Francis, 1970).

Beyond the need for health professionals to examine their attitudes toward the poor is their need to know the geography of poverty in their own community and to realize that these areas have a higher incidence of illness, substandard housing, inadequate education, and unemployment than the community at large (Lee, 1967). Once people from these areas of the city come for treatment, it is important that the health professional does not assume that the client is but a carbon copy of himself in values, knowledge, life style, etc. For example, the incorrect assumptions, often made, that the poor have regular meals or mealtimes, keep healthy, and plan for the future, lead to health advice and treatment prescriptions which cannot be followed, if, indeed, they are understood by the patient.

The lower socioeconomic-level individual's time concept has tended to focus more on the present than on the past or the future (Seward and Marmor, 1956), and if, as a patient, he becomes involved in therapy, it usually is for a short period (Hunt, 1960). All the studies on the lower socioeconomic-level patient convey the fact that the poor's response is different. Therefore, mental health personnel must be more in tune with the poor's expectations, needs, and life style. To this end, it is important to determine the patient's expectations and conception of therapy and the procedures involved. Hunt (1960) makes the point that present psychotherapeutic techniques have been drawn from research and treatment on middle- and upper-class patients, and he questions the validity of generalizing these principles to all classes, since they may be class-linked. He concludes that we must consider the possibility that psychotherapy as presently practiced may be effective only with the middle- and upper-class populations. Furthermore, if the therapist views his encounter with the lower-class patient or client from a traditional perspective, then he may unknowingly reject the patient when his expectations are not met. The results of one study (Overall and Aronson, 1963) indicated that these patients predominantly expected a medical-psychiatric interview with the therapist assuming an active but permissive role. In assuming this role, the therapist may find it necessary to deal with the patient's present and very concrete problems not only by listening to him talk about them but by actively assisting him to deal with them. For example, if the patient is about to be evicted from his residence, then his most pressing problem may be to find another place to live. In the long run, the effectiveness of any therapy for lower socioeconomic-level patients may be determined by the attitude of the therapist toward the patient's poverty and the therapist's willingness to become more active in helping him to solve not only his psychiatric problems but his mental health problems in the broadest sense of that phrase.

Health professionals tend to use a combination of standard middle-class English mixed with liberal portions of medical jargon when discussing health matters with patients. That this "second language" (Riessman, 1969) may not be easily understood by patients in general and even less so by the poor, who are in so many instances outside of the mainstream of information, radically affects what the patient and his family hear and what they understand. One of the best ways to deal with this communication problem is to explain in plain language and, more importantly, to listen to the patient and his family. The usual reason given for not explaining and listening is lack of time. Clear explanation and careful listening on the part of the mental health professional may take more time initially, but it may save time in the long run for both the professional and the patient, as well as prevent some health problems from becoming more serious than necessary.

In an attempt to effect structural changes, health professionals may participate in the ever-increasing so-called unorthodox facilities referred to earlier. Or they can join a growing number of other health professionals in such organizations as the Medical Committee for Human Rights, which publishes *Health Rights News* (Medical Committee for Human Rights). This publication presents the concerns of health consumers and workers and acts as a pressure group to bring about change. Within the traditional professional organizations, they can promote the formation of a citizen's advisory council. Such a council has recently been formed as an advisory group to the San Francisco Nurses' Association. And finally, one of the most potent means of change in a democracy is the vote. Like all citizens, health professionals need to keep abreast of the issues and to be informed as to the voting record on health issues of those in public office who represent us. Two sources of such information are: Americans for Democratic Action, which publishes not only voting records but also attendance records of those in the U.S. Congress, and Common Cause, spearheaded by John Gardner, former secretary, Department of Health, Education, and Welfare. Specific to California, *The Sacramento Report,* published by the Association for Better Health, provides members with information regarding bills before committees and elections in the state. Other states may have similar publications; if not, citizens have the opportunity and obligation to examine these records. For such information, the state's Republican Central Committee or the Democratic Central Committee may be contacted, since a representative's voting record is a matter of public record. Only when both the structural problems which impede the poor from seeking and receiving health care and the clinical problems which impede them from following through with a treatment program are recognized and eradicated will the poor be guaranteed adequate health care.

REFERENCES

Barker, Virginia (1972): "Baccalaureate Education in a Rural Setting," *Nursing Outlook,* May, pp. 335–337.

Bellaire, Judith (1971): "Teenagers Learn to Care About Themselves," *Nursing Outlook,* December, pp. 792–793.

Bradley, B. H. (1964): "Public Impressions of the Mentally Retarded," *Mental Retardation Abstracts,* January–March, p. 47.

Bullough, Bonnie, and Vern Bullough (1972): *Poverty, Ethnic Identity, and Health,* Appleton-Century-Crofts, Inc., New York.

Clausen, John A., and Melvin L. Kohn (1959): "Relation of Schizophrenia to the Social Structure of a Small City," in Benjamin Pasmanick (ed.), *Epidemiology of Mental Disorder,* American Association for the Advancement of Science, Washington, D.C., pp. 68–86.

———, and Judith R. Williams (1963): "Sociological Correlates of Child Behavior," in Harold W. Stevenson (ed.), *Child Psychology,* part 1, 62nd Yearbook of the National Society for the Study of Education, N.S.S.E., Chicago, pp. 68–100.

Connecticut Mental Retardation Project Report (1966): *Miles to Go,* Hartford.

Cooper, Isabelle (1971): "Health Care for Rockaway Children," *Nursing Outlook,* May, pp. 344–346.

Corbey, Janet H. (1971): "The Supervisor as Motivator," *Nursing Outlook,* December, pp. 801–803.

Curtis, Russell L., and Louis A. Zurcher, Jr. (1971): "Voluntary Associations and the Social Integration of the Poor," *Social Problems,* Winter, pp. 339–357.

Davis, Anne J. (1971): "The Poor Can Least Afford It: Poverty and Health in the United States," *International Nursing Review,* vol. 18, no. 4, pp. 360–366.

Dohrenwend, Bruce P. (1966): "Social Status and Psychological Disorder," *American Sociological Review,* February, pp. 14–34.

Dunham, H. Warren (1965): *Community and Schizophrenia,* Wayne State University Press, Detroit.

Dunn, Lloyd M. (1963): "Educable Mentally Retarded Children," in Lloyd M. Dunn (ed.), *Exceptional Children in the Schools,* Holt, Rinehart and Winston, Inc., New York, pp. 53–128.

Edgerton, Robert B. (1963): "A Patient Elite: Ethnography in a Hospital for the Mentally Retarded," *American Journal of Mental Deficiency,* November, pp. 372–385.

English, Joseph T. (1969): "The Dimensions of Poverty," *American Journal of Nursing,* November, pp. 2424–2428.

Erdman, Robert L., and James L. Olson (1966): "Relationships between Emotional Programs for the Mentally Retarded and the Culturally Deprived," *Mental Retardation Abstracts,* July–September, pp. 311–318.

Fantal, Berta (1964): "Preventive Intervention," in Frank Riessman, Jerome Cohen, and Arthur Pearl (eds.), *Mental Health of the Poor,* The Free Press, New York, pp. 362–370.

Francis, Davis R. (1970): "Deck Stacked Against the Poor?" *The Christian Science Monitor,* Nov. 30, p. 4.

Freeman, Howard, E., and Ozzie G. Simmons (1963): *The Mental Patient Comes Home,* John Wiley & Sons, Inc., New York.

Freeman, Ruth B. (1971): "Practice as Protest," *American Journal of Nursing,* May, pp. 918–921.

Gibson, Davis, and A. J. Butler (1954): "Culture as a Possible Contributor to Feeblemindedness," *American Journal of Mental Deficiency,* January, pp. 490–495.

Goddard, Henry H. (1914): *The Kallikak Family: A Study in the Heredity of Feeblemindedness,* The Macmillan Company, New York.

Goldberg, E. M., and S. L. Morrison (1963): "Schizophrenia and Social Class," *British Journal of Psychiatry,* November, pp. 785–802.

Gurin, Gerald, Joseph Veroff, and Sheila Feld (1960): *Americans View Their Mental Health,* Basic Books, Inc., Publishers, New York, pp. 384–385.

Haggstrom, Warren C. (1964): "The Power of the Poor," in Frank Riessman, Jerome Cohen, and Arthur Pearl (eds.), *Mental Health of the Poor,* The Free Press, New York, pp. 205–223.

Harrington, Michael (1962): *The Other America: Poverty in the United States,* The Macmillan Company, New York.

Harrison, Saul I., John F. McDermott, Jules Schrager, and Paul Wilson (1964): "Social Status and Choice of Treatment in Child Psychiatry," Paper presented at the annual meeting of the American Psychiatric Association, Los Angeles, Calif.

Henry, Sandra (1971): "Patient Advocacy and Community Involvement," *Nursing Outlook,* April, pp. 246–248.

Hollingshead, August B., and Fredrick C. Redlich (1958): *Social Class and Mental Illness,* John Wiley & Sons, Inc., New York.

Hunt, Raymond G. (1960): "Social Class and Mental Illness: Some Implications for Clinical Theory and Practice," *The American Journal of Psychiatry,* June, pp. 1065–1069.

Jackson, J. A. (ed.) (1968): *Social Stratification,* Cambridge University Press, Cambridge, England.

Jaco, E. Gartly (1960): *The Social Epidemiology of Mental Disorders,* Russell Sage Foundation, New York.

Joyce, Sister Carol Ann, and Barbara J. Lyso (1971): "People Who Need People," *Nursing Outlook,* July, pp. 470–472.

Klatskin, Ethelyn H. (1952): "Shifts in Child Care Practices in Three Social Classes under an Infant Care Program of Flexible Methodology," *American Journal of Orthopsychiatry,* January, pp. 52–61.

Knott, Maurice G. (1967): "Estimating the Number of the Retarded in New Jersey," in Monroe Berkowitz (ed.), *Estimating Rehabilitation Needs,* New Brunswick, N.J.

Langner, Thomas S. (1961): "Environmental Stress and Mental Health," in Paul H. Hoch and Joseph Zubin (eds.), *Comparative Epidemiology of Mental Disorders,* Grune & Stratton, Inc., New York, pp. 32–45.

Lee, Everett S. (1963): "Socio-Economic and Migration Differentials in Mental Disease," *Milbank Memorial Fund Quarterly,* July, pp. 249–268.

Lee, Philip R. (1967): "Creative Federalism and Health Programs for the Poor," *The Pharos,* January, pp. 2–6.

Lerner, Monroe (1969): "Social Differences in Physical Health," in John Kosa, Aaron Antonovsky, and Irving K. Zola (eds.), *Poverty and Health: A Sociological Analysis,* Harvard University Press, Cambridge, Mass., pp. 69–112.

Levine, Rachael A. (1964): "Treatment in the Home: An Experiment with Low Income Multi-Problem Families," in Frank Riessman, Jerome Cohen, and Arthur Pearl (eds.), *Mental Health of the Poor,* The Free Press, New York, pp. 329–335.

Levinger, Gloria, and Holly Billings (1971): "Nursing in a Low-Rent Housing Project," *American Journal of Nursing,* February, pp. 314–318.

Maxwell, Jane F. (1971): "Home Care for the Retarded Child," *Nursing Outlook,* February, pp. 112–114.

McDermott, John F., Saul I. Harrison, Jules Schrager, and Paul Wilson (1968): "Social Class and Mental Illness in Children," in W. Clayton Lane (ed.), *Permanence and Change in Social Class,* Schenkman Publishing Co., Cambridge, Mass., pp. 275–288.

Medical Committee for Human Rights: *Health Rights News,* the Committee, 710 S. Marshfield, Chicago, Ill.

Miller, S. M. (1964): "The American Lower Class: A Typological Approach," *Social Research,* Spring, pp. 1–22.

———(1964): "The Outlook of Working Class Youth," in Arthur B. Shostak and William Gomberg (eds.), *Blue-Collar World,* Prentice-Hall, Inc., Englewood Cliffs, N.J., pp. 131–132.

———, and Frank Riessman (1968): *Social Class and Social Policy,* Basic Books, Inc., Publishers, New York.

Mills, C. Wright (1956): *White Collar,* Oxford University Press, New York.

Mintz, Norbert L., and David T. Schwartz (1964): "Urban Ecology and Psychosis," *International Journal of Social Psychiatry,* Spring, pp. 101–118.

Murray, J. (1964): "Responses of College Men and Women to a Test of Knowledge of Mental Deficiency," *Mental Retardation Abstracts,* January–February, p. 46.

Myers, Jerome K., and Lee L. Bean (1968) *A Decade Later: A Follow-Up of Social Class and Mental Illness,* John Wiley & Sons, Inc., New York.

———, and Bertram H. Roberts (1959): *Family and Class Dynamics in Mental Illness,* John Wiley & Sons, Inc., New York.

Newman, Dorothy K. (1969): "Perspectives on Poverty," *Monthly Labor Review,* U. S. department of Labor, Bureau of Labor Statistics, February.

Orlansky, Harold (1949): "Infant Care and Personality," *Psychological Bulletin,* January, pp. 1–48.

Overall, Betty, and H. Aronson (1963): "Expectations of Psychotherapy in Patients of Lower Socioeconomic Class," *American Journal of Orthopsychiatry,* April, pp. 421–430.

Pasamanick, Benjamin (1962): "A Survey of Mental Disease in an Urban Population," *American Journal of Psychiatry,* October, pp. 299–305.

Pasquali, Elaine A. (1972): "Learning about a Poverty Budget," *American Journal of Nursing,* August, p. 1419.

Perry, Stuart E. (1965): "The Middle-Class and Mental Retardation in America," *Psychiatry,* May, pp. 107–118.

President's Panel on Mental Retardation (1962): *National Action to Combat Mental Retardation,* Government Printing Office, Washington, D.C., October.

Purcell, Theodore V. (1964): "The Hopes of Negro Workers for Their Children," in Arthur B. Shostak and William Gomberg (eds.), *Blue-Collar World,* Prentice-Hall, Inc., Englewood Cliffs, N.J., pp. 144–154.

Riessman, Frank (1969): *Strategies Against Poverty,* Random House, Inc., New York.

Rusk, Howard A. (1969): "Health in the Cities," *The New York Times,* Nov. 23, p. 60L.

San Francisco Chronicle, Jan. 18, 1971, p. 7.

Sarason, Seymour B., Thomas Gladwin, and Richard L. Masland (1958): *Mental Subnormality,* Basic Books, Inc., Publishers, New York.

Schutt, Barbara G. (1972): "Frontier's Family Nurse," *American Journal of Nursing,* May, pp. 903–909.

Seward, Georgene H., and Judd Marmor (1956): *Psychotherapy and Culture Conflict,* The Ronald Press Company, New York.

Sewell, William H. (1952): "Infant Training and the Personality of the Child," *American Journal of Sociology,* September, pp. 150–159.

Shortwell, Anna M. (1945): "Arthur Performance Ratings of Mexican and American High Grade Mental Defectives," *American Journal of Mental Deficiency,* April, pp. 445–559.

Shostak, Arthur B. (1969): *Blue-Collar Life,* Random House, Inc., New York.

Silver, George A. (1971): "National Health Insurance, National Health Policy and the National Health," *American Journal of Nursing,* September, pp. 1730–1735.

Srole, Leo, Thomas S. Langner, Standley T. Michael, Marvin K. Opler, and Thomas Rennie (1962): *Mental Health in the Metropolis: The Midtown Manhattan Study,* McGraw-Hill Book Company, New York.

Strauss, Anselm L. (1967): "Medical Ghettos," *Trans-action,* May, pp. 7–15, 62.

Svalastoga, Karre (1964): "Social Differentiation," in Robert E. L. Faris (ed.), *Handbook of Modern Sociology,* Rand McNally & Company, Chicago, pp. 530–575.

Thomas, Dorothy T., and Ben Z. Locke (1963): "Marital Status, Education and Occupational Differentials in Mental Disease," *Milbank Memorial Fund Quarterly,* April, pp. 145–160.

Underwood, Patricia R. (1971): "Communication through Role Playing," *American Journal of Nursing,* June, pp. 1184–1186.

United States Bureau of the Census (1970): "24 Million Americans—Poverty in the United States, 1969," *Current Population Reports,* Series P-60, no. 76, U.S. Government Printing Office, Washington, D.C.

Valentine, Charles, A. (1968): *Culture and Poverty,* University of Chicago Press, Chicago.

Wakefield, Robert A. (1964): "An Investigation of the Family Background of Educable Mentally Retarded Children in Special Classes," *Exceptional Children,* November, pp. 143–146.

Walsh, James L. (1969): "Nurses, Professional Striving, and the Poor," *Social Science and Medicine,* August, pp. 217–227.

Wilson, Patience, and Diane T. Fabric (1971): "Teaching Community Health Workers," *Nursing Outlook,* May, pp. 337–340.

19

SOCIAL FACTORS

Anne J. Davis

This chapter will discuss one social problem pertinent to mental health which, although not new, has recently attracted much public attention and has elicited strong and opposing points of view. Many other factors which play a role currently in determining the quality of life could have been considered, and their omission here does not imply their unimportance. Such social factors include changes in the family (Otto, 1970), in the church (Cox, 1965; Mudge, 1970), in education (Horowitz and Friedland, 1970; Roszak, 1968), and in the military (Bienen, 1971). In addition, complex social problems, such as crime, violence, pollution, invasion of privacy, racial conflicts, drug abuse, decay of the cities, and the population explosion, come to one's attention daily through the news media as well as other sources (Baily and Thayer, 1971; Bloomquist, 1971; Callahan, 1971; Duster, 1970; Ehrlich, 1968; Gil, 1970; Graham and Gurr, 1969; Greenberg, Milner, and Olson, 1971; Halleck, 1971; Kennedy et al., 1971; Marx, 1971; Meek and Straayer, 1971; National Advisory Commission, 1968; Pennock and Chapman, 1971; Rogers, 1971; Straus, 1971; Westin, 1967; Wheeler, 1969).

Rather than attempting to deal with this vast array of complex social problems, as important as they are, this chapter focuses on the role of women in the United States, examining their economic, legal, and educational position in society and indicating the way their social role can influence their well-being and their attempt at self-realization.

The contemporary women's movement in the United States has

historical roots which extend back to the earlier feminist movement of the nineteenth century. This earlier movement, remembered mainly as the one which finally resulted in the giving of the vote to women in the first quarter of the twentieth century, took as its task the reexamination of women's role and the relationship between men and women in the social, economic, cultural, and political institutions of society. This earlier feminist movement, as well as the present one, defined women as an oppressed group and traced the origins of women's role, in large part, to male-defined and male-dominated social institutions and value systems (Hole and Levine, 1971). The drive for suffrage in the earlier movement became the central focus only after decades of attempts to deal with an array of social issues affecting women. When women realized that they could not participate as political equals in the abolition movement of the 1830s, the political origins of the women's rights movement emerged. Women, barred from membership in many, if not most, organizations, had to battle for the right of public free speech. Sarah and Angelina Grimké, among the first women to speak out publicly on the abolition issue, came under severe attack and quickly surmised from this experience that the issue of slavery and the problems of women had many similarities. These women, along with others, challenged not only the concept of the natural superiority of men but also the institutions in society which functioned on that concept.

During the 1840 World Anti-Slavery Convention in London, women, relegated to the galleries and prohibited from taking an active part in the conference proceedings, learned that not only did society at large think it unnatural for women to be politically active, but so did the male radicals at the convention who were concerned with social inequality. Eight years after the London meeting, the Seneca Falls Convention, originated by Elizabeth Cady Stanton as a woman's rights convention, occurred. The convention participants wrote a Declaration of Sentiments and adopted twelve resolutions which vividly described the major social problems confronting women, such as (1) lack of profitable employment and scanty remuneration when employed, (2) lack of a voice in lawmaking and a lack of legal rights, (3) a subordinate role in church and state, (4) an unequal code or double standard of morals, and (5) the debasement of a woman's self-respect and the sanction against her leading an independent life. Specifically, these women wanted to gain legal control over their property and earnings, to have the right to divorce, and to secure the guardianship of their children. In short, they wanted to have economic, legal, and social rights befitting an adult. The Seneca Falls Convention is regarded as the official beginning of the women's suffrage movement. As the movement gained in strength, it came under even more vitriolic attacks than the Grimké sisters had experienced earlier. These attacks came from such sources as the press, the church, the legal profession, and the legislative bodies.

During the Civil War, the women's movement activities were in abeyance, although some women continued to work for women's rights. With the ratification of the Thirteenth Amendment abolishing slavery, sex distinction was introduced for the first time in the Constitution by the use of the word *male*. The women's movement saw this as a setback and made their first priority the drive for the vote. A woman suffrage amendment was introduced into every congressional session from 1878 until, with the ratification of the Nineteenth Amendment in 1920, 42 years later, women finally gained the right to vote in a democracy.

At present, the women's movement is in a state of flux. Comprised of a number of organizations, it serves both as a consciousness-raising mechanism and as an action-oriented group for social change. The literature on women's roles and the women's liberation movement continues to deal with many of the same issues over which women in the nineteenth century battled.

THE LITERATURE OF THE WOMEN'S MOVEMENT

Simone de Beauvoir's book, *The Second Sex* (1953), one of the first publications on women's liberation to reach a large, contemporary audience and now considered a classic, gives an account of women and their historical and present situation in Western society. Her central thesis, that since patriarchal times women have been forced to occupy a secondary place in the world, permits her to compare women's social position with that of racial minorities even though women constitute half of the world's population numerically. Furthermore, she believes that this secondary position has not resulted from the so-called natural or inborn feminine characteristics, but from strong environmental forces of educational and social tradition which are under the control of men.

In another widely read book, *The Feminine Mystique* (1963), Friedan describes the trapped woman inside the housewife and the social forces underlying the crisis in women's identity. A limited amount of literature on social factors and women has been available for some years. However, since the mid-sixties it has grown rapidly and ranges from the popular polemical to the meticulously researched presentation of issues. This literature includes such subjects as: sexual and social mythology (Ellmann, 1968; Figes, 1970; Janeway, 1971; Morgan, 1972; Reik, 1960; Roszak and Roszak, 1969), work and economics (Amundsen, 1971; Becker, 1971; Bird and Briller, 1968; Conference Report, 1955; Gilman, 1960; *Handbook on Women Workers,* 1969; Oppenheimer, 1970; Smuts, 1971), women and the family (Botts, 1957; Special Issue of the *Journal of Marriage and the Family,* 1971), education and careers (Astin, 1969; Astin, Suniewick, and Dweck, 1971; David, 1959; Epstein and Goode, 1971; Ginzberg, 1966; Komarovsky, 1953; Lever and Schwartz, 1971; Theodore, 1971; White, 1950), women's liberation movement (Adams and Briscoe, 1971; anonymous, 1971; Ellis, 1970; Epstein and Goode, 1971; Hobbs, 1970; Mitchell, 1971; Morgan, 1970; Stamber, 1970; Tanner, 1970; Thompson, 1970), and studies in power and powerlessness (Gornick and Moran, 1971). Several books deal with ethnic or cultural differences and women (Carson, 1969; Linner, 1967; United Nations, 1964; Ward, 1964). In addition, a vast number of publications on the historical perspectives of women and women's rights have poured off the presses (Beard, 1962; Catt and Shuler, 1923; Dingwall, 1956; Flexner, 1971; Grimes, 1967; Kradilor, 1968; Lerner, 1972; Lutz, 1968; O'Neill, 1969a; O'Neill, 1969b; Schneir, 1972; Scott, 1970; Scott, 1967; Sinclair, 1965; Smith, 1970; Wollstonecraft, 1967; Young, 1959). Two recent books which have received much attention deal with the bias toward women operating in our culture and reflected in our literature (Millett, 1970) and with the fact that neither men nor women are free from the social constrictions of sex roles (Greer, 1970).

SOME OF THE ISSUES UNDERLYING THE WOMEN'S MOVEMENT

Issues such as economic, legal, and educational discrimination against women, and abortion and child care receive high priority from the women's movement as social factors which must change to assure women full participation in society.

In March 1970, women headed 5.6 million families in the (United States Conference Report, 1970). Median incomes for this group did not exceed $4,000 in 1969, or approximately one-third the median income for husband-wife families in the same year. Furthermore, of this 5.6 million total, 2.4 million lived in poverty. Less than 30 percent of their income came from ex-husbands, late husbands, fathers, or other sources. Economists designated $4,855 as "near-poor" for urban families in 1969, which is above the median of $4,000 quoted above (Stein, 1970). Classified by race, white women in March 1969 who worked full time and were the main supporters of their families had median earnings of $4,855 while black women in the same situation had a median income of $3,235.

In 1970, more than 31.5 million women, half of all women between the ages of eighteen and sixty-four, were in the labor force (Flexner, 1971). The President's Task Force on Women's Rights and Responsibilities (1970) indicated that sex bias accounts for more discrimination than does racial bias. They support this statement with data which indicate that the median earnings for full-time workers employed year round for white men is $7,396; for black men, $4,777; for white women, $4,279; and for black women, $3,194. Women as a group earn approximately 58 percent less than men. The principal reason for this earning gap is that women most often work at unskilled, poorly paying jobs where unions have made no inroads to protect the workers. In 1940, women held 40 percent of the service jobs, e.g., hotel, hospital, and restaurant jobs; however, by 1970, they held 60 percent of these poorly paid types of jobs. In the same year, 7 percent of employed women with 5 or more years of college worked in service jobs or as clerical workers, salesclerks, or factory operators. In the professions also, an economic gap existed between men's earnings and those of women. According to Endicott (1970) the starting monthly salaries that firms expected to offer new graduates for the same job in 1971 differed as much as $52 based on sex.

Both fair employment practice legislation and equal pay laws require equal pay for equal skill, responsibility, and effort. However, no effective mechanism exists to enforce these laws, so compliance is voluntary. The federal Equal Pay Act of 1963 makes equal pay mandatory with some major exceptions. These exceptions, in the areas of farm and domestic workers, executives, administrative and professional employees including teachers, and the employees of small service or business establishments, tend to negatively affect women more than men in the labor force. In 1964, with the passage of the Civil Rights Act forbidding discrimination because of race or color but not of sex, only two states had statutes prohibiting sex discrimination in employment. By 1971, thirty-two states had such statutes which supplemented the federal act of 1963 (Flexner, 1971).

Representative Martha Griffiths from Michigan (1971) believes that discriminatory laws and practices reflect the bias of men, who tend to think of women only in the role of wife and mother, although, in fact, women constitute about 40 percent of the work force. She makes the following specific points to support her argument. Working wives pay into social security on the same basis as their working husbands; however, when a woman reaches the age to draw social security she must choose whether to draw the benefits as a wife or as a working woman. If both husband and wife have received fairly low incomes, they nevertheless pay as much or more in social security taxes as a man working as sole family earner. However, they draw less than the amount received by the man and his nonworking wife. Representative Griffiths estimates that to correct this inequity would require two and one-half billion dollars annually. This amount shows the extent to which working wives contribute to social security each year. She also indicates that her own government health insurance costs $2.80 more per month to cover herself and her husband than it costs a male colleague to cover himself, a wife, and two small children. She further reports that when Willard Wirtz, former Secretary of Labor, appeared before the Ways and Means Committee he used the phrase "secondary workers" to describe working wives and children. She thinks such rhetoric reflects attitudes toward these workers as individuals who have only secondary rights. Discussing the welfare laws, she indicates that more than almost any other type of legislation, these laws embody the myth of man as sole provider and women as homemaker and mother. In her opinion, welfare laws as they have appeared on the books have done more to drive men away from their families and reward women for rearing their children alone than any other single factor.

According to Kanowitz (1969) the legal position of women still remains essentially inferior to that of men in spite of progress to emancipate them under the law. He says that in one area of legal regulation after another, women continue to receive different and often less favorable treatment than men. Furthermore, he points out, judges and legislators continue to emphasize sexual distinctions which were the result of unequal legal treatment in the past, but now they use these same distinctions as justifications for unequal treatment of women in the future.

In the area of educational discrimination, data are more complex and open to different interpretations. Since the beginning of this century more girls than boys have finished high school every year, although in the past few decades this difference by sex has decreased. Beyond high school, however, the situation changes sharply. In 1969, 79 percent of boys completing high school entered college, while only approximately 60 percent of the girls with high school diplomas continued on to college. In addition, of those students entering college, more men than women, in proportion to the total number enrolled, completed a baccalaureate or first professional degree. This difference continues with the master's degree and becomes even more dramatic at the doctoral level. Women also tend to choose academic areas of concentration which in later life often lead them into less well-paying jobs. Part of the reason for this curriculum choice stems from the socialization process into sex roles which begins early in life and which perpetuates social norms regarding proper areas of interest for women. The social pressures to enter these less well-paying occupations come from many sources, such as the family, educational counselors, teachers, and numerous other significant people in a woman's life.

Although many women now have a college degree and/or professional training, a considerable number of highly trained women will not find positions where they can use their education and skills and must settle for jobs which offer fewer challenges and rewards, including money. Although a part of the problem may be attributed to the local employment factors confronted by men as well as women, the major reason seems to be discrimination on the basis of sex (Flexner, 1971). Writing about the educational establishment, Pullen (1971) says that graduate schools have had unwritten quotas to restrict the number of women enrollees, particularly in medical and law schools. Furthermore, in most colleges and universities, men have held the key administration positions even in the so-called women's colleges. Women must prove themselves more intelligent and must work harder to be admitted into certain university programs, and if they succeed, then they face the possibility of unemployment or accepting positions which do not fully utilize their abilities. Many women become discouraged and decide that the odds against them are too great.

Sex-typing which links occupations with sex roles makes the so-called traditional female occupations ones in which the occupational role becomes an extension of some aspect of the traditional female role, i.e., nursing, teaching, and social work. Such sex-typing can act to exclude both men and women from occupations thought of as characteristically either male or female. At the turn of the century, 80 percent of all health workers were physicians, predominantly male, whereas now the latter account for only 12 percent of the total. Manpower in the health field today is womanpower, since 75 percent of all health workers are women. Broken down into specific job classifications, women account for 98 percent of registered nurses, 74 percent of aids and attendants, 96 percent of practical nurses, 94 percent of nutritionists and dieticians, 95 percent of office workers, 80 percent of physical therapists, 75 percent of x-ray technicians, 90 percent of medical technologists, and 89 percent of medical social workers. In contrast, men account for 93 percent of doctors, 90 percent of chiropractors, 98 percent of dentists, and 80 percent of hospital administrators. Wages differ for the same employment position along sex lines, especially where women overwhelmingly predominate, e.g., the 145,942 women practical nurses receive on the average of $10 less per week than do their 3,350 male counterparts. Only in medical technology are salaries for men and women the same (Medical Committee for Human Rights, 1972). Sex-typed occupations, culturally defined, differ from country to country. For example, dentistry in Denmark and medicine in the Soviet Union are both considered female occupations. However, Epstein and Goode (1971) find that in all these cases, "popular rationalizations about the appropriateness of an occupation for men or women are nothing but post-factum explanations."

The issue that has probably caused more heated debate than any other in the women's movement is that of abortion. Basically, women who challenge the status quo of this legal, religious, and medical issue believe that a woman should have control over her own body and that the decision to have or not to have a child rightfully belongs to her. The argument goes that this decision is a personal one and should be confined to family and medical contexts and not be a matter for legal determination or ecclesiastical fiats. Lafferty (1971, p. 364), in reviewing the forces behind the proscription of abortion, says:

> Laws against abortion have remained in force because of certain myths that we have decided we want to perpetuate, certain views of what the good life is, which include ideas about the sanctity of fetal life, the religiosity of motherhood, the submissive and essentially maternal nature of women, the essential shameful nature of sex and sexual intercourse, and the natural superiority (physical and intellectual) of men.

The argument against abortion usually overlooks recent past data which indicate that 8,000 women or more have died every year from illegal abortions and that 90 percent of these abortions are performed on married women who have other children (Reiter, 1967). Also overlooked is the fact that the key to obtaining an illegal abortion is money, and that crime syndicates make approximately $350 million annually in the abortion business.

As with other issues, the position of the women's movement on abortion does not argue that every woman should hold the same ideas about abortion as every other woman, but that each must have freedom of choice without negative social consequences. Those who want abortion laws liberalized point to the fact that a number of countries in Europe and Asia, including Sweden, Norway, Denmark, England, Japan, and several Eastern European countries, have escaped moral decay despite their liberal abortion laws (Beaver, 1970). One writer (Hall, 1969) contends that the number of abortions performed in any given culture remains relatively constant and is related to the extent to which contraceptions are available and to the desire for a specific family size.

A recent study conducted by Kuntson *(San Francisco Chronicle,* 1972) shows that religion, and not education, is the major influence on health professionals' opinions regarding abortion. Variables such as sex, age, specific occupation, marital and parental status, and professional training in family planning have very little correlation with their value judgments on abortion, but rather ethical values established in childhood underlie these judgments.

The women's movement also speaks to the issue of child care centers by pointing out the number of working women with children and the fact that many nonemployed women also wish to enlarge their activities outside the home. This issue has long been under discussion by numerous groups. For example, the President's Commission on the Status of Women (Report, 1963) said that the gross inadequacy of present child care facilities is apparent. Child care services, needed in all communities for children from all kinds of families, are essential for women in a variety of circumstances if the status of women is to change. Eight years after the above report, Flexner (1971) states that although the need for child care facilities is no longer debatable, the United States remains abysmally far behind many other countries in providing this necessity. The fact that in 1970, 4.6 million women who were working or seeking work had children under six provides the data to support the establishment of inexpensive and competently run day centers. Although the Children's Bureau has indicated the urgent need for additional child care centers since at least 1958, and although some gains have been made toward establishing these centers, the need still remains great (*Handbook on Women Workers,* 1969).

These briefly sketched issues reflect some of the top priorities of the women's movement. As noted in the above discussion, a number of individuals and groups from the so-called "establishment" also place priority on social change to cope with these issues.

THE PSYCHOLOGY OF WOMEN

Many women resent the fact that past and present psychological studies of personality are totally inadequate in their knowledge and understanding of the psychology of women. Thompson (1964) points to a particularly basic fallacy in Freud's theory of penis envy in that he believed women to be essentially castrated males. This implies that girls start life with a "boyish outlook" which not only makes for a difficult reorientation at puberty but more importantly condemns them as women to lifelong envy of the male sex. Freud reached this conclusion without taking into consideration that many facts which led him to this belief were the product of cultural attitudes. Thompson takes the position that a woman's psychology "is something in its own right and not merely a negation of maleness" (Thompson, 1964, p. 41). She believes that the hostility between men and women does not differ from that found in any struggle where one group has definite advantages in prestige and position. Like differences in skin color, sex differences are obvious and can become convenient marks of derogation in competitive situations where one group wants to get and maintain power over another. In a patriarchal culture such as ours, the restricted opportunities afforded woman and the limitations placed on her development and independence provide a very real basis for envy of the male. Although progressive changes have occurred with regard to the status of women in many spheres of life, women still continue to be an underprivileged group. "They are discriminated against in many situations without regard for their needs or ability" (Thompson, 1964, p. 111). Freud, impressed with the biologic difficulties of women, "believed that all inferiority feelings of women had their roots in her biologic inadequacies. To say that a woman has to encounter certain hazards that a man does not, does not seem to be the same thing as saying woman is biologically inferior, as Freud implies" (Thompson, 1964, p. 126). Error in Freud's hypothesis stems from two major sources. First, "he saw the problem entirely from a masculine point of view"; and second, although he studied "only women from his own or closely related cultures," he assumed that what he observed was universal and relevant to all cultures. Cross-cultural studies now show that his assumption of the universality of penis envy in women was incorrect (Thompson, 1964, pp. 127–128).

It is not only culturally determined attitudes of men about women's sex role which have contributed to the lack of understanding of women, but, according to Thompson, "much which even woman herself may attribute to the fact of her sex can be explained as a result of cultural pressure" (1964, p. 129). This includes the acceptance by women that women's inferiority is based on biological facts. This has been part of society's prevalent attitude for many years, and until recently was accepted by both sexes. Such a concept has obvious advantages for men which make it more difficult for them to relinquish their beliefs, and, on the other hand, many women also have difficulties in freeing themselves from this idea, since their sex role socialization from childhood on has supported this attitude.

Weisstein (1970, 1971) maintains that when it comes to knowing what women are really like, psychology has nothing to say. It does not say what women want and need because it does not know, since the psychologists' research on human nature is based on the male model—woman as such has been ignored. Weisstein contends that an inspection of personality theory literature shows that much of this theory has developed from expensive clinical experience. She says that theories may arise from any source; however, no theorist may claim validity for his theory until it has been tested to see if the theory still holds true when numerous variables are considered. Much of the personality theory has not been tested as yet. Furthermore, psychologists do not tend to study the social context, with its expectations and pressures, in which people move, but limit much of their study to individual inner traits.

IMPLICATIONS FOR HEALTH CARE

One of the most persistent stereotypes of women pictures them as passive and dependent. The fields of psychology and psychiatry have tended to foster and perpetuate this image, since the assumption which underlies much of the literature from these two disciplines concerning women implies that "normal" women will find their identity and self-fulfillment completely in the role of wife and mother where they are dependent on, and maintain their identity through, others (Bettelheim, 1965; Engel, 1963; Erikson, 1964). One psychiatrist goes so far as to view the acceptance of the traditional women's role by women as a solution to societal problems (Rheingold, 1964). Much of the recent literature and debate on women, however, questions the validity of these assumptions, since they fit remarkably well with the common prejudice and serve to maintain the status quo of societal institutions. Weisstein (1970, p. 208) says that the real failure in psychology and psychiatry lies in the fact that these practitioners "have simply refused to look at the evidence against their theory and their practice, and have used as evidence for their theory and practice stuff so flimsy and transparently biased as to have absolutely no standing as empirical evidence."

Although for some women the roles of wife and mother as traditionally defined are sufficient for self-fulfillment, there is mounting evidence that for other women these roles, as historically defined, do not provide enough avenues for the realization of their true potential, nor do they reflect the present situation with regard to the functions which women are actually undertaking in society, such as work outside the

513

home. The debate centers on the fact that these disciplines view women in a one-dimensional fashion which measures their success in life only by examining their functions in the traditional sex role.

Health professionals, like everyone else, are greatly influenced by cultural definitions and attitudes as to what constitutes proper and appropriate activities for women. They, too, have been socialized into sex roles and most likely share similar views with society at large about sex-linked occupations, sex roles, and in general the "proper" place in society for women. Mental health professionals in particular need to be aware of their culturally derived values and attitudes regarding women and to examine their theory of and clinical practice with women, which may be based on outmoded and/or untested assumptions. These professionals also need to consider seriously the issues raised by the women's movement and to become familiar with the literature, much of which provides some startling factual data, as indicated earlier in this chapter. If mental health workers, willingly or unwillingly, feed into the discrimination against women in this society, then they limit their ability to effectively assist some women toward a fuller life. In clinical sessions with women, mental health workers must view some of their complaints as having a real basis in fact due to the economic, legal, and educational discrimination against women. Conditions such as those labeled "the housewife's depression" and "the empty-nest syndrome" also can be viewed not only as an intrapersonal disturbances but as reflecting aspects of the social world in which women find themselves. Rather than judging women who want a life style which extends the boundaries of the traditional female role, or who want or already have a life style at variance with the traditional sex role, as neurotic or maladjusted, health professionals may be more helpful to women patients if they view "the need or impulse to human growth as a primary human need, as basic as sex" (Friedan, 1963, p. 99).

In the final analysis, discrimination against any portion of the population, whether based on race, religion, age, or sex, weakens the fabric of society. If mental health professionals participate in the discrimination against women in our society, they greatly lessen their effectiveness with all clients, male and female.

IMPLICATIONS FOR HEALTH PROFESSIONALS
IN SEX-LINKED OCCUPATIONS

Within the health services in the United States, both medicine and nursing are sex-linked occupations. This essentially means that these occupations tend to define professional role behavior as an extension of traditional sex role behaviors. Within these traditional definitions, male doctors demonstrate aggressive behavior in a leadership role while, on the other hand, nurses, predominantly women, are expected to behave more in the typically female and passive role. Such narrowly prescribed behaviors based on traditional sex role definitions do not always allow individuals in the health delivery system to utilize the full extent of their knowledge, skills, and potential.

For many nurses who attempt to balance the traditional female role and remain "feminine" with professional competence, the real possibility of role strain emerges and can serve as one deterrent to job satisfaction. In addition, many nurses know from experience that to exhibit behavior considered to reflect so-called male characteristics, such as leadership, possibly invites criticism from both male and female colleagues.

As nursing continues to strive toward full professionalism, the problem of sex role–professional role strain may increase for the individual nurse unless the culturally held attitudes toward women and their role in society change. Moreover, this situation may be further strained by the attitudes and values held by colleagues whose view of women's role is based on a model which has more ties to the nineteenth century than relevance for today.

REFERENCES

Adams, Elsie, and Mary Louise Briscoe (eds.) (1971): *Up against the Wall, Mother,* The Glencoe Press, Beverly Hills.

Amundsen, Kirsten (1971): *The Silenced Majority: Women and American Democracy,* Prentice-Hall, Inc., Englewood Cliffs, N.J.

Anonymous (eds.) (1971): *Liberation, Now!,* Dell Publishing Company, New York.

Astin, Helen S. (1969): *The Woman Doctorate in America,* Russell Sage Foundation, New York.

———, Nancy Suniewick, and Susan Dweck (1971): *Women: A Bibliography on Their Education and Careers,* Human Service Press, Washington, D.C.

Baily, Gilbert E., and Paul S. Thayer (1971): *California's Disappearing Coast: A Legislative Challenge,* University of California Press, Berkeley.

Beard, Mary R. (1962): *Women as Forces in History,* Collier Books, New York.

Beaver, Janis (1970): "Antiquated Abortion Laws: Sexist Oppression of Women," *Guardian,* Apr. 14, p. 7.

Becker, Gary S. (1971): *The Economics of Discrimination,* 2d ed., The University of Chicago Press, Chicago.

Bettelheim, Bruno (1965): "The Commitment Required of a Woman Entering a Scientific Profession in Present-Day American Society," Paper presented at the M.I.T. Symposium on American Women in Science and Engineering, Boston, Mass.

Bienen, Henry (ed.) (1971): *The Military and Modernization,* Aldine Press, Chicago.

Bird, Caroline, with Sara Welles Briller (1968): *Born Female,* Pocket Books, Inc., New York.

Bloomquist, Edward R. (1971): *Marijuana: The Second Trip,* The Glencoe Press, Beverly Hills.

Botts, Elizabeth (1957): *Family and Social Networks: Roles, Norms and External Relations in Ordinary Urban Families,* Free Press Paperbacks, The Macmillan Company, New York.

Callahan, Daniel (ed.) (1971): *The American Population Debate,* Doubleday & Company, Inc., Garden City, N.Y.

Carson, Josephine (1969): *Silent Voices: The Southern Negro Woman Today,* Delacorte Press, New York.

Catt, Carrie Chapman, and Nettie Rogers Shuler (1923): *Woman Suffrage and Politics: The Inner Story of the Suffrage Movement,* University of Washington Press, Seattle (Republished by American Library Paperback, 1970).

Conference Report (1955): *The Effective Use of Womanpower,* U.S. Department of Labor, Women's Bureau Bulletin No. 257.

Cox, Harvey (1965): *The Secular City,* The Macmillan Company, New York.

David, Opal D. (ed.) (1959): *The Education of Women: Signs for the Future,* American Council on Education, Washington, D.C.

de Beauvoir, Simone (1953): *The Second Sex,* Alfred A. Knopf, Inc., New York.

Dingwall, Eric J. (1956): *The American Woman: A Historical Study,* Rinehart & Company, Inc., New York.

Duster, Troy (1970): *The Legislation of Morality: Laws, Drugs, and Moral Judgment,* The Free Press, New York.

Ehrlich, Paul R. (1968): *The Population Bomb,* Ballantine Books, New York.

Ellis, Julie (1970): *Revolt of the Second Sex,* Lancer Books, New York.

Ellman, Mary (1968): *Thinking about Women,* A Harvest Book, Harcourt Brace Jovanovich, Inc., New York.

Endicott, Frank S. (1970): *Trends in Employment of College and University Graduates in Business and Industry,* Northwestern University 25th Annual Report, Evanston, Ill.

Engel, George L. (1963): *Psychological Development in Health and Disease,* W. B. Saunders Company, Philadelphia.

Epstein, Cynthia F., and William J. Goode (eds.) (1971): *The Other Half: Roads to Women's Equality,* A Spectrum Book, Prentice-Hall, Inc., Englewood Cliffs, N.J.

Erikson, Erik (1964): "Inner and Outer Space: Reflections on Womanhood," *Daedalus,* Spring, pp. 582–606.

Figes, Eva (1970): *Patriarchal Attitudes,* Fawcett Publications, Greenwich, Conn.

Flexner, Eleanor (1971): *Women's Rights: Unfinished Business,* Public Affairs Committee, Inc., New York.

Friedan, Betty (1963): *The Feminine Mystique,* Dell Publishing Co., Inc., New York.

Gil, David G. (1970): *Violence against Children: Physical Child Abuse in the United States,* Harvard University Press, Cambridge, Mass.

Gilman, Charlotte P. (1960): *Women and Economics,* Harper Torchbooks, Harper & Row, Publishers, Inc., New York.

Ginzberg, Eli, with others (1966): *Life Styles of Educated Women,* Columbia University Press, New York.

Gornick, Vivian, and Barbara K. Moran (eds.) (1971): *Women in Sexist Society,* Basic Books, Inc., Publishers, New York.

Graham, Hugh D., and Ted R. Gurr (eds.) (1969): *Violence in America: Historical and Comparative Perspectives,* U.S. Government Printing Office, Washington, D.C.

Greenberg, Edward S., Neal Milner, and David J. Olson (1971): *Black Politics: The Inevitability of Conflict,* Holt, Rinehart and Winston, Inc., New York.

Greer, Germaine (1970): *The Female Eunuch,* McGraw-Hill Book Company, New York.

Griffiths, Martha (1970): "Women and Legislation," in Mary Lou Thompson (ed.), *Voices of the New Feminism,* Beacon Press, Boston, pp. 103–114.

Grimes, Alan P. (1967): *The Puritan Ethic and Woman Suffrage,* Oxford University Press, New York.

Hall, Robert E. (1969): "Abortion Laws: A Call for Reform," *De Paul Law Review,* Summer, pp. 584–592.

Halleck, Seymour L. (1971): *Psychiatry and the Dilemmas of Crime: A Study of Causes, Punishment and Treatment,* University of California Press, Berkeley.

Handbook on Women Workers (1969): U.S. Department of Labor, Women's Bureau Bulletin 294.

Hobbs, Lisa (1970): *Love and Liberation: Up Front with the Feminists,* McGraw-Hill Book Company, New York.

Hole, Judith, and Ellen Levine (1971): *Rebirth of Feminism,* Quadrangle Books, Inc., New York.

Horowitz, Irving L., and William H. Friedland (1970): *The Knowledge Factory: Student Power and Academic Politics in America,* Aldine Press, Chicago.

Janeway, Elizabeth (1971): *Man's World, Woman's Place: A Study in Social Mythology,* William Morrow & Company, Inc., New York.

Journal of Marriage and Family, (1971): Special Issue on Sexism in Family Studies, August.

Kanowitz, Leo (1969): *Women and the Law: The Unfinished Revolution,* University of New Mexico Press, Albuquerque.

Kennedy, Harold W., et al. (1971): *Symposium on Air Pollution,* DaCapo Press, New York.

Komarovsky, Mirra (1953): *Women in the Modern World: Their Education and Their Dilemmas,* Little, Brown and Company, Boston.

Kradilor, Aileen S. (ed.) (1968): *Up from the Pedestal,* Quadrangle Books, Chicago.

Lafferty, William (1971): "Abortion: Women, Men and the Law," in Elsie Adams and Mary Louise Briscoe, *Up Against the Wall, Mother,* The Glencoe Press, Beverly Hills, pp. 362–375.

Lerner, Gerda (ed.) (1972): *Black Women in White America: A Documented History,* Pantheon Books, New York.

Lever, Janet, and Pepper Schwartz (1971): *Women at Yale: Liberating a College Campus,* The Bobbs-Merrill Company, Inc., Indianapolis.

Linner, Birgitta (1967): *Sex and Society in Sweden,* Harper & Row, Publishers, Inc., New York.

Lutz, Alma (1968): *Crusade for Freedom: Women in the Anti-Slavery Movement,* Beacon Press, Boston.

Marx, Gary T. (1971): *Racial Conflict: Tensions and Change in American Society,* Little, Brown and Company, Boston.

Medical Committee for Human Rights, Bay Area Chapter (1972): "Health—Women's Work," *Bay Area Health Liberation News,* July–August, p. 3 (Reprinted from *Health/ PAC Bulletin,* April 1972).

Meek, Roy L., and John A. Straayer (eds.) (1971): *The Politics of Neglect: The Environment Crisis,* Houghton Mifflin Company, New York.

Millett, Kate (1970): *Sexual Politics,* Doubleday & Company, Inc., Garden City, N.Y.

Mitchell, Juliet (1971): *Woman's Estate,* Pantheon, New York.

Morgan, Elaine (1972): *The Descent of Woman,* Stein and Day, New York.

Morgan, Robin (ed.) (1970): *Sisterhood Is Powerful,* A Vintage Book, Random House, Inc., New York.

Mudge, Lewis S. (1970): *The Crumbling Walls,* The Westminster Press, Philadelphia.

National Advisory Commission (1968): *Report of the National Advisory Commission on Civil Disorders,* A Bantam Book, New York.

O'Neill, William L. (1969a): *Everyone Was Brave,* Quadrangle Books, Chicago.

——(1969b): *The Woman Movement: Feminism in the United States and England,* Barnes and Noble, New York.

Oppenheimer, Valerie Kincade (1970): *The Female Labor Force in the United States,* Population Monograph Series, no. 5, University of California Press, Berkeley.

Otto, Herbert A. (ed.) (1970): *The Family in Search of a Future,* Appleton-Century-Crofts, New York.

Pennock, J. Roland, and John W. Chapman (eds.) (1971): *Privacy,* Atherton Press, New York.

Pullen, Doris L. (1970): "The Educational Establishment: Wasted Women," in Mary Lou Thompson (ed.), *Voices of the New Feminism,* Beacon Press, Boston, pp. 115–135.

Reik, Theodor (1960): *The Creation of Women,* George Braziller, New York.

Reiter, Paul G. (1967): "Trends in Abortion Legislation," *St. Louis Law Review,* Winter, p. 269.

Report of the President's Task Force on Women's Rights and Responsibilities (1970): *A Matter of Simple Justice,* U.S. Government Printing Office, Washington, D.C., April.

Rheingold, Joseph (1964): *The Fear of Being a Woman,* Grune & Stratton, Inc., New York.

Rogers, David (1971): *The Management of Big Cities: Interest Groups and Social Change Strategies,* Sage, Beverly Hills.

Roszak, Betty, and Theodore Roszak (eds.) (1969): *Masculine/Feminine: Readings in Sexual Mythology and the Liberation of Women,* Colophon Books, Harper & Row, Publishers, Inc., New York.

Roszak, Theodore (ed.) (1968): *The Dissenting Academy,* A Vintage Book, Random House, Inc., New York.

San Francisco Chronicle (1972): "Religious Factor in Doctor's Attitude," Sept. 5, p. 2.

Schneir, Miriam (ed.) (1972): *Feminism: The Essential Historical Writings,* A Vintage Book, Random House, Inc., New York.

Scott, Anne Firor (ed.) (1967): *The American Woman—Who Was She?,* W. W. Norton & Company, Inc., New York.

——(1970): *The Southern Lady: From Pedestal to Politics 1830–1930,* The University of Chicago Press, Chicago.

Sinclair, Andrew (1965): *The Emancipation of the American Woman,* Harper & Row, Publishers, Inc., New York.

Smith, Page (1970): *Daughters of the Promised Land: Women in American History,* Little, Brown and Company, Boston.

Smuts, Robert W. (1971): *Women and Work in America,* Schocken Books, New York.

Stamber, Sookie (compiler) (1970): *Women's Liberation: Blueprint for the Future,* Ace Books, New York.

Stein, Robert L. (1970): "Women at Work," *Monthly Labor Review,* June, p. 17.

Straus, Nathan (1971): *Addicts and Drug Abusers: Current Approaches to the Problem,* Twayne Publishers, New York.

Tanner, Leslie B. (ed.) (1970): *Voices from Women's Liberation,* Signet, The New American Library, New York.

Theodore, Athena (ed.) (1971): *The Professional Woman,* Schenkman Publication Company, Cambridge, Mass.

Thompson, Clara M. (1964): *On Women,* Mentor Books, The New American Library, New York.

Thompson, Mary Lou (ed.) (1970): *Voices of the New Feminism,* Beacon Press, Boston.

United Nations (1964): *Civic and Political Education of Women,* Department of Economic and Social Affairs, New York.

Ward, Barbara E. (1964): *Women in the New Asia,* UNESCO, United Nations, Paris.

Weisstein, Naomi (1970): "'Kinder, Küche, Kirche,' as Scientific Law: Psychology Constructs the Female," in Robin Morgan (ed.), *Sisterhood Is Powerful,* A Vintage Book, Random House, Inc., New York, pp. 205–220.

———(1971): "Psychology Constructs the Female, or the Fantasy Life of the Male Psychologist," in Elsie Adams and Mary Louise Briscoe (eds.), *Up against the Wall, Mother,* The Glencoe Press, Beverly Hills, pp. 176–192.

Westin, Alan F. (1967): *Privacy and Freedom,* Atheneum Publishers, New York.

Wheeler, Stanton (ed.) (1969): *On Record: Files and Dossiers in American Life,* Russell Sage Foundation, New York.

White, Lynn, Jr. (1950): *Educating Our Daughter,* Harper & Brothers, New York.

Wollstonecraft, Mary (1967): *A Vindication of the Rights of Women,* W. W. Norton & Company, Inc., New York.

Young, Agatha (1959): *The Women and the Crisis: Women of the North in the Civil War,* McDowell, Obolensky, New York.

20

CULTURAL FACTORS

Anne J. Davis

THE NATURE OF CULTURE

Each society has its own culture or, more simply put, its way of life. The terms *society* and *culture* are not interchangeable, since *society* refers to an organized group of people whereas *culture* refers to an organized group of beliefs, morals, laws, customs, habits, ideas, and conditioned emotional responses shared by those in a given society. In reality, of course, society and culture are always linked, since without culture, a group of people cannot be a society but remains only an aggregate. The organization of all societies, and the existence of any one society, depends upon culture, since the sharing of ideas, attitudes, habits, etc., makes it possible for a group of people to organize and function as a society. Both societies and cultures persist over time and usually have a longer life span than an individual, and both are, to a large extent, self-perpetuating. The training or socialization of individuals, who must learn the shared attitudes, habits, customs, etc., has much to do with the persistence of society and culture; therefore, in any attempt to correlate personality and culture, the learning mechanisms become of paramount importance. Culture, in short, is the man-made part of the environment and is learned (Linton, 1956). It is what remains of our past working on our present to shape our future (Montagu, 1962).

Each culture has four basic conceptions or assumptions which have allowed man to order events, to organize experience, and to give meaning to his life and the world around him. All people in a culture view and interpret objects and events in the light of these four basic conceptions or assumptions, which are (Frank, 1950):

1. The nature of the universe, how it came about, how it functions, and who or what makes things happen, and why
2. Man's place in that universe, his origin, nature, and destiny—his relationship to the world
3. Man's relationship to his group—the individual's rights, obligations, and interests
4. Human nature and conduct, his self-image, what he wants and should have, how he should be trained and socialized

To comprehend the fundamental nature of culture one must grasp the inherent paradoxes involved in it. Culture is universal in man's experience in that all groups have one, but paradoxically, each particular culture has unique manifestations. Culture is stable, while at the same time dynamic, undergoing constant and continuous change. Culture plays a major role in determining our lives, yet it rarely intrudes into our conscious thought because it remains at the commonsensible, taken-for-granted level of experience (Herskovits, 1960).

The universals of culture reflect the similarities found in all cultures and include such aspects of human existence as: technological equipment to sustain life, a distribution system of materials produced, kinship arrangements, such as the family, political systems, a philosophy of life usually expressed in a religious system, language to convey ideas, art forms for aesthetic satisfaction, and a system of sanctions and goals to provide meaning to life. The socialization of individuals into their culture through a process of conscious and unconscious conditioning helps them achieve functional competence in their particular culture. Anthropologists refer to this process as *enculturation.* The enculturation of a person during his earlier years provides the basic mechanism for culture stability, while the same process, as it operates on more mature individuals, becomes a major factor in inducing cultural change. By the time most persons reach maturity, they have been sufficiently conditioned so that they function without difficulty within the limits of accepted behavior set by their group. However, later in life, the individual's range of conscious acceptance or rejection of certain aspects of his culture expands, and this may induce culture change. It can be seen, then, that not only is the individual conditioned by his culture, but in turn he can condition it. There exists a ceaseless interplay between tendencies toward standardization and tendencies toward variation.

Culture and the Individual

The enculturative experience attempts to mold the individual into the kind of person his group views as desirable. The group rarely achieves complete success, since some people are more pliant than others who resist this process to a greater or lesser degree. Yet, generally speaking, all people in a given culture become sufficiently alike so that differences between cultures become apparent. Two classic portraits of our culture during the early nineteenth century come from two astute observers and social critics: one, a Frenchman (de Tocqueville, 1945); the other, an English woman (Trollope, 1949). The whole field of cultural anthropology, subdivided into *ethnology,* the comparative study of culture, and *ethnography,* descriptive studies of individual cultures, provides us with rich and systematic data. To detail these many studies remains beyond the scope of this chapter; however, the bibliography includes selected titles for further reading (Benedict, 1934; Yang, 1945; Mead, 1949; Arensberg, 1968; Lewis, 1960; Kluckhohn and Leighton, 1942; Hostetler, 1963; Kuper, 1963; Yoors, 1967). Basically, the cultural influences exerted on the individual early in life can be grouped into three categories:

1. What others in the culture do to the individual, including child care and child training practices
2. What others in the culture consciously teach the individual, which includes all those activities referred to as instruction, e.g., manners
3. The behavior of others in the culture as observed by the individual, which includes the emotional tone characteristic of the adult performing the culturally standardized child training (Linton, 1956)

Whether the initial enculturation process begun in childhood does or does not receive support by subsequent experiences becomes an important factor in the adult's acceptance or rejection of new cultural items such as new ideas, changes in societal institutions, etc. In a stable culture these later experiences tend to reinforce the already established personality patterns and cultural norms. By contrast, in a rapidly changing culture, such as ours, the change in influences and the differences experienced between the personality-shaping early influences and those arising in adulthood resulting from rapid cultural change can serve as a disorganizing factor for both the individual and the culture itself.

Culture and Mental Illness

Discussions focused on the relationship between culture and mental illness do not tend to revolve around whether culture does or does not have an effect, since no person lives in a noncultural world. Rather, interest lies with the mechanisms by which the effect occurs and the degree to which cultural effects are significant. Some hold the opinion that culture has only minimal effects on the etiology, incidence, and symptomatology of mental illness. One typical comment from a psychiatrist in this camp maintains that reactions of Ghanian mental patients can be diagnosed according to Western psychiatric categories since the basic illness and reaction types do not differ. He believes that environmental, constitutional, and tribal cultural backgrounds serve merely to modify the symptom constellation, since the disorders of thinking, feeling, willing, and knowing remain basically the same across all cultures (Forster, 1962). Many persons, if not most, who work with and study mental health problems grant culture a much larger role in mental illness and health than is generally acknowledged. Indeed, many people in psychiatry and the social sciences believe that culture goes a long way in determining not only the amount of mental illness in a society but also the kind of disorders found there. Another point of agreement among this group is that the meaning of mental illness in a society results from that society's culture. They realize that both the researcher and the clinician are products of their own culture, which affects their view of themselves and others in, as well as outside, their own culture.

Beyond these general opinions and much rather fragmented research data, a great deal of uncertainty surrounds the complex interplay of culture and mental health. Despite a vast accumulation of research examining mental illness in various cultures around the world, the task of systematically collecting data that would specifically link culture and mental illness remains for the future. However, it has become generally accepted that no form of behavior can be judged as abnormal outside of its cultural context.

SOCIAL PSYCHIATRY AND THE RELATIONSHIP OF CULTURE TO MENTAL ILLNESS

Social psychiatry holds as its central concern the impact of social and cultural environment upon the development of personalities. To this end, it investigates the larger vista of people over the globe, including those in remote places, since these groups constitute the laboratory for the study of how culture relates to mental health and illness according to various living patterns. Social psychiatric research examines a number of factors, e.g., the extent to which the cultural environment can be said to play an active role in determining stress systems, family typologies, and the kinds of personalized meanings which operate within a cultural setting. This research takes as its point of departure the fact that culture includes traditional systems transmitted as methods for regulating behavior, ethics, and attitudes; that this transmission does not occur with perfect regularity; and that the cultural elements ultimately incorporated into personal functioning may produce problems which have become known as mental illness.

Historically, psychiatry has been greatly preoccupied with descriptive tasks of classifying mental illness on the basis of Western European and North American practice. At present, culture-personality analysis from anthropology has been incorporated to a larger extent as an essential part of the method and theory of social psychiatry, and future research most likely will continue this analysis in order to provide a framework for diagnostic and therapeutic purposes. Such a framework will include factors functioning in human existence, e.g., cultural, social, and experiential factors which play a major role in making the person what he is. Such research assumes that a person is not simply a product of historically derived diagnostic categories, but rather that the structure of evolving processes is basic to an understanding of an individual as a biological, social, and cultural being. Descriptive labels, such as "schizophrenia," have not always provided room for exploration of these essential processes and relationships in the world where man lives his life. Such labeling requires more analysis, and the theoretical underpinning of those descriptive terms must be further enlarged from one based on intrapersonal premises. They should include the fact that mental processes and disorders have a social and a cultural setting which always and essentially relate to the resulting forms of behavior.

Social psychiatry also examines the variations among ethnic groups in a complex society, since differences in incidence, prevalence, and type of disorders provide a practical basis for planning mental health programs and also may give insights as to the necessary ingredients for preventive measures.

TYPES OF CULTURAL STUDIES

Research germane to social psychiatry can be divided into several distinct categories. First, cross-cultural studies compare Western industrial cultures with preliterate, tribal, or nonindustrial ones. For example, one cross-cultural researcher (Leighton, 1969) asked the question, "If we start with Western definitions and the criteria by which we recognize disorders, to what extent can comparable phenomena be identified in other cultures?" He deduced that cultural patterns are not infinitely variable and that personality is not infinitely plastic. He also made the corollary proposition that there probably exist common, limiting factors the world over in both culture and personality. However, he reasoned that cultural differences must, to some extent, enter into both the definitions and the perceptions of psychiatric disorders, and to explore this question he studied the Yorba tribe of Nigeria. During a 3-month period he collected psychiatric data on 262 villagers and 64 residents of a town in western Nigeria, all of whom belonged to the Yorba tribe. Methods of data collection included two types of interviews with the above sample and interviews with headmen and elders of the tribe. This study revealed a number of noteworthy findings, including the Yorba healers' familiarity with most of the symptom patterns found in Western psychiatry, which they view as either illness or, at least, as undesirable behavior. However, their concepts and nosology of causes precipitating these symptoms are in a framework so different from that of Western psychiatry as to make comparison difficult if not impossible.

For many years, cross-cultural studies dealing with the variable effect of culture or cultural stress on mental health have been undertaken. For example, cross-cultural research includes studies on the Saulteaux Indians of Canada (Hallowell, 1936), the Peruvian Indians (Fried, 1959), the Ifaluk of Micronesia (Spiro, 1959), the Polynesians (Beaglehold, 1969), the Algerians (DeVos and Miner, 1958), the Ghanians (Field, 1960), and the Ashanti (Kraus, 1971). The value of such research lies in the fact that the greater the contrast between our culture and those being studied, the greater the potential for differences in definitions and perceptions regarding mental illness and health.

Another category of research, cross-national, confines studies to Western nations, where many cultural similarities exist as the result of historical events and influences (Farber, 1953; Gillespie and Allport, 1955; Singer and Opler, 1956; Wylie, 1964; Malzberg, 1964). Yet another category includes studies conducted within one complex country such as the United States, characterized as a pluralistic society with many subcultures. At times these studies focus on regional differences (Davis, Gardner, and Gardner, 1941), religious differences (Malzberg, 1963; Srole and Langner, 1969; Snyder, 1955), or ethnic differences (Glazer and Moynihan, 1963: Crawford, Rollins, and Sutherland, 1962; Gans, 1962; Parker and Kleiner, 1966; Eaton and Weil, 1955). The following section will detail several studies which have investigated ethnic groups in our own society and the relationship between these ethnic subcultures and aspects of mental health.

ETHNICITY AS A SUBCULTURE AND MENTAL HEALTH

Before discussing selected studies on ethnicity and mental health, some preliminary remarks seem necessary. Much of our present-day knowledge of mental disorders has come from observing people after they have become mentally ill, and particularly after they became sufficiently deviant to have contact with mental health professionals. Therefore, little of this knowledge has been based on observations of this group within the setting in which they fell ill. When the laboratory in which data collection occurs is a cultural group and the research investigates a phenomenon such as mental illness or mental health by describing its frequency, characteristics, patterns, and distribution, this is referred to as an *epidemiological approach*. This approach views each group as a natural laboratory in which factors of illness and health maintain some degree of balance. If this balance in one group differs significantly from that in another, this difference becomes a clue for the scientist in his search for factors either promoting or inhibiting the disorder. Goldberger's early use of epidemiological clues to explain, control, and prevent pellagra is one of the best-known and most dramatic examples in the literature (Parsons, 1952).

The following selected studies focus on three ethnic groups, the Afro-Americans, the Mexican Americans, and the American Indians. Along with other ethnic and religious groups, they have historically experienced the impact of nationalism and ethnic prejudice in the United States (Grebler, Moore, and Guzman, 1970; Hingham, 1963; Jordon, 1968; Josephy, 1970). This literature review acquaints the reader with selected research of these groups rather than drawing conclusions as to the role of culture in mental health and illness.

The Afro-Americans

Like many things, the present situation of the Afro-Americans can best be understood from an historical perspective. Unlike most early immigrants, who came from Europe, blacks came from Africa and not by choice, but in chains, with a complete loss of freedom which uprooted them from their cultural moorings. Throughout this period of history, and continuing until now, Afro-Americans have been systematically excluded from participation and influence in this society's major institutions. Such movements as Garveyism and organizations such as the National Association for the Advancement of Colored People and Southern Christian Leadership Conference have been but a few attempts to remedy this situation of exclusion.

The effects of this exclusion on Afro-Americans have been monumental in such areas as education, employment, and health care. For example, the life expectancy figures shows a persistent gap between whites and nonwhites. In 1900, the life expectancy for whites was 47.6 years, for nonwhites, 33.0; in 1930, 61.4 and 48.1; in 1960, 70.6 and 63.6; and finally in 1967, 71.3 and 64.6 (U.S. Department of Health, Education, and Welfare, 1968). The gap has lessened between these two groups; however, a substantial difference still exists. Numerous factors have combined to create this difference, one of which— widespread medical discrimination and segregation—is reported in Myrdal's (1944) pioneering study of blacks in America.

Afro-American Culture   In their study of major ethnic groups in New York City, Glazer and Moynihan (1963) concluded that Afro-Americans have no values and culture to guard and protect. Although scholars do not fully agree about the impact of slavery on Afro-American culture, a consensus has emerged that as brutalizing and uprooting as this experience was, this group managed to retain some of their past tradition. For example, in two important studies, Herskovits (1941, 1966) compared African cultural traits and Afro-American cultural traits and found similarities in language, religion, music, and other cultural aspects. That Africa has many rich and diverse cultures must by now be common knowledge. One book (Drachler, 1963) presents some of the stories, poems, songs, and folk tales from Africa, revealing the rich cultural roots of Afro-Americans. Numerous books and journals detail African decorative arts and textiles, printmakers, sculpture, etc. Other books have recorded Afro-American culture and its role in music, theater, art, and literature (Butcher, 1956). Additional sources on other aspects of African culture and Afro-American culture can be found in anthropological, psychological, and sociological research. In addition, biographies give us personal accounts of individual Afro-Americans who can view that culture from the inside (Brown, 1965; Cleaver, 1968; Conrad, 1943; Ellison, 1947; Malcolm X, 1964; Moody, 1968).

Black Americans and Mental Health   The relationship of ethnic identity and mental illness is a matter of controversial debate. The controversial quality of this debate hinges on the fact that some persons use the data to support their notions of racial or ethnic inferiority while others use the same data to insist on needed reform in the social system and specifically in health care delivery. The data referred to above indicate that, as of the early 1960s, black admission rates were higher in state mental hospitals in proportion to the population than were rates for whites (Wilson and Lantz, 1963). However, in research where socioeconomic status is controlled, psychosis rates among whites and blacks appear similar, which implies that these rate differences have more to do with being poor than with being black (Pasamanick, 1963). Furthermore, other researchers (Dohrenwend and Dohrenwend, 1969) examined eight studies to compare the rates of psychological disorders among white and black populations, and found that four of the reports indicated higher rates for blacks while the other four indicated the reverse. Because much research in this area has encountered problems either in data collection or in their interpretation, the only conclusion which can be drawn is that no proved correlation between ethnic identity and types of psychosis exists at present (Bullough and Bullough, 1972).

One psychiatrist (Poussaint, 1970) discusses the difficulty that Afro-Americans have in maintaining a positive self-concept and explores some of the ramifications supporting the existence of a black psyche. He begins by saying that no one can deny that many blacks have feelings of self-hate; however, this thesis has obvious limitations. Even if blacks had all the self-love and self-acceptance in the world, they could not express it in a social system which suppresses black self-assertion. Historically, through systematic oppression which attempted to extinguish his aggressive drives, the Afro-American became abjectly compliant. The rage which accompanied such emasculation had to be repressed and suppressed, since to express it openly one ran great risks. This repression and suppression, tied to compliant behavior, cost Afro-Americans their psychic development. According to Poussaint, today the "aggression-rage" constellation, and not self-hatred, stands at the center of the Afro-Americans' social and psychological difficulties.

Two other psychiatrists (Grier and Cobbs, 1968) indicate that nothing reported in the literature or from clinical experience supports the hypothesis that blacks function psychologically differently from any other group. They maintain that the psychological principles which first evolved from the study of whites hold true regardless of a person's color, and that unique black experience constantly influences growth and activity and often is a focal point upon which these basic principles are seen to act. They plead for clinicians who can differentiate unconscious depression from conscious despair and who have the wisdom to realize the difference between a sick individual and a sick society.

Kenneth Clark (1965) says that evidence regarding the nature and extent of individual psychoses and neuroses in the ghetto is not readily available. The factors which relate to this lack have to do with the comparatively few psychiatrists in the ghettos and the lack of money and psychological orientation of ghetto dwellers to seek help. He also says that, in the absence of research into the extent of actual prevalence of emotional illness in the black urban communities, one can raise some research questions (Clark, 1965, p. 83).

> Is the pathology of the dark ghetto so pervasive that mental disturbance does not stand out as clearly as it does elsewhere? Is the city government less observant of deviant behavior in the ghetto because it is subconsciously less concerned to protect the community from threat? Is less illness reported—or even recognized as illness— by ghetto families and friends? Are people who are emotionally disturbed already institutionalized for other pathologies—drug addiction, delinquency, homicide—and hence not diagnosed or treated as ill? Does the pattern of violence in the ghetto provide an outlet for emotional release that would in another culture be turned inward into phobias and depression? Do ghetto residents feel too alienated from the clinics and social agencies to seek help? Do the agencies tend to prefer as clients those who are "reachable" and hence indirectly weed out prospective Negro patients?

These questions point to the great need for more and better-designed research on the mental health problems of Afro-Americans. Any such research must take into account the cultural components which serve as a backdrop for the understanding of these problems. In the meanwhile, better social and economic conditions for Afro-Americans, combined with more and better health care, will go a long way toward lessening the gap between the haves and the have-nots. A number of issues surrounding, and possible solutions to, this problem have been suggested (Norman, 1969).

The Mexican-Americans

The preponderance of the literature on Mexican-Americans dates from the early twentieth century, and more recently numerous authors have written about some aspect of this culture (M. Clark, 1970; Crawford, 1961; Hanson and Beech, 1963; Hanson and Saunders, 1964; Heller, 1966; Humphrey, 1945; Leland, 1940; Loomis, 1945; McLemore, 1963; McWilliams, 1968; Madsen, 1964; Moore, 1970; Mott, 1945; Moustafa and Weiss, 1968; Romano, 1965; Rubel, 1960; Samora, 1961; Samora, Saunders, and Larsen, 1961, 1962; Saunders, 1954; Schulman, 1960; Sommers, 1964; Swickard and Spilka, 1961).

In one recent study, Madsen (1969) undertook a comparative analysis of the relationship between culture and mental illness among Mexican-Americans and Anglo-Americans in south Texas to examine the sociocultural determinants of mental health and illness in two ethnic groups belonging to the same society but maintaining different cultures. The researcher, following contemporary psychiatric theory, assumed that anxiety-producing stress constitutes a predisposing factor in most mental illness. He hypothesized that differences in the mental health of these two groups relate to differences in the stresses and anxieties produced within their respective cultures. Jaco's (1959) research, which presented the provocative proposition that Mexican-Americans suffer less mental illness than Anglo-Americans, served as the departure point for this study by raising the methodological question as to whether the total picture of mental health in any ethnic group can be obtained only by counting patients treated for mental illness. To extend earlier research, Madsen gathered ethnographic data for 5 years in order to examine the probability of dysfunctional behavior resulting from anxiety-producing stresses (1) within the traditional Mexican-American cultural context and (2) within the traditional Anglo-American cultural context, and (3) the context where the values of these two groups meet. He dealt with such cultural variables as world view; the place of the individual, the family, and society in each culture; male and female roles; the roles of parents and children; definitions of sickness and the meaning of death; and the concept of mental illness. He concluded that there is less mental illness among the Mexican-Americans than among the Anglo-Americans, and explained this finding by saying that Mexican-Americans have fewer role conflicts, since their rules of behavior are clearly defined so that they know what to expect of each other. The Mexican-American family also serves as an anxiety-sharing and anxiety-reducing mechanism in stressful situations, and in addition their world view enables them to blame external forces for their failures—which lessens guilt and self-doubt. In contrast, the Anglo-American's stresses fall directly on the individual, who tends to blame himself for failures and who does not experience the family as an anxiety-reducing mechanism. Among Mexican-Americans he found the highest area of anxiety occurring in those who actively strive for cultural transfer but have not been accepted by the Anglo-Americans. He also pointed out that Mexican-Americans have a cultural aversion to hospitals, since they see the hospital as a place to die and as a place of social isolation from their own group. Logically, then, it follows that this group will be less likely to seek treatment for any disorder, including mental illness.

Another study (Wignall and Koppin, 1967), conducted in Colorado, also noted Jaco's (1959) study. Jaco's earlier work showed that Mexican-American males in Texas had significant lower incidence rates for treated mental illness than did Anglo-American males. However, Mexican-American females had a higher rate of admission than did Anglo-American females and a slightly higher rate than their own males. This finding led to the hypothesis that the female role in Mexican culture is a stressful or vulnerable one. The Colorado study, however, found that Mexican-American males in that state have markedly higher rates of hospitalization for mental disorders than other males, whereas Mexican-American females have only slightly higher rates than other females and markedly lower rates than their own men. Alcoholic problems accounted for 28 percent of Mexican-American female admissions but for only 10 percent of other female admissions. This fact explains the difference between the two female populations, but the proportion of alcoholic disorders is not higher in Mexican-American males than in other males and therefore cannot be a factor in their high rate of admission to mental hospitals. One finding with cultural implications indicates that the greatest differences between Mexican-American males and other males occurs in the twenty to thirty-four age group, but only in areas, both urban and rural, where the Mexican-American community is small in numbers. Conversely, with a larger Mexican-American community, the male admission rates do not differ significantly from rates for other males and the female admission rates drop below those for other women. The researchers offer little discussion as to possible cultural explanations for these findings.

A number of investigators have examined the role of the curandero, or folk healer, in the Mexican-American community. Kiev (1968) focused on the impact of cultural factors on the form and content of Mexican-American folk theories and treatment and of the contribution of culture to personality formation and psychic conflict as well as to the development, patterning, perpetuation, and management of psychiatric illness. The researcher's rather loose approach presents many research design problems which have been noted in a research critique (Fabrega, 1968). More recently, another study (Edgerton, Karno, and Fernandez, 1970) using interviews and ethnographic investigations provides information about the beliefs and practices regarding folk psychiatry among Mexican-Americans in East Los Angeles. The researchers conclude that the importance of the curandero has greatly diminished in that area and the underrepresentation of Mexican-Americans in psychiatric treatment agencies cannot therefore be attributed to this folk practice.

One study (Stoker, Zurcher, and Fox) which may throw some light on the underrepresentation of Mexican-Americans in psychiatric treatment agencies found that while Anglo-Americans were more prone to use psychotherapy agencies, the Mexican-Americans relied on extended kinship groups to sustain their members. They also found that Mexican-American girls have fewer guidance problems in school and that at home they conform to the submissive female role of that culture, but that they tend to have more neurotic complaints and depressions, which the researchers say can be expected in family conflicts where there is more repression. Anglo-American girls are more compulsive and need to control the environment. Anglo-American mothers were described as "indifferent" and "continually rejecting," while Mexican mothers tended to be more "overprotective" and "restrictive," which leads to the daughter's dependency conflicts. According to these findings, Anglo-American dependency is accompanied by a lack of warmth, guidance, and support. Also, they found that the Anglo-American girls respond to therapy better than Mexican-American girls do, but they realize this may be due to the fact that the therapists are closer in cultural background to the Anglo-American patients and more distant from the Mexican-American patients.

Although more research, including replication of some of these studies cited, needs to be done on the Mexican-American culture and mental health and illness, several factors can be identified. First, the Mexican-American family serves an extremely important role in the individual's health and illness. Second, this group views the hospital not necessarily as a place to receive help but more as a place which isolates them from their major cultural and social group. Also, several questions can be raised regarding the future of this cultural group. If Mexican-Americans become acculturated more into the mainstream of American life, what effect will this have on the Mexican-American family? If the highest rate of anxiety occurs in those Mexican-Americans who strive for cultural transfer, and if there are significant changes in family patterns so that the family no longer serves to reduce anxiety, then will more Mexican-Americans need and/or seek psychiatric help? If more Mexican-Americans seek psychiatric assistance, will the health professionals understand the cultural context and its role in health and illness?

The American Indians

The voluminous literature on the American Indians comes from many sources, including diaries, journals, reports, and letters written by traders, colonists, missionaries, explorers, government agents, and others who had contact with different Indian tribes before the impact of colonization changed their lives. In addition, studies based on laboratory, field, and documentary research of anthropologists, historians, archeologists, and others have increased this source of information, if not everyone's understanding. To mention only a few of these studies, Berthrong (1963) has written about the Southern Cheyennes; Denig (1961) described the Sioux, Arikaras, Assiniboines,

Crees, and Crows; Hassrick (1964) depicted the Sioux; Heizer (1962) studied the California Indians; and Marriott (1945) gave an account of the Kiowa. Several paperbacks of interest include Wissler's (1966) recordings of his observations on Indian reservations at the turn of the century; a study of modern Messianic cults (Lanternari, 1963); and an account of five years in which a young anthropology student studied with a Yaqui Indian, Don Juan, known as a medicine man, a healer, and a sorcerer (Castaneda, 1968).

To speak of the American Indians as a homogeneous group overlooks the fact that, within the continental United States, eight cultural areas and tribal locations have been identified: the Indians of the Southwest, the California Indians, the Indians of the Plateau, the Indians of the Great Basin, the Plains Indians, the tribes of the Southeastern United States, the tribes of the Northeast woodlands, and the tribes of the Northwest Pacific Coast. Furthermore, twenty-one Indian language groups have been identified in North America, including Alaska, Canada, the United States, Mexico, and Central America, with approximately twelve of these groups being found in the continental United States.

Marginal Status and Personality Development of the American Indian
People who stand between two cultural worlds, influenced by two at times conflicting sets of values, often exhibit strong personality effects due to this situation. The *marginal man,* not only bicultural but frequently the recipient of prejudice as well, best describes the status of the American Indians. Numerous American Indian studies furnish information on the personality consequences of culture contact and the resulting marginal status (Hyde, 1957; Kroeber, 1961). As the white man came into contact with the Indians, he looked upon the native cultures as inferior and demanded rapid assimilation or segregation. The Indian leaders, subjected to the white man's authority, lost their people's respect and confidence. Most often, the white man condemned the native religions and made efforts to replace them with Christianity. All of this resulted in the loss of an integrated value system, which led to personal and social disorganization. MacGregor (1946) described the disorganizing effects of the reservation policy on the American Indians which continue even today to influence the personality development of Indian children. For example, MacGregor found among children of the Dakota Indians an anxiety which arose from not knowing how to behave. Results from Thematic Apperception Tests showed that these children thought of the world as a hostile and dangerous place and that they felt dissatisfied and deprived. However, one needs to examine some facts before jumping to any psychological conclusions regarding these test results.

A Special Senate Subcommittee on Indian Education called the American Indian situation a national tragedy of shocking proportions. They found that: Indians suffer a 40 percent unemployment rate, ten times the national average; they average an annual income of $1,500, which is 75 percent below the national average; on the average Indians die at the age of forty-four while the age for most Americans at death is sixty-five; the infant mortality rate is double that of the rest of the nation. This committee concluded that the American Indian is a lost and neglected citizen (*San Francisco Chronicle,* 1969). With these facts as background, the remainder of this section will focus on the Navaho Indians to illustrate the interaction of culture and health. The word "Navaho" has been anglicized from the older Spanish spelling, "Navajo"; however, this group refer to themselves as "Diné," or "the People." A detailed discussion of the cultural impact which the whites had on the American Indians will not be undertaken here; however, one historical account of this impact from the Indians' point of view can be found in Dee Brown's (1970) book.

The Navaho   The best-preserved original cultures of the United States occupy the area referred to as "the Southwest." In many respects, the fund of knowledge acquired by anthropologists about the people of this region exceeds anything known about any other similar area of like size.

The Navaho, who live in this area, form the largest Indian tribe in the continental United States, with their population of approximately 90,000. The Navaho today are threatened by two major factors: the pervasive and steady encroachment of the white's life style and the deterioration of the reservation land, resulting in increased poverty.

One of the most enduring accounts of the Navaho, a study done by an anthropologist and a psychiatrist (Kluckhohn and Leighton, 1942), hypothesized that the incomplete success of government programs in the past has been due to lack of understanding of certain human and cultural factors. They wrote their book to supply the background knowledge for those who hoped to effectively deal with the Navaho in human terms. Their account discusses the Navaho's past history; sources of livelihood and technology; housing arrangement, the hogan, and the personal relations within the hogan group and those that extend beyond it; how they view the world around them; their systems of government and religion; their theory of disease; their folk tales and myths; their language; and finally, their ethics and values. Specifically, and important for this discussion, the Navaho's fears primarily focus upon illness and death. Although they distinguish between disease, by which they mean mostly contagious infections, and generalized body fever or body ache; nevertheless, all illnesses, mental or physical, have supernatural origins. The idea of locating the cause of disease in physiological processes does not fit into the Navaho way of thinking. Any misfortune must be traced back to some deliberate or accidental violation of a taboo, or may be viewed as an attack by a ghost or witch. Treatment follows logically from this definition of causation and deals with these causative factors rather than with the injury or illness per se. The ultimate aim of every curing ceremony is the restoration of normal supernatural relationships. Such specialists as the hand-trembler and the singer use numerous techniques, including prayer, chants, self-induced trance states, etc., in the treatment process.

The Navaho do not believe in a happy-hunting-ground type of life after death, but view death as a horrible fate, seldom speak of it, and bury the dead as soon as possible. They regard the afterworld, located in the north and under the ground, as an uninviting place from which the dead return as ghosts to injure the living (Service, 1963).

The Navaho and Mental Health Research   In another earlier study, the authors (Leighton and Leighton, 1945) surveyed typical personality traits and explained these traits in terms of Navaho customs, child-rearing practices, and the pressure put upon the Navaho by the contemporary problems they face. The researchers concluded that the Navaho: (1) are a practical folk, (2) have respect for individuality, (3) are active and alert and show interest in the world around them, (4) have great capacity for control of their behavior, especially with whites and strangers, (5) have a language which expresses varieties of action rather than more static values, (6) maintain an outward poise and control but may be in turmoil inwardly, (7) are sensitive to criticism and ridicule, and (8) are moody sometimes but on the whole seem to enjoy life and have a keen sense of humor.

More recently, another study (Kaplan and Johnson, 1964), based on three years of field work, aimed at describing psychopathology and analyzing its meaning within Navaho society. The authors reached the conclusion that the Navaho example makes it clear that conception of illness and of cure go together; and furthermore, that it proves useless to attempt a cure with methods that do not fit the ill person's conception of the illness.

Two studies focus on one of the greatest mental health problems among the Navaho, excessive drinking. Ferguson (1968) indicates that Navaho tribal officials recognized this problem and established the Community Treatment Plan for Navaho Problem Drinkers in 1964. By way of background material, he says that although problem drinking is on the increase within the reservation, the most conspicuous type takes place outside the reservation where whole families drink together. Individuals receive much group pressure to enter into this behavior and are accused of group rejection if they refuse. The Navaho do not consider becoming drunk a social blunder nor do they consider being in jail for drinking a shameful experience; therefore, some of the social deterrents operational for whites do not function for the Navaho. Specifically, this study differentiates between characteristics of patients who responded to treatment and those who did not. The major characteristic of the successfully treated group was a lack of severe acculturation problems. This study concludes that the less acculturated patient suffers little anxiety because his identity is clearly Navaho, whereas the reverse holds true for the unsuccessfully treated group. The other study (Littman, 1970) describes the drinking pattern as episodic, explosive, socially disruptive, and nonaddictive. The Navaho, depicted as having a different time sense, a present-oriented life style, a lack of competitiveness, and a tendency to withdraw from challenges, responds best to drug treatment from an outpatient facility.

Wolman (1970) describes a year's work in group therapy using an interpreter with Navaho-speaking alcoholics. Prior to the coming of the white man, the Navaho culture had no familiarity with fermented drinks. This study points out the many problems for the therapist and the crucial role of the interpreter, who is ideally a professional who knows the languages of both cultures and is sensitive to cultural nuances.

IMPLICATIONS FOR HEALTH CARE

A number of potential problems stemming from cultural differences between the health practitioner and the patient can be identified. First, the possibility of communication problems looms large when people from different cultures confront one another (Adair and Deuschle, 1970; M. Clark, 1970; Parker and Kleiner, 1966). Part of this problem has to do with actual language differences. However, an even more complex aspect of communication misunderstandings has to do with the fact that people from different cultures place different meanings on objects, time, events, and behavior. Every health worker in the United States needs to realize the implication of living and working in a pluralistic society. One basic implication, which may sound abstract but which has very practical ramifications, is that there are multiple ways of thinking, perceiving, understanding, and behaving, all of which fit together logically within a given cultural context. When people from different cultures confront one another in a social, business, or medical transaction, the behavior of each is greatly influenced by his cultural background. The other may appear to think or act "strange" from one perspective but, if understood culturally, the thoughts or behavior may not only be understood but may prove to be perfectly natural and logical.

Sometimes patients from a different cultural or ethnic group cannot speak English, so arrangements for a bilingual interpreter are needed to assist the health worker in collecting necessary information about the patient, in discussing his health problem with him, and in attempting to allay some of his fears and anxieties. Even if patients speak English, they may not fully understand the nuances involved in the message. The task of getting the message across to the patient or his family falls to the health professional, and this involves much more than simply telling the individual what is going on or what something, such as a lab report, means. It entails taking the time and making the effort to receive some feedback from the patient or his family as to their understanding of what is being said or done to the patient.

In sections of the country where large numbers of patients from another cultural background seek medical care, the health professional may need to know the terms commonly used by this group to describe and explain health matters. Also, when patients speak a language other than English as their first language, such a simple device as having signs and directions available in that language enables the patient to find his way to the toilet, clinics, dining room, elevators, etc.

Without considering the cultural context of nonverbal behavior, health professionals may label behavior as deviant or abnormal. The patient's behavior may indeed appear to be abnormal, but the question is, Abnormal from what standard? In social psychiatry the question of normality invariably arises because of marked differences in values and beliefs and behavior found in various cultures. Although psychiatric illnesses may be labeled differently from culture to culture, they are functionally similar in that the patient's symptoms are either distressing to him or to the group with which he lives or to both, so that mental health problems must be situationally defined rather than judged against an absolute standard. This does not support the "cultural relativist" stand but suggests that it is not so much the content or character of the behavior but its compatibility with the individual or his group that indicates his need for help.

Another area of possible cultural conflict between the patient and the health worker may be that of folk beliefs and practices. Since folk cures fit logically in with the patient's cultural definitions of causative factors, the health professional who would dismiss these cures as unimportant or as inconsequential does so only out of his lack of knowledge or understanding of these matters. More health professionals working with patients from a different culture now view folk medicine as an important adjunct to their own medical approach. Wilford (1972), reporting on a federally funded school in Arizona for Navaho medicine men, said that often in the area in which "white man's medicine" had failed, especially the area of psychotherapy, medicine men had succeeded.

Clark (1970) identified problems arising in providing health care to the Mexican-American community which can apply to other cultural groups as well. One such problem area related to definitions of modesty and the taboos surrounding the invasion of privacy both by exposing the body and by discussing such sensitive topics as sex in a sexually mixed group, or with the mother of a male child, or vice versa. Other potential problems identified had to do with the manner in which health professionals approach patients and the response to hospitalization of patients from a culturally different group. The efficient, "Let's get right down to business" approach of many health workers may be offensive and foreign to these patients. To work effectively with them, one must realize this difference and modify his professional behavior based on an understanding of their culture. Hospitalization may be dreaded by many persons, but for those from a different culture, the fears and anxieties become exacerbated by such concerns as isolation from the cultural group, inability to communicate with others and to be communicated with, and unaccustomed routine and diet.

Health workers, particularly in the mental health field, need to learn about the cultures of their patients and, more importantly, to learn to use this knowledge in the care of these patients. Only then will health care, physical and psychiatric, become effective in reaching all the citizens in our pluralistic society.

REFERENCES

Adair, John, and Kurt W. Deuschle (1970): *The People's Health: Anthropology and Medicine in a Navajo Community,* Appleton-Century-Crofts, Inc., New York.

Arensberg, C. M. (1968): *The Irish Countryman: An Anthropological Study,* Natural History Press, Garden City, N.Y.

Beaglehold, Ernest (1969): "Pathology among People of the Pacific," in Stanley C. Plog and Robert B. Edgerton (eds.), *Changing Perspectives in Mental Illness,* Holt, Rinehart and Winston, Inc., New York.

————and P. Beaglehold (1946): *Some Modern Maoris,* New Zealand Council for Educational Research, Wellington, New Zealand.

Benedict, Ruth (1934): *Patterns of Culture,* Houghton Mifflin Company, Boston.

Berthrong, Donald J. (1963): *The Southern Cheyennes,* University of Oklahoma Press, Norman, Okla.

Brown, Claude (1965): *Manchild in the Promised Land,* The New American Library, New York.

Brown, Dee (1970): *Bury My Heart at Wounded Knee,* Holt, Rinehart and Winston, Inc., New York.

Bullough, Bonnie, and Verne Bullough (1972): *Poverty, Ethnic Identity, and Health Care,* Appleton-Century-Crofts, New York.

Butcher, Margaret J. (1956): *The Negro in American Culture,* A Mentor Book, New York.

Castaneda, Carlos (1968): *The Teachings of Don Juan: A Yaqui Way of Knowledge,* Ballantine Books, New York.

Clark, Kenneth, (1965): *Dark Ghetto,* Harper & Row, Publishers, Incorporated, New York.

Clark, Margaret (1970): *Health in the Mexican-American Culture,* 2d ed., University of California Press, Berkeley.

Cleaver, Eldridge (1968): *Soul on Ice,* Dell Publishing Co., Inc., New York.

Conrad, Earl (1943): *Harriet Tubman,* Paul S. Eriksson, New York.

Crawford, Fred R. (1961): *The Forgotten Egg: A Study of the Mental Health Problems of Mexican-American Residents in the Neighborhood of the Good Samaritan Center,* Good Samaritan Center, San Antonio, Tex.

———, G. W. Rollins, and R. L. Sutherland (1962): "Variations between Negroes and Whites in Concept of Mental Illness and Its Treatment," *Annals of the New York Academy of Sciences,* January, pp. 425–438.

Davis, Allison, Burleigh Gardner, and Mary Gardner (1941): *Deep South: A Social Anthropological Study of Caste and Class,* The University of Chicago Press, Chicago.

Denig, Edwin T. (1961): *Five Indian Tribes of the Upper Missouri: Sioux, Arikaras, Assiniboines, Crees, Crows,* University of Oklahoma Press, Norman, Okla.

de Tocqueville, Alexis (1945): *Democracy in America,* vols.1 and 2, Alfred A. Knopf, Inc., New York.

DeVos, George, and Horace Miner (1958): "Algerian Culture and Personality in Change," *Sociometry,* December, pp. 255–268.

Dohrenwend, Bruce P., and Barbara S. Dohrenwend (1969): *Social Status and Psychological Disorders,* Interscience Publishers, New York.

Drachler, Jacob (ed.) (1963): *African Heritage,* Collier Paperbacks, New York.

Eaton, Joseph W., and Robert J. Weil (1955): *Culture and Mental Disorders,* The Free Press, Glencoe, Ill.

Edgerton, Robert B., Marvin Karno, and Irma Fernandez (1970): "Curanderismo in the Metropolis: The Diminished Role of Folk Psychiatry among Los Angeles Mexican-Americans," *American Journal of Psychotherapy,* January, pp. 124–134.

Ellison, Ralph (1947): *Invisible Man,* New American Library, New York.

Fabrega, Horacio (1968): "Review of 'Curanderismo: Mexican-American Folk Psychiatry,'" by Ari Kiev, *Transcultural Psychiatric Research,* October, pp. 177–183.

Farber, Maurice L. (1953): "English and American Values in the Socialization Process," *Journal of Psychology,* October, 243–250.

Ferguson, Frances N. (1968): "Navaho Drinking: Some Tentative Hypotheses," *Human Organization,* vol. 27, no. 2, pp. 159–167.

Field, M. J. (1960): *Search for Security: An Ethno-Psychiatric Study of Rural Ghana,* Faber and Faber, London.

Forster, E. B. (1962): "The Theory and Practice of Psychiatry in Ghana," *American Journal of Psychotherapy,* January, pp. 7–51.

Frank, Lawrence K. (1950): *Society as the Patient: Essay on Culture and Personality,* Rutgers University Press, New Brunswick, N.J.

Fried, Jacob (1959): "Acculturation and Mental Health among Indian Migrants in Peru," in Marvin K. Opler (ed.), *Culture and Mental Health,* The Macmillan Company, New York, pp. 119–137.

Ganz, Herbert J. (1962): *The Urban Villagers: Group and Class in the Life of Italian-Americans,* The Free Press, New York.

Gillespie, James M., and Gordon W. Allport (1955): *Youth's Outlook on the Future: A Cross-National Study,* Doubleday & Company, Inc., Garden City, N.Y.

Glazer, Nathan, and Daniel P. Moynihan (1963): *Beyond the Melting Pot,* M.I.T. Press, Cambridge, Mass.

Grebler, Leo, Joan W. Moore, and Ralph C. Guzmán (1970): *The Mexican-American People: The Nation's Second Largest Minority,* The Free Press, New York.

Grier, William H., and Price M. Cobbs (1968): *Black Rage,* Basic Books, Inc., Publishers, New York.

Hallowell, A. Irving (1936): "Psychic Stresses and Culture Patterns," *The American Journal of Psychiatry,* May, pp. 1291–1310.

Hanson, Robert C., and Mary J. Beech (1963): "Communicating Health Arguments across Cultures," *Nursing Research,* Fall, pp. 237–241.

———, and Lyle Saunders (1964): *Nurse-Patient Communication: A Manual for Public Health Nurses In Northern New Mexico,* New Mexico State Department of Public Health, Santa Fe.

Hassrick, Royal B. (1964): *The Sioux: Life and Customs of a Warrior Society,* University of Oklahoma Press, Norman, Okla.

Heizer, Robert F. (1962): "The California Indians," *The California Historical Society Quarterly,* March, pp. 1–28.

Heller, Celia S. (1966): *Mexican-American Youth,* Random House, Inc., New York.

Hernandez, Luis F. (1967): "The Culturally Disadvantaged Mexican-American Student," *Journal of Secondary Education,* February, pp. 59–65.

Herskovits, Melville J. (1960): *Cultural Anthropology,* Alfred A. Knopf, Inc., New York.

———(1941): *The Myth of the Negro Past,* Beacon Press, Boston.

———(1966): *The New World Negro,* Indiana University Press, Bloomington.

Hingham, John (1963): *Strangers in the Land,* Atheneum Publishers, New York.

Hostetler, John A. (1963): *Amish Society,* The Johns Hopkins Press, Baltimore.

Humphrey, N. D. (1945): "Some Dietary and Health Practices of Detroit Mexicans," *Journal of American Folklore,* July, pp. 255–258.

Hyde, George E. (1957): "Indians of the High Plains," University of Oklahoma Press, Norman, Okla.

Jaco, E. G. (1959): "Mental Health of the Spanish-American in Texas," in M. K. Opler (ed.), *Culture and Mental Health,* The Macmillan Company, New York, pp. 467–485.

Jordan, Winthrop D. (1968): *White over Black,* University of North Carolina Press, Chapel Hill.

Josephy, Alvin M., Jr. (1970): *The Indian Heritage of America,* Alfred A. Knopf, Inc., New York, pp. 278–366.

Kaplan, B., and D. Johnson (1964): "The Social Meaning of Psychopathology and Psychotherapy," *Transcultural Psychiatric Research Review,* vol. 1, pp. 67–68.

Kiev, Ari (1968): *Curanderismo: Mexican-American Folk Psychiatry,* The Free Press, New York.

Kluckhohn, Clyde, and Dorothea Leighton (1942): *The Navaho,* rev. ed., The Natural History Library, Anchor Books, Doubleday & Company, Inc., Garden City, N.Y.

Kraus, Robert F. (1971): "Cross-Cultural Validation of Psychoanalytic Theories of Depression," *Transcultural Psychiatric Research,* October, pp. 164–166.

Kroeber, A. L., and Clyde Kluckhohn (1952): *Culture: A Critical Review of Concepts and Definitions,* Vintage Books, New York.

Kroeber, Theodora (1961): *Ishi in Two Worlds,* University of California Press, Berkeley.

Kuper, Hilda (1963): *The Swazi: A South African Kingdom,* Holt, Rinehart and Winston, Inc., New York.

Lanternari, Vittorio (1963): *The Religions of the Oppressed,* The New American Library, New York, chaps. 2 and 3.

Leighton, Alexander H. (1969): "A Comparative Study of Psychiatric Disorder in Nigeria and Rural North America," in S. C. Plog and R. B. Edgerton (eds.), *Changing Perspectives in Mental Illness,* Holt, Rinehart and Winston, Inc., New York, pp. 179–199.

———, and Dorothea C. Leighton (1945): *The Navaho Door,* Harvard University Press, Cambridge, Mass.

Leighton, Dorothea, and Clyde Kluckhohn (1947): *Children of the People: The Navaho Individual and His Development,* Harvard University Press, Cambridge, Mass.

Leland, R. G. (1940): "Medical Care for Migratory Workers," *Journal of the American Medical Association,* January, pp. 45–55.

Lewis, Oscar (1960): *Tepoztlan Village in Mexico,* Holt, Rinehart and Winston, Inc., New York.

Linton, Ralph (1956): *Culture and Mental Disorders,* Charles C Thomas, Springfield, Ill.

Littman, Gerard (1970): "Alcoholism, Illness, and Social Pathology among American Indians in Transition," *American Journal of Public Health,* vol. 60, no. 9, pp. 1769–1787.

Loomis, Charles P. (1945): "A Cooperative Health Association in Spanish-speaking Villages," *American Sociological Review,* April, pp. 149–157.

MacGregor, Gordon (1946): *Warriors without Weapons,* The University of Chicago Press, Chicago.

Madsen, William (1964): "The Alcoholic Argingado," *American Anthropologist,* April, pp. 355–361.

———(1969): "Mexican-Americans and Anglo-Americans: A Comparative Study of Mental Health in Texas," in Stanley C. Plog and Robert B. Edgerton (eds.), *Changing Perspectives in Mental Illness,* Holt, Rinehart and Winston, Inc., New York, pp. 217–241.

———(1961): *Society and Health in the Lower Rio Grande Valley,* University of Texas Press, Austin.

Malcolm X (1964): *The Autobiography of Malcolm X,* Grove Press, Inc., New York.

Malzberg, Benjamin (1964): "Mental Disease among English-born and Native-Whites of English Parentage in New York State," *Mental Hygiene,* January, pp. 32–54.

———(1963): *Mental Health of Jews in New York State,* Research Foundation for Mental Hygiene, Albany, N.Y.

Marriott, Alice (1945): *The Ten Grandmothers,* University of Oklahoma Press, Norman, Okla.

McLemore, S. Dale (1963): "Ethnic Attitudes toward Hospitalization: An Illustrative Comparison of Anglos and Mexican-Americans," *Southwest Social Science Quarterly,* March, pp. 341–346.

McWilliams, Carey (1968): *North from Mexico,* Greenwood Press, New York.

Mead, Margaret (1949): *Male and Female,* William Morrow & Company, Inc., New York.

Merton, Robert K. (1957): *Social Theory and Social Structure,* rev. ed., The Free Press, Glencoe, Ill.

Montagu, Ashley (1962): *The Humanization of Man,* Grove Press, Inc., New York.

Moody, Anne (1968): *Coming of Age in Mississippi,* Dell Publishing Co., Inc., New York.

Moore, Joan W., with Alfredo Cuellar (1970): *Mexican-Americans,* Prentice-Hall, Inc., Englewood Cliffs, N.J.

Mott, Frederick D. (1945): "Health Services for Migrant Farm Families," *American Journal of Public Health,* April, pp. 308–314.

Moustafa, Taher A., and Gertrude Weiss (1968): *Health Status and Practices of Mexican-Americans,* Advanced Report no. 11, Mexican-American Study Project, University of California, Los Angeles.

Myrdal, Gunnar (1944): *An American Dilemma: The Negro Problem and Modern Democracy,* Harper & Brothers, New York.

Norman, John C. (ed.) (1969): *Medicine in the Ghetto,* Appleton-Century-Crofts, Inc., New York.

Parker, Seymour, and Robert J. Kleiner (1966): *Mental Illness in the Urban Negro Community,* The Free Press, New York.

Parsons, Robert P. (1952): "Joseph Goldberger and Pellagra," in Samuel Rapport and Helen Wright (eds.), *Great Adventures in Medicine,* The Dial Press, Inc., New York, pp. 586–605.

Pasamanick, Benjamin (1963): "A Survey of Mental Disease in an Urban Population," in Martin M. Grossack (ed.), *Mental Health and Segregation,* Springer, New York, pp. 150–157.

Poussaint, Alvin F. (1970): "A Negro Psychiatrist Explains the Negro Psyche," in Robert V. Guthrie (ed.), *Being Black: Psychological-Sociological Dilemmas,* Canfield Press, San Francisco, pp. 15–25.

Romano, Octavio I. (1965): "Charismatic Medicine Folk Healing and Folk Sainthood," *American Anthropologist,* October, pp. 1151–1173.

Rubel, Arthur J. (1960): "Concepts of Disease in Mexican-American Culture," *American Anthropologist,* October, pp. 795–814.

Samora, Julian (1961): "Conceptions of Health and Disease among Spanish Americans," *American Catholic Sociological Review,* Winter, pp. 314–323.

———(ed.) (1966): *La Raza: Forgotten Americans,* University of Notre Dame Press, Notre Dame, Ind.

———, Lyle Saunders, and Richard F. Larsen (1962): "Knowledge about Special Diseases in Four Selected Samples," *Journal of Health and Human Behavior,* Fall, pp. 176–184.

———, ———, and ———(1961): "Medical Vocabulary Knowledge among Hospital Patients," *Journal of Health and Human Behavior,* Summer, pp. 83–92.

San Francisco Chronicle (1969): Editorial, Dec. 1.

Sapir, Edward (1949): *Selected Writings of Edward Sapir in Culture, Language and Personality,* David G. Mandelbaum (ed.), University of California Press, Berkeley.

Saunders, Lyle (1954): *Cultural Differences and Medical Care: The Case of the Spanish-Speaking People of the Southwest,* Russell Sage Foundation, New York.

Schulman, Sam (1960): "Rural Health Ways in New Mexico," in Vera Rubin (ed.), "Culture, Society, and Health," *Annals of the New York Academy of Sciences,* December, pp. 950–959.

Service, Elman R. (1963): *Profiles in Ethnology,* Harper & Row, Publishers, Inc., New York, pp. 159–184.

Simpson, George E., and J. Milton Yinger (1965): *Racial and Cultural Minorities,* 3d ed., Harper & Row, Publishers, Inc., New York.

Singer, Jerome L., and Marvin K. Opler (1956): "Contrasting Patterns of Fantasy and Mobility in Irish and Italian Schizophrenics," *Journal of Abnormal and Social Psychology,* July, pp. 42–47.

Snyder, Charles R. (1955): "Cultural and Jewish Sobriety," *Quarterly Journal of Studies in Alcohol,* December, pp. 700–742.

Sommers, Vita S. (1964): "The Impact of Dual Cultural Membership on Identity," *Psychiatry,* November, pp. 332–344.

Spiro, Melford E. (1959): "Cultural Heritage, Personal Tensions, and Mental Illness in a South Sea Culture," in Marvin K. Opler (ed.), *Culture and Mental Health,* The Macmillan Company, New York, pp. 141–171.

Srole, Leo, and Thomas S. Langner (1969): "Protestant, Catholic, and Jew: Comparative Psychopathology," in Stanley C. Plog and Robert B. Edgerton (eds.), *Changing Perspectives in Mental Illness,* Holt, Rinehart and Winston, Inc., New York, pp. 422–440.

Stoker, David H., Louis A. Zurcher, and Wayne Fox (1970): "Women in Psychotherapy: A Cross-Cultural Comparison," *Transcultural Psychiatric Research Review,* vol. 7, pp. 203–205.

Swickard, Don L., and Bernard Spilka (1961): "Hostility Expression in Spanish-American and Non-Spanish White Delinquents," *Journal of Counseling Psychology,* June, pp. 216–220.

Trollope, Frances (1949): *Domestic Manners of Americans,* Alfred A. Knopf, Inc., New York.

U.S. Department of Health, Education, and Welfare (1968): *Vital Statistics of the United States,* 1967, vol. 2, U.S. Government Printing Office, Washington, D.C., table 5–6.

Wignall, Clifton M., and Lawrence L. Koppin (1967): "Mexican-American Usage of State Mental Hospital Facilities," *Community Mental Health Journal,* Summer, pp. 137–148.

Wilford, John N. (1972): "A Federal School of Medicine Men," *San Francisco Chronicle,* Sunday Punch, July 16, p. 7.

Wilson, David C., and Edna M. Lantz (1963): "Cultural Change and Negro State Hospital Admission," in Martin M. Grossack (ed.), *Mental Health and Segregation,* Springer, New York, pp. 139–149.

Wissler, Clark (1966): *Red Man Reservations,* Collier Books, New York.

Wolman, Carol (1970): "Group Therapy in Two Languages, English and Navaho," *American Journal of Psychotherapy,* vol. 24, no. 4, pp. 677–685.

Wylie, Laurence (1964): *Village in the Vauchuse: An Account of French Village Life,* rev. ed., Harper & Row, Publishers, Inc., New York.

Yang, Martin C. (1945): *A Chinese Village: Taitou Shantung Province,* Columbia University Press, New York.

Yoors, Jan (1967): *The Gypsies,* Simon & Schuster, Inc., New York.

PART FIVE

Psychotherapy and the Nurse

21

INITIAL PATIENT ASSESSMENT AND EVALUATION

Eleanor M. White

The process of conducting the initial assessment of patients for both inpatient and outpatient treatment services is now a widely accepted practice for psychiatric nurses. The psychiatric nurse may fulfill this function as he engages in the practice of ongoing individual or group therapy, for crisis intervention, or for intake assessment and referral to other team members or treatment services. This is a decided change from the nurse's previous initial contact with patients on inpatient services, in which his functions were to decrease anxiety, provide an orientation to the unit, and facilitate the patient's developing relationships with staff (King, 1967, pp. 256). To fulfill these new functions the psychiatric nurse must be a skillful interviewer and must base his therapeutic decisions on a thorough understanding of a personality growth and development—structure, psychodynamics, and psychopathology. The initial therapeutic interview(s), although primarily aimed at assessment of the patient and his present emotional problems, has multiple purposes, the most important of which is the beginning establishment of a therapeutic relationship. This initial phase may involve only one interview or may take several sessions. Other important objectives of the intake assessment involve: the obtaining of essential data from the patient to identify current difficulties or reasons for seeking treatment, exploring present and past interpersonal and emotional difficulties, evaluating motivation for treatment, and making an assessment of ego-functioning. These data are necessary for determining a tentative therapeutic formulation, which includes a statement regarding the pathology present, a hypothesis regarding the intrapsychic dynamics of the problem, and constructs regarding the genetic development of the patient (MacKinnon and Michels, 1971, p. 44). From this therapeutic formulation a tentative diagnosis and treatment plan are identified and the appropriate method of therapy is suggested.

The initial contact between therapist and patient has been identified (Gill, Newman, and Redlich, 1954; Sullivan, 1954) as having great bearing on the development of the therapeutic relationship. First contact often occurs over the telephone when the patient calls to make an appointment. At this time the therapist can set the stage for the establishment of rapport by making the initial appointment himself and by making arrangements to see the patient as soon as possible, thereby indicating an interest in meeting and helping the patient. Often the patient will be calling on the basis of a referral by another professional, friend, or relative. If the therapist has had prior contact with the referring person, it is a sign of interest to note this by saying, "Yes, I understood you might be calling." The process by which the patient makes his initial appointment provides important data for the therapist as he begins his initial assessment. Does the patient sound highly anxious, confused, resistant, demanding? Is there a struggle around finding appointment times?

Gathering Information

In collecting, sorting, and collating the important information needed for achieving the purposes of the initial assessment the nurse must skillfully use himself in such a way that he gives messages of interest, concern, and support to the patient so that he does not perceive himself as a subject for research or study. The nurse also must structure the interview in a flexible manner by taking many of his cues from the patient rather than by following a rigidly structured psychiatric examination format. In providing initial structure, a guiding principle to follow is that the less organized the patient's current ego-functioning is, the more structure the interviewer must provide, both to elicit data and to decrease the patient's anxiety (MacKinnon and Michels, 1971, p. 42). Another important reason for providing structure in the interview is to clarify with the patient the purpose of the initial interviews and to note whether he will be seeing the interviewer for intake and referral only or whether he may continue treatment with him (Wolberg, 1967, p. 451).

Utilization of Questions in the Interview

In the interview the interviewer may need to utilize questions to obtain additional information from the patient, although as a general rule statements are preferable to questions. He should ask questions that will provide some focus or structure for the patient but still give him some room for answering, by asking, e.g., "Tell me about your family," "What is your work situation like?" "What seems to be concerning you right now?" rather than asking questions that may be answered by a simple Yes or No, ones that may confront the patient too directly with sensitive areas of his life, or ones that demand an explanation or "why" for what he is experiencing. In asking questions the therapist may gather data, clarify, or provide subtle suggestions to the patient (MacKinnon & Michels, 1971, p. 35). Questioning in the interview may proceed not only from the therapist to the patient but also from patient to therapist. The therapist should be prepared to answer questions regarding the process and length of therapy, probable diagnosis, and his own personal and professional qualifications for working with the patient. Wolberg suggests that the therapist deal with both the factual content of the questions and the latent messages by acknowledging and briefly exploring the concerns prompting the questions with an accepting-nondefensive attitude (Wolberg, 1967, p. 455). In relation to questions about diagnosis, the interviewer should avoid giving the patient a label or using technical jargon but provide answers that acknowledge the difficulties the patient is encountering.

Another function of the therapist in the initital interview is to clarify misconceptions regarding the process and expectations of psychotherapy. Frequent misconceptions are: that one must be "really disturbed" and "crazy" to seek psychiatric help; that an omnipotent medical person will magically cure the patient, or tell him what to do to be cured; that the patient will be seduced by the therapist to give up behavior, beliefs, or defenses that the patient does not want to give up. Wolberg notes that some patients fear that psychotherapy will rob them of their uniqueness, creativity, or talent (1967, p. 540).

Content and Process of Interviews

In the interview situation the therapist must be able to identify and deal with both the content and the process of the interview. The content is the factual data presented by the patient and the interventions and responses of the therapist, and is primarily verbal in mode; while the process is the developing relationship between the therapist and the patient and includes the implicit or latent meanings of communications between the two. The process will include the way information is provided or withheld—the manner in which both attempt to control or influence the interview situation (MacKinnon and Michels, 1971, p. 8).

Establishing Rapport and Therapeutic Alliance

As has been indicated, the focus on all that the therapist does during the initial assessment of the patient is aimed at the establishment of a sense of rapport and the beginning of a therapeutic alliance. Both the patient and the therapist approach the initial interview with varying degrees of anxiety. The patient's anxiety is generally related to his symptoms, the therapist's reactions to him, and the practical problems of therapy, such as fees and appointment times; and the therapist is generally concerned with his ability to help the patient or to provide an appropriate referral and to cope with the patient's reactions to the interview. In establishing rapport the therapist provides a sympathetic, attentive, accepting attitude and presents himself not as an aloof, detached observer, but as a real person who is truly encountering the patient. To facilitate rapport, Wolberg (1967, pp. 525–527) notes several don'ts for the therapist to be aware of, including:

1. Do not argue with, minimize, or challenge the patient.
2. Do not give false reassurance.
3. Do not make false promises.
4. Do not offer interpretations.
5. Do not offer a diagnosis.
6. Do not probe sensitive areas.
7. Do not attempt to sell the patient on therapy.
8. Do not take sides with the patient against significant others or previous therapists.

Initial resistance to psychiatric treatment is frequently encountered in early interviews, particularly if the patient has sought an appointment at another's request or insistence. When resistance is present, the therapist must be alert to his own defensiveness and meet this resistance with an acknowledgment and acceptance of these feelings. The therapist can identify for the patient areas that seem to be causing difficulty in his functioning or relationships, but stress with the patient that the matter of meaningful participation in therapy is truly the patient's own choice.

Early in the therapeutic process the therapist uses his "own genuine curiosity to awaken the patient's interest in himself" (MacKinnon and Michels, 1971, p. 57) and to initiate the beginning of a therapeutic alliance which is the relationship between the therapist's analyzing ego and the healthy and rational aspect of the patient's ego (MacKinnon and Michels, 1971, p. 11).

Essential Areas of Information

As noted previously, there are certain essential areas of assessment of the patient's life that the therapist focuses on and collates during the assessment process; this information either may be elicited in a fairly routine and straightforward manner or, perhaps more commonly, may be obtained by piecing together bits and pieces of information offered by the patient. A major shift in assessing individuals has been ~~has been~~ effected: from that of utilizing a rigid, medical model of assessment and the formulation of a traditional psychiatric diagnosis to that of delineating the psychodynamics at work in the patients' problems in living.

In gathering data it is important to remember that whatever data the therapist obtains from the patient will be incomplete even if he spends several interviews in the assessment process. The patient may withhold information because he screens out data he thinks is unimportant, because he fears exposure of certain sensitive material, or because he has not yet learned to trust the interviewer. Therefore, any clinical impressions reached by the interviewer must be viewed as tentative formulations (Wolberg, 1967, p. 457). Equally important is an awareness of cultural and ethnic differences in behavior that must be taken into consideration when attempting to get a picture of what is usual or "normal" for the patient.

Relevant areas of data to be gathered will include the following categories:

Identifying Characteristics: Name, age, sex, marital status, occupation, employment record, income, and ethnic and cultural origins.

Presenting Difficulties: (Here it is important to use the patient's own words in describing the problem.) This may be a fairly brief or concise statement of the problems facing the patient, particularly those causing the most distress, although not necessarily the most central in terms of the underlying dynamics. Questions to be asked in relation to this problem may be: "How long has this been a difficulty?" "What precipitated your seeking help at this time?" "How is this affecting your current life functioning?" After the patient has identified his primary complaint and spent some time discussing it, the therapist should then check for any additional emotional difficulties encountered by the patient.

Current Life Situation

Important cues as to what is happening in the life of the patient in relation to his seeking treatment may be gathered by asking the patient to describe to the therapist: the circumstances of his present life situation and the significant people in it; the way he spends his time and the activities that he enjoys; and any recent changes in his work or personal life. Patients who appear withdrawn or who have difficulty in giving details may be asked to detail a typical day for the interviewer. An important aspect of assessing the patient's current functioning is to note any signs of depression and to ask the patient whether he is subject to depression. This should be investigated in the first interview.

Family Constellation

The therapist needs to elicit both specific and general data in relation to the question, "Who are the members of your family, both presently and in the past?" Often important information in this area is omitted or recalled later, e.g., "Oh yes, my other brother is in Ohio," or some members are not mentioned and the therapist notes, "How about your father?" Members with whom the patient has maintained continued contact and support should be elicited as well as members who have left the family. In the interview in which the family constellation is discussed, it is wise to remember that the first feelings expressed may not be the most accurate ones, as the patient may experience difficulty in relating his feelings honestly. Helpful questions may include: "How would I know your mother (father, sister) from other strangers in a room?"

Psychosocial Development

The significant data may be gathered by assessing the patient's accomplishment of significant developmental tasks in his life, particularly in relation to the socialization process. This topic will include questions regarding what "growing up in your family was like," school experience, peer relationships, and close relationships with members of both sexes. The therapist will also be alert to signs of repetitious behavior problems in the past and present, but at the same time he should be alert for sudden or dramatic changes in the patient's patterns of behavior or quality of relationships.

History of Previous Emotional Difficulty and/or Therapy

The patient should be asked about a history of any previous emotional difficulty and whether or not he has received any previous therapy. This will include interviews with school counselors, outpatient or private therapy, hospitalization, and/or use of psychoactive drugs or other forms of therapy. It is wise to check into whether or not the patient has seen or is currently being seen by a general internist or other physician for treatment for "nerves" or other somatic symptoms, as this is not at all an unusual occurrence.

Drug and Alcohol Use or Abuse

An area of increasing importance is that of the use of alcohol or drugs by patients; and if the patient admits to their use, the therapist should try to determine how these might figure in the patient's difficulties. If the problem is primarily that of drug dependence and abuse, the interviewer must be alert to organic and psychic disturbances they may elicit. Attempts to control or otherwise cope with this problem should also be elicited.

Ego Assessment

An essential part of every personality assessment is the assessment of ego-functioning; making an ego assessment is an ongoing process in the interview which includes the areas of ego function (ability to cope with internal and external demands and realities) and ego strength (in relation to type and length of stress). Disturbances in ego-functioning are seen where there is poor tolerance of stress, dissociation, and failure to neutralize and sublimate drives. Five primary areas of ego-functioning and their related disturbances have been delineated by King (1967, pp. 258–160) and include:

Relationship to Reality This is defined as the individual's ability to adjust to daily relationships and experiences and to change roles subsequent to correctly perceiving and evaluating external data and the individual's ability to differentiate between self and the environment. Disturbances in this sphere may be seen by the adoption of rigid roles, delusions, hallucinations, denial, depersonalization, identity confusion, and an unstable body image.

Regulation of Drives This is the demonstration of an ability to allow for appropriate expression of feelings, to tolerate anxiety and frustration, and to sublimate, delay, and neutralize drives. Disturbances in the regulation of drives are seen in acting-out behavior or excessive control.

Object Relations This involves the demonstration of an ability to establish and maintain satisfying interpersonal relationships. Disturbances in object relations are seen in those who demand either excessive closeness to or distance from other people.

Thought Process   This is the utilization of a secondary thought process as the predominant mode of thinking, e.g., reality testing or logical thinking. Disturbance of thought process is seen in direct expression of drives, prelogical modes of thinking, excessive concreteness, use of florid symbolism, confusion of time and place referents, stereotypy, and paranoid thinking.

Defensive Functions   This involves the demonstration of the use of common defense mechanisms in an appropriate manner to handle anxiety. Disturbance of defenses is seen in excessive or inappropriate use with resultant distortion of reality.

Mental Status Examination

The mental status examination which is required in many institutions is fairly well standardized and is similar in scope and purpose to the above discussion. This examination attempts to give a standardized picture of the patient in terms of emotional and mental status and functioning (Sands, 1967, pp. 505–508). Data are gathered from the interview behavior and the therapist takes into consideration the above ego assessment plus general appearance, motor behavior, affect expression, thought processes, orientation, sensorimotor activity, memory, insight, and judgment. (For a more complete outline and discussion, see Thomas F. Graham, 1969, *Mental Status Manual.)*

Overall Assessment

It is of vital importance in viewing any potential patient to be alert to and attuned to his areas of wellness and to help him delineate his potential and operating strengths as well as his areas of difficulty. Here the therapist may need to provide some structure for the patient by asking questions about the patient's assets, talents, and personality strengths. Timing in the eliciting of this information is important and will take skill and finesse on the part of the interviewer, for most patients come with the expectation that they should focus on their problems (MacKinnon and Michels, 1971, pp. 10–11).

In evaluating the environmental factors impinging on the patient, the therapist must identify potential sources of support as well as sources of stress present in the familial, social, cultural, and socioeconomic interrelationships encountered by the patient. These factors are especially important when engaging in crisis intervention with patients and in making treatment decisions regarding the use of hospitalization or supportive therapy versus reconstructive therapy. Increasingly nurses are engaged in this form of psychiatric therapy and are involved in the identification and mobilization of resources within the patient's system.

Recognition and correction of physical illnesses are of paramount importance in the prevention and treatment of emotional disorders and demand that the therapist take into consideration an evaluation of the patient's physical health and status. In doing this the therapist must look for evidence of deprivations of basic bodily needs, such as oxygen, nutrition and fluids, sleep, and perceptual stimulation; all of these have relevance for today's culture, particularly in the young adult population, who may be involved in the practice of fad diets, the use of drugs, etc. (Kolb, 1973, p. 135).

A final element of assessment is that of the patient's motivation for therapy and change. Again, as in the other aspects of assessment, it cannot be made in a vacuum, but must take into consideration external factors impinging (threat of jail, a failing marriage, loss of job, loss of disability benefits), secondary gains of being in therapy, degree of dependency needs, the amount of discomfort the person is experiencing, and his capacity to tolerate discomfort while in therapy.

Other important questions to be asked by the interviewer of himself will be: (1) "How, or can, I work well with this patient?" (2) "Which type of therapy is best suited for this patient at this time, both in relation to whether it should be group or individual therapy, and in relation to differing models of either modality—supportive, reeducative, or reconstructive—brief or long-term?"

REFERENCES

Gill, Merton, Richard Newman, and Fredrick C. Redlich (1954): *The Initial Interview in Psychiatric Practice*, International Universities Press, Inc., New York.

Graham, Thomas F. (1969): *Mental Status Manual,* Sandoz Pharmaceuticals, Hanover, N.J.

King, Joan M. (1967): "The Initial Interview: Assessment of the Patient and his Difficulties," *Perspectives in Psychiatric Care*, vol. 5, pp. 256–261.

Kolb, Lawrence (1973): *Modern Clinical Psychiatry,* W. B. Saunders Company, Philadelphia, pp. 123–145.

MacKinnon, Roger, and Robert Michels (1971): *The Psychiatric Interview in Clinical Practice,* W. B. Saunders Company, Philadelphia.

Sands, William L. (1967): "Psychiatric History and Mental Status," in Alfred M. Freedman and Harold Kaplan (eds.), *Comprehensive Textbook of Psychiatry,* The Williams & Wilkins Company, Baltimore, pp. 499–508.

Sullivan, Harry S. (1954): *The Psychiatric Interview,* W. W. Norton & Company, Inc., New York.

Wolberg, Lewis, R. (1967): *The Technique of Psychotherapy,* 2d ed., Grune & Stratton, Inc., New York.

22

INDIVIDUAL PSYCHOTHERAPY

Marion E. Kalkman

Psychotherapy is a term with many meanings and many definitions. It has been defined very generally to mean any treatment which utilizes psychological methods rather than physical methods. According to Wolberg (1954, p. 3), "Psychotherapy is a form of treatment for problems of an emotional nature in which a trained person deliberately establishes a professional relationship with a patient with the object of removing, modifying, or retarding existing symptoms, of mediating disturbed patterns of behavior, and of promoting growth and development." Somewhat similar definitions include the following: "Psychotherapy is a formal treatment of patients distinguished by its dependence on psychological rather than physical or chemical agents . . . using principally verbal communication . . . [and] aims at ameliorative change of the patient by something done or said by the therapist" (Menninger, 1958, pp. 16–17); "psychotherapy is an interpersonal operation in which the total organismic adaptation of one individual is catalyzed by another individual in such a way that the patient's level of adaptive capacity is increased" (Whitaker and Malone, 1953, quoted in Chessick, 1969, pp. 13–14); and "psychotherapy is a deliberate attempt to apply psychological principles in an interpersonal setting to change the behavior of one so that he may be more comfortable in living" (Dellis and Stone, 1960, p. 131).

In the above definitions the latter two define psychotherapy as a treatment situation limited to one patient and a therapist. This type of psychotherapy may be more strictly categorized as individual therapy since psychotherapy is also used in the treatment of groups of patients and families. The following definition of *psychotherapy* is an excellent definition of individual psychotherapy: "Psychotherapy is a special kind of experience in which two people communicate with each other in a special way. It is a two-way communication designed to help one of them understand himself better and so be able to modify his behavior and achieve better comfort and health (Fleming, 1967, p. 416).

Before Freud, the only psychotherapeutic techniques available were suggestion, persuasion, and the giving of advice. These interventions were used haphazardly without any understanding of the therapeutic process and without a theoretical rationale for their application. Fromm-Reichmann writes, "It is to the immortal credit of Sigmund Freud that he was the first to understand and describe the psychotherapeutic process in terms of an interpersonal experience between patient and psychiatrist, and that he was the first to call attention to and study the personality of the psychiatrist, as well as that of the patient and their mutual interpersonal relationship" (Fromm-Reichmann, 1950, p. 3). In the course of exploring the working of his patient's minds, Freud developed the method of psychotherapy which he called "psychoanalysis." The techniques of the psychoanalytic method have proved so valid that they are utilized not only in other psychoanalytically oriented methods, but also in methods developed by psychotherapists who disagree with some of Freud's theoretical concepts or who may even reject them in totality. Moreover, these techniques have stood the test of time well. Greenson writes "It is an impressive fact that the fundamentals of psychoanalytic technique that Freud laid down in five short papers some fifty years ago still serve as the basis of psychoanalytic practice. No acknowledged major changes or advances have taken hold in standard psychoanalytic technique" (Greenson, 1967, p. 3).

COMPONENTS OF INDIVIDUAL PSYCHOTHERAPY

The three essential components of individual psychotherapy are: the patient, the therapist, and the setting in which the therapeutic interaction occurs. The requirements for each of these components are most specifically stated for psychoanalytic therapy, but many of them are also recommended in other methods of psychotherapy. Each of these three components will be discussed briefly.

What kinds of patients can benefit from individual psychotherapy? Chessick (1969, p. 201) replies, "When something has gone wrong on the road to emotional maturity and the individual is so in the grips of psychopathology that a reasonable and fruitful approach to life cannot be followed, it is time for psychotherapy." Fromm-Reichmann's answer is, "Anyone who consults a psychiatrist about marked emotional difficulties in living of which he wishes to be freed and who appears to be flexible and sincere, or shows the potentialities for both." In this category she includes character neuroses, neurotics, psychotics, and people with psychosomatic symptoms (Fromm-Reichmann, 1950, pp. 55–56). From Freud's time to the present most candidates for psychotherapy, especially individual psychotherapy, have come from the middle or upper class. Freud predicted that, in the future, "institutions or out-patient clinics will be started, to which analytically-trained physicians will be appointed, so that men who would otherwise give way to drink, women who have nearly succumbed under their burden of privations, children for whom there is no choice but between running wild or neurosis, may be made capable, by analysis, of resistance and of efficient work" (Freud, 1967, p. 9). Gould reports one step toward the fulfillment of Freud's prediction in his account of providing psychotherapy for blue-collar workers, members of an auto workers' union. Although the blue-collar worker has been considered a poor risk for psychotherapy because of lack of verbal skills, Gould found that this was not the case. However, he concludes, "Modified and new psychotherapeutic measures, adapted to suit the life style and value system of the blue collar worker, are necessary if the therapist is to be effective" (Gould, 1969, pp. 35–37).

THE THERAPIST

Who may practice psychotherapy and what are his requirements? According to Derner, "A psychotherapist is a person trained in psychotherapy. He may be a physician, psychiatrist, psychologist, social worker, minister, nurse, or other professional in terms of his disciplinary affiliation. However, if he is trained to do psychotherapy, he is a psychotherapist" (Derner, 1960, p. 131). In no other form of treatment engaged in by members of the health professions does the personality of the practitioner play such an important role in the success or failure of the treatment. At the present time, there is no agreement as to what the desirable personal characteristics of a psychotherapist should be. According to Knight, a good psychotherapist has "a fundamental liking for people, a conviction of the dignity, worth and potentiality of the individual, a curiosity regarding bio-psychological-economic factors influencing human emotions and behavior, a high sense of personal integrity, flair for empathizing with the

psychological experiences of others and a talent for verbal communication" (Knight, 1954, p. 68). Criteria derived from a study of therapists'
personalities by Strupp (quoted by Riess, 1960, p. 108) are:

> Psychotherapy is maximally effective when the therapist is able (a) to relate to the
> patient in a warm, empathic manner, so that the person of the therapist, as revealed
> in the relationship, will, in time, serve as a new, more mature, and more desirable
> model of reality than past interpersonal relationships; and (b) by appropriate
> technical devices to demonstrate . . . the self-defeating character of the patient.

Training of a Therapist

Since the personality of the therapist is of primary importance in
psychotherapy, most teachers of prospective psychotherapists recommend that trainees undergo a period of personal therapy. Riess states,
"The practice for which the person is to be trained involves intimately
the personality of the practitioner, and it is therefore imperative that
the training be accompanied by a personal analysis of the student"
(Riess, 1960, p. 106). Fromm-Reichmann also strongly endorses personal therapy for the prospective therapist. She states that the inner
security and self-respect which the therapist must maintain during the
stormy events which occur in the course of therapy require the
support derived from personal therapy. Personal therapy will also help
the therapist to handle his professional relationships with patients and
to keep his personal life apart from his professional life. By becoming
aware of his own dissociated and repressed experiences, the therapist
is better able to understand and help his patients to reveal repressed
elements in their lives. Fromm-Reichmann warns that because of the
interrelatedness between therapist's and patient's interactions, and
because of the interpersonal character of the psychotherapeutic process, any attempt at intensive psychotherapy is fraught with danger
when the therapist has not had personal therapy (Fromm-Reichmann,
1950, pp. 41–42).

A certain background in structured, academic courses is also
necessary. The specific courses may vary somewhat from training
program to training program, but essentially they must include psychology, human growth and development, and psychiatry. Riess
recommends psychology, human behavior, physiology, pathology,
social psychology and psychiatry, experimental design, and research
methology (Riess, 1960, p. 106). Recently, there is a beginning recognition that some content from the humanities is desirable in the training
program (Popper, 1965). Richness of life experiences is considered as
important as academic achievement by Bone (1960, p. 38). All teachers
of psychotherapy agree that supervised experience is the most valu-

able method for gaining knowledge and skill in practicing psychotherapy. Chessick writes, "Intensive individual long-term psychotherapy is a specific discipline that must be learned through supervised practice after one is healthy enough to at least hear what the patient is saying" (Chessick, 1969, p. 4). He also states that there are three generally accepted ways of teaching psychotherapy—individual supervision, case seminars, and reading—either alone or in seminars (Chessick, 1969, p. 161).

THE PSYCHOTHERAPEUTIC SETTING

Part of the formal aspect of treatment which Menninger referred to in his definition of psychotherapy is the psychotherapeutic setting or situation, that is, the climate and the conditions under which the interactions of the psychotherapy process take place. Great importance is placed on this component in psychoanalytic psychotherapy, in which the term used to define these conditions is *the analytic situation*. Greenson defines the analytic situation as the physical framework and the routine procedures of psychoanalytic practice which form an integral part of the process of being analyzed. He states that although one or more elements may be modified without interfering with the therapy, nevertheless, the setting does influence the various processes which occur in treatment. This is especially evident in the evolution of various transference reactions (Greenson, 1967, pp. 408–409).

Some of these elements include the development of an intense, emotional relationship between patient and therapist (the transference relationship); the development of a climate of security and trust in which the patient is able to reveal painful memories and in which he can regress without embarrassment, which is fostered by the use of the couch; the requirement that the patient follow the "basic rule" to speak whatever comes to his mind freely, to report somatic sensations, blanknesses, blocking, dreams, and so forth, and to obey the prohibition against acting out rather than discussing a problem. Some of the analyst's requirements are to observe and comment on the patient's behavior during the analytic session, to be able to empathize with the patient, to assure privacy and confidentiality of transactions in the therapy situation, and, the most important requirement, to be able to listen without being influenced by one's own experiences and values.

Fromm-Reichmann adds to this list the option that both therapist and patient have to agree or refuse to work with the other in therapy. However, once having accepted the patient, the therapist has the responsibility to continue to treat him in spite of unpleasant behavior or unexpected difficulties which may develop during the course of treatment (Fromm-Reichmann, 1950, pp. 39–42). Menninger comments that the "rules of the game" were worked out empirically by Freud, and they have been little improved upon or changed since his formulations of 1913 in "The Further Recommendations in the Technique of Psychoanalysis" (Freud, 1913), a paper which Menninger believes every student of psychoanalysis should almost memorize (Menninger, 1958, pp. 30–31).

THE CONTRACT

In addition to the above operational conditions, there are a number of reality-oriented conditions which must be discussed by therapist and patient. These include practical matters such as the setting of the fee and payment intervals; the time, place, and duration of the therapy sessions; the purpose for which therapy is sought; and the patient's expectations and the goals of therapy. The combination of the operational conditions and the physical or reality-oriented conditions makes up the content of the "contract." Mutual agreement as to what constitutes the contract can obviate much misunderstanding in later stages of the course of therapy and also save time which otherwise must be expended by the therapist to clarify and rectify vague or mistaken impressions of the patient.

Although the criteria for the three components of psychotherapy are rather rigidly defined in the psychoanalytic model, practitioners of other forms of psychotherapy have found it useful to incorporate many of the principles in their own practice, either directly or in a modified form, as, for example, substituting a comfortable chair for the analytic couch, or utilizing modified psychoanalytic techniques, such as some of the action techniques, to treat patients generally considered unsuitable for psychoanalysis, such as chronic schizophrenics, persons with personality disorders, and the aged.

The terms of the contract should be discussed with the patient either before or in the early initial sessions of treatment. This discussion should include the nature of the therapeutic relationship, the patient's role, and the therapist's role.

THE PROCESS OF INDIVIDUAL PSYCHOTHERAPY

Individual psychotherapy consists of a series of scheduled psychotherapeutic sessions of therapist and patient which roughly can be divided into three phases, (1) an introductory phase, in which a psychotherapeutic relationship is developed, (2) a working phase, which is utilized to achieve specific therapeutic goals, and (3) a termination phase, in which a gradual dissolution of the therapeutic relationship takes place. In actual practice a hard-and-fast line cannot be drawn between these three phases as the patient progresses in treatment. The length of time required for individual therapy varies according to the kinds of problems encountered during the course of therapy, the degree of severity of the patient's problems, the therapist's skill, and many other factors. Depending on the particular circumstances, duration of treatment may be long-term, i.e., six months to one or more years, or brief, i.e., limited to less than twelve sessions.

Phase I. The Introductory Phase

The first phase of psychotherapy is primarily one of the therapist and the patient getting to know one another and establishing a therapeutic relationship. As in the beginning of any relationship, each needs time to observe the other person, to become acquainted with his characteristic ways of expressing himself, and to make the first tentative exploratory moves in finding out what the other is like as a person. Ruesch says that the first contact has to be made through whatever media and channels will reach the patient—conversation, play, or work (Ruesch, 1961). If the patient is able to talk, the therapist, in responding to him, uses the same terminology that the patient uses. With mute patients, the therapist may need to use nonverbal as well as verbal communication to establish contact with the patient.

After the contact has been established with the patient, the therapist focuses his attention on observing the patient's behavior, listening to him in order to learn as much as possible about him from his own words, and trying to understand the nature of his difficulties. He also begins to build up the personal ties between the patient and himself by accepting him as a person and engendering in him a feeling of security and trust. One of the mistakes an inexperienced therapist is prone to make in his eagerness to develop a good relationship with the patient is to allow the relationship to become a social one. Regarding this tendency, Fromm-Reichmann (1950, p. 46) writes:

> Deep down in his mind, no patient wants a nonprofessional relationship with his therapist, regardless of the fact that he may express himself to the contrary. Something in him senses, as a rule in spite of himself, that an extra-professional relationship with his psychiatrist will interfere with a patient's tendency toward change and improvement in his mental condition. Moreover, the psychiatrist who enters into a social relationship with his patient may easily become sufficiently involved himself in the nonprofessional aspects of this relationship to be rendered

incapable of keeping control over the professional aspects of the doctor-patient relationship.

In the early stages of developing a relationship, a great deal of flexibility is needed. Each patient must be approached differently. For example, with highly verbal, psychoneurotic patients, one can move in rapidly. Shy, defensive, or withdrawn patients may need to be seen many times before they show any signs of response to the therapist. Often such a patient needs to become accustomed to the appearance and physical presence of the therapist before any interaction can take place. Some patients initially can tolerate only very brief sessions. Such patients include the suspicious, fearful patient, the very anxious patient, and the patient with a short span of attention, such as the acute or chronic brain-damaged patient, the mentally retarded, and the physically weak, debilitated patient. Interactions with these patients may have to be short and frequent. Later on, the duration of the interactions or sessions may be increased gradually as the patient improves. The therapist learns to terminate any interaction before the patient becomes fatigued or restless. Except for some unusual circumstance, it is generally not advisable for a therapeutic session to last longer than an hour.

The tasks that the therapist should accomplish in the first phase are: (1) facilitate the patient's ability to communicate his difficulties verbally; (2) develop a bond of trust and a feeling of security in the patient; (3) become aware of the main difficulties which interfere with the patient's successful functioning; (4) assess his strengths and weaknesses; and (5) determine what aspects of the patient's problems the therapist can be most helpful in resolving or ameliorating. The first task is to facilitate communication. For a number of reasons many patients initially find it difficult to talk freely. Some patients are unaccustomed to talking about themselves; others would rather do something about their problems than talk about them; and still others, such as schizophrenic patients, distrust words. Whatever the reason, the therapist should encourage, and even at times teach, patients to express themselves verbally. In this introductory phase of treatment therapy, sessions should be relatively unstructured, with the patient allowed maximum freedom to talk about anything he wishes. The therapist, playing a passive and permissive role, is primarily interested in observing the patient and in creating a climate in which the patient feels comfortable to talk.

Development of the Relationship As the patient continues to meet regularly with his therapist, it becomes easier for him to talk. He begins to experience the gratifying feeling of being accepted, of having someone genuinely interested in him as a person and who is concerned about his problems—an experience which most patients rarely, if ever, have previously encountered. The patient also begins to know and trust his therapist. However, shortly after this unaccustomed but highly pleasurable phase of the relationship, it is not uncommon to have the patient engage in some testing-out behavior to determine whether the therapist is actually as trustworthy as he appears to be. The therapist's truthfulness, sincerity, and reliability are all called into question at this time. This period of testing-out behavior on the part of the patient is often a difficult one for the therapist to endure. However, it is a necessary step in the development of the bond between patient and therapist. When the patient has resolved his doubts and ambivalent feelings, the relationship is on a firmer and often more realistic basis. Even after the initial period, some patients will continue to test the therapist from time to time during the course of the relationship, but usually briefly, and in a much milder form. Toward the end of the first phase of the relationship, the therapist attempts to gauge the strength of the therapist-patient bond in order to determine whether it is strong enough to tolerate the stresses which will be placed on it during the working phase of the relationship therapy.

Appraisal As the patient talks, the therapist listens and mentally begins to organize the data which the patient provides. Knight (1954, p. 68) describes this mental process as follows:

> The salient elements of the model (for appraisal of the patient) come to be automatically included, and comprehensive observations in a sequence arise from the spontaneous unfolding of the patient's account of himself. . . . With a great deal of intent listening and skillful questioning the examiner follows the unfolding material, noting significant elements, making and testing hypotheses as he explores the psychopathology, the adaptive capacities or ego strengths, the nature and strength of the motivation toward recovery, the external life factors which may operate for or against recovery, the kind of communication of which the patient is capable, and the capacity he shows to observe himself and to reflect retrospectively upon his feelings and experiences in their psychological aspects.

In making an appraisal of a patient, the therapist tries to determine in what ways the patient is not able to function adequately. Functional areas which should be appraised include the patient's intrapersonal or self-system, that is, how well his body functions physically and psychologically; his primary interpersonal system, or how well he is able to relate to the people and objects in his immediate environment, i.e., the members of his family, his intimate friends, his pets, and his home; and his secondary interpersonal system, indicative of how well he functions in his work relationships, in the community, and in the world in which he lives.

Other areas which should be evaluated include the strength of the patient's motivation to get well, the factors which help or hinder his ability to function more adequately, and the suitability of the therapy for this paricular patient. Some patients are strongly motivated to get well. These are often the patients with a great investment in their careers or in their family relationships. However, many psychiatric patients lack motivation to get well—some because they have been ill for a long time and have lost hope, some because the secondary gains of illness provide advantages they would not have if well, and some because they would have to face a life situation so bleak that if they recover, they would have no incentive to continue living.

The patient's assets and liabilities should be determined by evaluating his general health, physical energy, impulse control, ego strength, general intelligence, and ability to communicate, as well as external factors such as supportive family members and friends, economic resources, work or professional opportunities, and social and cultural interests. These data would enable the therapist to determine what factors are working in the patient's favor that could be utilized in planning the strategy of treatment, and what factors would need to be counteracted. During the first phase of therapy, therapist and patient test whether the patient responds well to this type of psychotherapy. For example, after working with a patient for a number of weeks, the therapist may reach the conclusion that the intimacy of a one-to-one relationship is too threatening to him. Again, he may discover that another patient whose impulse control is very weak cannot tolerate the permissiveness of this form of therapy.

Phase II. The Working Phase

The second phase of individual psychotherapy begins when the patient and therapist have achieved a good working relationship which is strong enough to enable the patient to face unpleasant and painful aspects of his problems and to accede to the inherent demands of therapy to change his behavior. It may take weeks or even months to reach this stage with some patients; with others it may be achieved in a relatively short time. Once a relationship has reached this stage, every effort should be made to move the patient along in the therapeutic process; that is, the patient is expected to work at his problems. One of the important goals at this time is to help him to make more effective contact with reality. Schmideberg (1958, p. 193) writes:

> The therapist should act as the patient's reality sense; decide which aspects of the patient's personality are normal or potentially normal, which should be developed,

and which discouraged. His ideas of magic and manic reactions must be curbed. We should try to give him a more realistic idea of his assets and limitations without hurting his feelings. We must try to modify his environment if possible or teach him to do so, and get him to accept what cannot be changed. He must be taught how to get on with people, how their minds work, how they react to him, to connect cause and effect, and to cope with his own moods, get over unhappy feelings and get more enjoyment from what he has.

Other goals include helping the patient to achieve a sense of his own worth, adequate feelings of security, and the ability to express or control his emotions appropriately, within reasonable limits, and without fear or guilt; also, to facilitate his ability to relate to others and to encourage work habits. Schmideberg (1960) states that employment gives him some hope and purpose and a sense of continuity and also forces him to suppress, at least temporarily, abnormal and antisocial reactions. Fromm-Reichmann's goals for therapy go beyond that of solving the patient's difficulties in living and relieving his symptoms. She believed that "self-realization" is a practical psychotherapeutic goal of paramount importance. She defined "self-realization" as an individual's ability to use his talents, skills, and powers to obtain personal satisfaction according to his own set of values, and his ability to reach out for and fulfill his needs for satisfaction (biological needs) and security (psychological needs) insofar as these needs could be satisfied without infringing on the rights or well-being of others. It is also Fromm-Reichmann's thought that the psychotherapeutic experience should provide the patient with the tools for the maintenance of his emotional stability during subsequent periods of uncertainty, frustration, and unhappiness (Fromm-Reichmann, 1950, pp. 34–35).

Goals for each patient should be individualized. Priorities should also be determined. These are arrived at in a number of ways. For example, goals aimed at preserving the patient's life would take precedence over all others. Another high-priority goal would be one that aims to change behavior which makes the patient unacceptable to others or which constitutes an environmental hazard. The patient's willingness to work on a particularly troublesome problem also holds high priority. Often it is helpful to ask the patient what aspect of his life he is most dissatisfied with and would like most to change. Goals may be short-term or long-term: short-term goals are those which generally pertain to immediate problems, often of a practical nature; long-term goals are those concerned with complex or chronic problems. Goals need to be evaluated from time to time and changed as necessary.

Coping with Specific Problems After the goals have been determined and priorities set, therapist and patient then begin to focus their attention on one specific sample after another of the patient's behavior or difficulty in functioning. They may begin with a topic or item with a high-priority goal, or a current problem that requires immediate attention. The therapist encourages the patient to talk about the topic as fully as possible. Ruesch (1961, p. 216) characterizes this middle period as consisting of detailed work, in which daily events are scrutinized and anecdotes of the past are avoided. Together therapist and patient try to understand the problem and to find ways of coping with the difficulty other than the one which the patient has been using unsuccessfully.

Testing New Patterns of Behavior Ruesch (1961) believes that true life experience is an important prerequisite for improvement. He writes, "Unless the patient can experiment and test reality in the areas of his difficulties, no amount of insight, discussion, and reconstruction is capable of altering repetitive behavior patterns." He must replace destructive behavior with adaptive behavior. He must expose himself to problem situations and practice coping with them. In order to integrate his new behavior it is most important that he have a "good" experience or response to give him a feeling that the new behavior will be successful (Wolberg, 1954). Schmideberg (1960) writes, "I use every device I can think of to push, or let the environment push him [the patient] into normal situations, and afterward, make him aware of having acted normally and having derived satisfaction from this."

Some patients need to be warned about too easy a victory, and others of possible disappointments. Therapeutic work on a given problem is not complete until the solution has been successfully applied a number of times and in a variety of situations. This is the "working through" process. Wolberg writes, "Therapeutic progress is gauged by the ability of the patient to apply what he has learned toward a more constructive life adaptation (Wolberg, 1954). When the working-through process has been completed with one problem, therapist and patient are ready to select another problem to work on. This process, repeated over and over again, constitutes the main task of the middle period.

Nurse-Therapist as Educator In the course of helping the patient to solve his difficulties in everyday life, the nurse-therapist often becomes involved in a considerable amount of education and reeducation of the patient. In Ruesch's words, "That which was traumatic and repetitive has to be undone. That which was not learned at home has to be acquired" (Ruesch, 1961). In nurse-patient psychotherapy, it is often possible for a patient to undergo a corrective emotional experience which may counteract previous unhappy experiences with parental figures early in life. For example, a person may learn how it

PSYCHOTHERAPY AND THE NURSE

feels to be accepted instead of rejected, to be regarded as worthwhile instead of to be ignored, to experience human closeness instead of loneliness. Mere exposure of a person to a beneficent influence does not constitute a corrective emotional experience. According to Alexander (1948, pp. 256–257) the underlying principle of corrective emotional experience "is a consciously planned regulation of the therapist's own emotional responses to the patient's material (countertransference) in such a way as to counteract the harmful effects of the parental attitudes."

Ruesch (1961) speaks of the "lacunae in life experiences," that is, the gaps of knowledge and experience so frequently encountered in many psychiatric patients. These gaps often contribute to the patient's poor comprehension of reality, problems in communication, immature judgment, and inappropriate behavior. Lacunae or gaps are not always apparent in encounters with the individual in ordinary social situations. Frequently they are revealed only during the course of a sustained relationship with a trusted and observant therapist. Sometimes these gaps are due to lack of information or knowledge necessary for successful functioning in everyday life, as, for example, inadequate sexual or other anatomical or physiological information.

Another kind of knowledge commonly found lacking in patients relates to basic knowledge about getting along with people. It is also surprising how many patients are ignorant of many practical details of everyday living. Without much difficulty the nurse-therapist can generally supply the patient with the missing factual data, or else refer him to sources where he can obtain it for himself. However, the missing emotional experiences in the patient's life are more difficult to remedy. Nevertheless it is often possible to overcome, to some degree, the effects of emotional deprivation in childhood through the positive emotional bonds which have been built up between patient and therapist over a period of time. The best-known illustration of this is the favorable effect of therapeutic mothering on children deprived of maternal affection in early life (A. Freud and Burlingham, 1944).

The Therapeutic Situation as Laboratory Several other therapeutic opportunities occur during the course of this middle working period. One is the utilization of what Fromm-Reichmann refers to as "the vicissitudes of the mutual interrelationship" between therapist and patient, that is, the happenings, behaviors, and interactions which develop in the presence of both therapist and patient during their contacts with one another. The therapeutic situation provides a wonderful laboratory setting in which not only isolated samples of behavior can be observed and investigated, but also the ebb and flow of the patient's progress over a period of time can be noted, including repetitive behavior, extinction or innovation of specific behaviors, characteristic behavior patterns, new coping mechanisms, and changes in direction of life goals. Insights obtained in this process of mutual observation, exploration, and understanding are more than intellectual achievements, they are also emotional experiences. The most valuable things in therapy, according to Reik (1948), cannot be learned; they can only be experienced.

Another experiential learning is the use of the therapeutic setting to provide an opportunity for the patient to explore new ideas, test psychological principles, and try out new behaviors by using the therapist as a sounding board or even as a sparring partner. In this protective milieu, the patient can gain confidence and develop some coping skills which will be later be useful to him in real life situations. Wolberg believes that the therapist should encourage such experimentation and suggests using role-playing techniques during the therapeutic session to facilitate the development of such skills (Wolberg, 1954). Consciously or unconsciously, the patient often uses the therapist as a model, especially in his attempts to improve his interpersonal relationships. Although most therapists scrupulously try to avoid imposing their own ethical and cultural values on their patients, undoubtedly many patients become aware of the therapist's personal philosophy and are influenced by it to the extent that they incorporate parts of it in their own life philosophy.

Phase III. The Termination Phase

Menninger speaks of a "turning point" in the course of therapy. The patient begins to experience a few successes both in therapy and in daily life. "It is an inescapable fact that if certain pressures are relieved, symptoms sometimes disappear and the sense of 'recovery,' or increased well-being and relative 'independence' force practical considerations to the fore" (Menninger, 1958, p. 161). The patient realizes that he has learned much from psychotherapy and begins to think that he may be able to go on learning by himself. The next consideration is termination of therapy, and with this consideration come the questions of whether the patient has made sufficient progress in therapy to warrant this and whether the patient is emotionally ready to give up his therapeutic relationship with his therapist.

Criteria for the termination of psychotherapy are not well defined in the literature. In fact, many writers do not discuss it at all. Fromm-Reichmann says that the patient is ready for termination when he can see people and situations as they are rather than as shadows of his past experiences; when he can manage his interpersonal relationships in ways appropriate to actual circumstances; and when he can place a realistic evaluation on his therapist and his relationship to him. "One criterion for tentatively appraising the success of treatment is brought about by the discontinuation of the patient's previous complaints and symptomatology, another means of evaluation may be given by the patient's sense of regained competence and the corroboration of this sense of competence in terms of actual accomplishment" (Fromm-Reichmann, 1950, p. 192). Menninger states that in a general way we can say that better relationships with himself, better relationships with others, and better utilizations of work, play, and other sublimations indicate such a satisfactory adjustment (Menninger, 1958, p. 165).

The decision to terminate therapy should be made mutually by both therapist and patient. "Patient and therapist should be satisfied with the results of their psychotherapeutic collaboration if and when the patient has gained a sufficient degree of lasting insight into his interpersonal operations and their dynamics to enable him, in principle, to handle them adequately" (Fromm-Reichmann, 1950, p. 188). In a similar vein, Menninger writes, "Ideally, of course, the situation is one in which the analyst is satisfied with the results of many months of work together, the patient is satisfied, and the reports from friends and associates are favorable" (Menninger, 1958, p. 163). When therapist and patient have agreed that termination is in order, it becomes necessary to set a specific date for termination. There are various ways of accomplishing this. Menninger writes (1958, p. 173–174),

> When I feel that the point of maximum benefit is approaching, based on criteria discussed, I begin to look for expressions of a similar opinion from the patient. If I get them, I incline to concur with him. Perhaps I answer with a, "why not, indeed." . . . If no "protest symptoms" appear, we gradually begin to speak in more definite terms as to just when it might be and I observe his reactions to this.

With such observation by the therapist and by allowing the patient the time to work through his feelings, a successful termination can be made. However, problems in termination often arise even when the patient is carefully prepared for it.

Problems of Termination   Termination is generally accompanied by two reactions that can interfere seriously with the successful resolution of the therapist-patient relationship if the therapist is not adequately prepared to deal with them. These reactions are (1) a marked change in the patient's attitude toward the therapist, and (2) a type of grief reaction. During this period the therapist may be surprised to note that the patient begins to make critical remarks about him both personally and professionally. These remarks may be both franker and more hostile than any previously made. Their purpose seems to be to help the patient achieve a more realistic evaluation of the therapist as a person, and also to promote a more social and peer-oriented relationship with him. This behavior helps the patient loosen the emotional bonds (transference) between himself and the therapist. It helps him to become emotionally independent in very much the same way that an adolescent frees himself from parental bonds by rebellious behavior. If the therapist is surprised by this behavior and does not recognize it as a sign of therapeutic progress, he is likely to react with hurt or anger and thus block the termination process.

The grief reaction is inherent in the termination of every meaningful relationship, including the therapeutic relationship. The therapist who is not aware of this may overlook signs of grief, particularly if the patient has difficulty in expressing his feelings or if his way of expressing grief takes a different form from the usual one. Therefore, the therapist should try to identify behavior which could have its origins in the patient's feelings of loss, and should validate these clues with him. Grief reaction at the termination of a relationship is essentially similar to that toward the loss of anything of great personal value. The patient must go through a mourning process in which the passage of time is one of the therapeutic factors. For this reason, a sufficient amount of time must be allowed in the termination plan. The process can be ameliorated by encouraging the patient to talk about the impending separation, about his feelings regarding it, and about his feelings regarding the loss of his therapist. When these areas have been thoroughly explored, it is helpful to focus his attention on the gains he has made during the relationship and on his plans for the future.

Because the relationship in psychotherapy is a mutual interrelationship, the therapist cannot emerge from the experience without also suffering from some feelings of loss at the termination of therapy. Many therapists are loath to recognize these feelings in themselves, and consequently cannot understand their own letdown feelings and mild depression. The mere acknowledgment of the reason for these feelings lessens the anxiety regarding them. However, it is most helpful at this time for the therapist to discuss his reactions fully with a consultant or some other understanding individual.

Specific Patient Reactions to Termination Common reactions to the termination of the transference relationship include (1) anger at the therapist openly expressed, (2) acting-out behavior, (3) regressive behavior, (4) repressive behavior, and (5) acceptance.

Anger. The patient who expresses his anger openly displays a very natural and healthy reaction. It speaks well for the relationship that the patient feels secure enough to do this. Such a patient is usually well along the road to recovery. Generally, after the patient has expressed his anger, he will have a change of mood and settle down to spend the remaining time in therapy working constructively on his problems. Not many patients are able to work through their problems as easily as this.

Acting out. Patients who act out their resentment are far more common and are more difficult to deal with. These patients may try to save face by rejecting the therapist before he can reject them by abruptly terminating therapy. The patient should be helped to understand his behavior and be given additional emotional support during this period.

Regression. Other patients may regress by reverting to symptoms or behavior which they once utilized but relinquished during the course of treatment. This regression is usually transitory and serves as a nonverbal protest against the termination of therapy. The response of the therapist to this behavior should be to give the patient understanding and support without becoming anxious or allowing the patient to become frightened or discouraged by his temporary setback.

Repression. Probably the most difficult to handle is the patient who gives no sign of response when the therapist mentions a definite date of termination. It is easy to interpret this as indifference. Actually, it represents a profound emotional reaction which the patient is unable to express. The patient attempts to avoid the reality of the dissolution of the relationship by means of repression and denial. The prospect of being left alone reactivates all the painful feelings centered about experiences of rejection in childhood when the patient could do nothing about the situation. He overreacts to this new "desertion" with the same feelings of impotence and despair.

The inexperienced therapist has difficulty in realizing that behind the bland and apathetic expressions of these patients are often profound depressions or hallucinatory states. To prevent such a reaction, the therapist should introduce the subject of termination repeatedly in conversations with the patient in order to give him an opportunity to express his feelings. Often the patient does not even hear or grasp the meaning of the words the first few times that the therapist tries to discuss termination; or the patient may hear and then promptly forget what has been said. The therapist should help the patient verbalize his feelings of resentment even though he implies that this is a preposterous idea and continues to deny such feelings. Sometimes it helps the patient if the therapist expresses the feeling that he will miss the patient. This often gives the patient tacit permission to admit that he, too, may have similar feelings. It may also help if the patient is told that on the termination of therapy the therapist will continue to be interested in his progress and in his efforts to get well.

Acceptance. Many patients are able to accept termination of the relationship realistically—that is, they express regret or even momentary resentment; however, they quickly adjust themselves to it. Such patients have achieved considerable emotional security. With the acceptance of termination the patient also accepts his new evaluation of himself as a person who can function independently of the parental figures in his past and who is confident that he can cope with the ordinary stresses and problems of daily life. "Patients should be prepared to meet the vicissitudes of their future life without anxiety or at least with sufficiently diminished anxiety that they can experience them without recurrence of the neurotic or psychotic responses which originally brought them into treatment" (Fromm-Reichmann, 1950, p. 190).

REFERENCES

Alexander, Franz (1948): *Fundamentals of Psychoanalysis*, W. W. Norton & Company, Inc., New York.

Bone, Harry (1960): "The Relationship between the Purpose of Psychotherapy and the Preparation for Practicing It," in Nicholas P. Dellis and Herbert K. Stone (eds.), *The Training of Psychotherapists*, Louisiana State University, Baton Rouge, pp. 27–42.

Chessick, Richard D. (1969): *How Psychotherapy Heals*, Science House, Inc., New York.

Dellis, Nicholas P., and Herbert K. Stone (1960): *The Training of Psychotherapists*, Louisiana State University, Baton Rouge.

Derner, Gordon F. (1960): "An Interpersonal Approach to Training in Psychotherapy," in Nicholas P. Dellis and Herbert K. Stone (eds.), *The Training of Psychotherapists*, Louisiana State University, Baton Rouge, pp. 130–145.

Fleming, Joan (1967): "Teaching the Basic Skills of Psychotherapy," *Archives of General Psychiatry*, April, pp. 416–426.

Freud, Anna, and Dorothy Burlingham (1944): *Infants without Families*, International Universities Press, Inc., New York.

Freud, Sigmund (1913): "Further Recommendations in the Technique of Psychoanalysis," in *Collected Papers*, vol. 2, Basic Books, Inc., Publishers, New York.

———(1967): "Lines of Advance in Psychoanalytic Therapy," in Harold Greenwald (ed.), *Active Psychotherapy*, Atherton Press, Inc., New York, pp. 1–9.

Fromm-Reichmann, Frieda (1950): *Principles of Intensive Psychotherapy*, The University of Chicago Press, Chicago.

Gould, Robert E. (1969): "Dr. Strangeclass or: How I Stopped Worrying about the Theory and Began Treating the Blue-Collar Worker," *Mental Health Digest*, vol. 1, no. 4, pp. 35–37.

Greenson, Ralph R. (1967): *The Techniques and Practice of Psychoanalysis*, vol. 1, International Universities Press, Inc., New York.

Knight, Robert P. (1954): "Evaluation of Psychotherapeutic Techniques," in Robert P. Knight and Cyrus R. Friedman (eds.), *Psychoanalytic Psychiatry and Psychology*, International Universities Press, Inc., New York, pp. 65–78.

Menninger, Karl (1958): *Theory of Psychoanalytic Technique*, Basic Books, Inc., Publishers, New York.

Popper, Hans (1965): "A New Curriculum," *Annals of the New York Academy of Sciences*, Article 2, vol. 128, pp. 552–560.

Reik, Theodor (1948): *Listening with the Third Ear*, Farrar, Straus & Co., New York.

Riess, Bernard F. (1960): "The Selection and Supervision of Psychotherapists," in Nicholas P. Dellis and Herbert K. Stone (eds.), *The Training of Psychotherapists*, Louisiana State University, Baton Rouge, pp. 104–124.

Ruesch, Jurgen (1961): *Therapuetic Communication*, W. W. Norton & Company, Inc., New York.

Schmideberg, Melita (1960): "Principles of Psychotherapy," *Comprehensive Psychiatry*, June, pp. 186–193.

———(1958): "Values and Goals in Psychotherapy," *Psychiatric Quarterly*, April, pp. 233–265.

Whitaker, C. A., and T. P. Malone (1953): *The Roots of Psychotherapy*, McGraw-Hill Book Company, New York.

Wolberg, Lewis R. (1954): *The Technique of Psychotherapy*, Grune & Stratton, Inc., New York.

23

GROUP PSYCHOTHERAPY

Eleanor M. White

DEFINITION OF GROUP PSYCHOTHERAPY

Group psychotherapy has been as broadly defined as any meeting of two or more patients with a therapist for therapeutic reasons, and as narrowly as the psychoanalytic definition which states that only psychoanalytically oriented group therapy in which there is strict adherence to analyzing transference and resistance in the group and resulting in basic personality changes in individual members can be called group psychotherapy. Yalom (1970, p. vii) states in fact that "group psychotherapy" is too narrow a term, and that the practice should be referred to as "group therapies." Most definitions in use today agree that *group therapy* is a treatment modality in which two or more patients and one or more therapists engage in a helping process designed to explore psychiatric and emotional difficulties in order to bring about relief or distress, increase of self-esteem, insight, and improvement of behavior and social relations. The specific goals of any group will: (1) determine the procedures to be followed, (2) indicate the intensity of therapy, (3) define the role of the therapist, and (4) focus attention on either here-and-now events or historical and intrapsychic material. According to Mullan and Rosenbaum (1963, p. 47), the two main elements in the development of group therapy are man's need for group communication and the intervention in this communication of psychological insight.

CURRENT PERSPECTIVES IN GROUP THERAPY

Whereas originally group therapy was instituted on a wide-scale basis to handle vast numbers of patients efficiently, as was the case in World War II, today it is viewed as a valid modality in its own right with distinct advantages over individual therapy. The following elements of group therapy are referred to as the *curative factors*: altruism, group cohesiveness, universality, interpersonal learning (feedback and disclosure), guidance, catharsis, identification, family reenactment, insight, instillation of hope, and existential factors (Yalom, 1970, pp. 60–82). With these factors in mind, Mullan and Rosenbaum (1963, p. 24) state that to place patients in group therapy for any other reason than because of its effectiveness is "unscientific, improper, and even destructive." Group therapy owes much of its acceptance as a treatment modality to the successful alliances of several disciplines, such as: psychiatry, nursing, psychology, education, social work, and sociology. This has helped to avoid "an overreliance on traditional medical points of view and psychiatric overconcern with pathological functioning" (Mullan and Rosenbaum, 1963, p. 66). It is now generally accepted that group therapy may take place in an unlimited variety of settings and with persons of all social classes, all types of mental illness, and varied age groups.

Recent philosophical and theoretical issues concerning the practice of group therapy include: (1) the utilization of group dynamics in the therapy of patients as a major vehicle of change versus the therapist's awareness of group dynamics without focusing on them in the group; (2) the implications and advantages and disadvantages of the therapist's full participation as a group member in the experience, as occurs within the experiential-existential framework in which the therapist is viewed as another human being facing the same existential quandaries (Durkin, 1964, pp. 249–272); (3) the use of nonverbal exercises and sensory communication, especially touch, in group therapy (Mintz, 1969); and (4) the relationship and consequences for group therapy and group therapists resulting from the "growth-enhancing groups" that have sprung up throughout the country in the past few years.

TYPES OF GROUP THERAPY

Traditionally, therapy groups have been classified according to the therapeutic goals of the group, such as: regressive-reconstructive (implying total restructuring of the member's personality); repressive-constructive (implying strengthening of defenses and repression of inappropriate behaviors and feeling, etc.); the activity level of the therapist (directive or nondirective); and the level of analysis in terms of insight achieved (superficial or deep). Recently, however, current practitioners are tending to avoid such narrow labeling and speak of group therapy in terms of five main approaches, including those cited by Wolf (1967, pp. 135–137):

1. Reeducative group therapy, which includes elements of lecture and/or discussion for primarily homogeneous groups of patients providing information, socialization, support, and strengthening of defenses
2. Psychodrama groups, which utilize psychoanalytic principles and theories combined with structured dramatization of a patient's intrapersonal and interpersonal emotional difficulties, providing more depth and breadth of experience than that available through usual verbal psychotherapies
3. Experiential-existential group therapy, with an emphasis on the experiencing of immediate feelings rather than the rational exploration of these feelings, with the therapist participating as a full member of the group
4. Group-dynamic group therapy, in which the central focus is the group rather than the individual members, and in which the exploration of group themes, relationships, interactions, and reactions takes place
5. Psychoanalytic group therapy, based on the philosophy and techniques of psychoanalysis, including the exploration of historical data, the uncovering of unconscious material, the use of dreams, and the analysis of transference phenomena and resistance as they occur in the group

A final category of group therapy to be discussed is one that incorporates elements of some of the above groups and that is increasingly being practiced today under the name of *intensive interactional group therapy* or *intensive group therapy* (Yalom, 1970). This method of group therapy is one which, although based on the major contributions of psychoanalysis and the dynamic formulations of personality functions, places primary emphasis on the utilization of the ongoing group process and on awareness of what is presently happening rather than the exploration of historical material, except as it is currently impinging on a member's experience. It has as its aims the correction of distortions, the development of more satisfying relationships, the use of consensual validation, and the development of interpersonal learning. It is the latter approach that will act as the model for therapy to be discussed further in this chapter.

THE NURSE AND GROUP THERAPY

Prerequisite for Group Leadership

Perusal of the group therapy literature in terms of expectations of the group therapist quickly alerts the reader to the fact that the group leader must possess several personal as well as technical or academic skills and attributes. In that the leader will be the most powerful norm setter in a therapy group, it is vitally important for any group therapist to be able to be aware of and to examine the effects of his behavior and beliefs on the group (Whitaker and Lieberman, 1964; Yalom, 1970). In addition, the therapist must be able to communicate a sense of acceptance, accurate empathy, honesty, and genuineness to the group members. Several authors note that in essence there is "no place to hide" for the leader in a therapy group, as his personality is apparent to the members, and he should not attempt to put on a "therapeutic mask" when engaging in group work (Mullan and Rosenbaum, 1963; Durkin, 1964).

As the proliferation of therapy groups has occurred, there has been an increase in the number and variety of professional disciplines of mental health personnel participating as group therapists. Only recently has there been an attempt to establish consistent guidelines for the training of these persons under the auspices of either a teaching or a clinical institution (AGPA, 1970; Gauron et al., 1970). The depth and breadth of training must be commensurate with the type of group therapy to be conducted. In terms of prerequisites for conducting intensive but not psychoanalytic group therapy, the following important elements have been identified:

1. A firm grounding in the principles and practice of individual psychotherapy
2. The therapist's previous participation in a personal psychotherapeutic experience, including a group experience as a member
3. Experience in coleadership and in leading supervised group therapy experiences, preferably with both inpatient and outpatient groups
4. Didactic seminars on the theories and principles of group dynamics and group psychotherapy
5. Exposure to research in relation to the field

For the psychiatric nurse or clinical specialist in psychiatric nursing, it is assumed that the preparation for becoming a group therapist will occur in the structure of an accredited graduate program in psychiatric nursing or its equivalent.

Issues for the Psychiatric Nurse as Group Therapist

The prominent issues encountered by the nurse as a group therapist are related to questions of changing professional roles, interdisciplinary territoriality, and the role of the nurse in relation to the burgeoning human potential movement. Yalom (1970, p. 378) notes that the increasing emergence of therapy and nontherapy groups, and the blurring of professional boundaries and roles in relation to the questions of training groups versus therapy groups, patient versus nonpatient roles, and leader as member of the group, have led to confusion about who is or is not competent and qualified to conduct group therapy. This confusion, in turn, has led to the establishment of two camps: (1) the traditionalists, who have reacted territorially with resultant tightening of qualifications and prerequisites for practice, thereby in effect excluding the psychiatric nurse (AGPA, 1970; Stein, 1971), and (2) anti-establishmentarians or nontraditionalists who see didactic training as being antithetical to the development of an effective therapist. At the same time Yalom notes that the field of group therapy has become "ideologically cosmopolitan," with members of a variety of disciplines practicing group therapy (Yalom, 1970, p. x). In the middle between these two camps are many professionals of all mental health disciplines, including this writer, who believe that properly educated and trained psychiatric nurses can function beneficially and effectively as group therapists in a variety of group therapy situations.

Increasingly the group therapy literature includes nurses as members of interdisciplinary teams and coleaders in therapy groups. Gauron and others note that after a decade of debate, nurses have become acceptable as group therapists, and they describe a multidisciplinary training program which accepts psychiatric nurses as students. Most nursing authorities are in agreement that accredited master's programs in psychiatric nursing prepare nurses who are competent to conduct psychotherapeutic groups with minimal or fairly high goals of change, although most nurses are not prepared to do psychoanalytic group therapy (Werner, 1970; Rouslin 1964; Mereness, 1963).

At this point a major responsibility of nurse group therapists is to participate in interdisciplinary experiences, workshops, and conferences, and to contribute to the literature by writing clinical reports on the practice of group therapy by psychiatric nurses, thereby making themselves visible. Recent attendance at an American Group Psychotherapy Association conference vividly demonstrated this fact as time after time it was made clear that professionals of other disciplines had no realistic concept of what a psychiatric nurse is and what he is prepared to do. There was also very little awareness of the professional abilities of nurses with different levels of nursing preparation and education.

In relation to the current group movement, the nurse must identify and articulate his own professional-ethical philosophy in deciding where and/or how he will participate in such group experiences.

ESTABLISHMENT OF GROUP

Even before meeting the group members, the group leader must take into account several basic considerations regarding the requirements of the agency, the potential members, and the therapist himself. While most of the psychoanalytically oriented literature on group therapy discusses only the ideal criteria for therapy, it is wise to remember that ideal conditions cannot always be met in the real world. Therefore, the nurse therapist must be able to take into consideration the actual factors he is dealing with and make appropriate adaptations. This section of the discussion will focus on the influences of the agency, the physical setting, the requirements of the group and its individual members, and the therapeutic process. These considerations include the following:

1. The composition of the group: the members and leaders
2. The structure of meetings
3. Open versus closed group format
4. The physical arrangements
5. The use of equipment
6. The group contract
7. The preparation of patients for a group experience

Selection of Members—Criteria

In selecting members for a group experience, the leader must ask himself: What administrative policies relate to admission of members, and what are the specific and general psychological needs of this group? Agency policies may be such that the leader does not have actual control over the selection of members for the group—for example, members are assigned by administrative staff. If the leader is faced with the task of evaluating and selecting patients for a group therapy experience, he must keep in mind two interrelated and complex questions: (1) Is the patient a good candidate for a group experience? (2) If so, what particular group? Psychiatric literature is rampant with such multiple, varied, and even conflicting criteria for assessing patient suitability for group therapy that the leader may feel like asking, "Why screen at all?" Yalom criticizes existing methods of classifying and diagnostically labeling patients for purposes of selection for a group experience. He notes that the potpourri of symptoms and characterological, behavioral, and folk nomenclature are evidence of the need for a system of classification which can convey relevant, predictive information about interpersonal behavior (Yalom, 1970, p. 157).

The individual interview still remains the most satisfactory and commonly used screening tool. It should focus on the person's life style and history, with the interviewer asking questions which will elicit information regarding interpersonal relationships and group relationships, both in the past and at the present time. Patients who during the screening interview exhibit a tendency to use denial and projection in relation to their problems, or who identify themselves as seeking therapy because of external pressures, are likely to do poorly in a group therapy experience. Moreover, patients who demonstrate a high level of conflict regarding interpersonal intimacy, in the direction of either schizoid withdrawal or excessive maladaptive self-disclosure (and a need for "instant intimacy"), may become overwhelmed by the group or may push group members away by placing unrealistic demands on them. Foulkes and Anthony (1957) and Bach (1954) suggest letting potential members attend a group meeting on a trial basis and then letting the group members join in the decision regarding selection. Other therapists have experimented with placing patients in a waiting group to test out the way they will interact in a group prior to joining an ongoing group (Abrahams and Enright, 1965). This test may be practical in large outpatient clinics or a private practice but is not usually feasible in most agencies.

Although there are contradictions and overlappings in the literature regarding suitable/nonsuitable characteristics of patients for group therapy, these preferences are usually related to the personality of the leader in terms of therapeutic orientation, experience, personality, and background. It is also true that the selection criteria should not be applied in a vacuum but must take into consideration the structure, procedural goals, and composition of the available groups (Yalom, 1970, p. 157). It is also important to note that while all patients may not be suitable for a heterogeneous, intensive group experience, they may be suitable for a more specialized or homogeneous group therapy experience. The unfortunate results of including inappropriate members in a group include: (1) premature termination of therapy by the member, leading to a sense of failure or alienation on the part of the patient; (2) assumption by the member of the role of the group deviant; and (3) the creation of a sense of failure and discouragement in the group. Premature termination usually occurs when the group is perceived to be too expensive in terms of time, money, energy, anxiety, frustration, discouragement, or rejection (Yalom, 1970, p. 173).

Certain general categories of patients have difficulty participating in a meaningful way in an intensive group experience and tend to spend their energies defending themselves, to the detriment of the group and themselves. Patients in these categories include:

1. The brain-damaged
2. The acutely psychotic
3. Those patients with weak egos and poor interpersonal relationships, such as chronic schizophrenics
4. Drug addicts and alcoholics
5. The acutely suicidal
6. Those patients with weak superego development, such as psychopaths and infantile characters
7. Those patients with severe oedipal disturbances, including hysterical personalities and homosexuals
8. The hypochondriacal and psychosomatic personalities
9. The rigidly paranoid patients
10. The extremely passive-dependent personalities
11. Those patients who cannot share the therapist with other members of the group

Criteria for including patients in an intensive group psychotherapy experience are even less well defined and more difficult to delineate than exclusion criteria. The only study delineating pretherapy personality factors in relation to successful outcomes in group therapy found only two variables as predictive of success: (1) the patient's attraction to the group, and (2) the patient's general popularity with the group (Yalom et al., 1967). Freeman and Sweet (1954) see group therapy as being beneficial for those patients who: (1) exhibit fears of becoming dependent upon the therapist, (2) are likely to evoke countertransference reactions in the therapist, or (3) have rigid social roles and demonstrate a capacity for interpersonal relationships and an ability to act as a catalyst in the group and are in good contact with reality. Psychoanalytically oriented therapists such as Slavson (1955) designate as criteria: need for ego strength, enough superego development to experience empathy, at least a minimal satisfaction in a primary relationship in childhood, and no severe oedipal disturbance.

Whatever individual criteria are used, the leader must always ask himself: (1) what will be the effect of this patient on specific individuals already in the group? (2) what will be the effect of this person on the total group? and (3) how will I react to and handle this patient in the group?

Composition of the Group: Homogeneous versus Heterogeneous

One membership variable that will influence the group's functioning—and, therefore, the role of the leader—is that of the homogeneous or heterogeneous composition of the group. Yalom notes that although there is only a beginning knowledge available on the effects of group composition on group effectiveness, most clinicians attest to the fact that some groups "jell" while others do not. He states that the "critical variable is some, as yet unclear, blending of the members" (Yalom, 1970, pp. 191–192). Actually a truly homogeneous group would be hard to establish, except under research conditions, for this would be a highly select and narrow population. For purposes of this discussion a *homogeneous group* will be defined as one in which leaders and the members themselves view one or more major identifying characteristics and/or purposes for being in the group as being common to all members, such as groups of: all women with weight problems; all adolescents with a history of drug abuse; all males with low back pain; or all patients who have been hospitalized with similar emotional difficulties. Authors such as Kadis et al. (1963) and Slavson (1955) have discussed the definition of homogeneity based on diagnosis of underlying psychodynamic characteristics. Whitaker and Lieberman (1964) focus on: similar conflict areas and patterns of coping; degree of ego strength and capacity to tolerate anxiety.

Advantages of a homogeneous group include the following factors:

1. Members quickly identify with commonalities among themselves, and this may hasten the inclusion and cohesion process.
2. The members may be able to confront each other on their interaction patterns, knowing each other's styles of coping well—this has proved to be particularly helpful with drug abusers and adolescents.
3. Members who produce anxiety in others and set up scapegoating roles for themselves in a heterogeneous group may work more beneficially in a homogeneous group, as, for example, patients with sexual identity problems, and patients with the same physical symptoms or psychosomatic conditions.

Groups currently operating within this framework include Alcoholics Anonymous, Weight Watchers, and groups for drug abusers. One drawback to such a group is that the members can bind together in resistance against the leader when threatened by change, and can support each other's denial and resistance. Such patients may also receive a positive or negative identification by membership in a specially designated group, e.g., heroin users referring to themselves as "junkies," and suicidal patients assuming a "suicidal identity" (Kobler and Stotland, 1964).

A *heterogeneous group* is one in which members demonstrate a variety of identifying characteristics but have the commonality of seeking help for some emotional and/or physical problems. Advantages of a heterogeneous group include: increased interaction of members, increased sense of individuality concomitant with a sense of commonality, and an enlarged view of the world and other people as the group membership more accurately represents the wider world. In forming a heterogeneous group, it is wise to keep the heterogeneity within certain limits, particularly in terms of age, life experiences, and ego strength. Groups usually work better if the age of group members does not span more than twenty years. Age, sex, occupation, diagnosis, and psychiatric difficulties may be mixed. However, any person who is defined as a member of a minority group or as a deviant from the general society should be offered the support of another such person in the group, for example, two males in an otherwise all-female group, or two ethnic-minority members in an otherwise homogeneous group.

Types of Leadership

The selection of a leader, or leaders, for a particular group experience is, again, often determined by agency policy or client needs. The leader selected for a particular group of patients should be skilled in group techniques and in tune with the group's needs. Although all group leaders may not work well with every type of patient or group, it may be possible to match one leader who is active with a fast-moving group and another who is content to work at a slower pace with a slower-paced group. The question of a single leader as opposed to coleaders or multiple leaders is a widely discussed one. In reading the literature and in talking with practicing group leaders, this writer found little middle ground on the subject. Some leaders prefer the coleadership or multiple leadership format, while others feel just as strongly that there should be only one leader in a group. Again, agency requirements may influence actual practice. In some teaching institutions it is a common practice for trainees or students to be placed in a group with a more seasoned leader, or two trainees may be paired together.

Advantages and Disadvantages of the Coleadership Model When considering entering into a cotherapy relationship, the following advantages and disadvantages (MacLennon, 1970) need to be considered in relation to both the leaders and the members involved:

Advantages:
1. Cotherapy is useful for the training of a new therapist, who can observe an advanced leader in action and at the same time gradually increase his own participation in the leadership role as he feels comfortable and gains experience. This arrangement helps to decrease the anxiety of the beginning therapist and provides increased support for him.
2. Cotherapy provides the new and inexperienced therapist with the opportunity for increased validation of group process by feedback from the other leader.
3. Cotherapists may act as role models for members in terms of cooperation, feedback, direct and clear communication, and ability to disagree.

4. Cotherapy may recreate the primary family constellation, with the therapists either playing different parental roles or being perceived in such by the members. It is particularly helpful if the leaders are of different sexes, although two leaders of the same sex may be perceived as fulfilling male and female roles. Bales has demonstrated that two leaders in a group evolve different roles, one the task leader and the other the socioemotional leader (Bales, 1953). Similarly, roles of the "good guy" and the "bad guy" may evolve.

5. Cotherapy situations may both evoke and define transference reaction, making them easier to handle; also, if countertransference occurs, it may be dealt with in the context of the cotherapy relationship.

6. One therapist may focus on the group process and the total group while the other therapist may be focusing on an individual member.

7. One therapist may act essentially as a nonverbal observer and provide feedback on the process during a postsession meeting.

8. Cotherapy is particularly helpful in groups composed of families, adolescents, and psychotics who may need more structure and limits.

9. Cotherapy provides opportunities for therapists to assume sole leadership during absences of one therapist without disrupting the schedule of meetings and the continuity of group process.

Disadvantages:

1. The "junior therapist" may never be perceived as an equal or true cotherapist, which may create group tension and uncertainty regarding the leadership roles.

2. Cotherapists provide opportunity for the leaders to be split by the group, and for subgroupings to arise.

3. Cotherapy is seen as an expensive use of leaders' time, as the group cannot necessarily double in size and remain effective.

4. Any strain or disagreement between leaders is quickly sensed and leads to a tense and inhibited group.

For cotherapy to be instituted in a group, the following important conditions should be met: the leaders should meet together prior to the first group meeting and gain a sense of each other as persons so that their relationship is one of openness and respect; they may differ in their approach to group interventions, but they must not be of such divergent theoretical, philosophical, and operational positions that they cannot work comfortably together. The goals of such a team are the development of mutuality and an open exchange of ideas and views. Heilfron, in an excellent article, stresses the development of a "we-ness" between leaders with an appreciation of each other's strengths and weaknesses and open interaction without a sense of separation or absolute dependence (Heilfron, 1969). Leaders also need to be aware of their own competitive needs. The roles that they assume in the group may be meeting their own gratification needs rather than the needs of group members. In addition to an initial meeting(s), the leaders ideally should meet immediately after each group session for the purpose of reviewing the group meeting. This postsession meeting provides an excellent opportunity for the leaders to focus on total-group process, to validate their perceptions of group events, to identify needs and dynamics of individual patients, and to check out their own interactions. This gives therapists the opportunity to identify and comment on their relationship and interventions with members and each other.

Disagreement between Leaders

The question of the way disagreement between leaders is to be handled is important and widely discussed in the literature. Traditionally any disagreement should be voiced only outside the group meeting. The premise is that open disagreement is apt to recreate the family scene with resultant group anxiety, and that it leads to splitting and subgrouping of the group members. More recently, however, writers cite the advantages of expressing such disagreements openly (Heilfron, 1969). The advantages are that the leaders can act as role models in allowing for differences in handling disagreement and can be perceived as human beings in interaction with each other. Such behavior affords members an opportunity to see the group leaders as unique individuals. As stressed previously, such disagreements must take place within the context of a relationship of trust and respect. Yalom (1970, p. 318) warns that disagreement during the early life of the group's development should be dealt with in the postsession meetings to prevent the group from becoming immobilized with anxiety before a sense of trust in the leaders and the group is established. Another way to prevent subgrouping of patients is to have both therapists interview patients together before placing them in the group. This decreases the likelihood of an initial contact fostering an identification with one or the other of the leaders as "my therapist." McGee and Schuman, in their article on the cotherapy relationship, stress that the cotherapists should function in a sense of mutual involvement with all aspects of the group's life (McGee and Schuman, 1970, pp. 25–35).

Open and Closed Groups

The terms *open group* and *closed group* are used to refer to groups in which members may or may not be admitted during the life of the group. The open group has the advantages of:

1. Providing for the needs of individual members by allowing them to enter or leave the group at an optimal time in their recovery
2. Recreating the family constellation, into which family members are born and die

3. Approximating the real world, in which people are always dealing with "comings and goings"
4. Placing responsibility on both individual members and the group for decisions regarding admission and termination of members

Precautions the leader needs to take in an open group include:

1. Preparation of new patients for the group
2. Preparation of the group for new members
3. Prevention of scapegoating new members by older members who are acting out their own conflicts regarding sibling rivalry
4. Avoidance of too much self-disclosure by a new patient during the first meeting
5. If possible, the admission of only one or two members at a time to the group, to avoid the possibility of a division between "old" and "new" members

Open groups are by far the most common occurrence, especially since the trend in psychiatric care is away from extended inpatient and outpatient treatment. One study focusing on short-term (one to ten visits) group psychotherapy demonstrated that an open, short-term group therapy experience can be helpful for patients (Curry, 1971), while another found that this format was helpful for crisis-oriented group therapy with lower socioeconomic-status patients, a major factor being that "older" group members act as role models for newer members in the group (Allgeyer, 1970). However, a pitfall in an open-group experience may include the danger of much of the group's energy being devoted to the comings and goings of group members, to the detriment of any other therapeutic work being done.

Closed groups offer the advantage of not having the group process interrupted by the admission and termination of members, thus avoiding the possible development of hostility and competition that these interruptions engender in threatened group members. This format is also helpful in developing a sense of cohesion and identification in the group. A disadvantage in a long-term closed group is that it may become "stale" without the addition of new members or may decrease in size to such an extent that it no longer functions as a group. The closed group is used most often for short-term or crisis therapy groups, group dynamics laboratories, and sensitivity training programs.

Another consideration regarding the open or closed nature of a group is whether the group will be open to observers and visitors. Some groups make the rule that a significant other (such as a spouse or parent) may be permitted to attend for one or two sessions to enable the group and/or a member to deal with some specific issue. Groups operating within a training institution are often under pressure to allow trainees to participate as observers either within the group setting or through an observation window. This should be permitted only with the knowledge and consent of the group. Matters of confidentiality, levels of group trust, and possible disruption of the group must be considered in making the decision. Each group will establish its own rules regarding the presence of observers. One group within a prison setting visited by this writer allowed professional observers to view the group interaction through a window as long as a viewer would join the group for the last 10 minutes of the session for purposes of mutual questions and feedback. Other groups may contract to allow the observers to attend for a certain number of sessions. Some groups may encourage verbal participation while others insist on no participation of the part of the observers.

Structure of Group and Meetings

Size Several interdependent variables need to be decided upon in establishing a group; these include the number of members, the frequency and duration of meetings, and the selection of the meeting site for the group. The ideal size of the group will be determined by such factors as the type of group therapy to be used (a superficial, supportive group can be larger than an analytic or intensive-interaction group), the skill of the therapist in working with a small or large group, the presence of a cotherapist, and the behavior patterns of the members (acting-out, adolescent, and psychotic patients need a smaller group size than those patients who are less anxious and less likely to act out during the group meeting). Most authorities believe that the ideal size for a therapy group is between five and ten members (Kadis et al., 1963). Groups of the ideal size promote a sense of participation and member importance, chance for consensual validation, and member-to-member interaction. When the number falls below five to seven, interaction decreases to the point that the group feels unable to develop or maintain itself as a group, and frequently the leader becomes engaged in individual therapy within the group. Yalom also notes that an additional disadvantage of too small a group is that the chance for broad consensual validation and for testing and analyzing one's behavior with a variety of individuals is lost (Yalom, 1970, pp. 215–216). This writer has also seen instances in which too small a group put pressure on the remaining members to "perform" and caused them to become highly anxious as increasingly personal and sensitive data were shared.

On the other hand, groups with too many members become too cumbersome for the leader to keep abreast of all the ongoing interactions and of the emotional and dynamic needs of each member. The amount of the leader's attention available to each member is also decreased, and this may create a climate where only the most verbal and aggressive members participate in the group process. Groups that operate on principles of group pressure, interdependence, and individual responsibility, such as Alcoholics Anonymous, Recovery, Incorporated, and self-government or therapeutic communities, may function well with twenty to eighty members.

Duration of Meetings   Another factor closely related to the group size is the duration of the meetings. Experience suggests that the longer the meeting, the larger the number of members who can be accommodated, up to a certain point. Likewise, the smaller the group, the shorter the length of the meetings. For example, if for some reason only one or two members attend a meeting, it may be necessary to decrease the length of the meeting so that the members are not put in the position of "filling time." Traditionally, the length of group meetings has been from 1 to 1½ hours; however, in the midsixties group therapists began experimenting with variations in the duration of meetings. It has been found that a group may need about 1 hour for warmup, establishment of themes, and the working through of issues, and that after about 2 hours the group tends to decrease in attention, efficiency, and energy (Yalom, 1970, pp. 210–211).

Marathon Groups   More recently, a great deal of attention and interest has been given to the development of "time-massed" experiences with group meetings varying from 4 to 48 hours at a time. The most widely acclaimed in such format is the "marathon group," originally developed by Frederick Stoller and George Bach (who originated the term) in working with hospitalized psychiatric patients (Stoller, 1968). Major premises of this approach are that by interacting together for an extended time, with little opportunity for sleep and escape from the group, the group process unfolds more quickly; the cohesion and identification of the members are speeded up; social facades and role playing decrease (Yalom, 1970, p. 211); and the member can view his "career" in the marathon as similar to his career in the world with a new awareness of his own potential for change (Stoller, 1968, p. 94).

Behavioral expectations or norms for these groups include intense interaction, intense involvement, honesty, self-disclosure, and constructive expression of aggression (Stoller, 1968, p. 94). Some practitioners have combined the marathon experience within the structure of an ongoing group format and have found that the intensive experience often provides an impetus for movement in a group that has reached a plateau and/or is demonstrating a need for a sense of increased cohesion. Several authors (Smith, 1970; MacLennon, 1970; McLaughlin and White, 1973) note that research into the effectiveness of time-extended formats has been poorly constructed and based primarily on anecdotal notes, and warn that therapists must differentiate between an emotional experience and a corrective emotional experience. It is also axiomatic that change requires the passage of time (Lorr, 1962), and that for this reason the marathon may be most effective when interspersed with ongoing regular sessions of group therapy.

Frequency of Meetings Frequency of meetings is another important and interrelated variable regarding the group structure. Most outpatient groups, depending on the needs of the patients, meet once or twice a week, while groups within an in-patient or day treatment setting usually meet two to three times a week. One advantage to meeting on a weekly basis is that it provides time between meetings for members to integrate and test out insights and new patterns of behavior. For certain patients it may be advisable to meet frequently for short periods of time to provide a place for socialization, contact, and support. Meetings that are spaced too far apart run the danger of allowing for covering over of conflicts and concerns.

Establishment of an Environment Several important variables must be considered when selecting a meeting site for a group. While the group leader may not always be able to obtain an ideal meeting site, he must take into consideration the way the physical factors may impinge upon and influence the group's functioning. The location of the room in relation to the rest of the building is an important factor to consider, as almost any group leader can readily recall past instances when a group session was interrupted at a critical moment in the interaction. Only recently this writer was conducting a "guided fantasy" experience in a classroom with group members lying on the floor with their eyes closed, when suddenly outside the room several students charged up to the door, yelling, "No one's in here!" Needless to say, the group was disrupted. Privacy of location is important in terms of both freedom from external disruptions, as well as freedom from concern about disturbing those outside the room, and freedom from embarrassment of being overheard while in the group. Content and depth of personal disclosure will be more superficial and inhibited if there are such disruptions as people walking through the room, members being called out, or nongroup members possibly overhearing the discussion. Other factors in relation to location of the meeting site are accessibility for members and availability of facilities such as restrooms.

Size of Room and Furnishings Room size is also important, and, of course, it must be related to the size of the group. If the leader wants to create an atmosphere of closeness and intimacy, then a smaller room in relation to the group size will be chosen; if the goals for the group are to decrease the sense of intimacy, then a larger room will serve better. Too large a room will tend to make a group feel lost or overwhelmed; too small a room often leads to a threat of too much closeness and can increase patients' withdrawal or aggression. This phenomenon is particularly apparent with adolescents. Another consideration is that in relation to the method of interaction that will be utilized in the group; a group which is primarily sedentary may utilize a smaller room than one in which there are experiences involving movement, e.g., role playing, psychodrama, or nonverbal exercises.

Although seemingly minor, as impinging factors, the furnishings and decoration of the room do play a part in creating a therapeutic atmosphere. In furnishing the room, components such as seating arrangements, presence of tables, ashtrays, rugs, pillows, pictures, lighting, and color of walls may affect the responses of group members. Recently on visiting two community mental health centers in different locations of the same city, this writer was struck by the vivid psychedelic appearance of the rooms at the center where many of the center's population are young and involved with the drug and "hip" scene, as contrasted with the sedateness and neutrality of the rooms in the center drawing upon a middle-aged, middle-class population.

Seating Arrangement Ideally a variety of seats should be provided, since some members prefer straight chairs while others prefer more comfortable ones. Couches are inefficient because they inhibit eye contact, mobility, and within our culture may have positive or negative values in relation to a sense of closeness or distance between members. The degree of closeness fostered by sitting on a couch also touches upon each person's sexuality, so that usually the two ends of the couch are occupied with the middle space remaining empty. Preferably, the chairs should be easy to move, so that members can control the degree of closeness to each other and to the group. Many times an individual member will "stake" out a seat, often without any verbal claim being made until perhaps a new member violates the other's territory and takes the other's seat. This situation happened to the writer several years ago while attending a staff meeting as a new psychiatric nurse. Just as she started to sit in a chair near the head of a table, another staff member loudly proclaimed with a horrified expression on her face, "That's Doctor X's chair!" Recently, while teaching an in-service education class for nursing personnel from this same unit, the former incident was recounted; smiles of recognition broke out as the staff amusedly acknowledged that the same seating pattern is still followed, although it was then 7 years later and many changes in staff had occurred. In a therapy group conducted by the writer, the self-esteem and mood of a particular member are very clearly tele-graphed by the place where he chooses to sit at each meeting, and this has become part of the process commented on by the members. Increasingly, large pillows are replacing chairs in group therapy rooms, to create an atmosphere of informality and casualness. If, however, the group is primarily composed of middle-aged women wearing skirts, they will probably not be comfortable sitting on the floor.

Audiovisual Equipment   The use of mechanical equipment such as tape recorders and videotape recorders within the group poses some technical and individual problems. Particularly within teaching institutions, where tape recorders are a common occurrence, they may in fact be treated in a casual manner by the leader, but not necessarily so by the group members. Tape recorders may be used by the leader for supervisory purposes or for teaching students, and they also may be used after the meeting, or for immediate playback during the meeting, to check on process or content. When introducing the use of a tape recorder, the leader needs to provide an opportunity for members to discuss their reactions. This writer has found it helpful to have the tape recorder somewhat visible but not prominent, so that it neither becomes a "state secret" nor a "star attraction." Sometimes it is helpful for a suspicious or hesitant member to have an opportunity to operate the tape recorder and hear himself on tape.

Videotape equipment is a fairly new addition to the armamentarium of the group therapist and evokes stronger reactions from therapists and patients alike, including a sense of "There's no hiding here." Initially, many individuals attribute much "power" to the camera and have fantasies about what the camera will pick up. One technique for handling these fears is again to permit the person to become familiar with the equipment by practicing being in control of it. It is also helpful to let each member "encounter" himself on the screen, for most people have never had such an opportunity and are ambivalent about what they see. This gives them a chance to deal openly with their own narcissism and self-concepts (Berger, 1970, p. 24). Most members are pleasantly surprised at what they see, although patients with low self-esteem and depressed mood will often state that they cannot stand what they see. Detailed discussion on the uses of video group therapy can be found in the recent literature (Berger, 1970; Wilmer, 1970; Robinson and Jacobs, 1970). Some of the most common uses of video for group members themselves is to help them get in contact with their own feelings about their physical appearance, to provide immediate feedback in terms of process, and to allow members to observe and identify their own incongruent verbal and nonverbal communication. One of the most prominent proponents of the use of video equipment, Milton Berger, cites the usefulness of video in providing feedback to highly disorganized or psychotic patients regarding their behavior when they use denial—e.g., that exhibited by the manic patient or the alcoholic (Berger, 1970, p. 25). The leader must make several decisions, such as location of the camera, who will operate it, and, of course, what use will be made of the tapes.

When any mechanical equipment is used, trust and confidentiality become considerations for the group; these concerns may become the first overt issue that the group uses to explore these themes and/or act out resistance to the leader, and must be dealt with accordingly. Many institutions require written releases to be signed by each member, detailing how the tapes are to be used and who will have access to them.

The Group Contract

The group contract, the basic operating agreement between the leader and the members, is intended as an explicit statement of group structure and expectations but frequently evolves on an implicit basis as well. Basic items included in the contract are:

1. The time, duration, and frequency of meetings limited or ongoing
2. Number of sessions
3. Open or closed group
4. Confidentiality—member and leader responsibilities
5. The use of mechanical equipment
6. Rules regarding observers, visitors, and addition of new members
7. Fees
8. Limits regarding:
   a. Attendance
   b. Extragroup socialization
   c. Contact with leader outside of group
   d. Use of physical force
9. General or specific expectations regarding participation.

The contract provides structure and safety for the group members as they enter the group experience. Yalom notes that patients enter a group with a "burden of procedural misconceptions and fantasies about what will happen in the group" (Yalom, 1970, p. 219). Verbalization and discussion of the contract by the therapist and the members help to create a climate of partnership in the experience and begin to establish group norms and expected role behaviors. In presenting the contract, the leader must be alert to the hazards of lengthy information giving, particularly since patients with high initial anxiety may selectively fail to attend to and/or distort specific items. Not all therapists believe in the expression of an explicit, detailed contract with a group; rather, some therapists view initial ambiguity in the group as desirable (Horwitz, 1964; Wolf, 1963). Recent investigation has shown, however, that "by subtle or subliminal verbal or non-verbal reinforcement even the most non-directive group leader structures his group" (Yalom, 1970, p. 226). While the group leader usually discusses all parts of the contract with the members in preparing them for therapy, reviewing the contract with the entire membership once the group is formed assists them to realize the operating principles underlying the group.

A group contract may be very general or quite detailed. The leader may open up certain items for group decision and certain ones he may decide prior to the first meeting are not to be determined by the group. Nevertheless, it is important to give members an opportunity to discuss their feelings regarding these items. In addition, leaders negotiate with each member regarding some new behavior he wishes to develop, or an old one he wishes to eliminate (Goulding, 1971).

PREPARATION OF PATIENTS FOR GROUP THERAPY

Closely intertwined with the selection of patients and the establishment of a group contract is the preparation of patients for group therapy. This preparation may be essentially nonexistent as part of the initial screening interview or may be an extended and extensive process. The purposes of such preparation are to help patients move smoothly enough into the group so that they identify with the group, its tasks, and the other members. Rabin (1970), in an excellent article on this process, comments that overall there is inadequate preparation of patients for group psychotherapy, and that the psychiatric literature is lacking in discussion or analysis of this process. He delineates five formats for preparing patients, including:

1. The giving of factual information, e.g., the contract
2. The use of written or recorded materials focusing on what to expect within the group experience
3. The presentation of a lecture to several patients at once, or an explanatory interview with a single patient focusing on anticipated member and leader roles, and the giving of a mental set for taking risks and showing feelings
4. A "pregroup" experience to be used both for diagnostic purposes and as a "holding action" while waiting to start an extended group experience
5. Individualized preparation to deal with specific fears and avoid premature placement

Adequate preparation of patients for the group experience may be reflected in a higher attendance rate, a decrease in target symptoms, increased faith in group therapy, and prevention of impulsive termination. Likewise, Janosik (1972) says that the leader can facilitate making the group experience a meaningful one by stressing, during the screening and preparation process, the rigorous pursuit of goals, serious commitment to the experience, and a sense of shared responsibility.

INTENSIVE GROUP THERAPY

The model for group therapy utilized by this writer is the previously cited intensive interactional group therapy which utilizes and focuses on ongoing group events and processes in relation to the individual members. The conceptual roots of this approach are to be found in psychoanalytic, interpersonal (Sullivanian), and group dynamics theories. Significant features of this model include the following beliefs: that transference analysis is not the primary vehicle for significant therapeutic change; that communication should be freely interactive rather than spokewheel or therapist-centered; that the group process is the major vehicle of change; that the crucial therapeutic experience is that feared consequences or catastrophic expectations do not occur; that genetic insight is not a prerequisite for significant and permanent personality change to occur.

Implications for Group Therapist

This view of the therapeutic process establishes specific tasks and functions for the therapist in such a group, as well as generating certain assumptions regarding his position and power in the group. The decreased focus on the establishment and analysis of transference relationships with the therapists sets the stage for the therapist to function as a participant observer in the group, and for the establishment of collaborative relationships between members and therapists with a sense of shared responsibility. This does not mean, however, that the therapist should attempt to shift positions entirely and become a full member of the patient group. He still maintains an ongoing sense of responsibility for being aware of the total group's process and functioning and of that of each individual within the group. The therapist maintains his position and responsibility in the group because of the academic and technical skills that he possesses and of the position and power that are given to him by the members "because he is therapist"—the private images they impart to him as a "healer" or "teacher." Within this framework the major overall tasks of the therapist are to encourage the development and maintenance of a group milieu which allows patients to experience their conflicts in a safe and growth-enhancing environment. The therapist works toward this end by assuming two primary roles with the group (Yalom, 1970, pp. 86–98): (1) as a technical expert who utilizes his skills to establish an open, interactive communication network, facilitate feedback and disclosure, monitor and influence the level of anxiety in the group, provide reinforcement for desirable behaviors and processess, and offer interpretations (on both the individual and group level; but this is not a primary task in this type of group); and (2) as a role model for group members in terms of interpersonal honesty and spontaneity, displaying a repertoire of interpersonal behaviors and acknowledging fallibility or limitations. By allowing his "self" to emerge in the group, the therapist helps patients to engage in the process of consensual validation, helping to decrease and remove parataxic distortions as they occur. In disclosing personal reactions and/or personal data, the therapist must always assess the possible effect on the group at any given moment, and must remember that a primary reason for this behavior is that of acting as a role model for such patient behaviors.

Within this framework for therapy, the therapist will tend to: (1) focus on the here and now of the group, (2) deal with process rather than specific content, (3) make group-level interventions rather than individually focused interventions, and (4) bring the group from indirect expression of wishes, fantasies, and impulses to explicit and direct expression. Whitaker and Lieberman (1964, pp. 198–199) note that errors in therapy are likely to occur on the basis of either nonunderstanding of the group and/or individuals at any given moment or the therapist's attempting to make the group viable for himself rather than for the members (similar to engaging in counter-transference behavior). It is important to stress additionally that what might be an appropriate therapeutic intervention in one stage of the group might well be inappropriate at another time.

Stages of Intensive Group Therapy

As therapist and patients gather for the purpose of participating in a group therapy experience, a certain sequence of events can be predicted to be set in motion. These events will constitute the stages of the group's life and the developmental tasks to be encountered by the group. The exact appearance and sequence of these events will vary from group to group but will center around the following: patients' expectations and concerns regarding the experience, anticipated patient behaviors, and the role of the therapist in the group. Three stages of group life are most commonly delineated: the initial stage occurs when the group goes through the process of establishing itself; the second is the working stage; and the third is the ending stage or termination. In ongoing, open groups it must be noted that once the group is established, the other stages will occur repetitively and even concurrently as members enter and leave the group.

INITIAL PHASE OF GROUP THERAPY

As noted previously, the process of therapy and the setting of the stage for a successful group therapy experience actually occur during the initial interviewing and preparation of patients for the group. The actual convening of the group for its first meeting is predictably an anxiety-producing experience for both therapist and patients. For the therapist, the anxiety will be related to questions such as: "How will this group mesh?" and "How can I most effectively utilize myself in this experience?" coupled with a sense of challenge and expectation for what will come and what might be. For the patients, the initial meeting is even more anxiety-producing, particularly for those patients who have not participated in a group therapy experience before.

Patient Assumptions

Patients will have fantasies, concerns, and expectations of self, the group, the other members, and the leader. These will be based on some accurate and some perhaps inaccurate assumptions. Whitaker and Lieberman (1964, p. 118) note that three of these assumptions are: (1) the patient's role is to disclose personal data, (2) the therapist is there to analyze these data and offer advice, and (3) other members are an audience. Operating on the basis of these general assumptions, patients are likely to enter the group at least somewhat ambivalently: they hope and wish to receive help but at the same time fear exposure with possible reactions of criticism, ridicule, or scorn. Other concerns of new members are: "How can I help anyone else when I feel so helpless?" and also, "Will there be anyone like me?" These concerns often lead to each patient comparing himself with the other members. In addition, other patients are often viewed as competitors for the therapist's attention, favor, and advice. Initial expectations of the therapist are that he will provide safety, protection, and advice and be all-knowing. It must be noted that many of these expectations are on the covert level and may be only partially recognized by the members (Whitaker and Lieberman, 1964, p. 143).

Because of the presence of these fantasies, assumptions, and expectations, certain characteristic patient behaviors may be anticipated to occur during the early life of the group. The first generalization regarding these behaviors is that in order to cope with the ambiguity of the situation and its resultant anxiety, patients will resort to their own usual ways of handling anxiety. Some patients therefore may attempt to seek structure and reassurance by demonstrating dependency upon the therapist and/or other members of the group by asking questions regarding the purposes, benefits, and procedures of the group, seeking advice for problems, or minimally participating, in the hope of prompting the therapist into action. Other patients may engage in pairing behavior in attempts to provide mutual support, identify similarities, and play out similar or complementary roles and needs. Some patients may engage in counterdependency behavior, such as negating any offers of the therapist and acting in a self-sufficient and/or "assistant therapist" role by focusing on others. Much of the initial discussion will include a recitation of problems and symptoms, or presentations of "life story," often on an intellectual-rational level rather than on an affective level. Communication is often stereotyped and follows the usual social norms operating in the broader community. This form of discussion often serves the purpose of allowing members the chance of sizing up each other, the therapist, and the total group. Additional group behavior involves the offering of advice for presented problems, and the making of interpretations for motivations of behaviors and/or feelings. All the individual and group behaviors must be viewed within the light of members attempting to make the group situation viable, which means avoiding or decreasing anxiety.

Early Themes

Prominent themes during the initial meetings will center on trust, safety, search for an ideal parent, and dependency/independency. One group that this writer has participated in has a handmade sign on the wall, inherited from a previous group, which says, "TRISK"—a coined word standing for trust and risk, two essential ingredients for having a beneficial group experience. As delineated by Schutz (1966), the first question of a group member must face is, "Will I be in or out?" The next question also occurring during this initial stage is related to the issue of control, "Where do I fit in the heirarchy of this group in relation to the other members and to the leader?"

Role of the Therapist and Therapeutic Tasks

During this stage of the group, the therapist must keep in mind two important considerations: one, that he will initially be the unifying force and connecting link for the rest of the group, and, two, that he will be the most significant or powerful norm setter in the group. These two facts are closely linked with the primary tasks for the therapist in this stage: to begin the work of developing a sense of cohesion and connectedness, to provide the needed amount of structure to keep anxiety at a tolerable level, and to delineate the basic norms for the establishment of the group.

Initial structuring of the group might include: a few introductory remarks on the part of the therapist regarding the contract (even though discussed with each individual previously, this group discussion helps patients to see this as a contract with the group not just as a contract with the therapist); a reiteration that this is a growth-focused and serious endeavor and that attendance and punctuality are important to help the group begin to establish itself as a group; and perhaps some exploration of what is coming to the group and what this first session will be like for each member and the leader. This type of structure begins again to set the stage for focusing on the now of the experience for the members.

Initial explicit norms likely to be set by the therapist include the above-mentioned ones plus one regarding confidentiality. Acting as a role model, the therapist can state what his responsibility is in regard to confidentiality and then allow the group to deal with this norm on their own when they are ready. Only as trust becomes an open issue will the group come to grips with this question and establish its own particular norm. Implicit norms will be established, often by what the therapist does not do as much as by what he says or does. For example, not providing answers or assuming "directorship" of the group in response to dependency behavior gives the message that the therapist wants the members to take responsibility and explore issues themselves. The presentation of a nonjudgmental attitude conveys acceptance and a message of safety—no one is to be ridiculed here. By focusing on the group process rather than the specific individuals, the therapist helps to increase a sense of interrelatedness and cohesion for this group of strangers who enter wondering what they have in common with each other. While eliciting initial impressions and concerns, the therapist needs to keep in mind that he does not want to focus on too direct expression of fears so that a sense of contagion sets in. In line with this caution, the therapist also needs to be alert for the overly anxious patient who enters the group and immediately discloses a great deal of personal data, keeping the focus primarily on himself;

although attempting to meet his own needs, this patient is also meeting needs of other group members to keep the time filled and the focus off them. The result of too intimate and early disclosure is often that the fears of the group members actually become magnified and the patient feels exploited. The therapist has a responsibility to provide some limits for this patient and to establish some safety in the group by indicating that he will provide structure and limits if need be. As the patients interact with the therapist and each other, they begin to assess and speculate on their own possible fate in this group in relation to the therapist and each other. During this time many of the therapist's interventions will be process comments on "what is" rather than giving interpretations of these behaviors. By providing only the minimally necessary structure, the therapist allows for the beginning development of this particular's group's constellations, conflicts, and initial solutions to emerge.

WORKING STAGE OF GROUP

Group movement into and through the middle stage of development is usually not as clearly identifiable as in the initial stage; however, there are certain aspects of group and individual behaviors that indicate that a shift has been made and that this stage is present. As the members resolve their concerns around position and control in the group, they then focus on concerns around intimacy, with such questions as, "How close do I really want to be with these people?" and "How much do I really want to reveal?" As these questions are resolved, the members begin to exhibit indications of being a cohesively working group. There is increased sharing of personal data, impulses, wishes, feelings, and reactions to each other and the therapist; interdependent rather than dependent behavior is demonstrated as members work collaboratively to identify themes, patterns, and conflicts and to appropriately deal with them; members show an increased sense of self-respect and respect and acceptance of each other. Group norms will continue to evolve to fit the group's current needs. Although the early life and history of the group will influence the current operations of the group, current internal and external events will impinge upon the group and call forth old conflicts or issues perhaps thought settled or worked through. Such events might be the addition of new members, illness or termination in either members or therapist, the therapist's absence or vacation, or community or family events (divorce, fire, murders, etc.).

During this stage the curative factors of the group are more prominent and operate more effectively. For the therapist, the task is to maximize the development and utilization of these factors by using the basic principles of group therapy previously noted. Three possible group phenomena or behaviors that are likely to occur and that will need attention from the therapist include the development of subgrouping, overt conflict between members, and acting out. Subgrouping may take place within the group or may involve socializing outside of the group. It may be identified by such behaviors as members frequently agreeing with each other but not with other members of the group, exchanging frequent glances, arriving and departing together and/or consistently sitting near each other, and the establishment of protective alliances. Effects of subgrouping are to stir up old conflicts related to inclusion and exclusion with possible splitting of the group and/or therapists into camps. It often arises as members perceive a subunit as being more viable for themselves than the total-group climate. In dealing with this, the therapist must make sure that he does not take sides but continues to make process comments, helping the group to see it as a group phenomenon and pushing for the exploration of what is happening. The therapist must be very careful also not to get caught carrying a secret that he feels he cannot share with the rest of the group.

Overt conflict between members may be related to the operation and development of parataxic distortions, presence of mirror reactions, the presence of a group deviant, or rivalry over the therapist. Rather than suppressing the expression of the conflict (which might have been done in the earlier stage), the therapist will need to monitor the affect, anxiety, and needs of the group to provide for controlled expression and exploration of the aggressive feelings, helping the members to learn the value for themselves and the group in doing this. Just as in dealing with subgrouping, the therapist must be careful not to get caught in the contest or take sides or make judgments as to "who is right."

Acting out is the behavioral enactment in the group setting or in relation to it (discharging the tension through behavior rather than through exploration and discussion) of internal conflicts, and may take the form of sexual relationships between members, threats of termination, actual termination, threats of suicide, and the establishment of subgroups. At times an entire group may engage in acting-out behavior, such as holding an alternate meeting without the therapist, or deciding to have a meeting become a party with members bringing food and wine, or establishing a pact to remain silent for an entire meeting. Any of these resistances must be explored in a nonjudgmental and firm manner.

TERMINATION STAGE OF GROUP

The process of termination in group therapy is always a group and individual task and may involve individual members or therapists leaving the group or the total group disbanding. In an ongoing open-ended group, the process is a repetitive one as members enter and leave, so that each member sees a cycle of being in the group: entering, belonging, and leaving. This reflects what occurs in everyday life, and the process of experiencing termination in a meaningful and healthy way can help patients to learn how to deal with this process in their lives. Particularly in today's mobile society, the ability to say goodbye in a rewarding manner is a valuable interpersonal skill.

In individual may terminate a group at any point in the experience, and the termination may be premature, well timed, abrupt, or fully explored. It is a common experience that early in the group's existence members may decide to leave for a variety of reasons. They may feel that they're not fitting in with this group; it may not be what they expected; they may have assumed the role of the deviant in the group; or they may be caught up in a subgroup that, unable to make the group viable, decides to leave. Sometimes a member will notify the therapist, outside of the group, of his intent to terminate. The therapist must decide whether to meet with the member individually or to urge his return to the group to explore and share his decision. No hard-and-fast rule can be set as to the most helpful procedure to follow. This writer has found it beneficial for both the individual and the group to make the leaving explicit and the good-byes direct rather than to have the member leave with no chance for unfinished business to be dealt with. Occasionally a premature termination may be averted by meeting with the member individually for a few sessions to explore the reasons for his wishing to leave. When the termination does occur, the therapist has the responsibility to help the member and the group look at the meaning of this for them and to see it not necessarily as a failure but perhaps as a result of nonfit, poor timing of entrance, external stress, or nonreadiness for the experience. At times it may actually be a healthy step for an individual to say, "I'm not ready; when I am, I'll be back."

Well-timed and valid termination will occur when there is a sense of mutual fit on the part of the member, other members, and the therapist. It is important to remember that what might be an appropriate time or level of functioning for one person may not be such for another. Such a termination does not come as a surprise to the group and is usually not abrupt but is dealt with by a few weeks of preparation.

Even under ideal circumstances termination is an anxiety-producing experience and one likely to evoke a variety of feelings and the reactivation of old themes, conflicts, and symptoms. For some people, doing the leaving is easier than being left; for others, the reverse may be true. Oftentimes feelings of abandonment, anger, sadness, and longing for closeness, as well as feelings of accomplishment and achievement, are activated. Each termination may be used by the group as a time of review—looking at where the member and the group have been and where they are now. This also is a time for members to get in touch with feelings connected with previous terminations and to engage in some working through and letting go of old attachments, It is important to view a member's leaving the group as not a graduation, but completion of one stage of growth in an ongoing process (Yalom, 1970, p. 278). Each therapist must also decide whether termination means a final good-bye or whether he or the group will allow a member to return at a later date if the person feels the need. With members who work well in the group, who are well liked and closely bonded to the group, it is important that the therapist recognize the evidence of subtle cues of "Stay, we need you," when in reality it is time for the member to leave and be on his own. This is exploitation of the patient and is to be avoided.

Two other forms of termination may occur: the therapist leaves the group, or the total group disbands. When either of these events occurs, the group as a whole is likely to have a stronger sense of separation anxiety, even if well prepared in advance and the ending is built into the structure of the group. It is important for the therapist to allow for and encourage the expression of these feelings, fantasies, and reactions in a nondefensive way. Many times the therapist must take the initiative with a group that is using avoidance or denial and start the process by sharing his own feelings and reviewing the experience for himself. This may give the group permission to join the process as he again, as in the beginning, shares of himself and perhaps provides a little more structure.

REFERENCES

Abrahams, D., and J. Enright (1965): "Psychiatric Intakes in Groups: A Pilot Study of Procedures, Problems, and Prospects," *American Journal of Psychiatry*, vol. 122, pp. 170–174.

AGPA (American Group Psychotherapy Association, Inc.) (1970): *Guidelines for the Training of Group Psychotherapists*, American Group Psychotherapy Association, Inc., New York.

Allgeyer, Jean M. (1970): "The Crisis Group: Its Unique Usefulness to the Disadvantaged," *International Journal of Group Psychotherapy,* vol. 20, pp. 235–240.

Bach, George (1954): *Intensive Group Therapy,* The Ronald Press Company, New York.

Bales, Robert F. (1953): "The Equilibrium Problem in Small Groups," in Talcott Parsons et al. (eds.), *Working Papers in the Theory of Action,* The Free Press, Glencoe, Ill., pp. 111–161.

Berger, Milton M. (ed.) (1970): *Videotape Techniques in Psychiatric Training and Treatment,* Brunner Mazel, Inc., New York.

Curry, Andrew (1971): "Short-Term Group Psychotherapy," Group Discussion at Golden Gate Group Psychotherapy Association Meeting, Berkeley, Calif.

Durkin, Helen E. (1964): *The Group in Depth,* International Universities Press, Inc., New York.

Foulkes, S. H., and E. J. Anthony (1957): *Group Psychotherapy—The Psychoanalytic Approach,* Penguin Press, Harmondsworth, Middlesex.

Freeman, M. B., and B. S. Sweet (1954): "Some Specific Features of Group Psychotherapy, and Their Implications for Selection of Patients," *International Journal of Group Psychotherapy,* vol. 4, pp. 355–368.

Gauron, Eugene, et al. (1970): "Group Therapy Training: A Multidisciplinary Approach," *Perspectives in Psychiatric Care,* vol. 8, pp. 263–267.

Goulding, Mary E. (1971): "The Marathon as a Method of Training Group Psychotherapists," Paper presented at American Group Psychotherapy Association Convention, Los Angeles.

Heilfron, Marilyn (1969): "Co-therapy: the Relationship between Therapists," *International Journal of Group Psychotherapy,* vol. 19, pp. 366–381.

Horwitz, Leonard (1964): "Transference in Training Groups and Therapy Groups," *International Journal of Group Psychotherapy,* vol. 14, pp. 202–213.

Janosik, Ellen (1972): "A Pragmatic Approach to Group Therapy," *Journal of Psychiatric Nursing and Mental Health Services,* vol. 10, pp. 7–11.

Kadis, Asaya, et al. (1963): *A Practicum of Group Psychotherapy,* Hoeber Medical Division, Harper & Row, Publishers, Inc., New York.

Kobler, A. L., and E. Stotland (1964): *The End of Hope,* Collier-Macmillan, London.

Lorr, M. (1962): "Relation of Treatment Frequency and Duration to Psychotherapeutic Outcome," in H. Strupp and L. Lubarsky (eds.), *Conference on Research in Psychotherapy,* American Psychological Association, Washington, D.C.

MacLennon, Beryce (1970): "Co-therapy," *International Journal of Group Psychotherapy,* vol. 15, pp. 154–164.

———, and Naomi Levy (1971): "The Group Psychotherapy Literature, 1970," *International Journal of Group Psychotherapy,* vol. 21, pp. 345–358.

McGee, Thomas F., and Benjamin Schuman (1970): "The Nature of the Co-therapy Relationship," *International Journal of Group Psychotherapy,* vol. 20, pp. 25–35.

McLaughlin, Frank, and Eleanor White (1973): "Small Group Functioning under Six Different Leadership Formats," *Nursing Research,* vol. 22, pp. 37–54.

Mereness, Dorothy (1963): "The Psychiatric Nursing Specialist and Her Professional Identity," *Perspectives in Psychiatric Care,* vol. 1, pp. 8–19.

Mintz, Elizabeth (1969): "On the Rationale of Touch in Psychotherapy," *Psychotherapy: Theory, Research, and Practice,* vol. 6, pp. 231–234.

Mullan, Hugh, and Max Rosenbaum (1963): *Group Psychotherapy,* The Free Press, New York.

Rabin, Herbert M. (1970): "Preparing Patients for Group Therapy," *International Journal of Group Psychotherapy,* vol. 20, pp. 135–145.

Robinson, Margot, and Alfred Jacobs (1970): "Focused Videotape Feedback and Behavior Change in Group Psychotherapy," *Psychotherapy: Theory, Research, and Practice,* vol. 7, pp. 169–172.

Rouslin, Sheila (1964): "Discussion . . . (On Meditations on Group Psychotherapy and the Role of the Psychiatric Nurse)," *Perspectives in Psychiatric Care,* vol. 2, pp. 16–17.

Schutz, William (1966): *The Interpersonal Underworld,* Science and Behavior Books, Palo Alto.

Slavson, Samuel R. (1955): "Criteria for Selection and Rejection of Patients for Various Kinds of Group Therapy," *International Journal of Group Psychotherapy,* vol. 5, pp. 3–30.

Smith, Robert J. (1970): "A Closer Look at Encounter Therapies," *International Journal of Group Psychotherapy,* vol. 20, pp. 192–209.

Stein, Aaron (1971): "The Role and Function of the Nurse in Group Therapy," Paper presented at the American Group Psychotherapy Association Convention, Los Angeles.

Stoller, Frederick H. (1968): "Marathon Group Therapy," in George Gazda (ed.), *Innovations to Group Psychotherapy,"* Charles C Thomas, Publisher, Springfield, Ill., pp. 42–95.

Werner, Jean (1970): "Relating Group Theory to Nursing Practice," *Perspectives in Psychiatric Care,* vol. 8, pp. 248–261.

Whitaker, Dorothy S., and Morton Lieberman (1964): *Psychotherapy through the Group Process,* Atherton Press, Inc., New York.

Wilmer, Harry A. (1970): "Television: Technical and Artistic Aspects of Videotape in Psychiatric Teaching," in Milton M. Berger (ed.), *Videotape Techniques in Psychiatric Training and Treatment,* Brunner Mazel, Inc., New York, pp. 211–232.

Wolf, Alexander (1967): "Group Psychotherapy," in Alfred M. Freedman and Harold I. Kaplan (eds.), *Comprehensive Textbook of Psychiatry,* The Williams & Wilkins Company, Baltimore, pp. 1234–1241.

———(1963): "Psychoanalysis of Groups," in Max Rosenbaum and Milton Berger (eds.), *Group Psychotherapy and Group Function,* Basic Books, Inc., Publishers, New York, pp. 273–328.

Yalom, Irvin, D. (1970): *The Theory and Practice of Group Psychotherapy,* Basic Books, Inc., Publishers, New York.

———, et al. (1967): "Prediction of Improvement in Group Therapy," *Archives of General Psychiatry*, vol. 17, pp. 159–168.

24

FAMILY PSYCHOTHERAPY

Ben H. Handleman

The genesis of family therapy cannot be attributed to any one person, specific group, or discipline. Social work has long played a role in offering services to the family; for example, traditional family service agencies exist in most major communities in the United States. Sociology and anthropology have looked upon the family as the primary unit from which personality is developed and social functioning is learned. Although the importance of the family unit was recognized, there was a tendency to look at individual and group behavior but not to focus on ongoing interaction between individuals within this primary group. Psychology, with its definite focus on the intrapsychic mechanisms of behavior of the individual, played an important part by concentrating on the individual. Freud, although aware of family influences, followed the traditional physician-patient relationship and treated only the patient. This two-person therapeutic structure, however, provided the beginnings of an interactional modality for the "working out" of personality problems.

Thus the individual was looked upon from different points of view by various disciplines; that is, (1) as a separate and distinct entity whose personality structure was only secondarily related to the family function, (2) as a clinical entity whose relationship with another person (the therapist) could be of therapeutic value, and (3) as an entity whose individuality was subordinated to, or whose personality was merged into, the identity of the family group.

It was only a matter of time before the overall family structure became the primary focus in attempts to understand the functioning of a given individual in the family. This focus was developed by investigators in different parts of the United States searching for answers to their specific questions regarding the family. Most research initially focused on the relationship between the family of the schizophrenic and its schizophrenic member, with special emphasis coming from the Bateson group (1956). The theory developed by that group was based on communication analysis which revealed tangential family communication patterns and led them to the development of the "double-bind" hypothesis. Other theorists, including Ackerman (1958), Bowen (1960), Spiegel and Bell (1959), Jackson (1957), Lidz et al. (1958), and Wynne (1958), began looking at the family as a total structure and attempted to influence each family member within the structure.

While some engaged in family therapy primarily for research purposes, a number of other early pioneers began treating families through the clinical modality of family therapy. These latter, who have confined their primary efforts to direct service and treatment, include Virginia Satir (1964), Charles Fulweiler, John Bell (1961), and Nathan Ackerman (1958). The important issue is not that they were the first to try family therapy, but rather that they possessed a strong enough personal conviction to attempt a therapeutic approach quite different from and contrary to prevailing views in psychiatry.

THE HISTORY OF FAMILY THERAPY

The beginning of the treatment method in which the entire family is interviewed together on an ongoing basis cannot be pinpointed to a definite date. In the early and midfifties, a few therapists openly began to discuss their views and experiences regarding their approaches to working with a total family on an ongoing basis. It was not until the latter part of the decade that published articles began to appear on this subject. Since then there has been a sharp and consistent rise in the numbers of family therapists and of articles regarding the treatment of families.

Early Difficulties

The idea of seeing an entire family together was once regarded as heretical, for psychopathology was primarily viewed as inherent in the character and personality of the individual. Consequently, much less importance was attached to the influence of family members—and the family as a unit—than on the behavior of the individual family member who was being seen as a patient. It was also difficult to involve family members in treatment, since the traditional psychoanalytic approach to psychotherapy was concerned only with the intensive patient-therapist relationship. Given the history of a therapist's difficulties in coping with the members of the patient's family, any other psychotherapist found it difficult to develop a family-centered psychotherapy. The therapist had to hurdle not only his own reluctance to treat families, but also the possibility of ostracism by his colleagues.

Another problem for those therapists who attempted family therapy was their uncertainty about the effectiveness of any specific technique. Lacking an accepted technique, they were wide open to criticism, since without this it would be impossible to validate the results of therapy. Although the difficulty of determining the effectiveness of a technique is a weakness common to the social sciences, and especially to the psychotherapies, it in interesting to note how frequently those who utilize an established and long-accepted method will expect, even insist upon, specific verified results from a different and untried method.

Another view regarding the difficulty in determining the beginning of the family therapy is that much of it was done in secrecy. Haley writes, "The secrecy about Family Therapy has two sources: Those using this method have been too uncertain about their techniques and results to commit themselves to print, and there has apparently been a fear of charges of heresy because the influence of family members has been considered irrelevant to the nature and cure of psychopathology in a patient (Haley, 1962).

Change in Attitude toward Family Therapy

The greater frequency in the literature of individuals and groups who are attempting family therapy and describing their efforts is marked evidence of the change in direction and attitude in the psychotherapies. With family therapy now being carried on in the open, the frequently raised issue is that it has not been a part of psychotherapeutic methodology all along. Those individuals doing family therapy find it difficult to understand why the family unit was not looked at more closely from interactional and transactional concepts rather than with sharp focus and heavy concentration on individual behavior, especially behavior of a pathological nature. In historical perspective it becomes clear that there were clashes of opinion with a definite swing away from family-oriented methods in the late 1930s. This trend continued until the advent of family therapy and community psychiatry, with their beginnings in the midfifties and early sixties.

Early Concepts Influencing Family
Therapy (from 1917 to 1930)

As early as 1917, Mary Richmond, a leading social worker, pointed out that a person's mental history was a result of his social relations, and that attempts to help a human being by influencing his mind would fail without knowledge of the family group of which he is a part. Friedman (1959) stated that in the 1920s Richmond "continued to see the family in the central focus of casework and she continued to view any essential changes in family experience as a change of adjustments in social relationships." The first large-scale research investigating middle-class families was initiated in the 1920s. Research then focused heavily upon the adjustments of individuals within the family, and this emphasis has dominated family sociology ever since. The beginning of this trend might arbitrarily be marked by Burgess's concept (1926) of the family as a "unity of interacting personalities" which minimized the importance of social structure, especially within the family context. Concomitantly with the development of Harry Stack Sullivan's interpersonal theory of psychiatry in 1927, the incorporation of psychoanalytical concepts into sociology fostered the beginning of "social psychiatry." Thus the emphasis was placed at the extreme ends of the continuum—on the individual or on the wider society.

Freudian theory became popular in the 1920s, as the helping professions were in need of a theoretical framework. Psychoanalysis was introduced into the social work school curriculum during this period. Mary Richmond and others in social work resisted the shifting of emphasis from the environment to the individual, feeling that what was needed was a more intensive understanding of family life. About this time, the child guidance movement had its beginnings. This development, initially an effort to treat delinquent children, evolved to include means to diagnose and treat neurotic and psychotic children. Treatment expanded to incorporate the mother, but the father's role was ignored. Only recently, through treatment and research of total families, has there been a focus on the shortcomings of the practice of seeing only the child and mother. However, in 1930 emphasis on the individual was in full swing. According to Bell et al. (1960), "Psychoanalytic notions were selected, simplified, and analytic notions were selected, simplified, and combined with the social psychological theories of G. H. Mead and others to give impetus to this movement. In short order, a very extensive literature was produced by psychiatry, social casework, and kindred professions; a literature in which correlations were established between . . . a piece of the child and a piece of the parent." The approach to the family included psychoanalytic theory and sociological theory. Parts of the family were dealt with, but the family as a whole was neglected.

Later Concepts Influencing Family Therapy (from 1930 to 1950)

One effect of the economic depression of the 1930s was that the family was less able to support its members, who in consequence suffered. The depression brought about a renewed interest in the family, although this interest was still within the framework of the study of personality, social structure, and external factors. For some unexplained reason, the family unit was not examined in the light of what was happening between the various members of the family in their daily life experiences. An exception to this was made by Oberndorf, who pioneered in marriage therapy. In 1938, Ackerman wrote "The Unity of the Family," in which he discussed the importance of viewing the total family when treating a disturbed individual. Others, including Sullivan, Fromm-Reichmann, Oberndorf, and Lidz, began examining the influence of people on each other.

Influence of Psychoanalytic Concepts

The influence of the psychoanalytic movement, with its emphasis on intrapsychic happenings, continued to gain momentum during the 1940s and 1950s. Although psychoanalysis is a system that focuses on the individual, there always remains the broader question of what influenced and continues to influence the individual, thus creating a specific personality. The emphasis on ego psychology tended to become more focused on the transactions and interactions that occur between a given person in psychotherapy and the people in his environment. The influence of others in the person's immediate environment became clearer and better understood as the idea developed that getting all family members together might prove a profitable and productive approach. Jackson and Satir (1961) point out that psychoanalysis has acted as both a positive and a negative force in expediting the family movement. They state that because most therapists in family diagnosis and therapy are psychoanalytically trained, psychoanalysis has contributed a vast fund of knowledge to personality theory and therapy. They also point out that the movement toward family studies may have indirectly stemmed from the disappointments individuals have had with the results of this expensive and time-consuming technique.

As therapists in the 1950s started working with total families, they began to find a vast area which had remained unexplored. It became clear that during a session with all family members present, things happened which a therapist could not be aware of when seeing only one or possibly two family members. In 1961, Dr. John Bell wrote his monograph *Family Group Therapy,* in which he described his work with a family and listed a six-step educational process that occurred in family group therapy. Around this same time Charles Fulweiler began to develop his specific approach with families. Shortly after this the move was on in the direction of beginning to understand what was happening within the context of the total family.

Beginning of Family Dynamics

With Nathan Ackerman's publications (1938; 1958), and Ruesch and Bateson's *Communication, the Social Matrix of Psychiatry* (1951), there was a trend toward understanding the family dynamics. Jackson, in 1957, wrote his paper, "The Question of Family Homeostasis," which portrayed the family as searching for a balance but constantly remaining in a static state. In 1956, Bateson, Jackson, Haley, and Weakland focused on communication and an advanced concept of the "double-bind" in formulating a theory of the etiology of schizophrenia. Other studies were undertaken which added to the knowledge of the contribution of family pathology to the interpretation of mental disturbance. By the late 1950s, there was considerable knowledge regarding families, and family therapy was on its way to becoming another important method of working with people having difficulty in coping with stress.

Concomitantly there was, and continues to be, a serious question on the part of some members of the helping professions as to the validity of family therapy. Although this doubt is decreasing, it will probably continue to exist until at some point family therapy will take its rightful place with individual psychotherapy, group therapy, casework, and other methods of helping and working with people. One of the essential by-products of this form of treatment is a greater focus on the healthy aspects and strengths which exist in the family and which can be further developed among family members, in contrast to the emphasis on the pathology of the individual who is the only one in treatment.

Family Therapy since 1950

The past decade has seen change and progress in psychiatric thinking and practice. The determinant of focusing on the transference phenomenon has kept psychotherapy focused on the psychodynamics of individual behavior. Psychoanalytic theory, with its basic intrapsychic frame of reference, concluded that allowing any other person to enter the patient-therapist relationship would contaminate the transference and thus delimit or nullify progress in the therapy situation. With the passage of time, focus was placed on including significant figures related to the identified patient. Therapists were careful to see the patient separately from the related person, or to have another therapist see that person.

The primary person focused upon was the mother, thus relegating the so-called seeing of families to interviews with child and mother on a separate basis. This approach was important in that the therapeutic focus was broadened to include interpersonal relationships. The next move was to a family-centered approach that could look at the interrelationships that exist within the transactional system of a specific family. This meant a definite shift from seeing the patient as the central problem to looking at the family structure, system, and relationships as playing a deciding role in the symptoms presented by the family member who was labeled as the identified patient.

WHAT IS FAMILY THERAPY?

Family therapy is a process, method, and technique of psychotherapy which recognizes and utilizes all family members by seeing the group in conjoint psychotherapeutic sessions on a regular and continued basis. The therapy process is centered not upon the individual who is identified as the patient, but rather upon the total family and family system that is utilized by family members in their ongoing interactional patterns. There are variances as to what constitutes "all family members." Thus far it is, and has been, the prerogative of the individual therapist to determine which family members he wishes to see in therapy sessions. Some therapists include the nuclear family of father, mother, child or children, as well as others who have played an important long-term role in the family—grandparents, uncles, aunts, boarders, etc.

Generally, the major focus is on the nuclear family, which includes the father-mother-child combination. Within this framework, there are variances as to the combinations of family members who should be seen. Some therapists include the children throughout all therapy sessions, while others drop the children after a few sessions. Some therapists will not see parents (marital couple) apart, while others believe it essential to give each person the opportunity to be seen separately. There are other possibilities, but the major factor is the importance of having knowledge about and working with the total family configuration as a central theme. Carroll (1964) relates that there is no movement in one segment of psychiatry away from working with the individual patient.

Types of Family Therapy

In viewing the field of family therapy, Carroll observes four kinds of operations (Carroll, 1964):

1. Those which are concerned with the primary patient and carry on individual observation and treatment in a multiple way and consider the family as a group of individuals. This approach is usual where the patient is hospitalized and work with the family is seen as an extension of work with the patient.
2. Those which consider and work with the family as a series of shifting dyads. This approach is congenial to Child Guidance Centers as a derivation of earlier work with the dyads of therapist-child, therapist-mother, and mother-child.
3. Those which see the referred patient only as the messenger for the family and who work with the family as a unit.
4. Those who work with the family and a segment of the community as an open system.

It becomes obvious that during a process of development and growth no specific approach can be clearly indicated as the best or only approach to family-centered psychotherapy. Each approach will have its merits and will tend to focus on different levels in attempts to describe and understand family processes.

Explorations in Family Therapy

Weakland (1962) points out that "in practicing family treatment at present one has only the choice between being cautious in overall attitude without having adequate guides to what appropriate caution specifically would be or being more frankly exploratory." Since 1962, when Weakland's paper was published, there have been more exploration and broadening of approaches to family therapy. What is important at the present time is extensive and exhaustive research which focuses on behavior and communication between individuals and between family members. As communication patterns between people are better understood, it is possible to be more definitive in therapy approaches to the family situation and setting.

Basic Theory

The basic knowledge and skill utilized in family therapy come primarily from individual behavior theory as developed in psychology and applied in the psychoanalytic approach to the treatment of individuals. Using this background, family therapy is now adding to this fund of knowledge and making further contributions to a human phenomenon: that each person is a reflection of the system of which he is a part. As the result of therapists' working with and studying the family sytem, the practice developed of looking at the total picture and fitting the individual into his natural schemata of personal development and ongoing living. Whereas individual psychotherapy offers the opportunity for change, family therapy also offers the opportunity for personal change in a manner which works in the direction of changing the system of which the individual is a part.

CONJOINT FAMILY THERAPY— THEORY AND PRACTICE

It is evident that family therapy did not spring into being as a complete entity but was an occurrence that evolved over a period of time from contributions by different professions with different conceptual frameworks. The major portion of the early work of developing the theory and practice of family therapy was done primarily by therapists who were looking for a clearer understanding of emotional illness and a more effective treatment technique or method for working with emotionally disturbed persons. The impetus for family therapy continues to increase at a gratifying rate, but, at this point, there is not yet a well-defined conceptual framework for conjoint family treatment. Toward the goal of developing a well-defined theoretical framework, therapists are using existing knowledge in their practice of conjoint family therapy to gain further experience and insight into family functioning. As research continues and relates more closely to clinical practice, family therapy will achieve recognition, by both practitioners and lay people, as a sound method of treatment. This recognition seems inevitable in view of the rapid growth of family therapy in the nearly twenty years of its existence.

Development of Family Therapy Centers

At the present time, there are only a few schools of family therapy, each with its specific manner of clinical treatment. The rapid growth of this treatment method has been due primarily to the development of family therapy centers. In addition, numerous therapists, whether or not affiliated with family therapy centers, have been using their own methods of doing family therapy. Accordingly, numerous approaches to working with families have been, and are being, developed. Like all other forms of psychotherapy, the theoretical principles of family therapy become functional only through application. The practitioner, on becoming a family therapist, brings to the method his own adaptations and therapeutic skills which make it his individual brand of therapy.

Definition of Conjoint Family Therapy

Among the centers studying family processes and treatment is the Mental Research Institute in Palo Alto, California, where the name *conjoint family therapy* is given to family treatment. Satir (1963) states, "Conjoint family therapy, as we have defined it, is a therapeutic approach in which the whole family, where there is an emotionally disturbed, a socially disturbed, or a mentally ill member, is seen together as a group. This is based on theory that the ill member, whom we designate as the Identified Patient (I.P.), by means of his symptom is sending a message about the 'sick' condition of the family of which he is a member." This message is an outgrowth of the communication pattern prevalent in the family. It is not the case of the identified patient being a victim of a pathological communication pattern and thus the "sick" one in the family, but rather a situation whereby communication and behavior on the part of family members elicit communication and behavior in other family members. These patterns then become the accepted family norm with little possibility for change.

Concepts of Conjoint Family Therapy

In a brief brochure, Dr. Don Jackson stated that the Mental Research Institute investigations were based on three unique concepts: (1) mental illness in the patient is almost always accompanied by emotional illness and emotional instability in other members of the family group, (2) effective treatment of illness in one member of the family often requires that the therapist work with the entire family as a treatment unit, and (3) human communication is a key to emotional stability and instability—to normal and abnormal health. The stress on the interrelationship of the family members is important in all three aspects, but the primary emphasis can be placed upon the final part of the statement "normal and abnormal health." Thus, the emphasis is on not only the problems in the family and the dysfunctional aspects of family life and living but also what might be a normal or generally acceptable pattern within a family context. Family therapy focuses a much greater degree of attention on the healthy functional aspects of individuals than on their dysfunctional or pathological functioning.

FOCUS ON FAMILY DYNAMICS

In any discussion of psychotherapy for the family, the first major factor to be considered is that more than one person is involved. The family unit may be just husband and wife, or it may include their children or other individuals who are closely related to the family. No matter what members the combination includes, the focus must be on what is going on between individuals and not only on what is going on inside each individual. The intrapsychic processes are utilized for diagnostic and treatment purposes within the framework of the interpersonal transactions. From this standpoint, conjoint family therapy is a communication-centered approach which looks at the transactions and interactions that exist when two or more people are together in psychotherapy.

Haley, in explaining the shift in psychiatry and psychology from a focus on the processes within an individual to a focus on his relationships with other people, states (Haley, 1963):

> If one could imagine the individual confined within his skin, all this terminology describes what is assumed to be going on inside that skin. As a result the language is inappropriate for describing the behavior of a psychotherapist and patient responding to each other. More important, the transactions between therapist and patient cannot be conceptualized with the theoretical models which are the basis for these terms. Yet, at this time, there is no adequate substitution for the usual psychiatric concepts. The analogies and terms necessary to describe different ongoing relationships are only beginning to be born. The first major step in this direction was taken by Sullivan who struggled to describe the relationships between people with the concepts and theories which had been developed for individual description. Others have continued in this attempt, but it would now appear that human relationships will only be described adequately if the individual-centered ideas are largely discarded. The ultimate description of relationships will be in terms of patterns of communication in a theory of circular systems.

This circular system deals with the give-and-take that goes on among individuals in their interpersonal relationships as they carry on transactions with each other.

Family Patterns of Behavior

Within every family the members are constantly dealing with each other in specific ways, for each family member knows full well how another family member will respond to a given form of communication. Because of these patterns of interacting, family members learn to behave toward one another and interact in a certain set manner rather than in a purely random fashion. This specificity of behavior helps to make things predictable and evolves into a known set of patterns, which in turn leads to what is called the family system.

FAMILY HOMEOSTASIS

Jackson, borrowing from the medical model of body homeostasis, put forth his concept of a family homeostasis. This theoretical construction postulates that there is a characteristic behavior among members of a family which continuously takes into consideration the rules with which a family must function. This constant awareness of the way in which a family operates brings about the "family balance." Jackson sees this balance or homeostasis of the family as a "dynamic steady-state system" which constantly exerts energy to maintain a status quo by reacting against any change in the status quo. A constant pattern of behavior operates within the transactional system of the family members to preserve and keep in balance the existing methods and patterns of interaction. Balance is kept within limits of an unstated but fairly specific range of interaction between family members. By staying within this known range of behavior, homeostasis is maintained, since any family member can then predict the behavior of others in the family (Jackson, 1957).

Shift in Family Homeostasis

The homeostasis of the family changes when one member shifts from what may be the expected pattern of behavior to an unexpected one. If one member makes a shift, the other(s) must move with the shift or behave in a manner which makes it clear that the shift is not acceptable. This latter maneuver leads to a move back into the traditional homeostatic pattern or to jockeying for change in the homeostasis in order to again attain a balance. For example, if in a given family a father and mother were frequently at odds with each other, their behavior might be acceptable up to a certain point; but if it went beyond that point, it might pose a threat to a child, or children, in the family and to themselves. At this point, a child could readily behave in a way to bring the situation back within the normal family limits by (1) getting in the middle; (2) starting a fight with a sib; or (3) performing a task that distracts the parents, thus forcing them to concentrate their attention on the child. There are many possibilities that could be expanded upon, depending on what elicits a reaction within a specific family context.

Restoration of Family Homeostasis

The intervention to restore family homeostasis will depend on what method has worked successfully in the past. If the child is successful in his maneuver, the original reason for the parental disagreement is overlooked; and though it still leaves traces of hurt for both parents, they nevertheless can now focus upon the behavior of the child. In a difficult situation, one member, in trying to achieve family homeostasis, may take on a symptom which could be defined as the family symptom. A child could engage in a delinquent form of behavior, since this might be his way of achieving a balance, and at the same time give a signal of the problems within the family setting. Even though this may be a rather painful tactic for the child, it nevertheless restores the family's traditional balance through their concentration on the child and the child's symptom. Unquestionably, this behavior may have further meaning and interpretation, but for the purpose of describing a homeostatic condition, this simplified interpretation will serve as an illustration.

The initial need for moving in the direction of family homeostasis is the need two people have for getting together and forming a relationship which has intimacy and duration. In a family, the pattern of relating to one another begins the moment two individuals who are later to become parents first see each other. From that moment on, a pattern of interacting begins which carries on to the point of deciding that they wish to set up a household and live together. This decision is usually reached when each individual in the relationship has certain hopes which he believes will be fulfilled by the other person. Accordingly, each person sets up the pattern of relating with the other person in order to fulfill his own hopes. At times, this is a successful venture; at other times, the partner does not live up to anticipation, thus leading to disappointment.

A hypothetical situation illustrates one portion of the interaction that could occur in this initial period of adjusting to each other while the courtship period was going on. If the female hoped to marry a man who was the type of masculine figure who could take charge and be dominant in the relationship, and the male was looking for a woman who was willing to take the feminine role and be somewhat submissive, thus preserving his masculine concept, this seems to be a well-balanced situation. However, if we look into the woman's family background, we might find that in her family it was the mother and not the father who was the dominant figure. Even though this woman hopes for a male to take care of her needs, she is uncertain how to behave and what to expect from a male, since she did not have this kind of experience in her growing-up years. Let us also assume that in the growing-up years of the male, he also had a mother who was a dominant figure. It would be difficult for him to learn the role of a male which would make him the dominant figure, because he would expect the female to be dominant since this was what he observed in his family during his formative years.

In this situation, we see that the two individuals involved will have to work out some combination of expected behaviors that will be satisfactory to both. If they function with each other on the basis of being unable to look at their own covert contribution to the relationship, they will soon find themselves disappointed and unable to trust each other. They will blame their being hurt on the other person as though they had no hand in the matter. The hurt develops because each individual's hopes are shattered because of his disappointment in the other person. Both will be unaware of their explicit roles in bringing about this disappointment because they will not have been able to understand the parental models upon which their behavior was based.

DEVELOPMENT OF INDIVIDUAL BEHAVIOR PATTERNS

Generally speaking, the male in a family develops his concept of maleness as he observes his father's functioning both in the relationship with his mother and as a father. The male's concept of a female is based upon his observation of his mother as she functions as a mother and a wife. The converse applies to the female. At times, other adults influence a person's behavior, but those individuals are of minimal importance and certainly do not dominate the situation. The direct attempts of any given person to change or modify his behavior so that it differs from the observed parental behavior are far more important. Unperceived behavior patterns cannot be changed, so the patterns continue.

The better each person understands the relationship between his patterns of behavior and his parental models, the greater his opportunity for developing a relationship which is overt and productive. If, as in the hypothetical example mentioned above, both individuals were aware of the wife's negative wish to be dominant and the husband's negative wish to be dominant, they might work out a pattern which could lead to greater fulfillment of their hopes rather than to disappointment. If, when choosing each other as mates, they had been able to discuss their concerns regarding their inadequacy in filling the male and female roles, they might have decided not to live together, or they might have gone on to develop a more open form of relating. There are many combinations possible in the relationship pattern of any two individuals; but this example gives an idea of the complexity of the relations between two individuals and points out that from this relationship a pattern or blueprint evolves which lays down the schemata for future additions to the family and for the potential method for functioning within the family. Satir (1965) writes:

> Because each person comes into the world without a blueprint for interacting in these ways, he must develop it as he grows from birth. The beginning of this blueprint will of necessity . . . be shaped by those who surround him. These are the adults who attempt to insure his survival . . . through nurture and economic support, through directing his actions, and through providing a model for what he can become.
>
> Most adults have little notion about their importance as models for the child. They behave as though the child sees and hears only that which he is directed to see and hear. If the way in which adults behave with each other and with the outside world, and the way in which a child is asked to behave are incongruent, the child will perceive this. Because the child is confined by the rules about what he may report, by his inability to judge and by his lack of a complete enough set of reporting symbols, the adult is deluded into believing that he is successfully labeling what the child sees and hears. The parent believes, in other words, that the child does not see or hear that which a parent does not directly direct him to see and hear. They believe that children's symptoms are distorted by obvious comment on the discrepancies which they have experienced and are experiencing. The child cannot grow if he must deal with important discrepancies upon which he may not comment openly. Clues to the nature of the discrepancies may be found in the way the family communicates.

THE ROLE OF COMMUNICATION IN
FAMILY THERAPY

Communication is the major thesis upon which conjoint family therapy is based. A general definition of communication might be that it is a process whereby an individual, through verbal and nonverbal means, transmits information to a second person who, in turn, receives the information and himself goes through the process of being the transmitter. In a continuing interaction there is the constant giving and receiving over a period of time. Watzlawick (1964) states three basic premises of the theory of human communication. The first basic premise is that "one cannot NOT communicate." Considered from the aspect of verbal and nonverbal types of communication, so long as someone communicates in some way to another person, his being on the scene is taken as a communication even if he does not speak. Silence does not mean that there is no communication, since on a nonverbal level a great deal can be transmitted to the receiver. Communication is behavior in its fullest sense and includes such manifestations as are expressed by the tone of voice, facial expression, body position, and manner of dress.

Watzlawick's second basic premise is that communication is a multilevel phenomenon. He views communication as essentially meaningless if it is reduced to one level, for two people are involved in communication—the sender and the receiver—each of whom has his own referent point. In addition, there is always a specific context in which to place the referent point. There are at least two portions to a communication: one is the content with its information value; the other, the portion that defines what the message is about and how its sender conceives of the relationship with the receiver.

From the moment two individuals make contact, their communication is such that there is a giving and a searching on the part of each one to determine the nature of the relationship to the other. Jackson (1957) relates the report-command theory of communication by pointing out that every message has both a content and a relationship aspect to it. The content communicates the factual and opinion level. While the facts, views, opinions, and feelings are being stated, communication at another level is concurrently attempting to influence and define the relationship. When two men meet, they may shake hands and utter a "Nice to meet you" or they may simply say, "How do you do." The content level is expressed in words that are as acceptable a mode of behavior as is the handshake.

At another level, or levels, there may be a number of other "messages" taking place. In what way did the handshake take place— who squeezed harder and what may have gone on in the mind of each individual regarding the other person? At the same time, at an eye contact level, what took place? Did eyes meet on an "equal" level, did someone drop his eyelids, look away, or look down? What facial expressions were manifested, or what did each one believe he saw in the facial expression of the other? These are questions put in a hypothetical vein, but in actuality similar thoughts do take place, depending upon the individuals and the context of the interaction. From the point of first meeting there is a sizing-up which leads to determining the relationship to follow. If the contact continues, the overt and verbal behavior will be only one aspect, along with the covert and nonverbal behavior which will indicate how this and future contacts will function for these two social beings.

The third premise of communication, that "the message sent is not necessarily the message received," has to do with the fact that there are differences in individuals. The production of one individual may be seen very differently by the observing person, since the person who is receiving the message has a different set of values, standards, and perceptions which, in turn, make his reality different from the reality of the person who sent the message.

Since there is a constant barrage of communication going on within the family context, it is the therapist's task to understand the patterns that exist and be able to analyze them with a high degree of accuracy. In the family context, it is of major importance that there is clarity in the communication of family members and that they are both efficient and effective in the means they utilize to communicate with each other. The clearer the transactions, the more certain are individuals of their position, since messages define the relationship of the person sending the message and the person receiving the message.

THE FAMILY AS A RULE-GOVERNED SYSTEM

Since members of families are constantly defining their positions by relationship messages, it soon becomes evident that everyone in the family attempts to program the relationships of other members, thus influencing them to function or think as he does. And because all family members participate in this venture, it leads to the members of the family putting behavior into an ordered format so that each may be aware of his respective position. Jackson (1965) postulates that the family is a rule-governed system; that its members behave among themselves in an organized, repetitive manner; and that this pattern of behavior can be abstracted as a governing principle of family life.

Jackson predicates that a rule occurs over a sequence of events which take place over a period of time, and that this rule is then reduced into a short, patterned sequence. It seems to be necessary to work things out in a relationship and break it down to as short a sequence of interactions as possible in order for communication not to be a lengthy and ever-repeating process. Jackson (1965) states, "Although the family as a unit indulges in uncountable numbers of different, specific behaviors, the whole system can be run by a relatively small set of rules governing relationships. If one can reliably infer the general rules by which a family operates, then all its complex behavior may turn out to be not only patterned, but also understandable . . . and, as a result, perhaps predictable." The adoption of rules by family members is a logical sequence, for if a rule is followed, there must be the same sequence of events each time with each individual according to the rule. If, in a family, the rule is that the father-husband is first in line for having certain needs filled, it puts the wife-mother in a very difficult position when an infant has needs at the same time that her husband does. If the rule is adhered to, then the wife-mother must function so that she fills the need of her husband first, since to break the patterns of expected behavior might mean unpredictable results which may prove untenable for the family.

METHOD AND TECHNIQUE IN CONJOINT FAMILY THERAPY

Therapeutic procedure is not the prerogative of an individual or of one specific group or school of thought. Even within a specific school of thought there must be variations, since each individual has his or her own unique way of functioning. In family therapy one of the primary considerations is the personality of the therapist. Since one of the qualifications of an effective therapist is his communication skill, the therapist plays an important role in the communication that goes on between him and the family members. The therapist who remains true to his own personality and values has the greater likelihood of becoming a successful family therapist. If he attempts to imitate another therapist or to adhere rigidly to a particular professional stereotype, he stands to lose his spontaneity and effectiveness as a family therapist.

UNDERSTANDING THE FAMILY'S FRAME OF REFERENCE

Families, like individuals, have their specific, idiosyncratic ways of behaving. Within a specific family each member operates from his own particular emotional frame of reference. This frame of reference, depending on the emotionality of the moment, influences the way he perceives the world around him. Thus, when there is an involvement in a relationship with another family member, each person selects clues from the other, depending on his own particular emotional frame of reference. By this means an individual in interaction will perceive from his point of view what the other person has communicated; and if this perception is revealed, it will indicate the nature of his subjective feelings.

Given two different emotional frames of reference, there can emerge an area of disagreement between the two people involved. In therapy, should each person come away from the same event with a different perception and conclusion, this could easily lead to arguments, which are a pitfall for the therapist. An essential principle of therapy at this point is that it is not important to determine who is right or who is wrong, but to get a factual picture of events so that each individual can reassess what has taken place and then get closer to finding out what fits in this situation. The therapist does not concern himself with the content per se, but rather how this content came to be and what are the covert and unspoken relationship messages which have evolved because of it.

Role Adjustment in the Family

The above paragraph indicated involvement between two people. Let us now look at a hypothetical family with four members: male adult, female adult, male child, female child. As each new member is added to the family, it has its effect upon the relationship of other members of the family. When a first child is born, the parents must adjust to the inclusion in the family of a new being whose needs are primary and total. This means that the mother and father will have less time for each other. Two possible effects of this can be (1) a ready adjustment or (2) disappointment or hurt leading to conflict, since each one of the parents will now be receiving less time and attention from the other than had previously been the case. Prior to the child's birth, they were in their respective roles of husband and wife, but now as father and mother they are expected to give more of themselves. It can be seen that adjustments must be made, with each partner finding his own way of accomplishing this.

Within our hypothetical family, there are four individuals, each having his own specific role as a male parent, female parent, male child, and female child. When we begin to look at the dyads within this family structure, there is the possibility of fourteen different combinations of interaction which could go on simultaneously within the family. At any given moment there can be the mother's perception of the father, son, or daughter; the father's perception of the mother, son, or daughter; the son's perception of the father, mother, or sister; the sister's perception of the father, mother, or brother; the wife's perception of the husband; the husband's perception of the wife. The important point is not what happens in a specific transaction between two members at any given moment, but what effect that transaction has on the two who are interacting and on the other family members.

624

Rigidity of Family Roles

For example, if the roles of the children are that the male child expresses most of the unruly behavior and that the female child must, at all costs, behave in an exemplary manner, there will be repercussions should the female child act in a way uncommon to her usual demeanor. Should she talk back to the mother, then the possibility arises that the mother could be upset and expect behavior from the father which, if not forthcoming, might make her feel unloved. In addition, the brother might begin to wonder about the usurping of his traditional role, and he could react, setting off a chain of reactions. The point is that if there is a change via one transaction within the family, there are simultaneously other interactional elements changed within the family system, thus altering the homeostatic balance. In practicing therapy, it is important to understand the varying interactional and transactional operations within a family system so that they can be examined together by the therapist and the family.

RATIONALE FOR TOTAL FAMILY IN THERAPY

A good case can be presented for seeing all family members together in family therapy, since the total picture of what goes on within a family cannot be presented by one family member. It is important for all family members to be involved so that the various perceptions can be pooled in order to make clear the manner in which each person in the family views a given situation. Leaving one person out eliminates an important part of the existing scene. This is why it is essential to involve all people who are important in the development of a family and not concentrate only on the person who happens to be the symptom bearer. The greater the focus on the person who develops symptoms, and by this means expresses the family distress, the less chance there is of clarifying the family situation and eliminating the dysfunction which produced the symptom.

INITIAL STEPS IN CONJOINT FAMILY THERAPY

The initial contact for treatment is usually made by one member of the family—to whom it must be made clear from the beginning which other family members are to be seen in therapy sessions. Therapists have varying ideas regarding which members should be seen, depending on their own experience or lack of experience in the past. Frequently the initial session, if this is a family with children, will involve only the parents, although it could just as easily involve the children. If the parents are seen in the initial interview, the interview is utilized to evaluate their interactions, validate their positions in the family, and clarify the therapist's plans as well as the parents' questions and concerns.

It is necessary to be clear about what will be done in family therapy and the process through which this will take place. The greater the therapist's ability to communicate clearly, the greater clarity the family achieves in their communication. Initially, the general concept that the therapist attempts to convey to the family members is his interest in the welfare of all the family members, not just one person. Thus, the therapist invites the opinions of everyone present about what seems to be the pain or hurt in the family so far as each person is concerned.

Negotiating the Contract for Therapy

The major theme in the initial interview is that of negotiating a contract or agreement. The greater the clarity in the agreement as to future functioning, the easier it will be for family members, since they will know what to expect, will have a concept of the ground rules, and will know that communication lines are open for any question anyone wishes to raise. The involvement of all the family members works as a safeguard for the therapist, making it possible not to become so involved in situations which would be detrimental to his functioning, e.g., having secrets with one member or forming a coalition with a single family member which could alienate others in the therapy session. If children are present at the first session, essentially the same procedure is followed, although it will take longer because more individuals are involved. If children are not present at the first session, they are told briefly when they do come in what took place when they were not in attendance. This brings the children up to date and enables them to start with the total family on an even footing.

The Family History

The concentration in conjoint family therapy is primarily on the here and now, but in order to understand present functioning, it is of value to know something about the family background. Any specific family begins at the point where the parents involved first made contact with each other. This is, of course, the period when they first saw and then met each other, carried on a courtship, and then decided to live together. This phase of their lives is looked into rather closely to get as clear a picture as is possible of their interactions. Their pattern of functioning had its groundwork laid during this period, and clues can be obtained regarding the potential resultant behavior in their children. This information is not wanted for the purpose of blaming either parent, but to get a picture of what took place at this period of their lives so that the individuals can be aware that their interactional picture started a long time ago and that they have been carrying on a similar pattern since that time.

A chronological history is obtained of the genesis of this family as a legal entity, including such items as the birth of children, moves the family has made, employment, deaths, handling of crises. It is important to synchronize these events in a chronological sequence in order to get at the family history, for example, second child born just after the father lost his job. In this way, each period of time will give a picture of all the events occurring within the family, and not as they happened to isolated individuals in the family.

The third historical entity obtained is the perceptual history of the two parents in the family. This means getting them to give their own perception of their growing-up experiences, information about their parents, their observations of marital interaction which took place between each of their parents, themselves, or their sibs. This is not done at extensive length, but does ask very specific questions to which both the parents in the family respond, thus giving the therapist clues such as how they each perceived their own family of origin.

Observation of Family Patterns of
Behavior

At the same time the historical material is being gathered, therapy continues (since the family members are constantly interacting), and the therapist is observing the patterns as they take place. The therapist is keenly alert to the interaction between the individuals and is looking for the patterns which exist to determine whether this is a functional family which can achieve a joint outcome or whether it is dysfunctional and in constant turmoil, confusion, and disagreement. In addition, the therapist notes which family members form coalitions, how homeostatic patterns are maintained, what the constant, repetitive patterns in the family are (here we start looking for the family rules), how spontaneous family members can be, what the breadth or restriction of their interactions is, and how they handle crises. These are some of the more important issues to look for while doing conjoint family therapy, although they are certainly not all-inclusive. A therapist must be constantly aware of the myriad issues going on in the fast and constant interchange of communication between family members.

Family Analysis and Diagnosis

The family therapist has as another major function the task of family analysis and diagnosis. This procedure is an accumulation of observations and specific tasks given to the family by the therapist in order to determine their pattern of functioning. Included in analysis and diagnosis is the analysis of communication patterns and determination of the ability of this family to make issues clear or leave them in a state of confusion, misunderstanding, and mistrust. Role-function discrepancy analysis helps to determine whether the function of each family member fits the role that that family member has within the family structure. For example, do wife and husband behave as equals as adults or do they interact on the basis of a parent-child relationship with one primarily taking the role of a child? If this is so, what does this mean in regard to the children, who frequently may see one of their parents in the position of a child in the family?

In analyzing the family situation the therapist must look for the degree of self-esteem that each individual has, because this will determine to what extent they are able to speak out and interact. Caution should be used regarding the family's meaning of words, since each family has its own meanings for certain words which are not known to the therapist until they are checked and clarified. Another important consideration is the family's expectation of the goals of therapy. That is, what is their preconceived notion regarding the possible success or lack of success in reaching a joint outcome?

Toleration of Individual Differences in the Family

Another issue of major importance in analysis is determining to what degree it is possible for individuals in the family to allow others to be different from them and to have differing perceptions. If individual differences are difficult or impossible in the family, then there will be a great deal of pain within the family since members will either struggle or give up their individuality to fit into the schemata of agreement and "sameness." The therapist should investigate how the family is able to handle decision making, whether it is possible for a member to make a decision and stay with it or whether decision making is difficult or impossible, based upon the member's experiences of previous attempts.

The general task of the therapist is to isolate, identify, and describe what is seen and heard during the therapy sessions and then to explain this behavior in terms which are understandable to the family members. The therapist also interprets the family behavior on the basis of rules, communication patterns, interactional ingredients, family history, family organization, process analysis, outcome analysis, and communication analysis. In order to do this, the therapist must be able to create a situation where people are willing to take the chance of looking openly at themselves and their actions.

THE THERAPIST AS A FACILITATOR OF FAMILY CHANGE

The central role of the therapist is to alter the perceptual world of family members so that it is possible for them to see that change is possible. The therapist does this primarily through interventions relating to the specific interaction that he sees in front of him. At the same time, the therapist uses some or all of the pertinent material that he has gathered and analyzed, waiting for the opportunity to present itself in the therapy session so that it can be used. With the change in the perceptual world of the individuals in the family and, consequently, the family itself, the responses ensuing between family members are quite different from reactions in the past. It is important, therefore, in doing family therapy, to get at the perceptions of each individual in relation to his or her survival significance, growth, and closeness and the end product of joint endeavors.

Goals of Family Therapy

Satir (1965) states:

> Our goals, in therapy, are also related to this analysis of family communication. We attempt to make three changes in the family system. First, each member of the family should be able to report congruently, completely, and obviously on what he sees and hears, feels and thinks about himself and others, in the presence of others. Second, each person should be addressed and related to in terms of his uniqueness, so that decisions are made in terms of exploration and negotiation rather than in terms of power. Third, differentness must be openly acknowledged, and used for growth.
>
> When these changes are achieved, communication within the family will lead to appropriate outcomes. "Appropriate outcomes" are decisions and behavior which fit the age, ability, and role of the individuals, which fit the role contracts and the context involved, and which further the common goals of the family.

THE ROLE OF THE THERAPIST

The role of the therapist is a very involved and intricate one, since he is dealing with voluminous happenings and messages. There is no specific sequence as to what takes place in therapy, since it depends on the given situation and the individuals involved. This does not mean that the therapist cannot have certain goals and a specific direction which he wishes to take, but he must remain flexible and be able to adapt to the occurrences in the family. Above all, the therapist must constantly be in control of the situation—with an awareness of what is happening and the skill and ability to move in at the appropriate time. The therapist does not take a back seat and remain an observer; he is an active participant who is clear on what should be done in the family situation and is not reluctant to do it.

The Nurse and Conjoint Family Therapy

Although public health nurses have always worked with families and provided the physically ill members of the family with necessary nursing care, it is only recently that nurses have become interested in (1) providing care for the emotionally disturbed members of the family, and (2) learning to regard the family itself as a possible patient in need of nursing intervention. Two factors have contributed to the expansion of the nurse's role in the community. Since the midfifties, new developments in psychiatric treatment, such as the introduction of the psychoactive drugs, the therapeutic community, day and night hospitals, and other new forms of social therapy, have resulted in the discharge of psychiatric patients to their homes and communities at a much earlier stage of their convalescence than had been possible in the past. These discharged patients are often far from completely recovered and require follow-up nursing care. Another factor is that sociopsychiatric studies in the area of community mental health indicated that families and communities could be "sick" as well as individuals (Spiegel and Bell, 1959; Hollingshead and Redlich, 1958; Faris and Dunham, 1939; Dollard et al., 1937). Nurses (who always have been well accepted by families and the community) are discovering a new and unparalleled opportunity not only to aid families in distress but also to promote better mental health attitudes in the family.

Conjoint family therapy provides the nurse with a suitable technique through which he can realize this opportunity. This method is not limited to a particular helping profession but can be acquired by persons whose professional education includes a background in the behavioral sciences, clinical experience in one or more methods of psychotherapy or social therapy, and an understanding of the responsibilities of the therapist-patient relationship. Courses in conjoint family therapy which include both theory and supervised clinical practice are available in a number of family therapy centers and in graduate programs in university schools of nursing and social work, as, for example, the Mental Research Institute in Palo Alto, California, and the University of California School of Nursing at San Francisco. At this latter institution a lecture and laboratory course in conjoint family therapy for graduate nurses at the postmaster's level has been offered since 1964. In this course, nurses carry families in treatment as individual therapists or as cotherapists under the supervision of a qualified preceptor in family therapy. Nurses are placed in facilities where they have previously worked with individual patients (Ketcham, 1966).

At the present time the number of nurses who are trained in the practice of conjoint family therapy is small. It is interesting to note that the nurses who have attempted to use family therapy have been individuals with a great deal of initiative and a desire to try a technique that is different from traditional nursing methods. Given adequate training, nurses have been able to move in readily into areas where they had not functioned previously because of the stereotyped concept of the role of the nurse held by many members of other professions. It was readily seen that the nurse with preparation in psychiatric and public health nursing can function on a team with other professionals in the treatment of families in a clinic setting or in the home, and on either an ongoing or an emergency basis.

More and more private and public mental health agencies are being developed where the well-prepared nurse is needed more as a clinician than in any other capacity. Another major role for the nurse prepared in conjoint family therapy will be as a psychiatric nurse educator in schools of nursing to teach conjoint family therapy to nurses. Nurses with research skills will also be needed to further the development of conjoint family therapy theory and practice, in particular as it relates to nursing. They will also be needed to engage in clinical research in family therapy, either as members of research teams where their acceptance by the community as workers in the home can assist in the involvement of families for research studies, or as independent investigators of their own research projects.

REFERENCES

Ackerman, Nathan W. (1958): *The Psychodynamics of Family Life*, Basic Books, Inc., Publishers, New York.
——(1938): "The Unity of the Family," *Archives of Pediatrics*, vol. 55, no. 138, pp. 51–62.

Bateson, Gregory, Don D. Jackson, Jay Haley, and John H. Weakland (1956): "Toward a Theory of Schizophrenia," *Behavioral Science,* vol. 1, no. 156, pp. 251–264.

Bell, John E. (1961): *Family Group Therapy,* U.S. Public Health Monograph, no. 64.

Bell, Norman W., and Ezra F. Vogel (eds.) (1960): *A Modern Introduction to the Family,* The Free Press, New York, p. 5.

Bowen, Murray (1960): "A Family Concept of Schizophrenia," in Don D. Jackson (ed.), *The Etiology of Schizophrenia,* Basic Books, Inc., Publishers, New York, pp. 346–372.

Carroll, Edward J. (1964): "Family Therapy—Some Observations and Comparisons," *Family Process,* March, pp. 178–185.

Dollard, John, et al. (1937): *Caste and Class in a Southern Town,* Yale University Press, New Haven.

Faris, Robert E. L., and H. Warren Dunham (1939): *Mental Disorders in Urban Areas,* The University of Chicago Press, Chicago.

Friedman, Natalie P. (1959): "The Changing Concept of the Family in Social Casework from Mary Richmond to 1959," An unpublished thesis, Columbia University School of Social Work, p. 21.

Haley, Jay (1963): *Strategies of Psychotherapy,* Grune & Stratton, Inc., New York, p. 4.

———(1962): "Whither Family Therapy?" *Family Process,* March, pp. 69–100.

Hollingshead, August B., and Fredrick C. Redlich (1958): *Social Class and Mental Illness,* John Wiley & Sons, Inc., New York.

Jackson, Don D. (1957): "The Question of Family Homeostasis," *Psychiatric Quarterly Supplement,* part 1, pp. 79–90.

———(1965): "The Study of the Family," *Family Process,* March, pp. 1–20.

———, and Virginia M. Satir (1961): "A Review of Psychiatric Developments in Family Therapy, in N. Ackerman, F. L. Beatman, and S. N. Sherman (eds.), *Exploring the Base for Family Therapy,* Family Service Association of America, New York.

Ketcham, Margery (1966): "Family Therapy—A Backward Glance," An unpublished paper written at the University of California School of Nursing, San Francisco.

Lidz, Theodore, Alice Cornelison, Dorothy Terry, and Stephen Fleck (1958): "Intrafamilial Environment of the Schizophrenic Patient, VI, The Transmission of Irrationality," *Archives of Neurology and Psychiatry,* March, pp. 305–316.

Ruesch, Jurgen, and Gregory Bateson (1951): *Communication: The Social Matrix of Psychiatry,* W. W. Norton & Company, Inc., New York.

Satir, Virginia M. (1964): *Conjoint Family Therapy. A Guide to Theory and Technique,* Science and Behavior Books, Inc., Palo Alto, Calif.

———(1965): "The Family as a Treatment Unit," *Confinia Psychiatrica* (Basel), vol. 8, pp. 37–42.

———(1963): "The Quest for Survival, A Training Program for Family Diagnosis and Treatment," *Acta Psychotherapeutica et Psychosomatica* (Basel), vol. 2, pp. 33–38.

Spiegel, John P., and Norman W. Bell (1959): "The Family of the Psychiatric Patient," in Silvano Arieti (ed.), *American Handbook of Psychiatry,* Basic Books, Inc., Publishers, New York, vol. I, pp. 114–149.

Watzlawick, Paul (1964): *An Anthology of Human Communication,* Science and Behavior Books, Inc., Palo Alto, Calif.

Weakland, John H. (1962): "Family Therapy as a Research Arena," *Family Process,* March, pp. 63–68.

Wynne, Lyman C., Irving M. Ryckoff, Juliana Day, and Stanley I. Hirsch (1958): "Pseudo-Mutuality in the Family Relationships of Schizophrenics," *Psychiatry,* May, pp. 205–220.

PART SIX

Psychiatric Nursing and Research

25

RESEARCH METHODS

Marion E. Kalkman

To do research, like undertaking inquiry of any other sort—filmmaking, art, political thought—is to go along a very black corridor, bumping from wall to wall, with the light hidden by a bend in the tunnel, thinking to set oneself a right question and at best finding out the answer to something else.

Penelope Gilliatt (1970)

Psychiatric-mental health nursing is a profession that requires some of its practitioners to go into the black corridor to engage in the difficult, frustrating, and often painful process of research, attempting to ask the right questions and, one hopes, finding some answers which will prove helpful in solving its many problems. Mere willingness to undertake the difficult task is not enough. Research requires certain qualities in the researcher. According to Wilson, these attributes include not only an inquiring mind and a deep love of learning—which are requirements in many disciplines—but also the ability to use words as instruments of precision and to invent new ones to express new concepts; to reason verbally by analogy to explain comparisons; to fit many resemblances into a single generalization; to think graphically in terms of dynamic models; to be able to take a fresh look at old knowledge; and, perhaps most importantly, to think creatively beyond logic to intuition (Wilson, 1970, pp. 104–106).

Where in nursing shall we find our nurse-researchers? One answer to this question comes from a paper of Martha Rogers: "The researchers will either come out of higher education or they are not going to exist. They do not come out of attics." She believes that "the creative, intelligent, independent, curious, skeptical, energetic, non-conformist student or practitioner" should be encouraged and must be provided with opportunities for continued study. Although investigative skill may begin in the master's program or even earlier, doctoral study prepares the university teachers, scientists, and researchers. "Not all doctoral students will become research scientists, but whereas there are research scientists who may not be good teachers, I have not known a good teacher whose competence was not increased by participation in some kind of productive scholarship" (Rogers, 1964).

THE CLINICAL RESEARCHER

A great need exists in psychiatric nursing for clinical research—for the careful observation and recording of clinical data and subsequent evaluation, conceptualization, validation, and publication of research results. Rioch (1955, p. 314) writes,

> Science may be considered as cumulative knowledge and, as such, requires primarily operational reports. In other words, the primary scientific task of the psychiatrist is to report his operations. From such reports in collaboration with his colleagues, he may then proceed toward elucidating which are the relevant operations; what are the relevant time intervals of the events studied; what is the extent of the relevant data.

Clinical research should be an integral part of good psychiatric nursing practice—that process which consists of observation, assessment, treatment, and evaluation of the results of nursing intervention. Clinical research problems emerge from the researcher's actual experiences in practice. Thus broad clinical experience becomes a prerequisite for clinical research. The clinical researcher also needs to know how to use a range of different research methods so that he can apply the appropriate method to investigate a given problem. The clinical researcher must also be aware of the two very different roles in which he functions, that of researcher and that of clinician. Although he is engaged in scientific research, he cannot forget his responsibilities to his patient-subjects as a therapist. Rioch gives a good description of the double role of the clinical researcher. He believes that the researcher in psychiatry must keep the whole treatment situation (therapist, patient, and setting) in mind during investigation, with all the implications that the research operations may have on the therapeutic process. Moreover, as a scientist, he must be able to view objectively and to evaluate the various factors and operations in the clinical situation which he is studying (Rioch, 1955, p. 316).

In the majority of instances these two functions must be performed sequentially, as the rate of therapeutic interaction is usually too great to permit differential handling of the input—that is, data—during the course of the interaction. Experience in both functions is necessary, not in the sense of learning two sets of jargons, ritualized actions, and beliefs, but rather in being a participant observer in one part of the total problem and a critical formulator in the other.

Rioch also warns against the use of one particular method of research. "There is . . . danger that a group [of researchers] limited by a special language—inevitably of highly condensed symbols—will exert pressure on its members to refrain from operations likely to evoke data inconsistent with the assumptions implicit in the language" (Rioch, 1955, p. 315). The psychiatric researcher should have adequate technical research skills in several research methodologies to be able to compare their concepts, evaluate their operations, and utilize them to review and revise the basic assumptions of his own research frames of reference.

There are a number of relatively new methodologies or approaches which have proved applicable or have been suggested as appropriate for psychiatric nursing research in addition to such well-known methods as clinical case reports, critical incident technique, participant observations, and structured and unstructured interview methods. Anne Davis recommends the phenomenological approach as one which is particularly applicable to nursing research. She writes (A. Davis, 1973, p. 225),

> The majority of students who enter the doctoral programs in nursing have arrived there by way of clinical preparation in their previous professional programs. It is this clinical approach which emphasizes observation, interviews, interaction, and interpersonal relations in an attempt to understand the patient's definition of the situation. In my opinion, this clinical research approach more perfectly fits conceptually the phenomenological approach.

A number of psychiatric nurses, including Marcella Davis (1970), have utilized the symbolic interactionism approach successfully in their nursing research. According to M. Davis, this approach places major emphasis on the way the self is shaped and altered through ongoing interaction with significant others in the person's interpersonal and social environment. This method requires the researcher to understand the person's situation from his own definitional perspective, so that insight can be gained into the way this perspective influences the person's behavior and self-concept (M. Davis, 1970, pp. 6–7). Blumer (1969, p. 47) describes *symbolic interactionism* as "a down-to-earth approach to the scientific study of human group life and human conduct. Its empirical world is the natural world of such group life and conduct. It lodges its problems in this natural world, conducts its studies in it, and derives its interpretations from such naturalistic studies." For further discussion on the nature and methods of phenomenology and symbolic interactionism, the reader is referred to the following: phenomenology: van den Berg (1955), Natanson (1969, 1970), Spiegelberg (1965), Strauss (1964); symbolic interactionism: Blumer (1969, pp. 1–60), Manis and Meltzer (1967), Mead (1934, 1964), McCall and Simmons (1966).

Psychiatric nurses may find general system theory useful as a method in nursing research. Such research could include exploration of the gaps in psychiatric nursing knowledge, inventories of psychiatric nursing resources, and research relative to the delivery of psychiatric nursing services to the public. For this type of research, some competence in operational research and systems analysis could prove helpful. Examples of problems for which research is needed include: alternate methods of providing psychiatric nursing care for chronic schizophrenic patients other than long-term hospitalization; preparation of nurses for, and appropriate roles of nurses in, community mental health programs; development and testing of models for preventive mental health programs; and methods for bringing psychiatric nursing care to segments of the community with special problems such as are found in slum areas, non-English-speaking enclaves, and isolated communities.

General systems research methods can also be utilized to explore problems in psychopathology and psychotherapy and for research in personality theory. Bertalanffy sees personality theory at present as a battlefield of contrasting and controversial theories, and quotes Hall and Lindzey's statement (1952, p. 71) that all theories of behavior are pretty poor theories and all of them leave much to be desired in the way of scientific proof. Bertalanffy suggests that although general system theory cannot be expected to provide solutions where personality theorists from Freud and Jung to a host of modern writers were unable to do so, the theory will have shown its value if it opens new perspectives and viewpoints capable of experimental and practical application, as appears to be the case (Bertalanffy, 1968, p. 105). Other references on the application of general system theory in psychology and psychiatry are Bertalanffy (1952; 1966; 1967).

CONTRIBUTIONS OF CLINICAL RESEARCH

Herbert Zucker points out the great contribution of clinical research to human knowledge. He writes, "It cannot be a matter of chance that the concepts that have illuminated human behavior most have come from working clinicians—Freud, Jung, Horney, Fromm, Sullivan, for example. This has happened, I believe, because the clinical relationship provides such a favorable opportunity for combining and identifying with people" (Zucker, 1967, p. 18). Major concepts have also been tested by clinical methods. Although such methods are slow, difficult, and in need of refinement, nevertheless clinical methods have been effective in revealing flaws in a number of these concepts when exposed to direct trial, which led to their revision, redefinition, or diminished use. Zucker (1967, pp. 18–19) adds,

> Despite these contributions, clinicians have always been made to feel a little ashamed of their apparent lack of scientific sophistication and rigor (the absence of laboratories, instruments, clear-cut experimental situations, and so on). General psychology might have done better had it not lighted so eagerly on some of the untidy aspects of clinical work; it should rather have tried to see what is involved in procedures that help generate such contributions.

Sanford believes that clinical research could also make a contribution toward better teaching by making it more relevant and more human. He writes (Sanford, 1970, p. 33),

> We could try to organize research around problems and people rather than around variables, disciplines, or factors. If we could get research organized in this way, teaching would follow because teaching does follow research. . . . I think we can humanize what we do in the universities and in practical work by bringing together what has been separated in science and in practice—research from action, action from teaching, and teaching from research.

EXPERIMENTAL SOCIAL INNOVATIVE RESEARCH

Some nurses associated with community health programs or other community agencies have become aware that the clients with whom they come in contact have problems closely tied in with problems of the community which primarily stem from economic, social, and cultural factors. Such nurses need research methodologies which will enable them to investigate social and environmental problems in their real-life settings. This cannot be done by experimental methods which ignore the humanitarian values of both the researcher and his subjects. Fairweather maintains that scientific methods can be applied to social problems so that changes can occur in a society, in a systematic, planned, and orderly manner, that are not only compatible with, but essential to, humanitarian values. He sees these methods as a combination of scientific and humanitarian thought, utilizing components from the various social sciences and forging them into a multidisciplinary approach (Fairweather, 1967).

Fairweather also believes that our society needs a mechanism for the evaluation of various solutions to critical social problems. He states that a research methodology is needed to test these solutions prior to their adoption and implementation by society, and he has developed one such method which he calls *experimental social innovation* (Fairweather, 1967, pp. 20–36). In this method the testing and evaluation of solutions to social problems are accomplished by establishing new learning and living subsystems in a larger general system, as, for example, a therapeutic community as a new subsystem in a mental hospital system. The development of new subsystems constitutes only one component of the experimental social innovation method. There are in all eight requirements. These may be stated as follows (Fairweather, 1967, pp. 20–30; Kalkman, 1973, pp. 169–170):

1. It defines a significant social problem.
2. It makes naturalistic field observations in the actual community setting.
3. It creates different solutions in the form of innovated social subsystems.
4. It designs an experiment to compare these created solutions.
5. It implants the innovated subsystems in the appropriate social settings.
6. It allows sufficient time for the operation of the innovated subsystems to evaluate their outcome.
7. It assumes responsibility for the lives and welfare of participants in the subsystem.
8. It uses a multidisciplinary approach.

GROUNDED THEORY

Glaser and Strauss (1967) have developed a method for generating theory from qualitative data—theory which can be useful in investigating problems in specific areas of concern. This method has been called *grounded theory* by its discoverers. The term *grounded theory* refers to the fact that the theory evolves from the basic data collected in the field. The primary difference between this method of research and the traditional experimental method is that the latter starts research with a known theory and attempts to determine whether or not the data can be explained by this theory. On the other hand, grounded theory starts with data which have been systematically collected, coded, analyzed, and compared, from which the theory emerges. Because grounded theory utilizes data collected in daily life situations, with problems of real concern to the persons involved, it has attracted the attention of a growing number of nurses, both researchers and clinicians. Several nurses have utilized this method in their research efforts. One such nurse is Jeanne Quint (1967), who used this method in her study, *The Nurse and the Dying Patient*. For a description and discussion of this theory, as well as an outline of its operational steps, the reader is referred to Glaser and Strauss (1967), *The Discovery of Grounded Theory: Strategies for Qualitative Research.*

REFERENCES

Bertalanffy, Ludwig von (1966): "General System Theory and Psychiatry," in Silvano Arieti (ed.), *American Handbook of Psychiatry*, vol. 3, Basic Books, Inc., Publishers, New York, pp. 705–721.

———(1968): *General System Theory: Foundations, Development, Applications,* George Braziller, New York.

———(1967): *Robots, Men and Minds,* George Braziller, New York.

———(1952): "Theoretical Models in Biology and Psychology," in D. Krech and G. S. Klein (eds.), *Theoretical Models and Personality Theory,* The Duke University Press, Durham, N.C.

Blumer, Herbert (1969): *Symbolic Interactionism, Perspective and Method,* Prentice-Hall, Inc., Englewood Cliffs, N.J.

Davis, Anne J. (1973): "The Phenomenological Approach in Nursing Research," in Esther A. Garrison et al. (eds.), *Doctoral Preparation for Nurses*, Printed at the University of California, San Francisco, pp. 212–229.

Davis, Marcella Z. (1970): "Transition to a Devalued Status: The Case of Multiple Sclerosis," Unpublished doctoral dissertation, University of California, San Francisco.

Fairweather, George W. (1967): *Methods for Experimental Social Innovation,* John Wiley & Sons, Inc., New York.

Gilliatt, Penelope (1970): "Review of Truffaut Film, 'L'Enfant Sauvage,' " *New Yorker,* Sept. 12, p. 69.

Glaser, Barney G., and Anselm L. Strauss (1967): *The Discovery of Grounded Theory: Strategies for Qualitative Research,* Aldine Publishing Company, Chicago.

Kalkman, Marion E. (1973): "The Changing Character of Mental Health Care and Implications for the Doctoral Education of the Psychiatric Nurse," in Esther A. Garrison et al. (eds.), *Doctoral Preparation for Nurses*, Printed at the University of California, San Francisco, pp. 156–173.

Manis, J., and B. Meltzer (eds.) (1967): *Symbolic Interaction: A Reader in Social Psychology,* Allyn and Bacon, Boston.

McCall, George J., and J. L. Simmons (1966): *Identities and Interaction: An Examination of Human Association in Everyday Life,* The Free Press, New York.

Mead, George H. (1934): *Mind, Self and Society,* The University of Chicago Press, Chicago.

———(1964): *On Social Psychology: Selected Papers,* rev. ed. (ed. by Anselm L. Strauss), Phoenix Books, The University of Chicago Press, Chicago.

Natanson, M. (ed.) (1969): *Essays in Phenomenology,* Martinus Nijhoff, The Hague.

———(ed.) (1970): *Phenomenology and Social Reality,* Martinus Nijhoff, The Hague.

Quint, Jeanne C. (1967): *The Nurse and the Dying Patient,* The Macmillan Company, New York.

Rioch, David McK. (1955): "Psychiatry as a Biological Science," *Psychiatry,* vol. 18, pp. 313–321.

Rogers, Martha (1964): "The Researcher in Nursing for Tomorrow Today." Paper presented at Graduate Symposium, University of North Carolina, Jan. 8.

Sanford, Nevitt (1970): "The Decline of Individualism," *Mental Health Digest,* vol. 2, no. 8, pp. 29–33.

Spiegelberg, H. (1965): "The Essentials of the Phenomenological Method," in *The Phenomenological Movement: A Historical Introduction,* vol. 2, Martinus Nijhoff, The Hague.

Strauss, Erwin (1964): *Phenomenology: Pure and Applied,* Duquesne University Press, Pittsburgh.

van den Berg, J. H. (1955): *The Phenomenological Approach to Psychiatry,* Charles C Thomas, Publisher, Springfield, Ill.

Wilson, Mitchell (1970): "On Being a Scientist," *The Atlantic,* vol. 226, no. 3, pp. 101–106.

Zucker, Herbert (1967): *Problems of Psychotherapy,* The Free Press, New York.

NAME INDEX

SUBJECT INDEX